Family
Medical
Dictionary

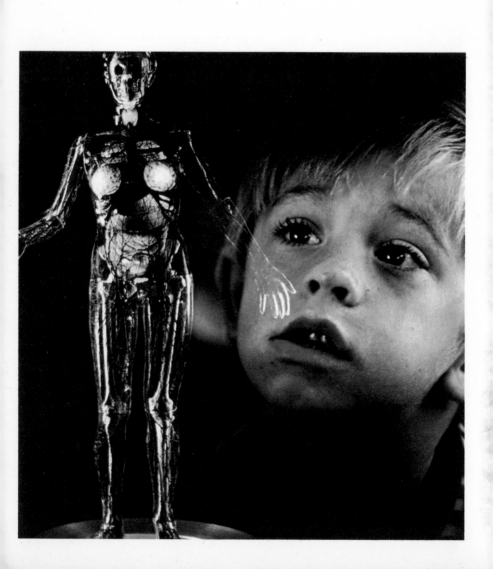

THE HAMLYN
Family
Medical
Dictionary
IN COLOUR

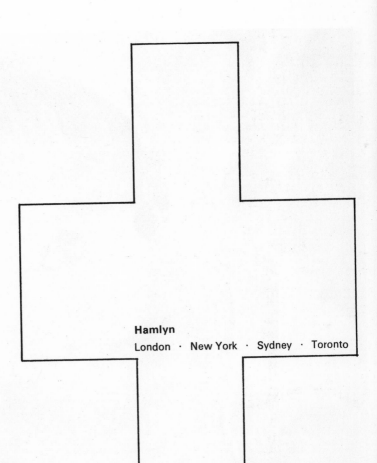

Hamlyn

London · New York · Sydney · Toronto

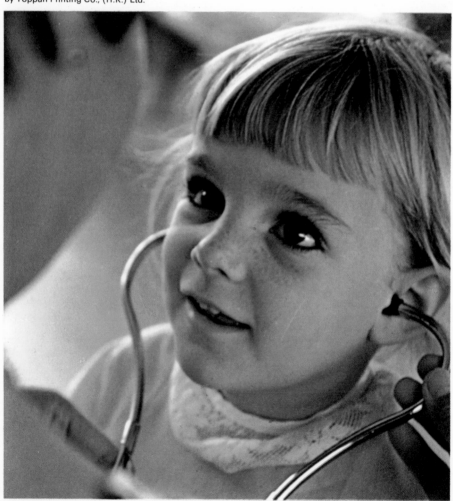

Dr. Trevor Weston
M.D., M.R.C.G.P.
Editor, Family Doctor Publications

Introduction

Medical knowledge has grown so rapidly that it is almost impossible for any one person, even a doctor, to know all of it. At the same time more and more people want to know about and understand the workings of their own bodies and minds. There is an increasing interest in how the various systems and parts of the human machine work; and in what can go wrong, and why, and how doctors set about putting it right again.

Doctors welcome this great upsurge of interest that people are taking in the way they are put together, because anybody who has some knowledge about what is going on inside them is able to co-operate much more sensibly and fully with the doctor and can thus contribute far more to their own treatment and recovery.

It used to be thought that all the body's workings were so complex that only people with special training could understand any of them. This is certainly not true today. It may be the rise in general standards of education or the large number of medical programmes on radio and television that has made the difference. But, whatever the cause, it is clear that – provided the subject is properly presented – there is no limit to what the average man and woman can follow and understand, no matter how apparently technical and specialized it may seem.

So the crucial factor is not really in people, provided that they are interested, but in the way the subject is presented to them. This is what really makes the discovery of oneself so rich, rewarding, compelling and entertaining – a saga of personal exploration. The adventure one wants to continue no matter how difficult and complex it becomes.

How should it be presented, then ? Firstly, accurately. Secondly, in language that people can readily understand – rather than in terms that are comprehensible only to the specialist who has spent 20 years using them. Thirdly, in coloured pictures and diagrams – for, properly used, they can explain more than any words.

What then, will you gain from this *Family Medical Dictionary* ? Information and entertainment, certainly; but also the fascination of special knowledge, the excitement of exploring fields new to you, the satisfaction of mastering ideas that you might have imagined to be too difficult for you, and – from a more practical point of view – a banishment of old wives' tales, and a deeper personal understanding of yourself and your family that cannot help being of continuing service to you.

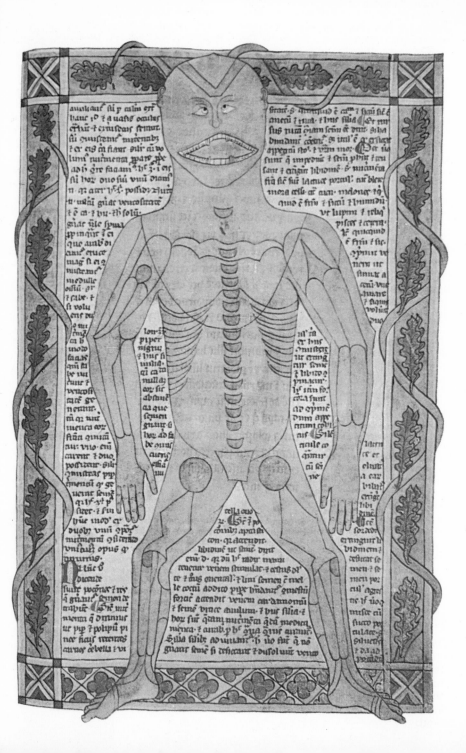

ABDOMEN is the part of the body which is bounded above by the diaphragm, separating the abdomen from the thorax (see **diaphragm, thorax**) and below by the floor of the pelvis (see **pelvis**). In front it is covered by the abdominal musculature, and behind it is bounded by the lumbar and spinal muscles. It contains the organs of digestion (stomach, intestines, pancreas and gall bladder), the organs of excretion (kidneys, ureters and urinary bladder), the organs of reproduction in women (ovaries, Fallopian tubes, uterus and vagina), certain other organs such as the liver, spleen and prostate, together with the arteries, veins, lymphatics and nerves supplying all these organs.

Like other parts of the body, the abdominal organs are subject to diseases and injuries. These include perforations, inflammations, obstructions and new growths. Many abdominal diseases are a combination of more than one of these. Cancer of the bowel, for example, is a form of new growth which may cause an obstruction.

New growths in the abdomen may be benign or malignant (i.e., cancerous). Colic occurs when any of the tubes within the abdomen tries to remove an obstacle by pushing it further along. Colic can be caused by a stone in the duct (tube) leading from the gall bladder, or a stone in the ureter (the tube from the kidney to the urinary bladder), or when there is any kind of temporary hold-up in the bowel (such as an attack of 'wind'). Perforations may be due to external injury (from car accidents, for example); or to the swallowing of sharp indigestible fragments such as

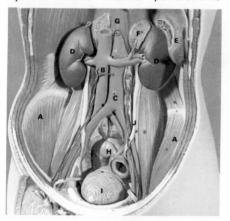

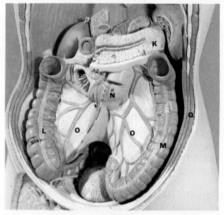

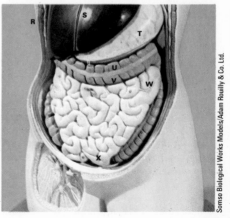

Main organs of the abdomen shown in this model are: a, the levator ani (muscle). b, the inferior vena cava (vein). c, the abdominal aorta (artery). d, the kidneys. e, the spleen. f, the suprarenal gland. g, the oesophagus. h, the rectum. i, the urinary bladder. j, the ureter. k, the pancreas. l, the ascending colon. m, the descending colon. n, the duodenum. o, branches of the superior mesenteric artery. p, interior of the duodenum. q, abdominal musculature. r, the liver, right lobe. s, the liver, left lobe. t, the stomach. u, the large intestine. v, the transverse colon. w, the jejunum. x, the ileum.

Somso Biological Works Models/Adam Rouilly & Co. Ltd.

bones; or to the rupture of an ulcerated stomach or intestinal wall.

ABLATION is a detachment or removal. Examples are the premature separation of the placenta or afterbirth (see **afterbirth**); and detachment of the retina (see **retina**), the back of the eye where the 'picture' of the outside world is formed.

ABORTION (also see **miscarriage**) is the miscarriage of the product of conception before the foetus (child) is viable, i.e., capable of separate existence. An **abortifacient** is a drug or instrument which can be used to produce a miscarriage. **Criminal abortion** is the use of any method to produce an illegal miscarriage. Nations differ in their laws covering the legality of abortion. In Britain for example, the Abortion Act, 1967, made legal the abortion of a woman, carried out in good faith to save the life or health (including mental health) of the mother; or in the case of a substantial risk of a malformed foetus; or to preserve the continued good health of any existing children. Such abortions must be carried out in institutions recognized for the purpose by the Secretary of State for Social Services, and must be notified to his department. The recommendation of two doctors is also required.

ABRASIONS are areas denuded of skin or mucous membrane. Minor external abrasions may be treated by washing the injured part with soap and water and the application of a covering, such as a plaster. Internal, and serious external abrasions need medical attention. In dentistry, abrasion means the mechanical wearing down of teeth.

ABREACTION, in psychiatry, is the process of freeing from the mind emotionally-charged but repressed material. It is used in cases where an experience, probably unpleasant, is lost from the conscious memory but remains in vivid form in the subconscious, causing hysteria, anxiety or amnesia for which there is no apparent reason.

Abreaction is a process of bringing these memories into the open — by hypnosis, by drugs such as L.S.D. or by 'free association' discussions with a psychiatrist — and, by discovering the cause of the condition, eliminating it.

ABSCESS means a localized collection of pus (see **pus**) in any part of the body, an example being a boil (see **boil**). Pus is formed when the blood supplies white corpuscles to defend the body against an 'invader', so that an abscess — a collection of dead corpuscles — forms on the battlefield between the invader (be it a bacterium or a bullet) and the body's defences. If the abscess is acute, or hot, it shows that the battle is continuing. In cases of external abscess, poulticing with hot fomentations may bring the abscess to a head and it may burst on its own or subside. It may need help by lancing, but for this medical advice should be sought. In certain parts of the body the abscess may become chronic (i.e. smouldering) or cold where the cavity filled with pus, after the battle is over, fails to clear. In thus occupying space, it presses on other organs and needs surgical intervention to help it drain, or heal.

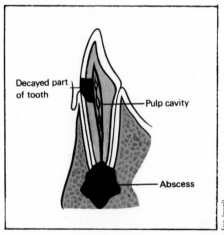

Decayed part of tooth

Pulp cavity

Abscess

Eric Jewell

An abscess at the base of a tooth, caused by decay exposing the sensitive central pulp cavity, is a common cause of toothache. Rinsing with bicarbonate of soda may bring temporary relief.

4

A.C. (abbreviation for **ante cibum**) means before meals. It is used on prescriptions to indicate when medicines should be taken.

ACARINA is the medical name for ticks and mites, which are carriers of many diseases. They are an order of the arachnida, a class which also includes spiders.

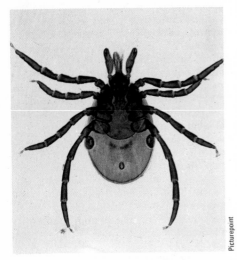

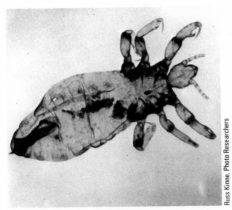

Ixodes (above) is a member of the acarina class of ticks, all disease carriers. Acarophobia is morbid fear of small creatures such as the louse (below).

ACAROPHOBIA is the term for the morbid fear of small mites, or even of small inanimate objects. It is also used for fear of 'the itch' **(see next entry)**.

ACARUS SCABIEI is a mite (sarcoptes scabiei) which causes 'the itch' or scabies (see **scabies**), a common complaint easily transmitted by infested clothing, dirty bedclothing or towels, or through crowded conditions. The mite is barely visible to the naked eye, but its burrow raises a small and very irritating spot on the skin, the irritation being particularly noticeable during the night.

ACCOMMODATION means alteration of the convexity of the crystalline lens of the eye in order to bring light rays to a focus on the retina (see **retina**). This alteration is brought about by a tightening of the suspensory ligament (which holds the lens) in order to 'flatten' the lens and thus bring distant objects into focus; or, alternatively, by relaxing this ligament to allow the lens, by its natural elasticity, to resume a more rounded (convex) shape and bring nearer objects into focus. Loss of the natural elasticity of the lens in middle age can leave it permanently more 'flattened', which explains why many people need reading glasses as they become older, though for distant vision no such assistance is necessary.

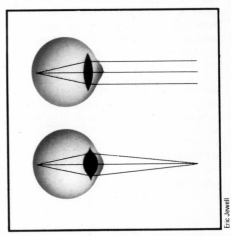

How the lens of the human eye adjusts to focus on faraway (above) and nearby (below) objects. Loss of elasticity in the ligament controlling this function is the reason why many middle-aged and elderly people need reading glasses.

5

ACCOUCHEMENT means childbirth. An **accoucheur** is an obstetrician.

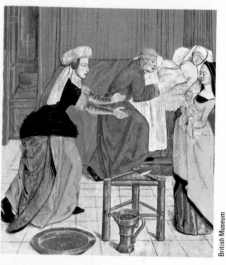

British Museum

Medieval view of an accouchement — in this case the baby has been delivered by a Caesarean section.

ACETABULUM means the cup-shaped depression on the outer aspect of the hipbone. It is the socket into which the head of the femur (see **femur**) fits. In diseases such as osteoarthritis, the socket and the ball-like head of the thigh-bone (femur) may become partially fused, causing pain and difficulty in walking. The name acetabulum comes from the Latin words acetum (vinegar) and bulum (a vessel); the socket was once thought to resemble a small vinegar cruet of Roman times.

ACETONE (dimethyl ketone) is a colourless, volatile liquid with a distinctive smell like that of many nail-varnish removers. In the body, it is a by-product of the faulty oxidation of fats, found especially in diabetics (see **diabetes**). Measurement of these ketone bodies in the blood or urine, which is called **acetonuria**, may give an indication of the severity of the disease. A smell of acetone emanating from a diabetic is a warning to call for medical advice. Acetone is sometimes used externally as an antiseptic.

ACETYLCHOLINE is believed to be the chemical substance which, on receiving 'messages' from the brain, causes muscle fibres to contract — thus allowing the body to perform both voluntary actions, such as walking, and involuntary ones, such as breathing. It is not yet fully understood, but scientists studying nerve functions believe that an impulse passes down the nerve from the brain, going through various junctions called synapses (see **synapses**) to the nerve endings in various organs. Whether this impulse is electro-chemical or electro-physical is not yet clear; however, the result is known to be the release of a chemical substance — in many instances, but not all, acetylcholine. Because the body could not function if muscles were able only to contract, it needs some other means of allowing them to expand again. It seems to have two means — the first, anticholinergic substances which are released independently; the second, an enzyme (see **enzyme**) called cholinesterase which destroys acetylcholine, thus limiting its activity.

ACETYLSALICYLIC ACID is the drug commonly known as aspirin (see **aspirin**).

ACHALASIA means the failure of a hollow organ to relax. In medicine it is commonly used for a stricture (see **stricture**) of the lower end of the gullet (see **oesophagus**) where it joins the stomach. This prevents food from passing into the stomach and the person may starve while the oesophagus balloons to a considerable extent. Achalasia has to be treated urgently, usually by passing weighted tubes through the obstruction.

ACHE is a constant or fixed pain which is dull to severe in character but, by continuing for long periods, causes great mental and physical disability. It can be acute at times, as in earache, stomach ache or colic (see **colic**). Some simple procedures, such as the use of heat and rubbing, will temporarily alleviate the worst of the pain, but if an ache is persistent or recurring medical advice should be sought.

ACHILLES TENDON is the name for the tendon (see **tendon**) which connects the calf muscles to the heelbone, enabling the muscles to bend and straighten the foot. Unaccustomed vigorous exercise can sometimes strain or tear the tendon, the result being a painful condition in which walking is difficult and running often impossible. Application of heat (from a liniment, for example) and rest will cure minor cases; more serious ones need physiotherapy treatment. The name comes from the Greek warrior Achilles, whose mother held him by the heel while she dipped him in the River Styx to protect him from wounds. Because the heel was left unprotected, he eventually died when an arrow struck him there.

ACHLORHYDRIA is a term used to describe the complete absence of hydrochloric acid in the stomach. The acid, which is produced by special glands in the stomach wall, is used by the body in the initial stages of digesting food. Lack of hydrochloric acid is one cause of indigestion.

ACHOLIA means the absence of, or suppression of the flow of, bile (see **bile**). Typically it is caused by a stone or growth which obstructs the bile duct, leading from the gall bladder (see **gall bladder**) to the small intestine, preventing the bile from playing its important part in the digestion of food. Surgery to remove the obstruction is the normal treatment for this condition.

ACHOLURIA is a feature of certain cases of jaundice. It means the absence from the urine of the pigments which are normally found in the bile and which give bile its greenish-yellow colour. The pigments are normally re-absorbed from the gut (intestine) and excreted in the urine; their absence helps the clinician to diagnose the cause of the jaundice.

ACHONDROPLASIA is a deformity seen in some congenital dwarfs. In the foetus, the normal process of converting cartilage to bone goes awry, especially in the long bones of the body. Some bones, particularly those of the head, do not suffer this impairment and are normal. Hence the typical dwarf has a normal-sized head on an abnormally short body.

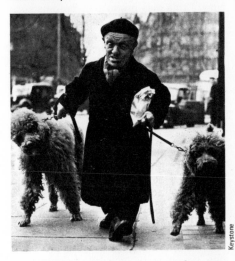

Keystone

An achondroplastic dwarf with typically stumpy body and relatively large head.

ACHROMASIA is the loss or absence of normal skin pigmentation, as in albinos (see **albinism**). It is also used in medicine to describe the extreme pallor associated with those near death. Achromatopsia means complete colour blindness.

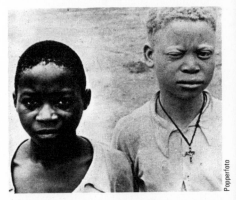

Popperfoto

Even among negroes, albinism occurs in about one person in 20,000.

ACHYLIA is the absence of *chyle* or digestive juices (see **digestion**).

7

ACIDITY is the medical term for an excess of acid in the system. The stomach normally produces weak hydrochloric acid as a digestive aid. Excessive production of this may produce symptoms such as sourness, heartburn and even pain. The remedy is usually correction by an alkaline mixture, such as sodium bicarbonate (bicarbonate of soda) which neutralizes the excess acid.

ACIDOSIS is a condition in which there is a general reduction of the alkali reserve of the blood because of an excess of acid. It occurs in some conditions, such as diabetic coma, where the level of bicarbonates in the blood drops because the body uses them to combine with, and dispose of, acid products produced when the disease is not controlled. (See **diabetes**).

ACIDS are substances containing hydrogen which is replaceable by metals to form salts. A common equation is HCl (hydrochloric acid) + NaOH (sodium hydroxide, an alkali) = (yields) NaCl (sodium chloride, or common salt) + H_2O (water). In a watery solution, acids dissociate; that is to say, the hydrogen atoms are free in the solution. 'Strong' acids are those in which the dissociation is most complete. Not unnaturally, strong acid solutions such as those used in industrial processes are dangerous to handle, and will cause burns if they come into contact with human skin. First aid for acid burns: first wash with copious quantities of water, to dilute the acid, then use a weak alkali (common washing soda and sodium bicarbonate are the most readily available) to neutralize the acid. Conversely, vinegar (acetic acid) is useful as an antidote for burns by strong alkalis such as caustic soda, which are equally dangerous.

ACNE is a skin condition in which the hair follicles, sweat glands and sebaceous glands (see **sebaceous**) of the skin become infected by the bacilli (germs). It usually affects the skin of the face, back and chest. It is commonest at puberty (see **puberty**) and up to 30 years of age. The

essential lesion (see **lesion**) is the comedo or blackhead, which develops into a pink papule, pustule or nodule. The unsightly rash which follows can produce great psychological distress, especially in adolescents. There is undoubtedly some connection between the occurrence of acne in adolescents and the increase of sex hormones (see **hormones**) circulating in the bloodstream at the time of puberty. These hormones affect the skin, making it more fruitful soil for invasion by the bacilli. Treatment includes scrupulous cleanliness in skin toilet and the use of antiseptic skin lotions. In some very resistant cases, antibiotics have to be used and even abrasive methods which pare off the outer layers of the skin. Among recent advances is the use of the contraceptive pill for young women with acne. Acne is a term also applied to other skin conditions with widely differing causes. Apart from the common type described here (acne vulgaris), a similar looking eruption can occur in people who have digestive disturbances (acne rosacea) and in people who take, or are in contact with industrially, such things as bromides (acne coagnimata or medicamentosa). However, these are not commonly seen.

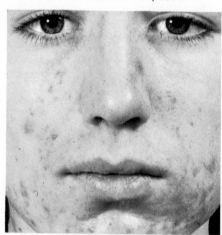

Acne, a common affliction of adolescence.

ACONITE is an extremely poisonous drug obtained from the plant aconitum napellus, or monkshood. It is now rarely used in medicine.

ACOUSTICS, from the Greek word *Akoustikos* (pertaining to hearing), is the science of sound. The **acoustic nerve** is the eighth cranial nerve, which serves the organs of hearing and balance.

ACRIFLAVINE is a commonly-used antiseptic.

ACRO- is a prefix meaning pertaining to an extremity (such as the limbs) or to heights. **Acrocyanosis** is blueness of the hands or feet. **Acrodermatitis** is inflammation of the skin of the hands or feet. **Acrohyperhidrosis** is excessive sweating of the hands or feet. **Acroparasthesia** means numbness or tingling in the hands or feet. **Acrophobia** means fear of heights.

ACROMEGALY (see **acro**) literally means an increase in the size of the extremities. It is caused by a malfunction of one part of the pituitary gland (see **pituitary**) resulting in overgrowth (see **adenoma**). This produces an increase in the size of the hands, feet, and face and some internal organs. It also disturbs the functions of other glands and may lead to a form of diabetes (see **diabetes**). X-ray therapy or surgery on the pituitary gland are the usual treatments.

ACROMIO CLAVICULAR JOINT is the joint which connects the **clavicle** (collar bone) with the upper and outer process of the scapula (shoulder blade) called the **acromium.**

A.C.T.H. In full, adrenocorticotrophic hormone (see **hormone**) is manufactured by the pituitary gland and travels in the bloodstream stimulating the cortex of the adrenal gland to produce cortisone and related compounds (see **cortisone**). A.C.T.H. extracted from the pituitary glands of animals is used in the treatment of rheumatoid arthritis, and other diseases.

ACTINIC means pertaining to the sun's rays or rays of the spectrum. **Actinotherapy** is treatment by the use of rays, for example, sunlight, ultra violet and infra red. **Actinomycosis** is a disease caused by a fungus **actinomyces** (ray fungus) in cattle and pigs which is sometimes communicated to humans and commonly attacks the jaw and lungs.

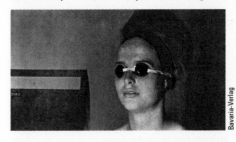

Health, and sometimes beauty, are maintained by the use of actinic rays.

ACUITY is sharpness, distinctness or clearness as of vision or hearing.

ACUPUNCTURE is an ancient Chinese treatment which consists of piercing the tissues with needles. Detailed maps were drawn to show lines of puncture for various symptoms in different parts of the body. It is a method seldom used in Western medicine, although it is sometimes successful in treating obstinate sciatica.

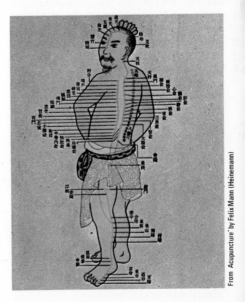

The Chinese method of acupuncture relieved pain in different parts of the body.

ACUTE means sharp; severe. It is used in medicine to describe pronounced symptoms of rapid onset. Usually these symptoms appear and disappear rapidly.

ADACTYLIA is a congenital malformation consisting of an absence of fingers or toes.

ADAM'S APPLE is a prominence in the neck of the larynx (voice-box) and its cartilages. It commonly appears in men particularly after puberty. Its name is derived from the legend that the apple which Eve gave to Adam became stuck in his throat.

ADAMSITE is the name of a poison gas used in chemical warfare.

ADAPTATION is a term used in biology and medicine to describe any change in structure, form, or habits to suit a new environment. Visual **adaptation** is the normal ability of the eye to adjust to varying intensities of light.

ADDICT is a person who has become completely dependent on a drug. Certain narcotic drugs such as cocaine, opium, and heroin taken either for relief of pain or for 'kicks' can cause addiction. The addict is unable to give up the use of the drug, and needs increasing doses to achieve the desired effect.

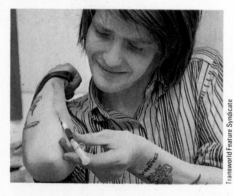

An injection provides euphoria to a drug addict, then acute depression.

ADDISON'S DISEASE In the middle of the nineteenth century an English physician, Thomas Addison, described two diseases which were given his name. The first, **Addison's anaemia**, is now called pernicious anaemia and is due to a lack of Vitamin B_{12}. The other, which is still called **Addison's disease** is due to an underproduction of cortisone by the adrenal glands (see **cortisone**). It is characterized by muscular weakness and changes in skin pigmentation. **Addison's disease** may be treated by oral doses of cortisone.

ADENITIS is an inflammation of a gland or lymph node. A common complaint in children is **cervical adenitis** where there is swelling of the glands of the neck, usually secondary to some acute infection in the mouth, throat or ear. Generalized swelling of the lymph nodes may occur in diseases such as glandular fever.

ADENOID, has particular reference to a patch of lymphoid tissue in the passages at the back of the nose. The **adenoids** are a protective device to trap harmful bacteria. They may become enlarged and cause obstruction to the airway. This condition most frequently appears in children. The common treatment is surgical removal called **adenoidectomy** (see **tonsil**).

ADENOMA is a benign tumour of glandular tissue. Its exact nature can usually only be determined by surgical removal and examination.

ADENOVIRUS is one of a large group of viruses, which have been found to be the cause of many respiratory diseases. It was first isolated in 1953 in **adenoids** surgically removed from children.

ADHESION literally means the force which sticks two surfaces together. In medicine it refers to the union of structures which should normally be separate. During the process of healing, a sticky fluid is produced which causes the damaged parts to adhere to surrounding tissues. In the abdomen, this may lead to bands of tissue called **adhesions** which contract as they dry and may cause obstruction of the gut.

ADIPOSE derives from *adeps* meaning fatty, fatlike, corpulent or obese. It refers to excessive accumulation of fat in the body either locally or generally. **Adiposis dolororosa** or Dercum's disease is characterized by deposition of symmetrical masses of fat in various parts of the body and accompanied by pain.

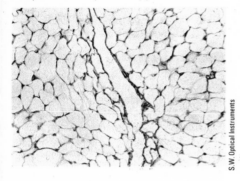

Adipose tissue is a loose fibrous tissue which stores fat globules in its cells.

ADJUVANT is an auxiliary medication, one which assists the action of a drug.

AD NAUSEAM means to the point of producing nausea or sickness.

ADNEXAE are accessory parts of an organ. They refer particularly to uterine tubes and ovaries.

ADOLESCENCE is the period extending from puberty to adult maturity.

ADRENAL is a ductless gland, sometimes called the suprarenal, which is located above the kidney. It produces two important groups of hormones, which it discharges directly into the bloodstream. One portion of the gland produces noradrenalin and adrenalin, which have a profound effect on the nervous system, the heart, the respiratory tubes, and the muscles. Another part of the gland (the cortex) produces cortisone and many related compounds (steroids) which affect the immunity system of the body, inflammatory processes in general, the metabolic balance of the body, and secondary sexual characteristics.

ADSORPTION is the property of attracting fluids. It also refers to the ability of certain solids to hold molecules in a thin layer on their surfaces.

ADULT is a person of mature age.

ADULTERATION is the addition of an inferior or impure substance to another.

ADVENTITIOUS, meaning accidental or acquired, refers to something occurring in an unusual or abnormal place.

AEDES, from the Greek for 'unpleasant', is a genus of mosquitoes. **Aedes Aegypti** carry yellow fever and dengue.

AEROBE is an oxygen breathing microorganism or bacterium which requires oxygen for life.

AEROPHAGY means swallowing air. It is a condition found in certain nervous patients who swallow mouthfuls of air.

AESCULAPIUS, according to Greek mythology, was the son of Apollo and was regarded as the god of medicine. His staff, with serpent and wings, is the emblem of many medical organizations.

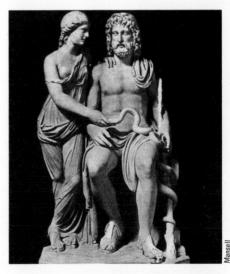

Aesculapius, the Greek god of medicine, holds his symbolic staff and serpent.

11

AESTHETIC pertains to the senses or feelings. It particularly refers to those associated with the perception of beauty.

AET. is an abbreviation from the Latin word *aetatis*, meaning 'of age'. (e.g. AET 6, six years of age).

AETIOLOGY means the origin or cause of any condition.

AFEBRILE means without fever.

AFFECT is a term used in psychology to describe the emotional mood. An affective reaction is an emotional response disproportionate to the apparent cause.

AFFERENT means carrying towards, as in the case of sensory impulses which are transmitted from the periphery towards the central nervous system.

AFFILIATION is the act of imputing the paternity of a child.

AFFINAL means connected through marriage or of the same genetic origin.

AFFINITY is inherent attraction. Chemical affinity is the force of attraction between atoms.

AFTER BIRTH is the placenta and membranes expelled from the womb after the birth of a child.

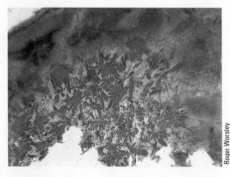

The sponge-like tissue of the placenta is dispelled from the womb as the after birth.

AFTER PAINS result from contractions

of the womb following the delivery of a child. They are usually of short duration.

AGAR-AGAR, of Singhalese origin, is a gelatinous substance obtained from seaweed, used in bacteriology to solidify culture media. Medically it is used as a laxative as it becomes bulky when moist.

AGEING is growing older or ripening (See Geriatrics, the care of the ageing).

AGGLUTINATION is the aggregation of suspended particles into clumps. It is used in medicine to describe the grouping together of cells suspended in fluid or of bacteria circulating in the blood stream by an antibody or **agglutinin**. As the body produces different agglutinins to fight particular diseases, their appearance can reveal the presence of specific diseases. Such is the purpose of the Widal test for typhoid. The determination of blood groups and of Rhesus factor is made by means of agglutination tests. A blood transfusion from a donor of an incompatible blood group will cause agglutination in the blood of the receiver. If a woman with a Rhesus negative blood group has an anti-Rhesus-agglutinin circulating in her blood stream agglutination may occur in the blood of a Rhesus positive baby in her womb.

AGGRESSION is an act or attitude of hostility which commonly arises from frustration or feelings of inferiority.

AGITATION is restlessness characterized by violent motion. **Agitated depression** is a mental disturbance characterized by continual activity and despondency.

AGONIST is a contracting muscle engaged in movement in opposition to another muscle, the **antagonist.**

AGNOSIA is a condition denoting the total or partial loss of the perceptive faculty by which persons and things are recognized. It is usually classified according to the sense affected, for example, optic or tactile **agnosia.**

AGORAPHOBIA, from the Greek words **agora,** 'market place', and **phobia,** 'fear', is the fear of open spaces. Its opposite, **claustrophobia,** is the fear of confined spaces.

AGRANULOCYTOSIS is a disease marked by the diminution or absence of the type of white blood cells called granulocytes. It is commonly caused by certain classes of drugs, or by radiation, which among other things may cause destruction of the bone marrow, where the majority of white blood cells are formed.

AGRAPHIA is the loss of ability to write.

AGUE is an archaic term for an attack of malaria. It is also used to denote a recurrent chill with shivering, a rigor, or a neuralgia.

AILING means indisposed, not well. An **ailment** is a disease, sickness, or a complaint.

AIR consists of nearly 80 parts of nitrogen and about 20 parts of oxygen, a small amount of carbon dioxide, and even smaller amounts of the inert gases such as argon and neon. The oxygen in the air sustains respiration in almost all living things. The carbon dioxide is used by plants in photosynthesis. Nitrogen compounds help make up body proteins.

AIRWAY is a device used in anaesthesia (see **anaesthesia**) to maintain a clear and unobstructed respiratory passage. The word also refers to the respiratory passages themselves.

ALBINISM, ALBINOISM is the congenital lack, either total or partial, of pigment in the skin, hair and pupil of the eye.

ALBUMIN is one of a group of protein substances, the chief constituents of animal tissues. It is soluble in water, and coagulable by heat. **Serum albumin** is the chief constituent of blood plasma. **Albuminuria,** the escape of serum albumin into the urine, is usually a sign of some kidney disfunction.

ALCOHOL originally meant powder. After the fifteenth century, it was applied especially to chemical powders or essences. Its modern usage is derived from the phrase 'alcohol of wine'. The alcohols are derivatives of the hydrocarbons. **Ethyl alcohol** (C_2H_5OH) is the product of the fermentation of fruit or grain and exists in many drinks, notably wine, beer, whisky, brandy, rum, gin, sake and liqueurs. It acts as a depressant on the central nervous system, although its initial ingestion gives rise to euphoria, increased pulse rate and a sense of warmth. These effects were responsible for the belief in the value of alcohol as a stimulant. Large doses cause muscular incordination, stupor, and even death. In medicine it is used for its fuel value in the debilitated. It is also an effective skin antiseptic and can be used for the antiseptic storage of instruments.

ALCOHOLISM, when chronic, is a state of addiction to alcohol. It may eventually have various effects on the nervous and digestive systems, principally constant depression and even death of brain and nerve cells, and irritation of the lining of the stomach which causes a gastritis and cirrhosis of the liver. Injuries to heart and arteries from alcohol are not uncommon.

ALDOSTERONE is a very important hormone produced by the cortex of the adrenal gland (see **adrenal**). Under its influence the body excretes potassium and retains sodium. Only in recent years has it become clear that retention of sodium causes retention of water in the body. Therefore, people who produce too much aldosterone tend to get 'waterlogged'. This occurs, for instance, in certain cases of heart failure. New diuretics (see **diuretics**) can combat aldosterone and relieve this accumulation of fluid.

ALEXIA is word-blindness (see **word-blindness**).

ALIMENTARY CANAL means the entire length of the tract through which food passes on its way through the body. It begins at the mouth and ends at the anus. In between are the pharynx (throat), oesophagus (gullet), stomach, small intestine, and large intestine.

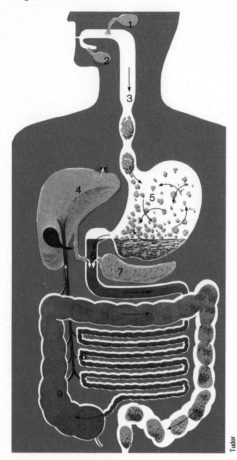

1 Salivary gland. 2 Salivary gland. 3 Oesophagus. 4 Liver. 5 Stomach. 6 Duodenum. 7 Pancreas. 8 Small intestine (ileum). 9 Large intestine (colon).

ALKALI is a chemical which can neutralize an acid. Alkalies can, therefore, be regarded as the chemical 'opposites' of acids. Mild alkalies, such as bicarbonate of soda or aluminium hydroxide, are used to counteract the effects of stomach acidity. Strong alkalies, like ammonia and caustic soda, are as dangerous as strong acids and can burn delicate tissues. If they are taken internally, they may be lethal. The antidote is a weak acid, such as vinegar or lemon juice. It is, however, more important to

14

irrigate the tissues at once with as much water as possible. When an alkali has been swallowed, *on no account make the patient vomit.* Get him to hospital immediately.

ALKALOSIS means an upset in the body's internal chemistry in which conditions become alkaline rather than acid. This can result, for example, from a massive overdose of an alkali, (see **alkali**) which is absorbed into the blood stream.

ALKAPTONURIA is an unusual congenital disorder (see **congenital**) in which a dark pigment is deposited throughout the body and excreted in the urine.

ALLANTOIS is a structure which grows out from the embryo (see **embryo**) early in its life within the womb. Eventually, it forms the afterbirth (see **afterbirth**) and umbilical cord.

ALLERGY means a type of hyper-sensitivity to certain substances outside the body. These substances (**allergens**) may be pollens, secretions of biting insects, animal hairs, or even common foods, such as eggs. Frequently, allergens are protein in nature. Even household dust may frequently be an allergen, but recent research suggests that this may be because dust often contains the bodies of microscopic mites, which are themselves largely protein. Very often it is impossible to decide which foreign substance is responsible for a particular allergy. Among the symptoms of allergy are rashes, profuse catarrh, swelling of the larynx (voice-box) which produces choking and wheezing in the chest. Among the diseases often related to allergy are asthma, eczema and hay-fever.

ALLOPATH is a term used by homeopaths to describe an orthodox doctor.

ALOPECIA means baldness (see **baldness**). The term is most often used in relation to the condition known as **alopecia areata** in which large tufts of hair fall out, leaving bald patches on the scalp.

AMENORRHOEA means absence of the

periods. The common causes are pregnancy, anaemia and the menopause.

AMENTIA is mental deficiency.

AMINOPHYLLINE is a drug whose principal value is in the treatment of asthma, and as a diuretic (see **diuretic**).

AMMONIA is an extremely irritant gas. If the eyes or nose are exposed to it, they should be washed thoroughly with water. Liquid ammonia is a strong alkali. For treatment of ammonia poisoning, see **alkali.**

AMNESIA means loss of memory. Contrary to popular belief, total amnesia is not likely to follow a blow on the head; it is much more often of psychological origin. Head injuries do, however, tend to produce amnesia for the events which occurred immediately before (and sometimes immediately after) the blow.

AMNION is the 'bag of waters', that is, the membrane which contains the fluid in which an unborn baby floats. It contains between one and two pints of fluid.

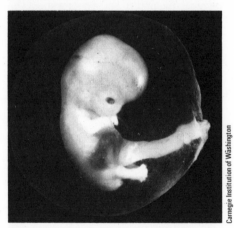

The foetus floats freely in the amnion, attached only by the umbilical cord.

AMOEBIC DYSENTERY is a serious disease which occurs in tropical and subtropical countries. It principally affects the bowel and liver and is caused by infection from an organism called *entamoeba histolytica.*

AMPHETAMINES are a group of drugs which were once used as 'slimming pills'. They were more or less useless in this capacity, and doctors now rarely prescribe them.

AMPICILLIN or 'Penbritin' is one of the semi-synthetic penicillins, (see **antibiotics**).

AMPUTATION is the cutting off of any part of the body.

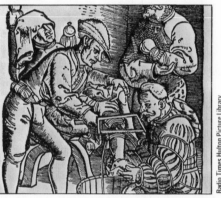

Early amputations were endured without an anaesthetic.

ANAEMIA is weakness of the blood. There are several basic types. By far the commonest is **iron-deficiency anaemia**, which may be caused, as the name implies, by the lack of iron in the diet, or by loss of iron in bleeding. It may occur in women during heavy periods: among men the bleeding most likely results from an ulcer.

A much less frequent kind is **megaloblastic anaemia**, the commonest form of which is pernicious anaemia (see **pernicious anaemia**). A similar anaemia occurs in some pregnant women, but this can be prevented or cured by the taking of folic acid tablets.

Rare types of anaemia include **aplastic anaemia** in which the bone marrow fails to regenerate the red blood cells, and **haemolytic anaemia**, in which there is an

15

unusually high rate of destruction of the red cells.

ANAEROBES are bacteria which can live without oxygen, for example, *'tetanus bacilli'.*

ANAESTHESIA means absence of feeling. **Local anaesthesia** was first produced by using the drug cocaine, but this proved to be so dangerous that it was replaced by newer compounds, such as lignocaine and procaine.

General anaesthesia was probably first discovered in 1800, when Sir Humphry Davis anaesthetized animals and himself, with nitrous oxide. Incredibly enough, no-one paid any attention to his discovery. In the early 1840's, several Americans began using either nitrous oxide, or ether, to extract teeth. The first operation in Britain on an 'etherized' patient was carried out by Liston on 21 December 1846. The following year, Sir James Simpson discovered the anaesthetic properties of chloroform.

Chloroform is very rarely used today and the common general anaesthetics are nitrous oxide, halothane trichlorethylene, cyclopropane and sometimes ether. *The essential thing to remember for any patient having a general anaesthetic is never to have anything to eat or drink beforehand.* Disregard of this rule may have fatal consequences.

ANALGESICS are pain killing drugs.

ANAPHYLACTIC SHOCK is an extreme, often fatal form of allergy following injection of foreign material into the body.

ANEURYSM is a swelling of a blood vessel. Aneurysms in the blood vessels around the brain may burst and cause strokes (see **strokes**).

ANGINA PECTORIS is chest pain caused by disease of the arteries supplying the heart muscle.

ANKYLOSIS means restriction or fusion of a joint.

ANTHRAX is a bacterial disease caught from sheep, cattle or from their hides or wool — hence its popular name 'woolsorter's disease'.

ANTIBIOTICS are drugs used against germs. By convention, the term is applied only to drugs derived from organisms such as fungi. Examples are the penicillins, the tetracyclines, streptomycin and erythromycin.

ANTIBODIES are internal products of the body which attack and destroy foreign substances, such as invading bacteria.

ANTISEPSIS is the technique of killing germs. It was developed by Lister, following on the work of Pasteur.

AORTA is the largest artery of the body.

APPENDICITIS is an inflammation of the **appendix vermiformis.** The cause is unknown, but the symptoms are pain which settles over the appendix (see **appendix**) and persists for many hours, loss of appetite and fever. Vomiting is usual. For such a condition, nothing should be given by mouth, and a doctor should be called immediately. On no account give a purge. There have been unfortunate consequences when children with tummy aches were given laxatives when the actual cause of the trouble was, in fact, appendicitis.

Acute appendicitis is normally treated by removal of the appendix (appendicectomy or appendectomy). The recovery rate from this operation is now practically one hundred per cent, even though it was considered a difficult and dangerous procedure when it was first carried out.

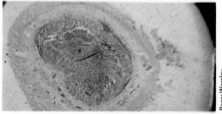

Roger Worsley

A normal appendix is seen here in section

APPENDIX literally means something added on. It is a term applied to a number of anatomical structures. The most well known, of course, is the **appendix vermiformis** (meaning 'worm-shaped appendix'), the structure which becomes inflamed in acute appendicitis (see **appendicitis**). It is an appendage to the ascending colon (that part of the large intestine which lies in the right side of the abdomen), which means that in most people it lies under the region of McBurney's point. The latter is an anatomical landmark which lies on a line drawn between the navel and the front prominence of the hip bone; it is the classical site of greatest tenderness in appendicitis. The appendix, which is about the thickness of a worm, and about the length of a finger, has no function whatever. It is present only in man, in certain apes, and in the Australian wombat.

APPETITE is desire for food. It is customary to draw a distinction between appetite and hunger, which provides a much more powerful stimulus. We do not yet have a clear understanding of the cause of either appetite or hunger.

APPROVED NAME is the official name for a drug, as opposed to its trade name or its chemical name.

APRAXIA means loss of the ability to carry out purposeful movements, for instance combing the hair or picking up an object, despite the fact that no paralysis is present.

AQUEDUCT is the canal along which fluid passes. There are two of these in the inner ear which communicate with the sub arachnoid space (see **arachnoidea**). The **aqueduct of Sylvius** or **cerebral aqueduct** is the cavity of the mid-brain through which cerebrospinal fluid circulates.

AQUEOUS or aqueous humour is the transparent fluid of the anterior chamber of the eye.

ARACHNIDA are one of the classes of Arthropods (see **arthropoda**), which includes scorpions, spiders, mites, and ticks. They usually lack wings and antennae, but some can live on the surface of the body, particularly in the hair. Both ticks and mites are the agents of disease. Ticks suck human blood.

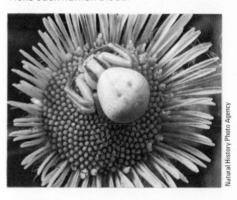

The crab spider, a member of the class arachnida, is a relative of ticks and mites.

ARACHNOIDEA is the central of the three membranes, also called meninges, which surround the brain and spinal cord. Between it and the innermost layer, the pia mater, is a space, the **sub arachnoid space.** When blood vessels rupture blood may flow into this space. The condition is called **sub arachnoid haemorrhage,** and surgery may be needed both to arrest the haemorrhage and to remove any clots.

ARCHES are structures resembling an arc or bow. There are many arches in the body, but those of the aorta and the foot are the most common examples. They are also found in the backbone and the skull.

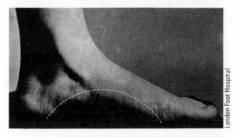

The high arches of the human foot enable man to walk upright on two legs.

17

ARCUS is a white ring around the cornea of the eye. It is common in the aged.

AREA is an anatomical term used to describe a particular surface or region of the body. In particular, the surface of the brain is described as divided into many areas which are responsible for ordering various functions such as speech, hearing, sight, smell and voluntary muscular activities.

AREOLA is any minute interstice or space in a tissue. It also relates to the coloured or pigmented ring surrounding the nipples of the breasts and the part of the eye's iris which encloses the pupil.

ARGYRIA is a bluish discoloration of the skin and mucous membranes caused by the prolonged administration or application of preparations of silver.

ARM is the upper extremity, reaching from the shoulder to the wrist joints. In Man the adoption of the upright posture frees the arm from weight bearing and allows it to be used for the myriad purposes of throwing, digging, lifting and so on. The arm and hand have played a major role in constructing Man's environment.

ARNICA is applied to sprains and bruises. It is extracted from the dried heads of the plant **Arnica montana.**

AROMATIC compounds have a ring-like structure. They are related to benzene and many having a spicy odour.

ARROWROOT is a variety of starch. At one time it was widely used to treat intestinal upsets and diarrhoea, especially in children and the aged.

ARSENIC is metal, but displays some non-metallic properties. It has held a place in history as a medicine, a poison, and as constituent of yellow pigments. Its poisonous qualities suit it for use as an insecticide and as a constituent of poison gas. Relatively easily available, it has for centuries been a favourite choice for murder. When given in small quantities over a long period of time it produces symptoms that resemble natural gastro-enteritis. Today, laboratory tests make arsenic easy to identify, but even before such tests it could be detected in the hair and nails where it is stored. A combination of arsenic and iron, was at one time a popular ingredient of tonics. In medicine arsenic has been valuable in the treatment of syphilis. **Arsphenamine** (bob or salvarsan) was one of the first drugs used to treat a specific disease.

ARTERIOSCLEROSIS is a thickening of the wall of the artery, causing loss of elasticity and blocking of the passage. Blood flow through the **sclerotic artery** may be seriously curtailed. The increased pressure required to force blood through the smaller pipes may be reflected in raised blood pressure which in turn may cause the heart to become damaged and enlarged. The cause of the thickening and degeneration is not yet known but research into ageing and disorders of the body's metabolism may provide the clue. The **sclerotic artery** becomes brittle and may burst, or pieces of the thickening may break off and block the artery completely.

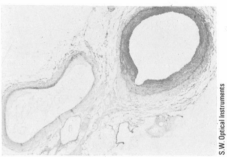

S.W. Optical Instruments

The artery, right, and vein, left, shown in section, carry blood throughout the body.

ARTERY is a blood vessel conveying blood from the right and left ventricles of the heart to the tissues. In all but one case, **arteries** contain blood which is freshly oxygenated. The exception is the **pulmonary artery** which takes the venous, deoxygenated blood from the heart to the lungs, where it is oxygenated.

ARTHRITIS is the inflammation of a joint. The symptoms are usually pain, redness, swelling and stiffness of the joint. Some types of acute **arthritis** may spread and cause severe pain. In its chronic forms it may involve particular joints. Rheumatoid **arthritis** is a chronic inflammation in most cases of the smaller joints of the hands and feet. **Osteo-arthritis** is a condition in which the joints crumble and degenerate and is common to joints which bear large weights – hips, knees or spine.

ARTHRODESIS, the fusion of a joint to make it stiff by removing its articular surfaces, is an operation sometimes performed to restore stability or to relieve pain.

ARTHROPLASTY means the making of an artificial joint, or a plastic operation on a joint which is diseased or damaged.

ARTHROPODA is the largest division or phylum of the animal kingdom and includes insects, crustaceans, spiders. The members have segmented bodies and an external skeleton with jointed appendages. Many **arthropoda** are pests or agents of disease.

ARTICULATION literally the joining together of sounds, is used in medicine to denote the movement of joints.

ARTIFICIAL INSEMINATION is the fertilization of the egg or ovum of the female by means other than intercourse. The sperm is artificially introduced into the uterus by an instrument such as a syringe. Widely used in veterinary fields, it enables large numbers of females to be fertilized by a relatively small number of selected males. In medicine A.I.H. (**artificial insemination by husband**) is practised and allowed when there is reason to believe that there is obstacle to fertilization in the normal way. A.I.D. (**artificial insemination by donor**) is practised in certain parts of the world in cases where the male is completely infertile.

ARTIFICIAL LIMBS (see **prostheses**) are used by patients who suffer amputa-

tion and by the congenitally malformed.

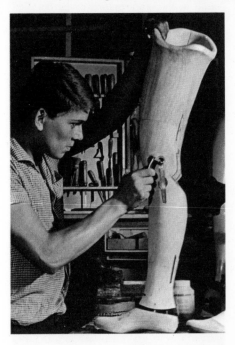

Artificial limbs enable the handicapped to walk with little disability.

ARTIFICIAL RESPIRATION is the promotion of normal breathing by artificially forcing air in and out of the lungs. (Intermittent pressure of hand or machine on the rib cage simulates normal breathing and maintains the flow of oxygenated blood to the lungs, artificial respiration is most commonly needed in cases of drowning, electric shock, asphyxia from smoke or asphyxia in the new born, and the first stages of diseases such as poliomyelitis. In this case there is paralysis of the muscles of respiration and permanent **artificial respiration** by an iron lung machine is required.

ASBESTOSIS (see **silicosis** and **pneumoconiosis**).

ASCARIS is a roundworm sometimes nearly a foot long which can infest man.

ASCITES is a condition commonly known as dropsy, which results from the collection of fluid in the abdomen. It is associated with heart failure or cirrhosis of the liver.

ASCORBIC ACID or Vitamin C is found in citrus fruits and green vegetables. Several centuries ago the disease scurvy caused by a deficiency of **ascorbic acid**, used to be common among sailors. But it was found that eating limes and citrus fruit during long periods at sea prevented outbreaks.

ASEPSIS is the complete absence of bacteria or any other organisms which cause infection. It was developed from antisepsis, the removal of bacteria by the use of antiseptic fluids. **Asepsis** implies that bacteria are not present. Modern operative techniques in surgery rely on the achievement of an **aseptic** milieu.

ASEXUAL REPRODUCTION is reproduction without sexual union. It occurs in some of the lower forms of plants.

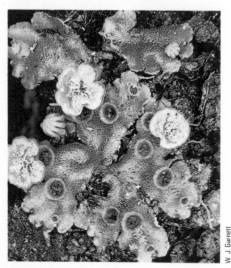

W. J. Garnett

The liverwort reproduces when a raindrop explodes the cups on its surface.

ASPHYXIA which literally means absence of pulse, is the name given to the symptoms which result when the action of the heart and lungs is stopped. The most common cause is suffocation

20

resulting from deprivation of oxygen.

ASPIRATOR is a negative pressure apparatus which is used to withdraw liquids from cavities — a process known as **aspiration**. An **aspirator** is used in surgery to keep the field of operation clear of blood and other fluids.

ASPIRIN, the name commonly used for acetylsalicylic acid (see **salicylates**), is a drug which has immense value in the relief of pain and fever. It is, however, an acid, and it should not be taken by those subject to stomach trouble. Overdoses are highly dangerous, and care should be taken in its use.

ASSOCIATION, apart from its usual meaning of 'joining' or a 'society', has a special connotation in psychology — a mental linking of objects, persons or events, with ideas, thoughts and sensations. **Free association**, a spontaneous association of mental images with little rational sequence or continuity, is used by psychiatrists to elicit thoughts repressed by patients.

ASTEREOGNOSIS is the inability to recognize objects by the sense of touch. It is found in certain kinds of nervous diseases.

ASTHENIA is a term used in medicine to describe a general loss of strength, which may be the result of psychological or physiological causes. Rest and a good diet. are the best methods of treatment.

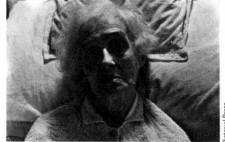

Pictorial Press

Asthenia is common to hospitalized patients, particularly to the elderly.

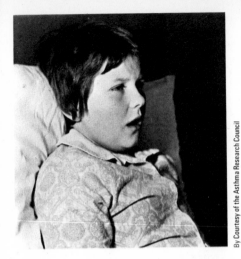

'Paroxysms of dyspnoea' is the medical term — but this young asthmatic knows only that breathing is very difficult. She feels she is suffocating.

ASTHMA is an allergic condition (see **allergy**), in which wheezing and difficulty in breathing occur at more or less frequent intervals. It develops rather more frequently in childhood than in adult life, and affects men more than women. Three factors may be involved in the precipitation of an attack of asthma; these are respiratory infection, psychological factors (such as anxiety or depression), and allergy. It may be impossible to trace the cause of the allergy. Regardless of the cause, the end result is contraction of the smaller bronchi and bronchioli (the passages through which air passes through the lung), swelling of mucous membranes and the over-production of mucus within the lung. Thus starved of a proper oxygen supply, the sufferer forces air into his lungs, but because of their blocked-up state has difficulty in exhaling. Attacks may be brief or last several hours. Some relief may be obtained by sitting the patient up and loosening his clothing, and by the use of various drugs. Longer-term treatment includes breathing exercises; isolation from any allergen (allergy-producing agent) by, for example, a change of occupation; and desensitizing the patient by inoculation against the allergen. Drugs must be prescribed carefully. Bronchial asthma developed in childhood often lessens in frequency or severity during adult life, but susceptibility to attacks, which is probably inherited, never ends entirely. So-called *'cardiac asthma'* is a completely different condition, being, in fact a form of heart failure. Although the treatment is entirely different, the symptoms, including 'gasping' for air', are similar to those of bronchial asthma. An attack of cardiac asthma calls for immediate medical attention.

ASTIGMATISM is a defect of vision caused by an irregularly-curved cornea (outer layer) of the eye. Instead of being curved equally in all directions, for example, from top to bottom and from side to side, the cornea has 'meridians' of varying radius. This means that instead of focusing at a point on the retina (the area at the back of the eye which transmits visual messages to the brain), light rays entering the eye are diffused over a wider area. In the same way that an out-of-focus camera produces a blurred picture, this produces blurred vision. A small degree of astigmatism is found in nearly everybody; a more serious degree can be corrected by spectacles whose lenses are curved to compensate for the defect in the eye itself.

ASTRAGALUS is the ankle bone. It is also called talus.

ASTRAPHOBIA is a morbid fear of lightning and thunderstorms.

ASTRINGENTS are substances used in medicine to help stop secretions or discharges, especially bleeding or the flow of mucus (see **mucus**). Some act by shrinking blood vessels, some by helping blood to coagulate and form a scab, and some by extracting from an organ the water which would help form mucus. The most important are the metallic astringents, including copper sulphate, silver nitrate, zinc sulphate, mercurous perchloride and calcium carbonate. In concentrated form, most of these are extreme

21

irritants, if not acutally corrosives, but in highly diluted form they are useful coagulants. Typical uses are in the treatment of diarrhoea (see **diarrhoea**), which in its simplest form is the production and discharge of copious quantities of mucus in the bowel; in the treatment of external ulcers; and in stopping the flow of blood from wounds. Adrenalin is widely used as an astringent in cases of bleeding from the throat or nasal passages. The body naturally produces adrenalin in the adrenal glands near each kidney. The adrenalin, together with its related compound, nor-adrenalin, simultaneously increases the rate of breathing, speeds up the heartbeat and contracts blood vessels. Synthetic adrenalin, applied externally, merely shrinks surface blood vessels. The vegetable astringents, containing gallic acid or tannic acid, have been known for centuries but are not now widely used.

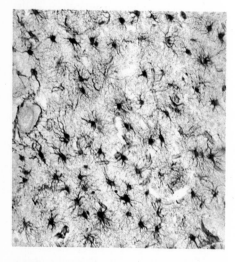

The dark nuclei and multiple branches of astrocytes, nutrient cells of nervous tissue in the brain and spinal cord.

ASTROCYTE is the name of the main cell of the neuroglia, the fine web of fibrous tissue, blood cells and so on which is the supporting tissue of the central nervous system. In cross-section it can be seen to have many processes (i.e., branches) giving it a star-shaped appearance. Along these processes, in both the white and the grey matter, flows nourishment for the nerve cells.

ASTROCYTOMA (see **astrocyte**) is the name for one of the commonest tumours of the brain or nervous system. It is malignant, but relatively slow-growing and has a fairly good prognosis (see **prognosis**), or outlook for life if found early and removed by operating. It is difficult to diagnose because it causes relatively few symptoms, being often in a part of the brain where pressure on the surroundings is unlikely, and hence failing to attract attention.

ASTROID means star-shaped (see **astrocyte**).

ASYLUM means a sanctuary, a place offering refuge from the outside world. It is correctly used of institutions for people unable to care for themselves — for example the paralysed or the blind. However, by becoming associated largely with hospitals for mentally disturbed people — especially the gaunt, prison-like hospitals of earlier centuries — it has lost much of its earlier meaning.

ASYMMETRY, in medicine, means a variation in the size, shape or position of organs on opposite sides of the body; or the lack on one side of the body of an organ found on the other.

ASYMPTOMATIC means without symptoms. For instance, many apparently healthy women have asymptomatic urinary infections. Although they have no symptoms, it is essential that they receive treatment until tests show the infection to be gone.

ATARAXIA means complete tranquillity, calmness or peace of mind. Hence **ataraxic, ataractic,** meaning a tranquillizer used in speaking of drugs such as reserpine and azacyclonal.

ATAVISM means the reappearance in an individual of remote ancestral characteristics which have not appeared in the intermediate generation. The everyday expression is 'a throwback'.

ATAXIA means lack of co-ordination of muscular action in various parts of the body. It is usually applied to difficulties in co-ordinating the movements of walking. Similarly, **ataxaphasia** means the inability to produce words in their proper order, and **ataxaphemia** the inability to co-ordinate the muscles producing speech. **Locomotor ataxia** is an old name for one of the stages of syphilis which produces difficulties in walking. The modern name is tabes dorsalis (see **tabes dorsalis**).

ATELECTASIS means imperfect expansion of the lung. It is used to describe two distinct conditions. The first is an uncommon (and usually fatal) condition in which the lungs of a new-born baby fail to expand. (Most babies expand their lungs with a deep cry soon after being born.) The second is a condition in which a blockage of one of the bronchial tubes carrying air into the lung 'starves' the lung of air and causes it to collapse. The blockage may be caused by mucus, as in bronchitis or inflammation of the lung, or by a foreign body. Children, in particular, are apt to get small objects like peanuts 'down the wrong way'. This may need urgent attention, because the objects can obstruct the air passages and prevent proper breathing.

ATHEROSCLEROSIS is a disease of the arteries in which deposits of lipids, which are fatty substances, build up on the artery walls. The lipids form in rough clusters or plaques, called **atheromata** (from which the Greek word *athare*, meaning porridge). By damaging the bloodstream substances which cause blood to clot, the plaques can become enlarged with clotted blood. Thus the bore of the artery is narrowed, producing higher blood pressure, and sometimes a clot will break free and block an artery — i.e., cause a thrombosis (see **thrombosis**). Atherosclerosis is believed to result from faulty diet, or tension, or both. It begins in early adulthood among a large proportion of people and may reach a dangerous state only after many years, or not at all. Thrombosis is more prevalent among peoples with advanced standards of living than among primitive peoples, but it has not been established whether this is because advanced people have a more faulty diet, or simply because more of them live to an age where the atherosclerosis becomes serious. In its earlier stages, the effects of atherosclerosis can be relieved by drugs. It is a form of arteriorsclerosis (see **arteriosclerosis**).

ATHETOSIS is a disorder of movement and posture, usually caused by brain damage in the early years of life. The patient makes intermittent movements which he is unable to control, and movements which he makes deliberately are clumsy and unco-ordinated. In trying to control his unwanted movements he may take up an odd posture. He may also make grimaces. Athetoid movements occur also in a condition called chorea (see **chorea**).

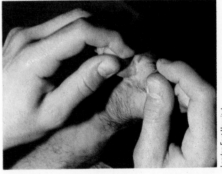

London Foot Hospital

Splitting, peeling skin — an intensely irritating result of athlete's foot.

ATHLETE'S FOOT is the everyday name for the infection of the feet by a fungus which is correctly described as tinea pedis. It is one of a number of plant parasites or dermatophytes (see **dermatophytes**) which can grow on the skin. Tinea normally occurs after contact with an infected person at a swimming pool or public bathhouse, or by using the same bathmat or laundry as an infected person. It can easily become prevalent at schools, military camps or sports training sheds. Tinea appears as little vesicles (blisters) be-

23

tween the toes. These are intensely irritating and, when scratched, are apt to break and attract infections of other types. As the area on which the fungus breeds may be moist, and is usually away from the air, tinea is difficult to eradicate once it takes hold – indeed, it may lie dormant and recur throughout adult life. Of the many ointments, paints, lotions and powders on the market for the treatment of this condition, most contain either salicylic acid or undecyleuric acid, both effective fungicides. However, trial and error testing of several preparations may be necessary before the individual finds one to suit him, and medical advice may have to be sought if the tinea-covered area becomes extensive or is infected by bacteria. Tinea also occurs on other parts of the body, notably between the legs (**tinea cruris**) and in the beard area (**tinea barbae**). The word tinea is the Latin word for a gnawing worm; like the word ringworm (see **ringworm**) it reflects ignorance of the true cause of the condition.

ATLANTO-OCCIPITAL JOINT is the name given to the joint between the Atlas (see **atlas**) and the base of the skull, the Occiput (see **occiput**).

ATLAS is the first cervical vertebra linking the skull to the spine. The second vertebra, the axis (see **axis**), fits into it like a peg, so that the head can rotate.

ATOMIZER is the name for a device which breaks up a liquid into a fine spray. A household example is the scent spray. A medical example is the aerosols used to combat such conditions of the lung as asthma and chronic bronchitis; these emit drug solutions in a fine spray, which is inhaled by the patient.

ATONY means a lack of tone (see **tone**) in the muscles to the point where they cannot perform their proper functions. An example is **atonic bladder**, where loss of muscular function makes it impossible to pass the urine.

ATOPY is a generic name for a group of

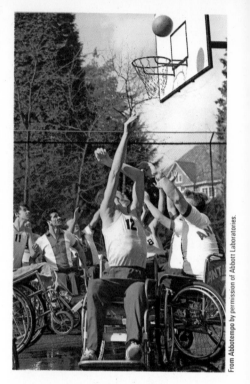

From Abbotempo by permission of Abbott Laboratories.

Stoke Mandeville Games help in the rehabilitation of paraplegic patients, whose legs are paralysed by spinal injury.

allergies (see **allergy**) which can be inherited and were at one time considered to be unique to Man. They include hay fever, asthma and atopic dermatitis. Recent research has shown that the atopic group can occur in animals too and also that, since most other allergies can also be inherited, this group differs little, if at all, from the allergies generally.

ATOXIC is a term used to describe a non-poisonous substance or a substance from which the poison or toxin has been removed.

ATRESIA is the closure of a normal opening such as the anus, vagina or auditory canal. It is found in new-born babies, sometimes in association with other abnormalities. It can usually be easily corrected by modern methods of plastic surgery.

24

ATRIUM means a cavity, entrance or passage. It is used anatomically to describe the two upper chambers of the heart where the blood from the veins collects (see **auricle**). Sometimes in heart disease the atrium beats out of phase with the part of the heart pushing out the blood to the body (see **ventricle**). Depending on the nature of the abnormal rhythm, the heart is then said to be fibrillating or fluttering.

ATROPHY is used in medicine to mean a reduction in the size of an organ or cell which has been, or which is, in disuse. It can also be used of the wasting of organs or muscles and of degeneration. Examples are: **Progressive muscular atrophy**, an uncommon chronic disorder of the nervous system which results in wasting of the limb muscles. **Atrophy of the liver,** a cellular degeneration; it occurs, for instance, where the cells actually degenerate, in cases of acute poisoning by substances (such as cleaning fluids) which are inadvertently swallowed.

ATROPINE – see **BELLADONNA**

A.T.S. is the common abbreviation for anti-tetanic serum. Until recent years this serum, which contains antibodies, called antitoxins, against tetanus, was given routinely as a protection for wounds and abrasions which might have come into contact with infected soil. It confers a 'passive immunity' (see **immunity**) – that is, one that is not produced by the patient's own body. However, it also tends to cause side effects (see **side effects**). Now, the usual procedure is to try to make the body produce its own antibodies by stimulating it with a vaccine (tetanus toxoid) thus producing 'active' immunity.

ATTAR is a general name for any of the volatile oils. **Attar of roses** is used in lotions and mixtures to make them smell and taste better.

ATTENUATION means a thinning, weakening or diluting. In medicine it is used especially to describe the reduction of the virulence of a virus or other micro-organism. This may be achieved by the continuous culture of several generations of the organism in the laboratory; the repeated inoculation of a culture through animals (this is referred to as *passage*); exposure to excessive light, heat or air; or the introduction of a weakening agent into the culture where it grows. Attenuated organisms are important because they will produce the same antibodies in the human body as will the more virulent organism; thus they can be used for vaccines.

ATTIC is the name for part of the middle ear, a cavity above the main chamber. Sometimes an infection in the attic will perforate the eardrum – an **attic perforation**.

ATTITUDE, in medicine, is the term used to describe the posture, or the position of the body and limbs; for example, the position of the foetus in the womb and how it is lying.

ATYPICAL means not typical, or irregular. One condition it is used to describe is a form of pneumonia, **primary atypical pneumonia**, due either to a virus infection or to another organism known as 'Eaton agent' and presenting symptoms different from the 'classical' attack.

AUDIBILITY means ability to be heard. Human beings can detect sound waves only of certain frequencies. The lowest frequency, or pitch, that the human ear can detect is approximately 30 vibrations per second (corresponding to a very deep vibrating rumble). The highest is in the region of 30,000 vibrations per second (corresponding to a piercingly shrill sound). Some animals can hear sounds outside the human range.

AUDIOMETERS are instruments for measuring the acuity (see **acuity**) and range of hearing. An **audiogram** is a record, in graph form, of the variations in the acuity of hearing of an individual as shown by the audiometer.

AUDIOVISUAL means relating to the ear and eye. It is used of apparatus which requires the use of both sight and hearing – for instance, television, as compared with radio (ear only) or the printed word (eye only). In education, audiovisual aids such as closed-circuit television are used for more rapid teaching than would be possible by lectures alone or by reading.

AUDITORY means relating to hearing, or to the organs of hearing. The **auditory canal** carries sound waves from the outer ear to the eardrum (see **ear**). The **auditory nerve** transmits the signals from the eardrum via the bones of the inner ear to the brain. A part of this nerve is also concerned with balance, and when damaged can cause giddiness.

AURA is most commonly used in medicine to describe the peculiar warning symptoms of an attack of migraine (see **migraine**) or epilepsy (see **epilepsy**). These warnings may be visual (wavy lines or a bright light), acoustic (a noise such as 'ringing bells') or olfactory (a sensation of a smell not necessarily connected with one's immediate surroundings). The Latin word *aura* means a breeze, odour or gleam of light.

AURIS is the medical name for the ear (see **ear**). **Auricle** is the lobe of the ear, but is also applied to the appendages of the upper chambers of the heart (see **heart**) because they bear a rough likeness to ears. An **auriscope** is an instrument, sometimes incorporating a light, for examining the ear. An **aurist** is an otologist, a specialist in diseases of the ear. **Auristillae** are eardrops. *Auris* is the Latin word for ear.

AUSCULTATION is listening to the sounds made by internal organs, such as the heart, lungs and intestines, through the chest or abdominal wall. Usually this is helped through the use of a stethoscope (see **stethoscope**), although the noises can be heard by the direct application of one's ear. Auscultation has a wide variety of uses, ranging from the detection of heart and lung disease to the monitoring of the baby's heartbeat in the womb during pregnancy and labour.

26

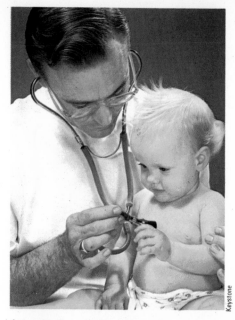

Keystone

Auscultation helps determine whether this child's heart is developing normally. The doctor is using a stethoscope.

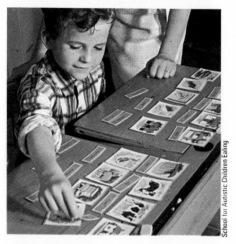

School for Autistic Children Ealing

Picture games help these autistic children develop rational thinking patterns, instead of being lost in their own world.

AUTISM means the state of being withdrawn from other people. **Autism of early childhood** is a condition affecting 4 in 10,000 children which begins from birth or within the first $2\frac{1}{2}$ years of life.

The development of the ability to use and understand speech, gestures, facial expressions and other forms of language is severely delayed, often leading to screaming as a means of communication. Characteristic disturbances of behaviour include fear of harmless objects while real dangers are ignored; an urgent need to keep wearing the same clothes, clutch the same toys, follow familiar routines, and so on; and retention of the babyhood habit of examining new objects by tasting and licking. The children can be greatly helped by special education similar in some ways to that used for deaf and blind children.

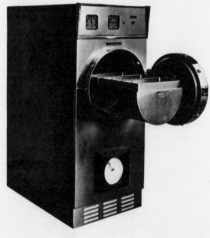

Steam sterilizes surgical instruments in a hospital's autoclave.

Drayton Castle

AUTOCLAVE is an apparatus for sterilization by steam under pressure. It consists of a strong, closed boiler containing a small quantity of water, and in a wire basket or perforated tin, the articles — surgical instruments, for example — which are to be sterilized. Because it operates under pressure, the water can be raised well above its normal boiling temperature, effectively killing bacteria over a period of time. Hospitals make extensive use of autoclaves.

AUTOHAEMOTHERAPY is a form of treatment by which blood is withdrawn from the patient's own vein and re-injected into his own muscles elsewhere.

Once used widely, in the belief that it would stiffen resistance to disease, it has now fallen into disuse.

AUTOIMMUNIZATION is the process by which the body, in overcoming an attack of a disease, retains its immunity against further attacks. Most, but not all virus diseases (see **virus**), such as ordinary (as distinct from 'German') measles, chickenpox and mumps, produce auto-immunization.

AUTOLYSIS is the self-digestion of cells within the living body, or the chemical breaking down of the tissue of an organ by an enzyme (see **enzyme**) peculiar to that organ. Sometimes this process is quite normal as when injured tissue is digested and replaced. But sometimes, enzymes escaping through a wound to areas where they are not normally present cause destruction. An example is the escape of pancreatic enzymes (see **pancreas**) into the stomach through a fistula (see **fistula**).

AUTOMATISM is the performance of acts by a person who knows nothing of what he is doing. It occurs, for example, in somnambulism (sleep-walking), after an attack of epilepsy, after concussion, and in some forms of hysteria such as fugue (see **fugue**). A person suffering from such a condition should be watched in case he injures himself or others.

AUTONOMIC from the Greek words *autos* ('self') and *nomos* ('law') means independent in origin, action or function; self-governing. In medicine it is applied to that part of the nervous system which controls bodily functions not requiring conscious thought — the heartbeat, for example, the movements of the intestine, and respiration. A complete network of nerves exists for these purposes. Normally one is quite unconscious of its workings, but it can be influenced by the higher nervous system, producing such reactions as blushing (see **blushing**), 'nervous stomach' and palpitations.

AUTOPLASTY is the repair of a defect (such as a non-healing burned area of

27

skin) by grafting tissue from another area or portion of the person's own body. Plastic surgery is one sort of autoplasty.

AUTOPSY is the correct description for the *post-mortem* (after death) examination of a body. It may be asked for by the relatives or by the attending doctors to ascertain exactly the cause of death, or to see whether some underlying condition has remained undiagnosed. It may be required by law if death is sudden or if the subject has not been recently examined by a doctor. In this case it is usually carried out on the orders of the coroner (see **coroner**). Except in remote places, the examination is usually carried out by a pathologist, who takes great care of the remains to enable a proper burial or cremation to be carried out. Some religions, notably orthodox Judaism, have a great aversion to such examinations, particularly the removal of any organ for further testing, such as microscopy. However, the practice has won wide approval for the light it has shed on bodily disease processes. In cases of suspected foul play, the autopsy result is vital in the compilation of evidence that a crime such as murder has been committed.

AUTOSUGGESTION means the acceptance of an idea, mainly from within one's own mind, which produces in oneself some change of bodily or mental state. It can be the persistence in the mind of ideas received while in a highly suggestible or hypnotic mental state. It is seen most dramatically after accidents, where a very slight injury may produce bizarre results — even paralysis.

AVASCULAR is the term for a bloodless area or part. Making an area temporarily avascular by compression can be of great service during operations on places like the middle ear.

AVICENNA, Ibn Sina (980–1036) was a famous Persian physician who wrote in Arabic a great compendium of medical knowledge, the *Canon*, which was the accepted authority in the Middle Ages. He was the first recorded person to des-

cribe the preparation of alcohol and of sulphuric acid. He noted that the urine of diabetics was sweet, and described anthrax (see **anthrax**).

AVOIRDUPOIS, strictly, is the English system of weights and measures. Colloquially it is used of those putting on excess fat.

AVULSION, in surgery, is the destruction of a nerve — for example, to paralyse the diaphragm and rest a diseased lung.

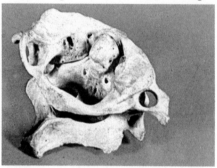

Shown together and apart: the atlas and the axis vertebrae in the neck

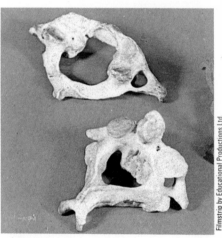

AXILLA is the anatomical name for the armpit. In the human the axilla is one of the few remaining sites of body hair.

AXIS — the line about which a rotating body turns — is used in medicine to describe the second cervical vertebra, around which the first, the *atlas*, turns.

28

BABINSKI is the name of a famous neurologist (a specialist in disorders of the nervous system) who gave his name to a reflex (see **reflex**). The Babinski reflex is elicited when a doctor scratches the soles of a patient's feet with a pin, or other sharp object. This procedure is a routine part of every full medical examination. In a healthy person, the toes should curl at the stimulus of a scratch on the sole of the foot, unless, of course, the skin is too thick for the sensation to get through. Sometimes, also, the patient is 'tensed up' and his toes do not curl as they should — again this is of no significance.

However, if the toes (and, more particularly, the big toe) go *upwards*, then this is referred to as a 'positive Babinski response' or 'upgoing planter reflex'. As a rule, this is a sign of trouble higher up in the central nervous system — for instance, a positive Babinski sign is often present after a stroke has taken place, and may provide valuable confirmatory evidence of the diagnosis.

These remarks, incidentally, do not apply to infants. In babies the central nervous system is immature, and the response to various stimuli is therefore at variance with what occurs in adults. Scratching the sole of a baby's foot will usually result in the toes going upwards, instead of curling, but this is perfectly normal. A normal child over the age of two, however, should have the same reaction as an adult.

BACILLI is a Latin word meaning 'little rods.' Bacilli are, therefore, rod-shaped-bacteria (see **bacteria**) — for instance the bacillus of tetanus or lock-jaw (see **tetanus**), the bacillus of anthrax (see **anthrax**), the bacillus of plague (see **plague**), the bacillus of tuberculosis (see **tuberculosis**), and so on. (See also **bacteriology**.)

BACK is the name generally applied to the part of the body which extends from the neck to the buttocks. It includes some of the most powerful muscles in the body; it also contains the vertebral column, which may be regarded as the main support of the whole trunk.

The muscles of the back consist of various layers, each running in a different direction. In addition, the spinal column has many ligaments attached to it, again running in all directions.

Thus the back is a complex structure consisting of a great many bones, joints, muscles and ligaments, and it is easy to see how readily the function of any of these structures can be interfered with, thus producing backache (see **backache**).

The expression 'a broken back' means in fact, a fracture of the spinal column. Fractures of the spine may or may not be of great seriousness, depending on where they occur. This is because the spinal cord (see **spinal cord**), which carries nerve impulses to and from the brain, runs inside the spinal column as far as the lumbar region. Therefore, a spinal fracture below the level at which the spinal cord ends is not likely to be all that serious. In addition, it is perfectly possible to have minor fractures of parts of the spine — for instance the 'processes' which stick out of the bones — without causing any severe damage. A typical example of this would be the 'stress fracture' suffered by men who do a lot of shovelling in their work;

Modern medicine has now curbed the deadly effect of the bacillus tuberculosis.

S. W. Optical Instruments

their muscles are believed to break off a 'process' of bone from a vertebra. (See **vertebra**.) Major fractures of the spine which damage the delicate tissue of the spinal cord ('complete fractures') are much more serious and must always be treated with the greatest care. They are really a combination of fractures and dislocation, and the effect may even be to shear right through the nervous connections between the brain and the body. If this occurs fairly low down (for instance in the chest or upper lumbar region) the results will include a paralysis of everything below the level of damage. However, if damage occurs in the neck, the results may be even worse — paralysis of respiration, or even death. This is the mechanism of judicial hanging, in which the jerk of the rope dislocates the topmost vertebrae of the neck, and cuts through the cord.

Never move a patient with a broken back, except when absolutely vital (e.g. to carry him to an ambulance). Even then, treat him with the utmost gentleness, moving the spine as little as possible, and carrying him *face downwards*.

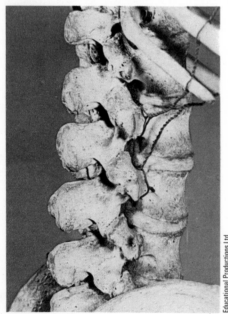

Educational Productions Ltd.

The five lumbar vertebrae form the lower part of the spine.

BACKACHE is one of the most common of all symptoms dealt with in a doctor's surgery. Unfortunately, it is only rarely that it is possible for him to come to a definite diagnosis, largely because the back itself is so complicated in structure (see **back**). Most of the population suffers from backache at one time or another, and many lay people come to the conclusion that they suffer from 'fibrositis', 'lumbago', 'chills in the back', 'rheumatism' or other ailments. In fact, these so-called conditions do not have any scientific evidence to support their existence. One only has to think about the immense complexity of the arrangements of bone, muscle, cartilage and ligament in the back to realize how easily painful minor strains can be produced, and also how easily the slight degree of arthritis (to which most of us are subject after the age of 40) can produce backache.

Apart from strains and arthritis, there are various other causes. Congenital deformities may sometimes produce pain in children and young people, blows or muscular effort may produce minor fractures of the spine, and protrusion of cartilages between vertebrae ('slipped disc') may be a cause of agonizing pain running from the back down the leg. Backaches may also result from spinal disease.

BACTERIA are germs. The word has been rather loosely used in the past, but, in general, germs (or 'microbes') are either *bacteria*, which are relatively large organisms or *viruses* (see **viruses**), which are considerably smaller. Among the important differences between the two groups is the fact that antibiotics can be used against bacteria, but are almost completely useless against viruses.

Bacteria were first seen by man in 1687 (although not associated with disease until the 19th century) when Leeuwenhoek observed them through the newly-invented microscope; viruses, being much smaller, were not visible until the invention of the electron microscope in the twentieth century. The bacteria are divided into two main groups — the bacilli (see **bacilli**), or rod-like bacteria, and the cocci, which are round. (See also **bacteriology**.)

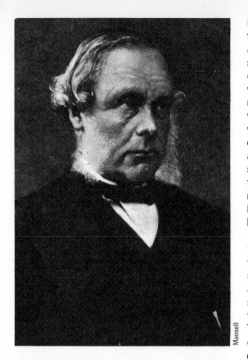

Mansell

Joseph Lister, the founder of antiseptic surgery, based many of his experiments on the work of Louis Pasteur.

BACTERIOLOGY is the study of germs and other microscopic forms of life, mainly those responsible for disease. (Owing to a confusion in terminology which has grown up over the years, bacteriology is not, as the name would seem to imply, just the study of bacteria.) Although germs had been observed through the microscope as long ago as 1687, it was nearly two hundred years before men began to suspect that micro-organisms were the cause of many diseases. Among the most important pioneers in this field was Semmelweiss. He was appalled by the high death rate in maternity wards, due to what was called 'puerperal fever'. A high proportion of newly-delivered mothers went down with this fever, and never recovered. It now seems incredible that it was not realized that the fever was due to infection by germs. Semmelweiss had little experimental basis for his theories, but in 1847 he decided to introduce strict measures of cleanliness in his wards

in an attempt to combat the spread of fever. Such was the ignorance prevailing at that time that he was subjected to the scorn and ridicule of his colleagues. However, within a very short time, Semmelweiss was thoroughly justified – the death rate among the mothers under his care fell with astonishing swiftness. Little interest was taken in Semmelweiss' work. A quarter of a century later, Louis Pasteur attempted to convince the world, by a series of brilliantly designed experiments, that germs caused infection. Again, the response was ridicule, from both the public and the medical profession. Eventually, however, Pasteur's work achieved recognition among the more open-minded scientists of his day – notably Lord Lister, who was at that time a relatively unknown surgeon in Scotland. Lister resolved to apply Pasteur's germ theory of disease to surgery, and thereupon developed the technique of antisepsis (see **antisepsis**). This had a remarkable effect on the results of his operations – the death rate fell dramatically, due entirely to the virtual abolition of post-operative infections. Lister brought his methods to King's College Hospital, London, where he taught them to the world. Although many of his fellow surgeons persisted to the end of their lives in their old ways (doggedly refusing to wash their hands before operations, never washing their instruments, and so on), their results were so disastrous, compared with those of surgeons who recognized the occurrence of infection by germs, that eventually the views of Semmelweiss, Lister and Pasteur triumphed. The new science of bacteriology was established.

Robert Koch developed bacteriology into a more exact science during the latter part of the nineteenth century. He found ways of growing micro-organisms in the laboratory, and laid down the first clear classification of them. They are grouped as follows: (a) *bacteria* (see **bacteria**), which are largish germs, visible under the microscope; (b) *viruses* (see **virus**), which are much smaller, and, in fact, so minute that they can be filtered through porcelain; (c) *Rickettsiae*, which are intermediate-sized organisms responsible for typhus and certain other fevers; (d) *yeasts*; (e) *fungi*, a small number of which cause disease in man, and (f) protozoans, which are minute single-celled organisms and probably members of the animal rather than the plant kingdom.

The list of disorders which are caused by micro-organisms is very long. The *bacteria*, for instance, are variously responsible for boils and similar infections of the skin (see **staphylococci**); sore throats, erysipelas and rheumatic fever (see **streptococci**); lobar pneumonia (see **pneumococci**); gonorrhoea (see **gonococci**); cerebrospinal fever (see **meningococci**); anthrax; diphtheria; tetanus; gas gangrene; botulism; tuberculosis; whooping cough; brucellosis; cholera; food poisoning; typhoid; plague; and a number of other infections.

Viruses are also responsible for numerous ailments, including the common cold. They are parasites which depend for their existence on the cells which they invade. Through their activity, the host cells are damaged or destroyed. Among the diseases caused by viruses are: influenza, mumps, measles, chicken-pox, smallpox, German measles, polio, and yellow fever. *Rickettsiae*, which are usually transmitted to man via ticks, fleas and similar parasites, are nowadays very rarely responsible for disease in this country; however, in other parts of the world, they are the cause of dreadful epidemics of typhus, Q fever, trench fever and Rocky Mountain spotted fever. Among the *fungi* which cause disease in man are those responsible for ringworm, athlete's foot, actinomycosis (see **actinic**) and other fungal infections of the lung, and moniliasis (thrush). Finally, *protozoans* are the cause of such diseases as malaria, sleeping sickness and amoebic dysentery.

BACTERIURIA means the presence of bacteria in the urine. A few germs in a urine specimen are of no importance, being due usually to contamination only. However, when there are more than a certain number of bacteria in the urine, this is called *significant* bacteriuria. When a hospital laboratory reports significant bacteriuria, this is a certain indication of the presence of infection (see **urinary infection**).

32

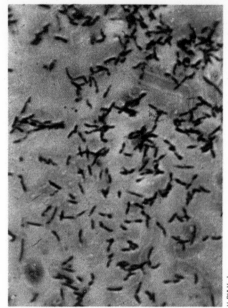

The *vibrio cholerae*, the bacillus responsible for the disease of cholera, was first discovered by Robert Koch. Bad sanitation and flies are the main causes for the spread of the disease.

BALANITIS means inflammation of the foreskin (prepuce) and often· of the glans penis, which underlies it. Balanitis sometimes occurs in small boys. Among adults, it is common in two categories of person. The first group is those who have neglected normal hygiene when washing. Balanitis of this type can become chronic and eventually lead on to cancer. Thus, it is obvious that boys should be taught at an early age to wash the genitals properly. The second group of people in whom balanitis tends to occur are diabetics. This is because of the fact that they pass sugar in the urine over a long period of years; it is believed that this encourages the growth of germs at the lower end of the urinary passage. In fact, this is probably not the whole story – diabetics are prone to infections of many kinds, for reasons that are not fully understood. (See **diabetes mellitus**.)

Balanitis is very frequently an indication for circumcision (see **circumcision**).

BALDNESS is absence of hair from parts of the body where it should normally be present — usually, of course, it implies baldness of the head. A very small number of cases are associated with specific diseases, but in the vast majority of instances, male baldness must, unfortunately, be regarded as part of the ordinary process of ageing. This type of baldness is often referred to as 'frontal' baldness, since it usually starts with recession of the hairline above the forehead; at the same time, there is often enlargement of the 'bald patch' on the crown of the head. Frontal baldness is very often inherited, from father to son; so, regrettably, it is the case that those whose fathers are bald stand a very good chance of going bald themselves. There is, at the present time, very little that can be done about this condition. It is quite certain that men who go to expensive 'hair-restoring' clinics, or who put themselves in the hands of barbers purporting to be able to cure baldness, are wasting their money. People describing themselves as 'trichologists' frequently make a great deal of money in this particular line of business, but readers would be well advised to have nothing to do with them.

In order to understand why frontal baldness cannot be cured, it is first essential to have a grasp of a few facts about the growth of hair on the scalp. There are about 100,000 hairs on the average man's head. Each hair arises from a minute follicle (or pit) in the scalp, and each grows about 0.35 millimetres a day in length. At any one time, about eighty-five per cent of these hairs are actually growing; the remainder are in a resting phase. Each hair goes through a growth phase of several years before entering the resting period. The 15,000 or so resting hairs will remain in their follicles until they either fall out, are pulled out, or are forced out by new hairs growing up from underneath. The hair shaft within the follicle is an entirely dead structure. Nothing whatever rubbed into or put on it will have the slightest effect as far as making it grow is concerned. It may be that at some date in the future it will be possible to give some sort of treatment, probably by mouth or by injection, to *prevent* hairs from going into the resting stage and subsequently falling out. This might be practicable, firstly because it is already known that the proportion of resting phase hairs varies a lot with the general health of the person in question — increasing, for instance, when a man is seriously ill. Secondly, the process of going bald is believed to be in some way related to the level of male sex hormones circulating in the body, and it might be possible to influence the survival of hair through hormone treatment. It should be made clear, of course, that baldness is quite definitely *not* caused by deficiency of male sex hormones — indeed, there are a good many people who believe that baldness is associated with masculinity and increased virility. So balding men can take comfort from that. The best thing a man can do, therefore, in order to avoid becoming bald, is to maintain his scalp in as healthy a condition as possible (see **dandruff**) by frequent washing and thorough drying. It is not advisable to use a sharp comb or brush. A hard hat should not be worn. In the rare instances where baldness is due to generalized illness, treatment of the disease should help the baldness. (See also **alopecia.**)

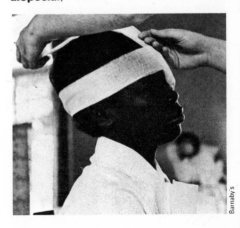

This patient is having an eye bandage fixed by the correct method.

BANDAGES should be available in every home's first aid kit (see **first aid**). Indeed, a knowledge of simple principles of bandag-

33

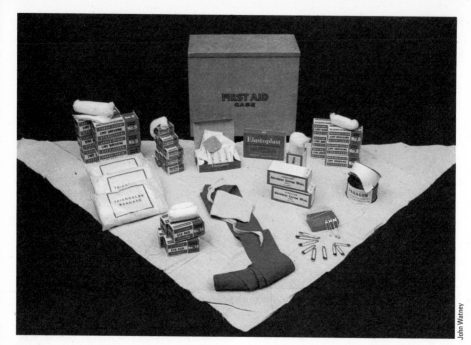

Every home should contain an adequate supply of bandages for emergencies. A sensible collection would include one large triangular bandage of unbleached calico; small, medium and large unmedicated dressings; a spool of adhesive plaster; a packet of absorbent sterilized cotton wool; a sterilized eye-pad with a bandage in a sealed packet; and 6 safety pins of assorted sizes for various purposes.

ing is extremely valuable; basic instruction is available through the first aid courses of various charitable groups and the Red Cross Society, and similar organizations, and these courses cannot be too highly recommended. Bandages may be of various materials. One or two ordinary *crêpe bandages* should be included in a first-aid kit. These are utility bandages — they are broad and strong, and can be used in an emergency for lashing splints to a limb, or as a simple sling, or for keeping a dressing on a limb. It is a good idea to have in stock a variety of *cotton bandages* of different widths, suitable for anything from a child's little finger to father's forearm. At least one long roll of wide *adhesive bandage* is a useful invest-

ment — this type of bandage is extremely suitable as a temporary expedient in sprains. In the case of a sprained ankle, for instance, it may be some time before a doctor can get to see the patient. In the meantime, support can be provided by applying a strip of adhesive bandage down one side of the calf, under the instep of the foot, and up the other side of the calf. The rest of the bandage is then applied in a cylindrical manner down the calf, with a figure-of-eight at the ankle to give further support under the instep. Also very useful are *tubular gauze bandages*, which can be bought with a special applicator that makes bandaging unbelievably quick and convenient. The applicator, which may be a wire or plastic frame, varies in size, depending on what part of the body is to be bandaged. The tubular gauze comes in the form of a long cylinder of bandage which is slipped over the frame of the applicator. The applicator is passed back and forth over the limb or finger to be bandaged, while a series of layers of gauze are fed out from the frame, producing a very neat dressing. Plaster bandages are applied by a doctor when rigid support is required.

34

BARBER'S ITCH, or **sycosis barbae,** is the name applied to a troublesome condition which affects the beard area in men. The whole of the shaving area becomes reddened and inflamed, with raised lumps (papules) and pustules around the hair follicles. There may also be a silvery-looking sheen on the skin. These features primarily result from infection by the germ known as **staphylococcus pyogenes** (see **staphylococci**), a common pus-forming bacterium present in boils, carbuncles, and similar infections. There may, however, be secondary infection caused by ringworm (see **ringworm**), and this is responsible for both the silvery scales and the intense itching. The sufferer may scratch the beard area and make the condition much worse. Shaving, too, makes **sycosis barbae** worse, and it is for this reason that it was originally known as 'barber's itch' since people believed that it was contracted at visits to the hairdresser. In these days, when most men shave themselves, it is obvious that barbers' utensils can rarely be the cause of infection.

Treatment may be prolonged but is usually successful. It is often necessary to stop shaving, since the razor cuts the tops off the little bumps in the skin, and this aggravates the condition. Otherwise, treatment is directed toward clearing up the staphylococcal infection and toward getting rid of ringworm. Antibiotics are usually the most effective method.

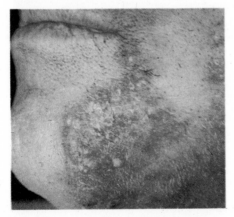

Barber's Itch causes a reddening and inflammation of the beard area.

BARBITURATES are sedative drugs used, among other purposes, to relieve anxiety and to promote sleep. They have played an increasingly important part in medical prescribing since the early 1940s, to the extent that it is widely felt that too many people have become dependent on large daily quantities of barbiturates.

Nevertheless, these drugs are immensely useful. They are classified according to the length of time in which they are believed to exert their effect in the body. Ultra-short acting barbiturates include Brietal and Pentothal. These drugs have an immediate effect of such a short duration that they can be used as general anaesthetics. An injection given into a vein in the arm reaches the brain in about 10 seconds, and immediately produces unconsciousness. From the effect of a single injection of Brietal or Pentothal the patient will remain 'out' for several minutes, but in most operations, it is the practice to administer, in addition, an anaesthetic gas. Pentothal is widely referred to as 'truth serum'. Of course, it is nothing of the kind, and the belief that people who are anaesthetized with it suddenly divulge their innermost secrets is nonsense. All that can be said is that if a *dilute* solution of either of the drugs is injected into a vein it will produce great mental relaxation. In such a state of relaxation, it is possible that a person might be more willing to answer awkward questions. This property of producing relaxation is an important effect of all the barbiturate drugs, and, in fact, it has now been found possible to use even the ultra-short acting barbiturates in this way. Psychiatric patients who have some particular irrational fear (such as claustrophobia), or who are paralysed with fright in certain situations, can be given dilute intravenous injections of barbiturates. During the few minutes of the drug's action, the patient is encouraged to imagine himself in the feared situation (e.g. riding on the underground, or going in a lift). The injection of barbiturate takes away the anxiety, and, after a few weeks of this treatment, the patient is often greatly improved.

Barbiturates of intermediate duration of action include Seconal, Soneryl, Nembutal and Amytal. These drugs have an effect which lasts for sufficient time to provide a night's sleep, and they are therefore widely used as hypnotics (sleeping pills). There is no reason, of course, why patients should not take these drugs under medical supervision, but it is important to remember that, as they are barbiturates, they are dangerous. The prescribed dose should therefore never be exceeded, and it is also vital to avoid taking them with alcohol: the combination of the two may have fatal results.

The longest-acting group of barbiturates includes Veronal and Gardenal (phenobarbitone). These drugs are mainly used for daytime sedation in various conditions, and for the suppression of epileptic attacks.

BARIUM ENEMA is a type of X-ray study of the lower bowel in which radio-opaque barium sulphate is injected into the back passage and a series of radiographs is taken.

BARIUM MEAL is an X-ray study of the upper parts of the gastro-intestinal tract, and, in particular of the stomach and duodenum. The patient is given barium sulphate to swallow, and a series of X-rays are taken. Such conditions as gastric ulcer, duodenal ulcer, and hiatus hernia (see **hiatus hernia**) may be demonstrated.

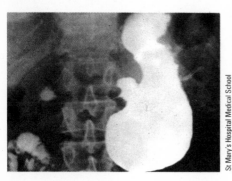

Barium meal indicates an ulcer in the left-hand wall of the stomach.

BARLEY WATER is a drink given to children which once enjoyed a great vogue. It is made from pearl barley, lemon and sugar. The ingredients are simmered in water for several hours and then strained.

36

BARRIER CREAM is a cream intended to prevent damage or infection. **Water repellent barrier cream** is used by those whose work involves getting skin wet. **Nasal barrier cream** (usually impregnated with an antibiotic) prevents transmission of nasal infections.

BAT EARS, or jug ears, are ears which are naturally prominent. They are not caused, as many people believe, by sleeping with the ears turned forward during babyhood. Taping the ears back to the head does not improve the condition. If such ears are a real embarrassment, simple plastic surgery will cure the condition.

B.C.G. is a vaccine against tuberculosis; its full name is *Bacille Calmette Guérin*. It is given to young children whose environ-

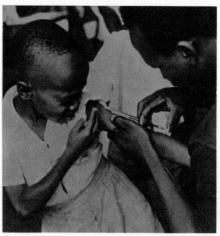

B.C.G. vaccine protects a Nigerian boy against TB, a major African disease.

ment renders them likely to fall victim to TB, and to doctors, medical students and nurses (who are also, of course, more likely than other people to get the disease). In Britain, it is frequently given to school-children of about 13 years of age. It has probably significantly reduced the incidence of TB. B.C.G. is the only vaccine which provides effective immunization against TB and which, at the same time, is safe enough for human use.

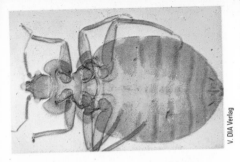
The wingless, blood-sucking bed bug is parasitic on Man. It remains hidden during the day and bites during the night.

BED BUGS are minute blood-sucking insects. They remain hidden in mattresses and blankets during the day. At night, when the unfortunate occupant of the bed goes to sleep and the bed warms up, the bugs emerge and begin to bite. When bed bugs are suspected, it is usually best to treat all bedding with D.D.T. It may also be advisable to treat adjacent furnishings and cracks in walls.

BED SORES are skin inflammations which tend to ulcerate. They can be extremely troublesome for those who are confined to bed for long periods. They rarely occur in young, fit people (for example, a young man with a broken leg) when reasonable care is observed. In the old and debilitated, however, bed sores often occur despite preventative measures. They usually develop on the buttocks, the shoulders, the backs of the heels, and the elbows, that is, on those areas which support most of the weight when a patient is lying flat on his back.

Prevention is, of course, better than cure, and when anyone is confined to bed for more than five or six days, care should be taken to avoid the development of sores. The bed-ridden patient's back, buttocks, elbows, and heels should be washed, dried, and carefully powdered once or twice a day. He should be encouraged to change his position regularly. If immobile or unconscious, he should be turned from his left side to his right, or vice versa, every two to four hours. If the skin over any of the pressure areas appears red and inflamed,

consult a doctor for advice. He will probably suggest the application of a protective cream and the provision of a 'ripple bed' or other special mattress.

BEE STINGS are seldom serious, but in a small number of cases they can result in anaphylactic shock (see **anaphylactic shock**). Individuals in such a condition, should be taken to hospital rapidly; artificial respiration should be applied if necessary. Bees sometimes leave a part of their sting, as well as poison, in the skin, and for the ordinary case of bee sting, it is only necessary to remove any sting which remains. Many people feel that bathing with bicarbonate of soda is helpful.

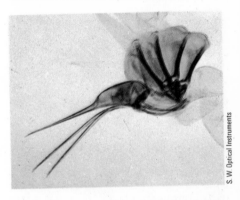
The bee's sting and poison (carried in the sac) may be left in its victim's skin.

BEEF TEA is made by simmering water into which beef has been shredded. It was once popular as a food for invalids.

BELLADONNA, or Atropa belladonna, is a poisonous plant known as the 'deadly nightshade' which grows on wild and chalky soils. The name 'belladonna' (or 'beautiful woman') comes from the alleged fact that the plant was once used by Italian girls to make their eyes seem large and beautiful. **Atropine,** the most important alkaloid of the plant, dilates the pupils. But it also makes it impossible for the eye to accommodate, that is, to focus on close objects. Other effects of atropine include quickening of the pulse and dryness of the mouth and respiratory tract.

Atropine is an extremely useful drug

37

as a premedication (see **premed.**) for general anaesthesia: it dries up the secretions which might otherwise cause difficulty during the anaesthetic period. Atropine is also effective in decreasing the activity of the gut in certain stomach and intestinal troubles. It is used in ophthalmology and as an antidote to certain poisons. *Poisoning by belladonna or atropine:* the warning symptoms are dryness of the mouth and enlargement of the pupils, together with a fast pulse rate. If the dose has been very large, unconsciousness and paralysis may result. Make the patient vomit and get him to hospital at once. If possible, take the plant or berries along for identification purposes.

get to a doctor or a hospital immediately.

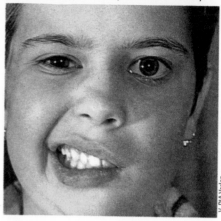

In Bell's Palsy, the muscles of the face are paralysed, the mouth is drawn to the side, and the eye cannot close.

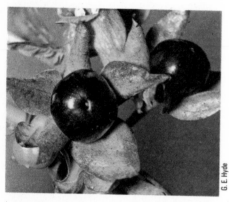

The berries and leaves of belladonna contain the poisonous juice atropine.

BELL'S PALSY, or 'wry face', is quite a common condition in which the mouth is drawn sharply to one side and the whole face becomes asymmetrical. Occasionally the sense of taste is impaired if the nerve passing through the skull is injured. The condition results from a paralysis of the seventh cranial nerve which supplies the muscles of the face. The cause of the paralysis is not known. Fortunately, however, a high proportion of sufferers recover spontaneously. The first effective treatment for Bell's Palsy was discovered in 1966, when it was shown that immediate injections of A.C.T.H. (see **A.C.T.H.**) produced remarkable results. It is essential to have this treatment at once – within 24 hours, if possible. Anyone with the condition should

BENDS (caisson disease) is an affliction of skin-divers, deep sea divers and others, such as tunnellers, who breathe pressurized air. When an individual works for a time at increased pressure, the nitrogen from the air he breathes dissolves in his tissues. If he 'decompresses' gradually, that is, undergoes a slow reduction of air pressure, he will be perfectly safe. If, however, he decompresses rapidly (as in the case of a diver or an escaping submariner who quickly rise to the surface), he is likely to experience the bends. Bubbles of nitrogen form in the tissues and produce excruciating pain and even paralysis, headache and dizziness. In certain cases death can suddenly result. The condition can usually be remedied if the patient is recompressed for a period, and decompressed slowly.

BENEDICT'S SOLUTION is used in medicine to test the sugar content of urine.

BENZEDRINE is a highly dangerous drug of the amphetamine group (see **amphetamines**). It produces an elevation of mood and wakefulness, which make it popular with some young people. Its non-medical use should be avoided at all costs, as many people who have taken benzedrine have progressed to the use of even more dangerous drugs such as heroin.

38

BENZYL PENICILLIN, also known as crystalline penicillin or penicillin G, is the most commonly used form of this antibiotic. (See **penicillin**.)

BERI-BERI is a disease caused by lack of vitamin B_1. It is common throughout the Orient and certain parts of the tropics, mainly because the diet of poorer people in those areas consists largely of rice. When rice is milled, the husk, which is the only portion containing vitamin B_1, is removed.

There are several forms of beri-beri. The principal manifestations of the 'wet type' are similar to those of heart failure – the body becomes grossly swollen and waterlogged (oedematous). The symptoms of the 'dry' type of beri-beri are like those of a very severe neuritis (inflammation of the nerves); thus, there may be paralysis and complete loss of feeling over areas of the skin. These changes occur because one of the normal chemical breakdown processes in the body is blocked in the absence of vitamin B_1. The physical changes caused by 'wet' beri-beri are not so clearly understood, and it has recently been suggested that some other deficiency may be involved in this form of the disease.

BERRIES which grow wild are often

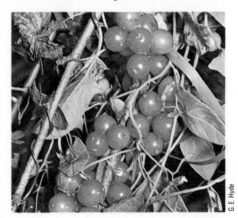

Berries of Black Bryony are among the many poisonous fruits of the countryside.

poisonous to small children, and, indeed, to adults. As most poisonous berries are either red or black when they have ripened, they may be distinguished by their colour. Among the most dangerous of berries are the woody nightshade (red), the deadly nightshade (black) (see **belladonna**), the cuckoo-pint or lords-and-ladies (red) and the Yew (red).

When a person has swallowed berries which may be poisonous, it is advisable to make him vomit, and get him to a hospital immediately. Take the berries for identification.

BEZOAR is any kind of solid body which forms in the stomach or intestines. **Trichobezoars** are masses of hair that form in the stomachs of cats who have swallowed a lot of their own hair and occasionally in human stomachs (for instance, children or deranged persons who may eat large amounts of hair). Trichobezoars may be removed by operation.

BICARBONATE OF SODA (sodium bicarbonate or baking powder) is a mild alkali (see **alkali**) widely used to neutralise stomach acidity. The carbon dioxide released from the soda is used in cooking to make cakes 'rise'.

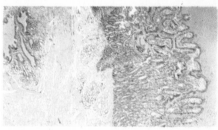

The gall bladder, shown here in detail, is a reservoir for bile in the body.

BILE is a fluid secreted by the liver. It aids in the digestion of fats and the absorption of nourishment from the food passing through the intestines. It flows from the liver, down the bile ducts and into the gut, where it acts on the intestinal contents, and changes their colour from pale to brown.

Bile is usually golden yellow in colour, but it may be greenish. About a pint of bile flows down the bile ducts and into the duodenum each day. Part of it is stored in

39

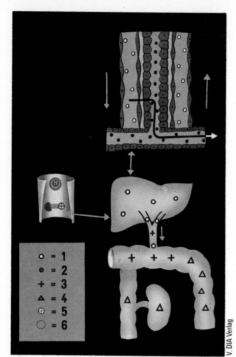

V. DIA Verlag

Bile, formed in the liver, assists in digestion by emulsifying fats. Chemicals, 1, 2, 3, 4 are its active ingredients. They are being manufactured at the top of the picture. In the centre, bile is entering the digestive tract. Bile contains the remnants of red blood cells, 5, 6, which are being broken down on the left (in blue).

the gall bladder, which acts as a reservoir, contracting and emptying when a fatty meal is eaten. When anything obstructs the common bile duct (e.g. a gall stone, a growth, or a cyst), the bile is dammed up within the liver. If this continues, the skin begins to turn yellow and the motions become putty coloured. These symptoms indicate obstructive jaundice (see **jaundice**).

A bitter yellow or green liquid which is vomited is always bile. In an adult, this may not be of great significance, as it sometimes accompanies dyspepsia. But in a newborn baby it is usually the sign of an intestinal obstruction beyond the point where the common bile duct enters the duodenum.

40

BILHARZIA, or schistosomiasis, is a parasitic disease of certain tropical countries. There are three principal species of the parasite which causes this disease: *Schistosoma mansoni* (found mainly in Egypt), *Schistosoma haematobium* (found mainly in East and Central Africa), and *Schistosoma Japonicum* (found in the Orient). The victim is infected when he bathes in infested water. The schistosomes penetrate his skin, and later mate and produce eggs in the veins within his abdomen. The eggs pass to either the intestine or the bladder where they cause bleeding and tissue destruction. Many eggs are passed out in the urine or the faeces. In areas where hygiene is poor, these discharged eggs are often eventually emptied into a river or lake containing snails, which act as an intermediate host for the parasite until it is mature enough to infect another passing swimmer.

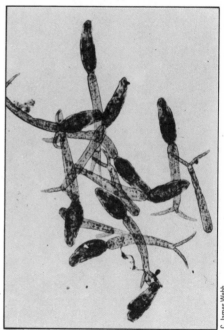

C. James Webb

Infective schistosomes of the disease bilharzia penetrate the skin of a swimmer, mate and produce eggs in his abdomen.

BILIRUBIN is the yellow pigment of jaundice (see **jaundice**).

BIOPSY means removing a small piece of tissue for examination under the microscope as an aid to diagnosis.

BIRTH (see **labour**).

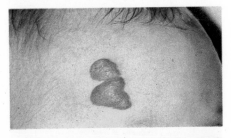

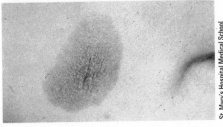

St. Mary's Hospital Medical School

The birthmark, *top*, is common and usually falls off, quite naturally, soon after birth. The more complex kind, *above*, may require removal by surgery.

BIRTHMARKS are skin discolorations of various kinds which are present on all of us from birth. Generally they are small and unobtrusive. *Moles*, or raised pigmentations, are the commonest type and rarely require treatment (see **moles**). More troublesome are the types of birthmark known as *naevi*, which may be disfiguring. *Capillary naevi*, which usually occur in the region of the head, are composed of dilated capillaries (see **capillaries**), or tiny blood vessels. Carbon dioxide snow may be used to destroy small naevi of this type; larger ones can be dealt with by radium therapy or excision. However, not all cases are suitable for treatment, and many plastic surgeons prefer not to remove them. In such instances, cosmetic preparations may be used to cover the naevus. *Cavernous naevi* are purplish swellings which consist of dilated veins from which blood can be forced out by pressure. Where practicable, cavernous naevi are excised

or burnt away. Sometimes, it is possible to shrink them by injecting liquid to thrombose (clot) the veins inside them.

BISMUTH is a metal which was once widely used in the form of injection for the treatment of syphilis. It has now been superseded by penicillin for this purpose. Medicines containing bismuth are still frequently employed for stomach disorders.

BITES are abrasions, punctures, or lacerations of the skin caused by animals. Ordinary **dog-bites** usually only require thorough cleansing with an antiseptic and a small dressing. It is, however, advisable for those who are not fully immunized against tetanus (lock-jaw) to receive the necessary injections. The risk of rabies, or hydrophobia, (see **rabies**) following a dog-bite is non-existent in countries where there are strict laws governing the quarantining of dogs.

Members of the cobra and viper families are largely responsible for the approximately 30,000 deaths each year from **snake-bites**. The vast majority of these occurs in India, and snake-bites are rarely fatal elsewhere.

The viper or adder may be distinguished from the common and completely harmless grass-snake by the dark line down its back and the 'V' on the top of its head. It is usually a benign reptile, which is frightened of human beings and makes off when it hears them approaching. During the spring, however, when the viper is drowsy, it may not hear the approach of human feet and, in self-defence, attack those who tread on it.

Bites from its fangs are unlikely to give serious trouble to an adult, or even to a child, unless the injection of venom goes into a vein, or anaphylactic shock results (see **anaphylactic shock**). However, it is wise to suck the bite out and wash it carefully. A doctor should be consulted to decide if an injection of snake-bite serum is required. Do *not* follow the dangerous practice of making a cut in the skin near the puncture wounds. This is useless and may lead to complications. If the patient develops severe shock of the anaphylactic type, he should be given artificial respira-

41

tion, if necessary, and rushed to hospital.

The effects of **spider-bites** have been greatly exaggerated. Although many tropical spiders are 'poisonous' (in the sense that they carry venom), the number that can actually kill is small. One of the most dangerous members of this group is the *Latrodecta*, the female black widow spider. She is glossy black and has a characteristic red hourglass mark on her belly. In the U.S.A., she spins her web in woodsheds, disused buildings, and outdoor lavatories. Many patients are bitten on the buttocks or genitals while going to the toilet. The agonizing pain which shortly follows is principally abdominal and may thus be mistaken for an entirely different illness. An anti-serum is used for treatment. However if an abscess forms it is treated in the normal way. The number of deaths attributable to the black widow spider probably do not exceed two or three per cent of those bitten.

(For stings, see **bee stings, hornet stings,** and **wasp stings**.)

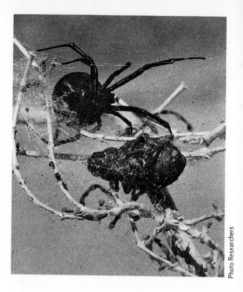

The Black Widow spider spins its web in disused buildings. Its bite is extremely dangerous, and sometimes fatal.

BLACK DEATH is another name for the bubonic plague (see **plague**) which ravaged Europe in the Middle Ages.

BLACKHEADS are dark spots in the skin caused by sebaceous glands blocked with dust or dirt. They are common among adolescents and those with acne. Blackheads may be pressed out with the fingers, but they must be scrupulously clean. It is, however, better to use an instrument which is easily obtainable for the purpose. A doctor's advice should be sought if blackheads are troublesome.

BLACK MOTIONS usually indicate bleeding in the intestines. They are normal if iron tablets are being taken; in other cases, consult a doctor.

BLACK VOMIT, or 'coffee-ground vomit', is generally caused by bleeding in the stomach. Consult a doctor at once.

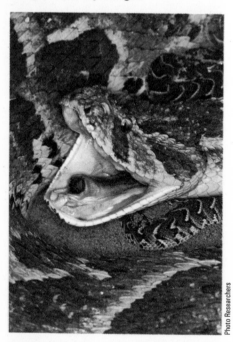

When the African Puff Adder bites its victims, it injects venom from poison glands connected with its teeth.

BLACKWATER FEVER is a severe phase of malignant tertian malaria (see **malaria**). The blood pigment haemoglobin (see **haemoglobin**) is not retained by the kidneys, but goes through the kidney

42

filter and into the urine. The urine which is then passed is black in colour.

BLADDER is a muscular sac capable of powerful contraction. In humans it usually refers to the **urinary bladder**, but it also applies to the **gall-bladder** (see **gall-bladder**). The urinary bladder is situated in the front of the pelvis. In men, it is immediately in front of the rectum; in women, in front of the uterus and the vagina.

Urine leaves the bladder and reaches the exterior through a tube called the *urethra*. In the female in particular, this tube is so short that it is relatively easy for germs to enter the bladder from the outside and cause a *cystitis*, or bladder infection. Recent research has shown that urinary infections are potentially serious and should be treated with antibiotics until laboratory tests indicate that the bladder and urinary tract are free of infection (see **urinary infection**). Otherwise, such infections may spread up the *ureters* (the two tubes which carry urine to the bladder) as far as the kidneys, where they may do great harm.

When there is a stoppage of the urine, the bladder accommodates a rather larger volume of urine than the approximate pint which it customarily holds. In such cases, the bladder would eventually burst if the stoppage were sufficiently prolonged. Such an occurrence, however, is very rare indeed: firstly, because the patient usually receives medical aid in time, and secondly because the kidneys probably secrete less urine into the bladder once the retention has started. (See also **urine, stoppage of**).

Other conditions which may affect the bladder include diverticula (pouches which form in the walls), stones (which must usually be removed by operation, either by cutting the abdomen open or by passing a crushing device up the urethra), and growths (both benign and malignant). All these conditions may be inspected, without cutting the abdomen, by passing a thin telescope-like device called a cystoscope up the urethra. Some types of cystoscope have special devices on the end which make it possible for them to grasp stones and crush them, to remove small stones, or to cut pieces from the prostate

gland (see **prostate**), which lies at the neck of the bladder. (See also **cystitis, ureter, urethra, urine**).

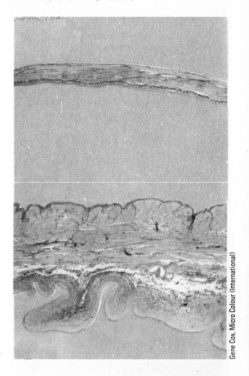

Gene Cox, Micro Colour (International)

The bladder wall, distended, *at top*, relaxed, *below*, consists of four layers: mucous membrane, epithelial cells, muscular coat, and serous membrane.

BLEEDING, or haemorrhage, means any kind of blood loss, whether external or internal.

Bleeding from an artery is characterized by bright red spurts in time with the pulse. Such bleeding may be dangerous, especially if the large femoral artery, which supplies blood to the leg, is opened. Arterial bleeding in the arm is much less serious. **Bleeding from a vein** is indicated by the 'welling' of dark blood. It is not usually of great seriousness but often does require medical attention – a stitch or a pressure dressing may be needed. **Bleeding from capillaries** (tiny blood vessels) occurs when the skin is slightly cut or grazed. The area should be carefully cleansed; it is also important to ensure that tetanus immunization is up to date.

Treatment of severe bleeding. Apply *very* firm pressure over the site of the bleeding, preferably using a thick clean pad of tissue, such as a large wad of cotton wool, or several clean handkerchiefs; a wide bandage, firmly wound over the pad, may help. The pressure must be *constantly* maintained until medical help arrives. If this does not arrest the bleeding satisfactorily, move the pressure pad slightly nearer the heart. Elevation of the part is helpful.

The most efficient method of stopping bleeding from an artery is to apply pressure directly to the point of bleeding, or fractionally above it. The main exception to this principle occurs when the bleeding point is inaccessible in the deep muscles of the thigh. In such cases, the femoral artery (which is felt beating firmly at the groin) should be compressed backwards against the head of the thigh-bone.

(For bleeding diseases, see **haemorrhagic disorders**; for bleeding nose, see **epistaxis**; for bleeding from the back passage, see **bowels** and **haemorrhoids**; for bleeding from vagina, see **periods**; for bleeding in the urine, see **haematuria**).

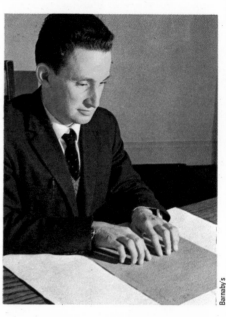

BLINDNESS is a condition which involves the total or partial loss of vision. Common causes include retinal diseases (see **retina**), glaucoma (see **glaucoma**), cataract (see **cataract**), and diabetic retinopathy (see **diabetes mellitus**).

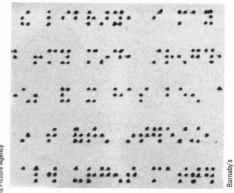

The use of a tourniquet to control arterial bleeding, once standard First Aid procedure, is now believed to cause damage to blood-starved tissues.

The blind man, *top*, reads with his fingers. The raised pattern of dots which form the braille alphabet, *above*, was invented for the blind in 1834.

BLEPHARITIS is inflammation of the eyelid.

BLIND SPOT is a tiny area on the retina of the eye which is insensitive to light.

BLISTERS (see **scalds**).

BLOOD consists of a fluid (plasma) which contains red corpuscles, white corpuscles, blood platelets, and dissolved salts, hormones and other chemicals. Red corpuscles (or red cells) are tiny biconcave discs which contain the pigment haemoglobin, whose remarkable chemical properties enable them to carry oxygen (see **haemoglobin**). When haemoglobin is lacking a condition of anaemia (see **anaemia**) is present.

The white cells are basically concerned with the defence of the body. One particular group, the neutrophils, increase rapidly in number whenever the body is invaded by bacteria. If the infection is generalized, these neutrophil white cells circulate in the blood stream and attack the invading bacteria. If it is a localized infection, such as a boil, they congregate around the infection zone, wall it off from the rest of the body, and thus prevent the spread of the infection. There are other types of white cells, and they have their own specialized functions in protecting the body against attack. For instance, one group, the eosinophils, increases rapidly when the body develops an allergic response to any foreign substance.

Platelets, which play a vital role in the process of clotting of blood, are also present in the blood.

Blood circulates throughout the body, bringing the tissues nourishment and oxygen and carrying away carbon dioxide and other waste products. Blood is pumped by the left side of the heart, through the arteries, into the tissues where the oxygen in the blood is exchanged for carbon dioxide and waste products. The transfer of gases is effected through the walls of microscopic vessels called capillaries. The walls of these tiny tubes are partly permeable, that is, they allow essential materials to flow in and out, to and from the tissues. When the blood has passed back through the capillaries, it flows on into the smallest branches of the veins, or venules. These gradually combine to form larger and larger veins, which eventually reach the right side of the heart. From here, the blood is pumped to the lungs where it receives a fresh supply of oxygen before it returns to the left side of the heart, where the cycle restarts its life-giving processes.

The blood flowing through the arteries contains oxygen and is therefore said to be oxygenated; this is why it is red. Because the oxygen is taken up in the tissues, by the time it reaches the veins it is deoxygenated and is therefore much darker and almost bluish in colour.

The heart normally pumps about ten or twelve pints of blood every minute, but this amount increases sharply during exercise or strenuous activity. The amount of blood in the body varies greatly from person to person, and even in the same person on successive days. Generally, however, there is rather less than one pint of blood for every 14 pounds of bodyweight.

Blood is constantly being manufactured in the marrow of the small bones, in some glands, and, probably, in the spleen.

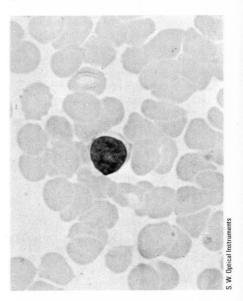

The small white cell, or lymphocyte, stained here is one of the body's defenders.

BLOOD DONATION is an almost painless and completely harmless procedure which involves the taking of blood from a vein in the arm. The blood can then be safely stored at a temperature of 2° to 6°C. for three weeks before use.

A brief initial health check is the only

requirement for becoming a blood donor (see **transfusion**).

BLOOD GROUPS are classifications made according to the ability of the blood of one person to agglutinate the red corpuscles of another's (see **agglutination**). The most important systems of blood grouping are the ABO and the Rhesus systems. In the ABO system, people are classified into group A, B, AB, or O. Blood groups A and B each contains a different antigen (a substance which causes antibodies to form against the antigens which may be present in other blood). If group A blood is given to someone of group B, or vice versa, the antigens cause agglutination and the results may be disastrous. Group O blood, known as the 'universal donor', contains no A or B antigens, and could, if necessary, be given to a person of any blood type provided there were no Rhesus incompatibility. AB blood, the 'universal recipient', contains both A and B antigens and no opposing antibodies, therefore, people with AB blood could in emergency receive blood from type A, B, or O. (See **transfusion**; for Rhesus blood grouping, see **Rhesus factor**.)

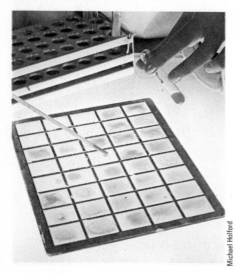

Before blood can be given in transfusion, the laboratory must check that the blood groups of donor and recipient are compatible.
46

BLOOD POISONING usually refers to a condition known as septicaemia in which a person is poisoned by germs which circulate in his blood. If the bacteria deposited from the blood cause abscesses to develop over his body, it is known as pyaemia.
Blood poisoning was once a common and often fatal infection. Today, however, it is usually curable by antibiotics if it is caught in reasonable time.

BLOOD PRESSURE is the pressure exerted by the blood on the walls of the arteries. (For high blood pressure, see **hypertension**.)

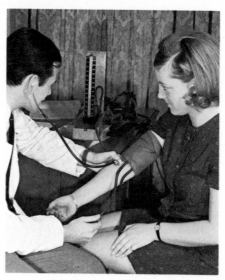

Michael Holford

A sphygmomanometer is the instrument used to measure blood pressure. Pressure raises mercury in a column.

BLOOD SPITTING, or haemoptysis, is the bringing up of blood from the lungs. It can have a variety of causes, some serious and some trivial. However, all patients with this symptom should see a doctor at once.

BLUE BABY is the non-medical term used to describe babies who are born with certain types of heart defect. The blueness (cyanosis) is an indication that the blood is not being properly oxygenated; and it is normally seen around the face and extremities.

BLUENESS, or cyanosis, is a common sign of certain disorders of the heart or lungs (see **blue baby**). The blueness appears when a proportion of the haemoglobin (see **haemoglobin**), the pigment which carries oxygen around the body, is insufficiently oxygenated. The appearance of cyanosis is an indication to consult a doctor, since it may indicate the presence of chronic pulmonary disease or of various kinds of cardiac disabilities (see **lung** and **heart**).

BLUSHING, the rushing of blood to the skin, is an extremely common phenomenon among girls, and, indeed among young people generally. The psychological mechanisms which cause blushing are not entirely clear. It is probably significant that a clothed person usually blushes only in the exposed areas (the face and neck), while a naked person blushes much more extensively. Feminine blushing is usually quite attractive to the male, and this, perhaps, explains at least part of its function. It may, however, be a source of great embarrassment to adolescents, and in such cases a reassuring word and some mild sedation from the family doctor may be helpful.

BOIL is an infection of a hair follicle usually caused by the bacterium known as *Staphylococcus aureus* (see **staphylococci**), an extremely common micro-organism which is often present in the nose and in many infected cuts, styes, and pimples. Staphylococci are easily transmitted from person to person. If they manage to get down a hair follicle blocked by sweat, skin oils, or other debris they may form a boil. In such circumstances, the bacteria rapidly multiply and pus is formed around them. Because the internal volume of the hair follicle is small, the pressure becomes so great that the boil is usually extremely painful. In some cases, however, the body's defences overcome the infection and the boil 'resolves'. More frequently, the boil bursts, or has to be lanced by a doctor, and pus flows out. The emergence of the 'core' marks the end of the condition.

Some boils, however, develop into a large abscess, and incision, preferably in an operating theatre, is essential. A boil may also develop into a carbuncle (see **carbuncle**) if it spreads more widely into the tissues.

It is essential *not* to touch boils or the pus from them with one's fingers, as this may well lead to the spread of infection elsewhere. The development of crops of boils is often caused by touching. In such cases, a doctor will usually send a specimen of pus to the laboratory and, in the meantime, put the patient on an antibiotic. As crops of boils are occasionally an indication of diabetes, the doctor will generally also check the urine for sugar.

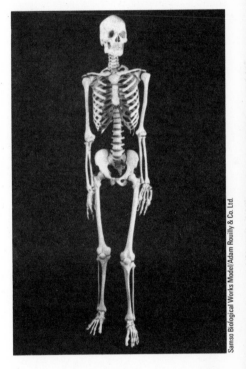

Samso Biological Works Model/Adam Rouilly & Co. Ltd.

Some 212 bones form the human skeleton, framework of the body.

BONES are the framework of the human body. There are about 212 bones in the body, although the number may vary slightly. Many people have tiny extra bones called **sesamoid** bones. The largest bone in the body is the **femur** or thigh bone. The smallest are the six small auditory ossicles (three on each side of the middle ear), which conduct sound waves. Bone consists of a basic **matrix** which has been impregnated with calcium and phosphorus in the form of calcium phosphate and calcium carbonate. Bones show up on X-rays, because heavy elements like calcium slow down the rays and cause a 'shadow' to form on a sensitive screen.

The outer layers of a bone are hard and compact. The inner portion of long bones consists of marrow. The marrow of children's bones is red, because it is involved in the production of blood. In adults, the red marrow of the long bones is largely replaced by fatty yellow marrow. In times such as severe illness where there is need for increased blood formation, the red marrow increases in size again. The whole bone is sheathed in a membrane called the **periosteum** in which run both blood vessels and nerves. Because of the presence of nerves, the periosteum can be immensely tender when a bone is bruised or fractured. The long bones of the body can only elongate at special regions near each end called the **epiphyseal cartilage** or **epiphyseal plate.** Injury or disease in childhood which affects this plate may lead to failure of the bone to grow.

The bones of children are generally strong, and many children who are claimed to have 'fragile bones' have nothing of the kind — they merely put themselves to the risk of fractures more often than others. After middle age, bone decreases in thickness, becomes demineralized, and the fibrous tissue which composes it becomes less resilient. The bones of old people are, therefore, often brittle. This explains why they are especially liable to fracture, as a result of even moderate strain, and are sometimes slow to heal (see **fractures**).

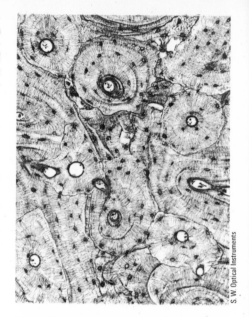

Through the canals (the white spaces) in the bone run blood vessels and nerves which maintain and repair it.

BORACIC ACID (or boric acid) is a mild antiseptic, which can be bought without prescription, and is suitable for the bathing of delicate tissues such as the eyes. A very small number of young babies are violently hypersensitive to it, however, and if any untoward reaction occurs, its use should be discontinued.

BORNHOLM DISEASE, epidemic pleurodynia, or 'Devil's grip', is a relatively harmless virus illness which tends to occur in epidemics. The symptoms are rather similar to those of 'flu'. A characteristic feature is sharp, gripping pain over the tops of both shoulders.

BOTULISM is a rare but highly dangerous form of food poisoning caused by the toxin (poison) produced by the bacterium *Clostridium botulinum*. It is usually associated with the growth of the bacterium in prepared foods. This toxin is probably the most poisonous substance known to man. It has been suggested that 1/6000 of an ounce could wipe out the entire human race.

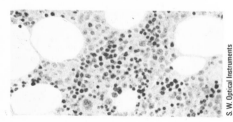

Red bone marrow, shown microscopically, produces the blood's red corpuscles.

BOWELS are the intestines (see **alimentary canal**). The human intestine is a continuous tube about 28 to 30 feet long. The phrase 'large bowel' is commonly used to mean the large intestine, while 'small bowel' means the small intestine. The term 'having the bowels open' is frequently used by both lay people and doctors to refer to the process of evacuation of faeces. Regularity of the bowels is not as vitally important as most people imagine (see **constipation**). What *is* important, however, is any *change* in bowel habit. The sudden onset of constipation (or of looseness of the bowels) should be regarded with suspicion, particularly when it occurs in middle-aged or elderly people.

If you have this symptom, you should consult your doctor right away — he may want you to see a specialist who can arrange bowel X-rays. *It is of the greatest importance not to delay.* This is particularly true if the symptom is combined with *abdominal pain,* with *black motions,* or with *bleeding* from the back passage. All these can be symptoms of serious disorder within the bowel which must be treated immediately.

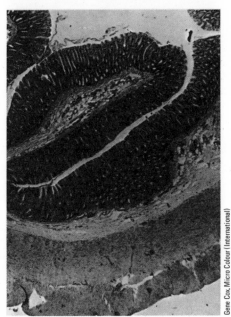

The bowel's four-layered structure is shown in microscopic section.

BRACHIAL means pertaining to the arm. The **brachial artery** is the main artery supplying blood to the arm; and the **brachial plexus** is the complex of nerves serving the arm.

BRADYCARDIA means slowness of the pulse. Its opposite is tachycardia (see **tachycardia**). A pulse rate considerably slower than the normal 72 beats per minute is not necessarily reason for concern — it may be associated with perfect health. Many highly-trained athletes have a bradycardia of as low as 45 or even 40 beats a minute. Other people with bradycardia may, however, have disease of the heart.

BRAIN and spinal cord together make up the central nervous system. The human brain is the most complex structure in the world. It controls all the conscious and unconscious functions of the human body, and is capable of the most intricate feats of reasoning and calculation. The brain weighs about three pounds and is greyish-white in colour. It has a firm and slightly rubbery consistency. Nevertheless, it is a relatively fragile structure which can be very easily damaged by blows to the head.

The front part of the brain consists of two large hemispheres (the cerebral hemispheres), which are divided into various lobes: the frontal, temporal, parietal, and occipital. Each lobe is sub-divided by fissures into many separate areas, and the deepness of these fissures is such that the actual surface area of the brain is very great in comparison with its size. The surface is formed by a thin layer called the cortex.

In the frontal lobes, the cortex is believed to play an important part in the higher intellectual functions. In the temporal lobes, which lie at the sides of the brain, the cortex is concerned, among other things, with hearing. It is even possible to mark out a musical scale in this region, so that electrical-stimulation of a particular spot makes the subject hear a particular musical note. The cortex of the occipital lobes (at the back of the cerebral hemispheres) controls the sense of sight. It is quite easy to confirm that certain areas of this part of the cortex are linked with specific parts of the field of vision.

Gene Cox, Micro Colour (International)

Running down each cerebral hemisphere is the deep fissure of Rolando. Behind this, slightly towards the back of the head, the cortex is associated with sensation in general. Electrical stimulation of this part of the brain makes the subject feel, for instance, as if he is being touched on the foot or the hand. In front of the fissure of Rolando is the motor cortex, which regulates movement in all parts of the body. The lowest part of the motor cortex deals with movement of the tongue and the face; immediately above is the area related to movement of the neck; next comes the arm, the trunk and the leg. Finally, at the very top, is a small area of the cortex which controls all movement in the toe.

From the motor cortex of the cerebral hemispheres, hundreds of thousands of nerve fibres relay 'instructions' downwards through the mid-brain and the hind-brain to the spinal cord, where they reach their final destinations in the muscles which carry out movement. This network is complicated by the fact that most of the descending fibres actually cross over within the brain, so that the left cerebral hemisphere controls the right side of the body, and vice versa. This is an important consideration, because it means that bleeding in the left half of the brain, from a stroke or a head injury, is likely to cause a paralysis of the right side of the body.

There are various other parts of the brain, among the most important of which is the cerebellum (see **cerebellum**). The entire brain is surrounded by three membranes — the dura, the arachnoid and the pia — which play an important part in protecting it from injury. The blood supply of the brain is from four arteries — the two internal arotid arteries and the two vertebral arteries. These join at the base of the brain so that if (as very often happens) one or other of them is affected by disease, the work of supplying the blood can, to some extent, be carried on by the others.

Brain injuries depend in their extent upon both the force of the blow and its direction. This is why quite a slight blow to the head in a particular place may have serious, or even fatal, results. It cannot be emphasized too strongly that the popular conception that a blow on the head produces only

a short and harmless period of unconsciousness is dangerous nonsense. Any blow to the head severe enough to cause unconsciousness invariably causes some degree of brain damage, whether slight, moderate, or serious. Unconsciousness, dizziness, or confusion after a blow on the head is always an indication to go to hospital.

Brain diseases are generally indicated by defects in sensation, disturbances of normal bodily movements or abnormalities in mood and behaviour. If insufficient blood is reaching the brain, for some reason, such as arterial disease, there may be fainting attacks, headaches and perhaps ringing in the ears. A sudden arterial blockage may result in the death of a part of the brain, and prove crippling or fatal.
(See also **Cerebral abscess, cerebral tumours, encephalitis, epilepsy, hydrocephalus** and **stroke**.)

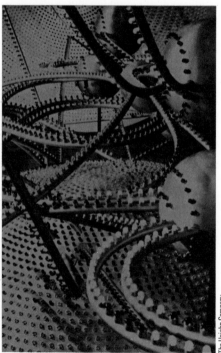

The complex system of the human brain is simulated by a computer model. The functions of its 600 million nerve cells are simplified by electronic 'cores'.

50

BRAN provides 'roughage' in the diet. It is meal from the outer covering of grain.

BRANDY is an alcoholic drink obtained by distilling wine. It was widely used as a 'stimulant' in medicine in former times, though, in fact, like all alcohol, it is not a stimulant at all. In Victorian novels, the doctor is often pictured as responding to all emergencies by 'stimulating' the patient with brandy — Sherlock Holmes' Dr. Watson, for instance, seems to have known of no other treatment, whatever the cause of the patient's illness! Brandy, of course, is a depressant of brain function; this property may, however, be useful in promoting sleep (especially in the elderly), and in giving a feeling of drowsy well-being to worried and anxious patients. Sometimes it is useful in the treatment of fainting.

BREAD, 'the staff of life', is the staple carbohydrate (see **carbohydrate**) food of much of the Western world, in the same way as rice is the staple carbohydrate of the Orient. Bread is prepared from various types of grain; for instance, rye bread is very popular in many parts of Europe, and elsewhere bread is made from maize or oats. In Britain, however, bread is almost always made from wheat. If the entire grain of the wheat is ground up, the flour which is produced is called 'whole meal'. Whiter flours contain less bran (see **bran**), or none at all, and, though they produce bread which is more digestible, it is nonetheless not so nutritious. This is because there is less 'wheat germ', the part of the grain which contains vitamin B_1. Bread contains only a minute amount of fat, and a small quantity of protein, but more than half its content is starch (see **starch**). It is believed that bread is fattening because of its starchy nature; brown and white bread are not particularly different in this respect, and there is no point in eating one in preference to the other when trying to slim — the best thing is to eat neither. Similarly, there is no point in trying to slim by eating toast instead of bread; toast is just bread from which the water has been driven off by grilling. It is just as fattening as ordinary bread.

Recently flour has been required by law to contain a certain minimum of a number of essential chemicals. But many people feel that there has been a decline in the tastiness of bread generally. There may, however, be no connection between these facts, and it may just be that modern mass-production methods are responsible.

BREAST is the name applied to the mammary gland. It is the structure whereby

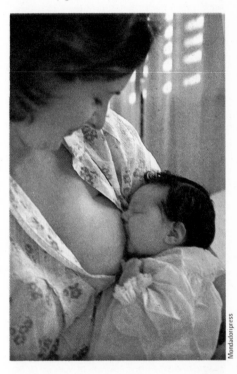

Mondadorpress

The milk from his mother's breast gives the baby all the nourishment he needs for the first vital months of his life.

every female mammal is capable of feeding her young with milk. In addition, in humans it plays a part in the process of sexual selection (see **sexual selection**), one of the most important evolutionary mechanisms. In most human societies, the bosom is to some extent the equivalent of the bright plumage of birds — in other words, as a secondary sexual characteristic, it attracts the potential mate, and hence helps to ensure the continuance of the

51

human species. Even in the days of ancient Greece, for instance, it was recognized that the superb bosom of the Venus de Milo was not only an object of immense beauty and attraction, but was a feature ideally suited for motherhood.

Nipples are present in both sexes, but they only become fully developed in the female. The nipples lie on what is called 'the milk line', which runs from the collarbone down to the groin. In animals, there may be nipples all down this line, and indeed humans very often have small (rudimentary) nipples along the same line, below the breasts.

Around the nipple is the wide disc of the areola (which many people confuse with the nipple itself). The areola varies greatly in size, and also in shade, depending on the colouring of the person. It also darkens in pregnancy, and usually remains rather darker than the virginal areola thereafter.

On the apex of the nipple are the openings of the lactiferous ducts — 15 to 20 in number. Each opening leads back to a little milk reservoir (the ampulla) and thence to a large number of lobules. These lobules form the bulk of the breast, though there may be a quantity of fat, particularly in more mature women.

Cancer of the breast is a common illness; its results are often tragic, but what is not generally appreciated is that the vast majority of cases could be cured if caught early enough. Furthermore, the public has not yet been educated to realize that the only way to catch breast cancer early is for *every* woman to examine her own breasts quite briefly every couple of weeks or so. This can readily be done by running the flat of the hand over the bosom. Any lumps present should be reported to the doctor next day, and it should be possible to arrange an examination of the lump by a surgeon within a few days at most. Although many breast lumps are not cancerous, the procedure described should be followed *whenever* a lump is found. The surgeon can, by a simple and painless test, ensure whether the trouble is malignant or not. It cannot be emphasized too strongly that many unfortunate women find lumps in the breast and hide them away, out of fear. Never do this — see

52

your doctor or a surgeon right away.

There are many other conditions which can affect the breast. Various forms of **mastitis** are quite common: it may appear as an abscess, but more often it consists of swelling and pain in one part of the breast. A frequent condition is mastitis due to infection by germs (often occurring during lactation). This must be treated by antibiotics. A new form of mastitis which has occurred recently is that suffered by girls (such as topless waitresses) who have tried to increase the size of their busts by silicone injections. Mastitis may occur because of some disorder in the ovaries or the pituitaries. Cysts, abscesses and benign growths of the breast are all quite common, and often only a surgeon can distinguish between these conditions and cancer.

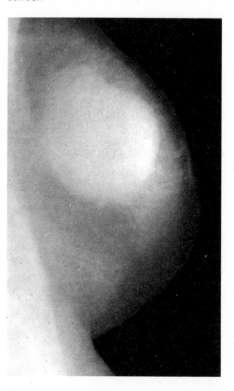

The hard lump of tissue within the breast shows clearly on this X-ray. If a lump appears, a woman should immediately check with her doctor in order to obtain speedy and effective treatment.

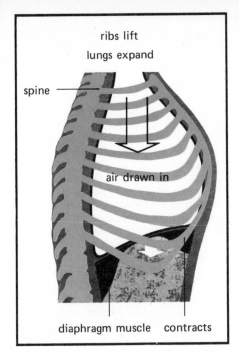

ribs lift	ribs lower
lungs expand	lungs return to original volume

spine

air drawn in

air expelled

diaphragm muscle contracts

diaphragm muscle relaxes

The mechanism of breathing: the first picture shows *inspiration*. The air is drawn in, oxygen extracted and passed into the bloodstream. At the same time the waste product carbon dioxide is passed from the bloodstream into the lungs. In *expiration*, air is pushed out of the lungs by muscular contraction.

BREATH is the air we breathe in and out during the process of respiration (see **respiration**). The inhaled breath is, of course, ordinary air, while the exhaled breath contains a lower amount of oxygen than air does, and a higher amount of carbon dioxide and water vapour.

Bad breath (halitosis) is an extremely common condition, and it would be fair to say that most people suffer from it occasionally, even if only on 'the morning after the night before'. In most cases, bad breath can be prevented by cleaning the teeth carefully and paying regular visits to the dentist. It is possible that the mouthwashes which are so widely advertized are of some value, but the popular remedy of taking chlorophyll pills is quite futile.

BREATH HOLDING is possible for varying lengths of time, depending on such factors as the physical fitness of the person. Many fit young men can easily hold their breath for two minutes or so, and trained skin-divers can manage considerably longer periods. Under no circumstances, however, should swimmers engage in underwater breath holding contests, which have had fatal results in the past. This has happened because people who try to stay underwater for longer than they should are liable to black out and drown. Particularly dangerous is the practice of prolonging breath holding time by 'overbreathing' beforehand. Although this is recommended in certain swimming manuals, it is potentially lethal, since it 'washes out' carbon dioxide from the blood stream. This removes much of one's desire to breathe, and frequently leads to complete unconsciousness.

Breath holding attacks are common in young children. They often occur when the infant is upset of frustrated about something; suddenly, he stops breathing, although he generally remains perfectly

53

conscious. The breath is held for periods of up to a couple of minutes, and the child may become quite blue in the face. During this time, of course, mother or father is usually getting desperately worried. In fact such attacks are rarely serious. They are believed to be simply a manifestation of anger or unhappiness, similar in nature to a tantrum. The parent's best course is to sit or lay the child down in a comfortable position. He will soon start breathing again. But it is always advisable to consult a doctor to discuss the best method of handling the child. Breath holding attacks usually go away altogether by the age of three or four. They should not be confused with fainting fits or convulsions, which are quite different (see **convulsions**).

BREATHLESSNESS is a symptom of many diseases. Its occurrence is always an indication to consult the doctor, and it should not be regarded as simply a symptom of advancing years. However, there are many conditions of no great seriousness· which cause breathlessness — the commonest, undoubtedly, being *obesity*. Very fat people cannot help but be breathless, even when their heart and lungs are in good condition. Among young people who complain of breathlessness, the common causes include *minor nervous upsets* and *anaemia*. Young people whose nerves are a bit upset often worry lest there is something wrong with their hearts, and this leads them to complain of breathlessness; anaemia (see **anaemia**) is a frequent occurrence among young women, especially if they have heavy periods.

Acute lung infections often cause breathlessness associated with fever (and often with cough). Among these conditions are bronchopneumonia and lobar pneumonia (see **pneumonia**), pleurisy (see **pleurisy**), acute bronchitis (see **bronchitis**), and bronchiolitis (see **bronchiolitis**). Other *respiratory tract infections* may produce partial obstruction of the upper airways, and hence breathlessness characterized by stertorous (noisy) breathing. These conditions include laryngitis (see **laryngitis**), diphtheria (see **diphtheria**), the group of childhood

disorders known as 'croup', and sometimes even severe colds, which can block a child's upper respiratory passages and make him breathless.

Chronic (long-standing) lung conditions also tend to produce breathlessness. There are too many to list fully, but among the most important are chronic bronchitis (see **bronchitis**), asthma (see **asthma**), pulmonary tuberculosis (see **tuberculosis**), and pulmonary fibrosis (see **fibrosis**). (See also **lungs**.)

Heart disorders may also cause breathlessness; where this occurs, it is most commonly a manifestation of failure of the left side of the heart (which receives blood from the lungs, and pumps it to the rest of the body). (See **heart**.) This left-sided heart failure causes considerable accumulation of fluid in the lungs, and hence breathlessness. It is characteristic of this type of breathlessness that the patient is considerably relieved by sitting up — when he lies flat again, he becomes short of breath once more.

BRIGHT'S DISEASE is the old name for nephritis, which was first described by Bright in 1827. Since nephritis is now known to be not one disease but a group of different diseases, the term is now dropping out of use.

BRITISH PHARMACOPOEIA is a volume published by an officially-appointed commission; it lists all important medical preparations used in Britain.

BRONCHIECTASIS is a chronic lung condition. Its characteristic feature is a shrinkage of the substance of the lung accompanied by a marked dilatation (widening) of the smaller air-tubes (bronchi) which carry air into the lung, (see also **lung**), and results in the secretion of large amounts of pus and the formation of balloon-like cavities in the lung. This widening is a structural change, and largely irreversible; however, the condition can be greatly helped by treatment. Bronchiectasis may follow whooping cough, measles or flu in childhood; it may also be the consequence of a failure to recover fully from bronchopneumonia.

BRONCHIOLITIS is an inflammation of the smallest tubes which lead into the lungs — the bronchioles. (See **lung**.) In its commonest form, it is an infection of young children, caused by a virus (see **virus**).

BRONCHITIS is an inflammation of the large air tubes which lead into the lungs — the bronchi. (See **lung**.) Bronchitis may be *acute* or *chronic*, and the two disorders are entirely different.

Acute bronchitis is a short-lived bronchial infection, usually over within a week or so. It is common in all age groups, and is rarely very serious, except in debilitated patients. It is usually caused by infection with a virus (see **virus**), and it is therefore not surprising that it may follow rapidly on a cold. As the bronchi become inflamed, a dry cough develops, and the patient complains of a raw feeling in the upper chest, made temporarily worse at each bout of coughing. Mild attacks of acute bronchitis may go no further than this and clear up spontaneously. Very often, however, the patient starts to feel rather poorly, and may even have to take to his bed. After a day or two, the cough may 'loosen', and sputum may start to come up. If this is green or yellow, it indicates that there is now bacterial infection of the bronchial passages (see **bacteria**), and a course of an antibiotic should help to cut the attack short. If acute bronchitis (or, indeed, any kind of acute chest infection) has not cleared up after a couple of weeks, *it is absolutely essential to have a chest X-ray, in case there is any more serious underlying condition.*

Chronic bronchitis is, as the name implies, a long-standing bronchial inflammation. It is exceptionally common in Great Britain, for reasons that are not entirely clear. Among the factors that are

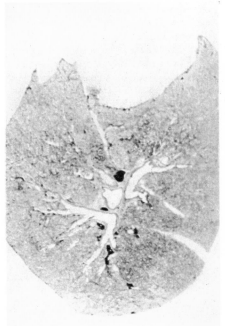

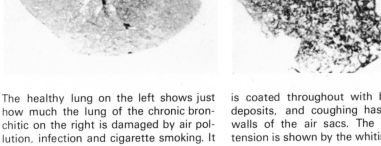

Diana Wyllie filmstrip 'Chronic Bronchitis'

The healthy lung on the left shows just how much the lung of the chronic bronchitic on the right is damaged by air pollution, infection and cigarette smoking. It is coated throughout with black smoke deposits, and coughing has broken the walls of the air sacs. The ensuing distension is shown by the whitish spaces.

important in causing the inflammation, however, are *smoking*, which causes irritation of the air passages roughly in proportion to the amount of tobacco smoked each day, and to the quantity of smoke which is inhaled; *air pollution*, which also irritates the bronchial tubes; and *repeated chest infections*, which are common in the winter in most industrial countries. The usual story of someone with chronic bronchitis is that he has always been a smoker, has always lived in a rather 'smoggy' area, and has tended to catch 'chest colds' every winter for as long as he can remember. At first, it was only a few chest infections each winter, but, over the years, the number of episodes increased, and the time needed for recovery lengthened. Eventually, the sufferer may have a continuous racking cough all winter through, with only a moderate respite in the warm summer months. It should be emphasized, of course, that this story does not apply to every case of chronic bronchitis, but the features described are common to most people with the condition. Many patients go on to develop emphysema (see **emphysema**) and obstructive airway disease (see **obstructive airway disease**).

The liability to serious lung conditions, such as bronchopneumonia, or even lung cancer, is increased in long-standing chronic bronchitics. It is obvious, therefore, that anything which can be done to prevent chronic bronchitis (or to alleviate it, once it has developed) is of considerable importance. Prevention can to some extent be achieved by encouraging the public to give up smoking, by cutting down air pollution, and by educating people to go along to their doctors for treatment, and, if necessary, X-rays, when they have chest infections. The treatment of chronic bronchitis involves, of course, persuading those patients who are still smoking to give it up, and treating the disorder with various drugs. These include dilators of the air passages, where necessary, drugs to affect the formation of sputum, and, of course, antibiotics when required. Furthermore, it may eventually be necessary to give heart stimulants (see **digoxin**). This is because the combination of chronic bronchitis and emphysema often leads to failure of the right side of the heart, which is endeavouring, against heavy odds, to pump blood to the diseased lungs. (See **heart**.)

BRUCELLOSIS is a fever caused by one of three types of bacteria. The first, *Brucella abortus*, is carried by cattle, and, in fact, causes them to abort — hence its name. As a rule it does not have this effect on human beings, however, to whom it is passed in infected milk; instead it produces *undulant fever*, a disabling but seldom fatal illness which is often difficult to diagnose. The disease is now something of a rarity in Great Britain, but a high proportion of veterinary surgeons have positive blood tests for it, so presumably there is still quite a reservoir of infection among animals in this country. The closely related germ *Brucella melitensis* occurs in Malta and other Mediterranean countries; it infects goats, and is passed to human beings in the goats' milk. The form of brucellosis it produces is known as Malta fever or Mediterranean fever. The third germ is called *Brucella suis*; it originates in pigs, and does not appear to occur in Britain. All types of brucellosis may be treated with antibiotics. This disease's existence is yet another argument for the universal pasteurization or sterilization of milk (see **pasteurization**) which would effectively prevent the spread of infection to humans.

BRUISES are contusions of the tissues underlying the skin. Bleeding into the cellular spaces of the skin produces the characteristic purple discoloration, which later changes to brown, and finally fades to a yellow colour as the blood pigments are absorbed as the broken blood vessels heal.

BURNS are injuries caused by dry heat. (For treatment of burns, see **first aid**). The old classification of burns into 'first-degree', 'second-degree', etc. is now rarely used. More important is to assess the *area* of a burn, as a percentage of the body's surface. This gives a much better guide as to seriousness, when coupled with a simple assessment as to whether it is superficial or deep.

C.S.F., or cerebro-spinal fluid, is a clear liquid which is found in the ventricles (cavities) of the brain and around the spinal cord which protects these areas from shock. Examination of the fluid gives much valuable information about the state of the brain and the spinal cord. C.S.F. is 'tapped off' for examination by means of a lumbar puncture, a procedure which involves pushing a needle into the small of the back, or lumbar region. (See **lumbar puncture**).

CAECUM is the structure, lying in the lower right-hand side of the abdomen, which forms the beginning of the large intestine. It is the part of the large intestine into which the contents of the small intestine are emptied. The appendix (see **appendix**) also opens into it.

In Man, the caecum is less than three inches wide, but in herbivorous animals, such as the rabbit, it is relatively larger, as it aids in the digestion of grass and similar foods.

CAESAREAN DELIVERY is the removal of a baby from the womb through an incision in the abdomen. It has been practised intermittently for several thousand years. Popular myth attributes the word 'Caesarean' to the method by which Julius Caesar was allegedly born. It is, however, far more likely that it derives from the *lex caesarea* (the Latin verb *caedere* means 'to cut'), a Roman law which required that the operation be performed on women expected to die before normal delivery and it was necessary to get the baby out rapidly in order to save it. It was not until the late 1800s that a Caesarean operation was developed which could be safely performed on a living mother.

Caesarean section, as it is often called, is now a common procedure. It is usually performed when there is any obstruction to the passage of the baby, such as a deformity of the mother's pelvis. Another common indication is *Placenta praevia* (see **placenta praevia**), a condition in which the placenta is so attached to the wall of the uterus that it lies across the neck of the womb. If the mother suffers from diabetes, the baby's chances of survival are considerably increased if it is removed from the womb by Caesarean about four weeks before the estimated date of delivery. At other times, a Caesarean section is required because there are signs of immediate danger to the baby, such as Rhesus incompatability or possible heart failure.

CAFFEINE is a mild stimulant, present in both coffee and tea, which tends to promote wakefulness. A small amount of caffeine is contained in certain proprietary pain-killing tablets.

CAISSON DISEASE (see **bends**).

CALAMINE is a zinc-containing lotion which is widely used to soothe inflamed skin. If any skin irritation develops, its use should be discontinued.

CALCIUM is a chemical element which is essential for the formation of healthy teeth and bones. Its main sources are milk and cheese, which account for the importance of these ingredients, particularly milk, in the diets of children.

The level of calcium in the body is principally controlled by the parathyroid glands (see **parathyroids**).

As calcium obstructs the passage of X-rays, bones and teeth appear dense on X-ray films and plates. (See also **rickets** and **tetany**.)

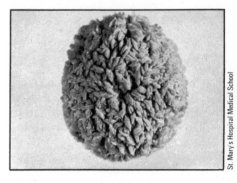

St. Mary's Hospital Medical School

This stone, three centimetres in diameter, was removed from a human kidney.

CALCULI are stones of various sizes, made of various substances which form in many parts of the body, for instance,

57

stones in the kidney and urinary passages or in the gall bladder and bile duct (see **stones**).

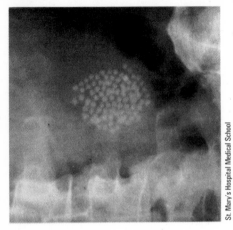

St. Mary's Hospital Medical School

X-rays reveal concentrations of minerals known as calculi, in the gall bladder.

CALORIES are units of energy. There are two units given this name: the standard calorie, and the kilocalorie, which is 1000 times larger. The kilocalorie, usually intended by the word 'calorie', is the amount of heat required to raise the temperature of one kilogram of water one degree centigrade. Dieticians use it to measure the energy taken in from food. The average adult requires about 2,000 to 2,500 kilocalories to carry out normal activities, but more may be needed for strenuous manual work.

CANCER is a malignant growth formed by the abnormally rapid reproduction of cells. Cancerous cells have two particular properties. The first, known as 'invasiveness', is the capacity to infiltrate and destroy adjacent organs — for example, a cancer of the bowel may spread into the bladder. The second is the ability to form *secondary deposits* in distant parts of the body. Cancer cells break off from the parent growth and are carried, usually in the blood stream, to another organ, where they begin to reproduce and form additional tumour masses.

It is not entirely clear why cancers occur. They principally affect two age

groups: children, and, to a much greater extent, people over the age of about 40. At present it is believed that cancerous growths in children are related to some form of developmental abnormality. And it is certain that chronic irritation is involved in the later development of cancer.

Treatment for cancer is often effective if the condition is brought to medical attention at an early stage. Surgery, X-rays, radium, and more recently chemotherapy are commonly used methods and often promote full recovery. Consult a doctor at once if you have any of the following symptoms:—

Any unusual lump, bleeding, or ulcer; any sudden change in bowel habit; any cough which persists after three weeks; any passing of black motions; any unexplained severe weight loss. (For specific cancers, refer to the entries on various organs of body. For cancer of the blood, see **leukemia**.)

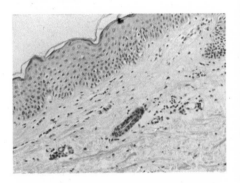

Normal cells, *above*, are aligned in neat rows. *Below*, the haphazard arrangement of cancerous cells.

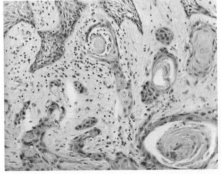

Ken Moreman

58

CANNABIS, Marijuana, or hashish, is an intoxicant prepared from *Cannabis sativa,* a plant grown in the Orient and in the West Indies. It is generally used in cigarette form. No *physical* ill-effects have been described in those under its influence. There is intoxication characterized by a feeling of euphoria, often with a distortion of the sense of time.

In the East, cannabis is widely available and its use is entirely within social and legal bounds. In several Western countries, such as Great Britain and the United States, both possession and use of the drug are unlawful. In these countries, controversy centres on the question whether the use of cannabis leads to the taking of dangerous and addictive 'hard drugs' like heroin and cocaine.

CANTHARIDES (see **Spanish fly**).

CAPILLARIES are the minute vessels which join the arterioles (the ends of arteries) to the venules (the ends of veins). Because the capillary walls are thin and semi-permeable, they allow nutrients and dissolved gases in the blood to pass through them to and from the tissues (see **blood**).

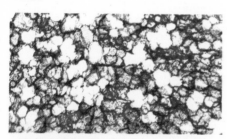
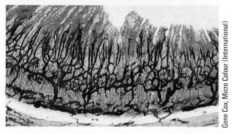

Sections of the lungs, *top,* and intestine, *above,* injected with red dye, show the capillary network in the body's tissue.

CARBENOXOLONE is a drug used in the treatment of ulcers. In the 1960s, it was isolated from licorice extracts and proved to be the first effective method of healing gastric ulcers. Previous remedies had only been able to provide relief of symptoms. The drug is manufactured under the name of Biogastrone.

CARBOHYDRATE is an organic substance consisting of carbon, hydrogen, and oxygen, in which the hydrogen content is twice that of oxygen. In chemical composition, carbohydrates are mainly sugars and starches. Common examples of carbohydrate foodstuffs are bread, potatoes, sugar, and rice. After these foods are digested, they are converted into sugar and absorbed by the body. It is generally believed that carbohydrates are more responsible for producing obesity than the other main types of food—proteins and fats.

CARBOLIC ACID, or phenol, is a coal-tar preparation. Its use as an antiseptic was popularized by Lord Lister in the 1860s when he introduced antisepsis into surgical practices, but it is now rarely applied to human tissues as it may cause irritation and serious damage. It is, however, widely used as a disinfectant. It is a most dangerous poison, and should be kept out of the reach of children.

CARBON DIOXIDE (or CO_2) is a gas which can be produced in the combustion (or burning) of carbon or carbon compounds. It is exhaled from the lungs in the process of breathing. Air which is inhaled contains a minute amount of carbon dioxide and about 21 per cent oxygen. The oxygen is carried by the blood to the tissues and is exchanged for the waste product carbon dioxide. The carbon dioxide is then carried back to the lungs through the blood stream and is released through the mouth (see **blood**).

The carbon dioxide which is exhaled by both Man and animals is used by green plants, particularly trees, in the process of photosynthesis. In this process, carbon dioxide is absorbed and oxygen is given off. This is the direct reversal of the respiratory process in animal life.

Gene Cox, Micro Colour (International)

CARBON MONOXIDE (or CO) is a highly poisonous gas which is a constituent of gas used for domestic purposes and is also found in the exhaust fumes of all combustion engines, such as automobiles and petrol motors. Carbon monoxide is dangerous because it combines with the haemoglobin in the blood to produce carboxyhaemoglobin and thereby deprives the tissues of oxygen. It is rendered more lethal because it is tasteless and odourless: a potential victim of a gas leak may not realize he is in danger of being poisoned.

As a result of carbon monoxide poisoning, unconsciousness may take place rapidly, depending on the concentration of the gas in the room or vehicle. The victim is often pinkish in colour because of the formation of carboxyhaemoglobin in the blood. Death or permanent brain damage is likely unless the victim is given immediate aid. He should be taken from the gas-filled room or automobile at once, given artificial respiration and taken straight to hospital. Damage to the nervous system can cause complications – such as blindness – which fortunately almost always clears up in time.

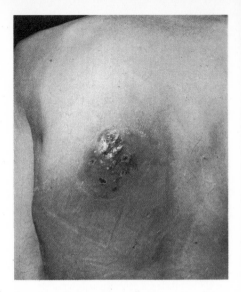

A carbuncle does not remain localized, but spreads over an area of the skin.

CARDIAC means pertaining to the heart.

CARDIAC FAILURE (see **heart failure**).

CARDIOLOGY is the branch of medical science devoted to the study of the heart and its disorders.

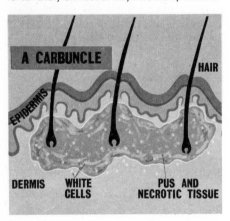

A CARBUNCLE

HAIR

EPIDERMIS

DERMIS   WHITE CELLS   PUS AND NECROTIC TISSUE

Infection of a hair follicle in the skin's dermal layer causes a carbuncle to form. The area is surrounded by pus.

CARBUNCLE is a skin infection, usually caused by staphylococcus bacteria, the same as are responsible for boils. A carbuncle is similar to a boil, but does not remain localized as a boil does and spreads more widely over the body (see **boil**).

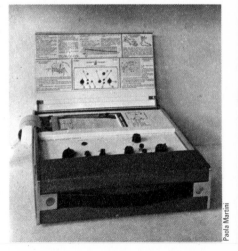

Paola Martini

An electrocardiograph is used in cardiology to record the variations in the heart as it contracts and relaxes.

60

CARTILAGE is gristle. It is a tough but pliant material which forms part of the human skeleton. It occurs at various sites in the body — notably in the nose and the ears, and at the joints of the large bones — where it is necessary to have strength combined with a certain amount of elasticity. In children, there is a layer of cartilage, the **Epiphyseal cartilage**, running through each of the long bones, and from this the bone grows in length.

The two cartilages of the knee are called **semi-lunar cartilages** because each of the pair is shaped like a half-moon. These form a cushion between the lower end of the thigh-bone, the femur, and the upper end of the shin-bone, the tibia. Injuries and strains may readily tear one or both of these cartilages, producing intense pain.

From an initial injury to the cartilage, often sustained in sporting activity, the patient may suffer recurrent episodes in which his knee suddenly 'goes'. In such cases the tear in cartilage may become more extreme each time. There is a violent stab of pain as the knee gives way. It may become locked, and, after each episode, there may be gross swelling. For this condition it is essential to consult an orthopaedic surgeon as soon as possible. Removal of the torn cartilage by surgical operation is often recommended and is extremely effective. Delay in obtaining medical advice may lead to the development of arthritis.

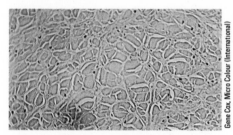

Gene Cox, Micro Colour (International)

The microscope reveals the crescent-structure of the semilunar cartilage in the knee.

CASCARA, an extract from tree bark, is a powerful laxative. However, like most purges, it is now prescribed infrequently by doctors (see **constipation**).

CASTOR OIL is a bitter-tasting laxative oil extracted from plant seed. It is now seldom used except as a preparatory agent before abdominal X-ray, where it is necessary to evacuate the bowels. It is also used in midwifery to try to start women off in labour, as violent contractions of the gut are sometimes believed to induce contractions in the uterus.

CASTRATION means removal of the sex glands, that is, the ovaries or the testes. In women, this operation, known as oophorectomy is required in a number of disorders of the ovaries. It may also be performed during a hysterectomy, at the same time as the uterus is removed. The operation does not impair the woman's ability to have, or to enjoy intercourse; it does, however, permanently prevent the possibility of conception.

In medieval times and, indeed, well into the eighteenth century, choir boys were sometimes castrated to preserve their boyish voices. These singers were subsequently known as *tenore castratti*. Today, removal of the sex glands in young adult males is rare except in the Middle East. It produces the condition known as eunuchoidism, which is characterized by the unusual deposition of bodily fat, and general loss of aggressive instincts.

In adult males, orchectomy, the removal of both testes, may be necessary when the bladder, and occasionally the testicle, is affected by tuberculosis, or when an irreducible hernia is being repaired (see **hernia**). The removal of both testes is likely to reduce sexual drive greatly.

Small children sometimes develop a fear of castration or sexual mutilation which Freud called a **castration complex**. According to Freud, a boy fears that his attachment to his mother will be punished by a 'jealous' father with the threat of castration. As a defence against the anxiety he experiences, the boy seeks to identify with his father.

CATARACT is a common condition in which the lens of the eye becomes opaque, making vision difficult. The centre of the lens hardens until eventually scarcely any light at all passes into the eye.

This condition is principally found among the elderly, among diabetics, and, less commonly, among babies, particularly those whose mothers have had German measles during pregnancy. In the first type, **Senile cataract,** modern surgical techniques are extremely successful in restoring sight. Unfortunately, surgery performed on diabetic cataract is not equally effective.

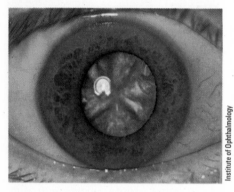

With a cataract, the lens of the eye becomes opaque, vision reduced. In the elderly, the condition is often reversible.

CATARRH is a liquid which flows from the mucous membranes of the upper respiratory tract and is often associated with an ordinary head cold, and this condition clears up spontaneously. If the liquid is purulent, that is, green or yellow in colour, it indicates the presence of bacteria (see **bacteria**). In such cases an antibiotic is often an effective means of treatment.

CATGUT is a material used for surgical stitching. It is made from animal intestines, not those of cats. Because it slowly dissolves in the body, and therefore does not have to be removed when the tissue has healed, it is used for internal stitching. Other materials are generally used for stitching the skin and the outer muscle layers of the body.

CATHETERS are thin tubes made of elastic, rubber, glass, or metal used to evacuate or inject fluid. **Bladder catheters** are passed up the urethra, the tube which connects the bladder to the exterior, to

facilitate the drainage of urine, for example, if there is acute retention of urine due to an enlarged prostate gland (see **prostate**). **Cardiac catheters,** which are pushed up a vein until they reach the heart, are used either to release X-ray dye inside the heart or to measure intra-cardiac pressures.

CAUTERIZATION is the burning of tissue by chemical or electrical means, for instance, burning away of warts.

CELLS are the basic units of the human body and of all living things. Each cell consists of a jelly-like fluid, protoplasm, and contains a kernel, or nucleus, which directs the activities of the cell.

Higher animals develop from a single cell, the fertilized ovum, which has been penetrated by the sperm. The fertilized ovum then divides into two cells, then into four, and so on; they arrange themselves into various layers and masses, and gradually change in shape and chemical composition to compose the organs of the foetus.

Cells are the building blocks of the human body. They have a vital function in repairing worn out and diseased tissues which are normally replaced by the multiplication of the remaining healthy cells. Growth and development result from the increase in the number of cells, and the differentiation of cells into different types of tissues, depending on the particular function the cell performs.

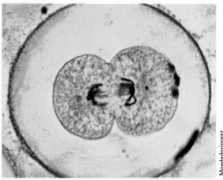

A cell, the basic unit of life, divides into two 'daughter' cells. Each daughter is a replica of the original, complete with nucleus and protoplasm.

CEPORIN is an antibiotic drug chemically related to the penicillins. It is, however, reserved for serious infections which laboratory tests have proved to be resistant to other antibiotics.

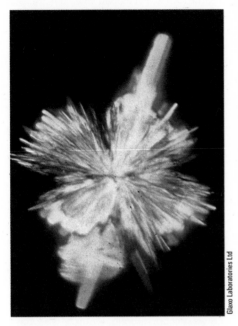

Ceporin, shown in its crystal form, is closely related to the penicillins.

CEREALS are grasses which have edible seeds, such as wheat, barley, and maize. All cereals are mainly composed of carbohydrates (see **carbohydrate**), that is, they are starchy foods. They are a valuable source of energy, but as they are largely deficient in protein and fat, cereals should be supplemented in the diet with foods rich in these substances, such as meat, milk, butter and eggs.

CEREBELLUM is the largest portion of the hind-brain. It consists of two lateral cerebellar hemispheres which, together, are about the size of a fist. The cerebellum governs such bodily functions as balance and muscular co-ordination. It is believed that alcohol has what is called a 'selective' effect on the cerebellum, which accounts for the fact that excessive consumption makes one stagger and fail to co-ordinate movements properly.

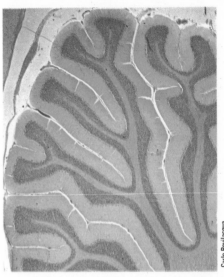

The cerebellum, seen in section, is vital in the control of muscular movements.

CEREBRAL ABSCESS is a collection of pus in the brain. It is one of the three types of abscess, known as **intracranial abscesses,** which may occur inside the skull as a result of germs entering from the exterior. The other types, subdural and extradural abscesses, affect the membranes covering the brain, rather than the brain substance itself.

An **intra-cerebral abscess** usually develops from some obvious focus of infection through which the germs pass into the brain, for instance, a mastoid infection, a dirty head wound, or occasionally a sinus infection. The patient becomes ill quite rapidly, complains of intense headaches, and experiences mental confusion. There may be vomiting. The temperature and pulse usually rise. And fits or paralysis may follow.

Special tests, including an electro-encephalogram (see **E.E.G.**), may be necessary to diagnose the condition. The patient is then treated with antibiotics to counteract the infection. It is not usual to operate immediately on cerebral abscess, as is the case with the other two types of intracranial abscess. The

63

surgeon often waits one or two days to enable the pus to localize and be more easily drained off.

Recovery from cerebral abscess is not always complete; unfortunately, it sometimes leads to the development of epilepsy.

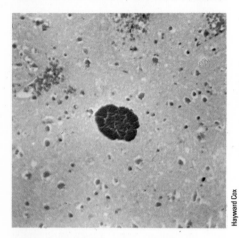

Hayward Cox

A section of brain tissue indicates a cerebral abscess produced by bacteria.

CEREBRAL TUMOUR is an abnormal growth of tissue in the brain. About one-third of all brain tumours are 'secondary' growths, that is, they are caused by cancer elsewhere in the body which spreads to the brain. Another third, known as *gliomas*, grow from the connective tissue of nerve centres in the brain. Some of these are highly malignant and result in early death, but others carry a better prognosis. Differentiation between the main types of glioma can be made by examining a piece of tissue under the microscope.

About 15 per cent of all cerebral tumours arise from the membranes, *meninges*, surrounding the brain. There is a high recovery rate for patients with these tumours, called *meningiomas*. The other major kinds of cerebral growths are tumours of the pituitary gland and of the auditory nerve (which emerges from the brain and runs to the ear). These also carry a good prognosis.

The symptoms of cerebral tumours are epilepsy, headache, personality changes and visual disturbances — though not all will necessarily occur in the same patient.

64

Before the age of 45 to 50, cerebral tumours are rare, although a substantial number do occur in small children. Fear of brain tumours is extremely common, particularly among persons whose father or mother have developed one, but there is no evidence whatever that these growths are hereditary.

The diagnosis of this condition may be difficult. The normal diagnostic aids are: special X-rays, examination of the cerebro-spinal fluid (see **C.S.F.**) and observation of the back of the eye with an ophthalmoscope, which enables the doctor to see if the pressure inside the skull has increased.

CERVICAL means 'pertaining to the neck'. The word refers, first, to the neck itself, and secondly to the neck of the womb (see **cervix**).

CERVIX means 'neck' and normally refers to the neck of the womb, or *cervix uteri*. It is rounded in shape, and about half an inch protrudes into the top of the vagina. The cervical canal, through which both the foetus and menstrual fluids pass, traverses the cervix.

The highest incidence of cancer of the cervix occurs among women who have borne children, and it normally appears after the age of 30 — between 10 to 15 years after the first delivery.

The commonest symptoms of cervical cancer are bleeding between the periods and bleeding after intercourse. A doctor should be consulted immediately if these symptoms occur.

The 'smear test' (see **smear test**) detects cervical cancer before the symptoms appear, and at a stage when it is normally curable. Many doctors believe that it should be routinely performed on all women over the age of 27.

Other conditions which affect the cervix include erosions and benign growths. Cervicitis, or inflammation of the cervix, is a common condition which may produce troublesome discharge. The cervix is likely to be torn in childbirth, and in such cases it must be sutured, or stitched. If the cervix happens to be malformed that is, long with a narrow mouth, it may cause pain during menstruation.

CETAVLON, also known as cetrimide, is a widely-used general antiseptic.

CHAFING is soreness and roughness of skin. It commonly occurs in small children, around areas where two skin surfaces rub together, for example, at the groin. Mild chafing can be treated by careful drying after washing, by frequent powdering, and when necessary, by the use of a cream or lubricant, such as vaseline. More severe cases should be seen by a doctor. (See **nappy rash.**)

CHAGAS' DISEASE is an infection, transmitted by parasitic insects, which is widespread in South America. It can affect the heart, and it frequently results in sudden death.

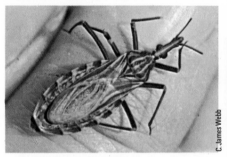

The reduviid bug (actual size) transmits Chagas' disease by biting its victims.

CHANCROID is a venereal disease, caused by the bacterium *Haemophilus ducreyi*. It is characterized by the formation of an ulcer in the genital area and by enlargement of the glands in the groin. In temperate climates, it seems to occur less frequently than gonorrhoea or syphilis. But in tropical countries, it is common. Treatment with sulphonamide tablets is usually curative.

CHANGE OF LIFE, or menopause, is the time when a woman's reproductive functions cease. It does not, however, mean that the ability to perform or enjoy sexual intercourse has ended. The ovaries cease to release eggs, and the hormonal balance of the body is altered. The periods should stop in one of three ways:

(a) they stop suddenly, and never return;
(b) the interval between the periods becomes longer and longer, until they cease altogether;
(c) the amount of blood lost at each period gradually decreases, until it ceases altogether.

In many women, menopause is normally accompanied by some emotional tension and physical discomfort such as hot flushes, weariness, and depression. An understanding family can do much to help a woman through such occurrences. Some comfort may be obtained from the fact that menopausal symptoms eventually pass off. In the meantime, hormone treatment, or mild sedation, may help.

Very heavy or irregular bleeding during the menopause is abnormal, as is any bleeding *after* the menopause. If such symptoms occur, consult a doctor.

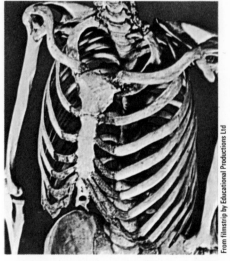

The chest is enclosed by bones of the ribs, 12 on each side of the chest cavity.

CHEST is the upper trunk. The framework of the chest consists of the ribs, the sternum (breastbone), and the vertebral column (backbone). Within the chest is a space known as the thoracic cavity, which is lined by an airtight membrane (the pleura). Within this cavity are the lungs and the heart. The lungs are supplied with air by the windpipe, which divides into the

65

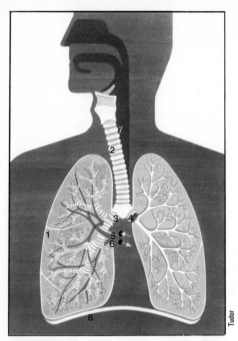

Tudor

The chest cavity contains the lungs which are enclosed in the pleural membrane, 1. Air enters through the windpipe, or trachea, 2, which divides into the bronchial tubes, 3 and 4. Arteries, 5, and veins, 6, carry blood to and from the heart. The oesophagus, 7, passes through the chest to the abdomen through an opening in the diaphragm, 8.

two bronchial tubes after it enters the chest.

The other main contents of the chest include: the upper part of the aorta (the great artery which carries blood away from the heart), the venae cavae or great veins (which bring blood back to the heart), and various nerves which supply vital structures. In children, a considerable volume of the thoracic cavity is taken up by the thymus gland. The function of this structure is unknown, but it is believed to play a major part in protecting the body against infection.

The term 'diseases of the chest' normally refers to diseases of the lungs alone, and not to diseases of the other structures in the thoracic cavity. The common symptoms of chest diseases are coughing, breathlessness, wheeziness, and chest

66

pain. Coughing may result from a number of lung disorders. If a cough persists for more than two or three weeks, or if it is associated with blood-stained sputum, a doctor should be consulted at once. If a cough produces green or yellow sputum, an antibiotic may well be an effective means of treatment.

A doctor should also be consulted for breathlessness, wheeziness, and severe or prolonged pain in the chest. Although these symptoms may not indicate a serious disorder, the doctor may decide to refer the patient for an X-ray or an electrocardiograph (see **E.C.G.**).

CHICKEN-POX is a mild infectious disease of childhood. As with many childhood illnesses, babies usually inherit immunity from their mothers. This natural protection is effective up to six months of age, but then gradually diminishes. The visible symptom of chicken-pox is an eruption of pustules which is centripetal, that is, largely affecting the trunk and thinning out towards the extremities.

The incubation period for chicken-pox is approximately 14 to 21 days, and the child is probably not infectious for longer than a week after the rash appears.

Because chicken-pox is caused by a virus, there is no medical treatment which is effective against it, and no treatment other than isolation is required, calamine lotion is often used to relieve itchiness.

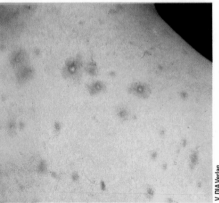

V. DIA Verlag

Between 11 and 21 days after infection from chicken-pox, the skin eruption appears.

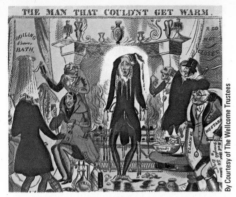

THE MAN THAT COULDN'T GET WARM.

Though there is no cure for the common cold, everyone has a favoured remedy.

CHILL is another name for a cold. Chills and colds are probably the commonest illnesses in the world. Though exposure to a draught of cold air, sudden immersion in water, or wetting of the feet on a cold day may be predisposing factors, the condition is caused by a virus. (See **virus**.) Antibiotics, therefore, have no effect on chills whatsoever.

A cold in the head is associated with nasal catarrh. The catarrh sometimes extends into the frontal sinuses causing headache, or, in children, it may spread up the Eustachian tubes causing inflammation of the middle ear and painful earache. When the throat is affected, the tonsils may become inflamed. If the virus spreads to the lower end of the respiratory passages, bronchitis follows. Coughing indicates that the air passages in the region of the larynx contain mucus. Coughing is a series of involuntary expirations which attempt to force the irritating mucus up into the mouth, where it can be expelled.

There is no cure for the common cold. For the relief of symptoms, bed-rest is often beneficial. Aspirin (or one of the many aspirin-containing proprietary remedies) may also be effective.

CHIROPODIST is a non-medical person who deals with minor disorders of the feet, such as corns, bunions, and callouses.

CHIROPRACTORS are practitioners of a system of medicine which is based on the belief that many diseases are simply caused by minor displacements of the spine and can be relieved by pressure. Chiropractors do not have medical degrees.

CHLORAL is a sedative. When taken in moderate doses it produces sound sleep. It is widely given to infants who need night-time sedation. Although it is effective in such cases, it may irritate the child's stomach and cause vomiting. In large doses, chloral is dangerous and the prescribed amount must not be exceeded.

CHLORAMPHENICOL or chloromycetin, is an antibiotic derived from a soil organism. It is now produced synthetically. It came into use during the 1950s and soon proved an extremely effective agent against a wide range of bacteria. However, it has very dangerous side effects – it may depress the function of the blood-forming organs so much that neither red blood cells nor white blood cells are produced. The former condition is called aplastic anaemia (see **anaemia**) and the latter is called agranulocytosis (see **agranulocytosis**). Both these conditions can be fatal.

Today, attitudes to chloramphenicol vary in different parts of the world. In many countries, however, it is felt that the drug is so dangerous that it should be reserved for certain uncommon indications, such as typhoid fever.

CHLORINE is a poisonous gas which, in liquid form, is commonly used as a bleaching agent and germicide. It is used extensively in the disinfection of water and in treatment of sewage.

CHLORODYNE is a patent medicine said to be of value in colds, chills, diarrhoea, neuralgia, and a variety of other ailments. It promotes a pleasant sensation in the abdominal region and, in moderate doses, is completely harmless.

CHLOROFORM is an anaesthetic gas which is inhaled to produce insensibility to pain during surgical operations. For the better part of a century, it was probably the most widely used anaesthetic. It was first introduced in medical practice in 1847, by Sir James Simpson, who was seeking a surgical anaesthetic more convenient in use than ether.

Chloroform effectively produces unconsciousness, but it has dangerous side effects. It may, for example, have a fatal toxic effect upon the heart. Many new anaesthetic drugs have been developed in the last 20 years, and these have almost entirely replaced chloroform.

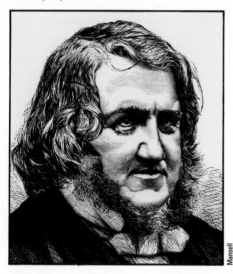

Sir James Simpson was the first man to use chloroform as an anaesthetic.

CHLOROPHYLL is the green pigment of plants, which acts as a catalytic agent in the process of photosynthesis. In photosynthesis, carbon dioxide, the waste product of human and animal respiration, is extracted from the air by plants and reacts with water from the soil to synthesize food stuffs and provide energy. Oxygen is given off as a result of this process. (See **carbon dioxide**.)

Chlorophyll has enjoyed a reputation as a breath deodorant but there is no evidence that it is of any value at all in this respect.

CHLOROQUINE is a drug used in the treatment of malaria. In recent years it has also been used to treat rheumatoid arthritis, but its value has been limited by the fact that it can cause blindness.

68

CHLOROTHIAZIDE is a diuretic (see **diuretics**) — a drug which increases the flow of urine. It is effective in such conditions as heart failure (see **congestive cardiac failure**) where changes in the circulation promote the retention of salt and water in the body.

CHOLECYSTECTOMY is removal of the gall-bladder. The operation is commonly performed on patients who have gall-stones (see **gall-stones**) and on some patients who have cholecystitis.

CHOLECYSTITIS is inflammation of the gall-bladder. *Acute cholecystitis* is quite sudden in onset. There is agonizing pain in the upper right side of the abdomen, usually accompanied by fever and vomiting. Many patients respond to conservative treatment in hospital, without the aid of surgery.

Chronic cholecystitis is a long-standing inflammation which most commonly affects women who are described as 'fair, fat, and fifty'. The characteristic ache in the right upper abdomen is associated with nausea and flatulence. Depending on the results of special X-rays, known as cholecystograms (see **cholecystogram**) removal of the gall-bladder may be indicated.

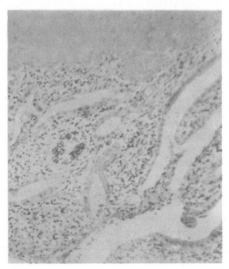

This cross-section of a diseased gall-bladder shows the inflamed tissue.

CHOLECYSTOGRAM is a type of X-ray of the gall-bladder (see **gall-bladder**). A special dye, opaque to the passage of X-rays, is injected into a patient suffering from a suspected chronic cholecystitis (see **cholecystitis**). As the dye should be concentrated in the gall-bladder, an X-ray film of the abdomen indicates the functioning of the organ.

CHOLERA is a severe and often fatal infectious disease of the gastro-intestinal tract, caused by a bacterium called the *Vibrio cholerae,* or *Vibrio comma* (because of its comma-like shape). The effects are profuse diarrhoea and vomiting, which rapidly produce severe, and potentially fatal, dehydration. Treatment consists of immediately replenishing the massive amounts of fluid lost and in killing the cholera bacteria with antibiotics.

Cholera, like most infectious gastro-intestinal diseases, is caused by poor hygiene. The bacteria are transmitted in food or water which has become contaminated by faeces from an infected person. Great epidemics of the disease still occur in Asia, but there have been no serious outbreaks in Europe or America since the First World War.

CHOLESTEROL is a chemical produced in the body by the breakdown of fats. It is important in body metabolism and is necessary for the formation of various hormones. In recent years there has been some evidence to connect a high level of cholesterol in the blood with arterial disease and heart disease.

Diets which are rich in 'saturated' fats (mainly animal fats and butter) are known to be associated with high levels of cholesterol and other related compounds. Low fat diets, and diets which contain only 'unsaturated' fats (corn oil, cottonseed oil, and fish oils) lower the levels of these chemicals.

Although individuals who have arterial disease and are prone to heart diseases often have a high level of cholesterol and related compounds, it has not yet been conclusively proved that eliminating from the diet the fats which are responsible for cholesterol formation actually reduces the

chances of developing these diseases.

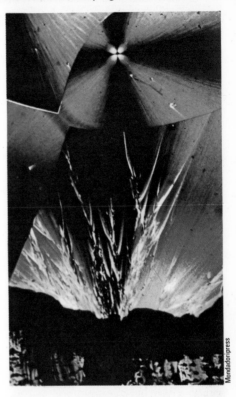

Mondadoripress

Pure cholesterol, extracted from the body tissue with alcohol or ether, is a complex alcohol which can be crystallized.

CHOREA is a disorder of certain centres in the brain. The two common forms are **Huntingdon's chorea,** which is an hereditary defect, and **St. Vitus' dance** (see **St. Vitus' dance**). These two disorders are completely unrelated; they do however affect the same brain centres and therefore both produce a very similar and characteristic writhing of the limbs.

St. Vitus' dance, or **rheumatic chorea**, is most common in children about 12 years old. Like rheumatic fever, it is believed to be related in some way to infection by the streptococcus bacterium. First, the child becomes 'fidgety'. Later, uncontrollable sinuous writhing movements usually appear in one arm. Fortunately recovery normally follows after several weeks' treatment in hospital.

69

CHRONIC means a disease or disorder of long-standing, as opposed to 'acute'.

CIRCULATION – (see **blood**).

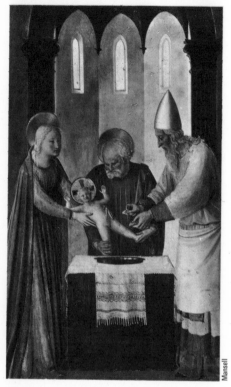

In some cultures and religions, circumcision is an act of ritual importance performed on infants shortly after birth.

CIRCUMCISION is removal of the fore-skin. In adults, the operation is occasionally performed in cases of balanitis (see **balanitis**). It is, however, far more commonly carried out on young babies. In the Jewish religion it is part of religious ritual. The operation was once fashionable in many parts of the world, but it is now much less frequently carried out except in the United States.

In many countries, doctors feel that circumcision (like tonsillectomy) was quite unjustifiably performed in the past. The arguments advanced in favour of the operation are that it is 'more hygienic', that it prevents likely trouble in the passing of

urine during infancy, and that it promotes sexual harmony in later life by diminishing the sensitivity of the penis thus delaying male orgasm. None of these has any validity. The theory that circumcision prevents the development of cancer of the penis in adult males is, however, true. But this condition is rare, and largely occurs in men who have consistently neglected to wash themselves properly.

The arguments against having a child circumcised are as follows. The operation is painful, and complications are frequent – a small number of deaths follow it each year. Painful ulcers on the tip of the unprotected penis may cause the child agony. Children may be terribly mutilated – by improper operations – a number of complete or partial amputations of the penis are accidentally performed at circumcision. Finally, the loss of sensitivity caused by removal of the protecting foreskin seems to have no advantage whatsoever.

CIRRHOSIS is a disorder of the liver in which fibrous tissue, similar to scar tissue, replaces normal tissue. There are several varieties of cirrhosis, but a common type is caused by alcohol.

CLAUSTROPHOBIA is the fear of being in confined spaces.

CLEFT PALATE – (see **hare-lip**).

CLIMAX, or orgasm, is the highest level of excitement in sexual intercourse. Until the late 1940's, understanding of the climax in both men and women was extremely vague. Before that time, some gynaecologists were declaring that between 25 and 50 per cent of women were 'constitutionally frigid', that is they were incapable of experiencing a climax. But the research of Dr. Alfred Kinsey and, more recently, that of Masters and Johnson, has greatly extended our knowledge.

In women, the climax is an extremely complex physiological reaction. After the clitoris and the vagina have been stimulated for a period of some minutes, the muscles surrounding the womb and the vagina contract, producing the pleasurable sensation accompanying orgasm.

Most women do not experience orgasm when they first make love. The length of time necessary for climax to be experienced depends on a number of factors — principally on the woman's sexual inhibitions and the ease with which her responses are aroused. It is quite often some months before the first climax occurs.

Once a woman starts to experience orgasm regularly, it can give her a sense of deep emotional fulfilment. Many (though not all) women find eventually that they have the capacity for *repeated* orgasms. Many women achieve three or four orgasms during love-making, and are frustrated with less. Some can experience twenty climaxes or so.

In men, orgasms, the ejaculation of sperm, is achieved by stimulation of the penis. Usually this is done by moving the penis, particularly the tip, against the corrugated walls of the vagina. The friction causes certain muscles connected with the male sexual system to contract and relax. These contractions force the sperm out of the penis. Orgasm is accompanied by exceedingly pleasant physical sensations which affect the entire body. They are, however, most intense around the genital area. These begin a few seconds before the first emission of sperm, reaching their peak at the first or second emission, and gradually diminish as the muscle-contractions cease. Repeated orgasms in men are not common over about the age of twenty.

Since the 1940's, a great deal has been written on the subject of *simultaneous climaxes*. Many couples are concerned because they cannot achieve sexual 'harmony'. Actually, simultaneous climax is far from essential — and not always possible. But generally, with time and experience, most couples are often able to achieve simultaneous climax (see **love-play; premature climax; intercourse**).

CLITORIS, one of the organs of the female genitalia, is a small mound of tissue lying in front of the pubic bone. Stimulation of it forms an important part of love play.

CLOTTING is the formation of a solid lump of blood, lymph, or other fluid. A clot,

or thrombus, in the blood may be undesirable, for instance, where clots form in the leg veins and are carried to the lungs. Clots may also form in the heart when the circulation is feeble and the blood flowing through the heart is slowed down. In general, however, clotting is an essential process which prevents the loss of vast quantities of blood when the skin is cut. In a 'clotting disorder', one of the necessary chemical ingredients is deficient — such a condition is present in haemophilia.

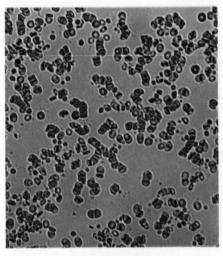

Within seconds of exposure to air, blood cells, *above*, begin to clump. After continued exposure, *below*, a clot forms.

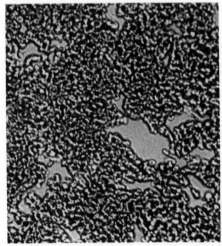

C. James Webb

71

CLUB FOOT, or *talipes,* is a deformity of the leg, usually present at birth. There are several varieties of club-foot, the commonest being *talipes equino-varus,* in which the sole of the foot is turned inwards, and the heel is off the ground. If this condition were allowed to progress untreated until the toddling stage, the child would be walking on the upper part of the side of the foot, immediately behind the little toe.

Treatment of club-foot involves training it to grow straight. For this purpose, strapping, splints or plaster-casts may be required. A small number of children eventually need an operation so that the foot may be brought to its natural position.

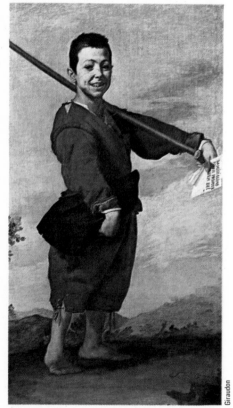

In *talipes equinus,* the foot is pulled up at the heel and the person walks on his toes.

COARCTATION is a narrowing. The term is commonly applied to a narrowing of the aorta — the great artery which carries

blood from the heart. This condition can be treated surgically.

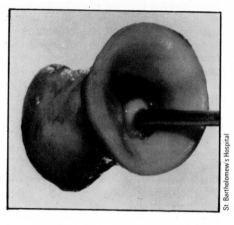

In coarctation, the aorta, the largest artery in the body, becomes narrowed.

COCAINE is a highly dangerous drug obtained from the leaves of the coca plant. It was formerly used as a local anaesthetic, but has been supplanted by newer drugs, such as lignocaine.

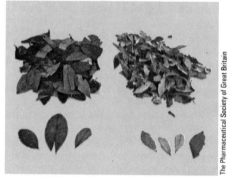

Dried coca leaves can be chewed to obtain the alkaloid cocaine, the anaesthetic.

CODEINE is a drug derived from morphine, but much less potent in the relief of pain, and with no addictive properties. It comes in two types of tablets — codeine compound tablets (which are actually largely aspirin), and codeine phosphate tablets, which are considerably stronger. A liquid codeine mixture is also available for the relief of a cough.

72

'COELIAC CHILDREN' are those who suffer from the disorder known as *coeliac disease.* The child is usually affected when he is about one year old. Until that time, he has been perfectly normal, but then he 'fails to thrive'. He loses his appetite, and his weight decreases. He passes bulky, pale, and ill-smelling motions during periods of digestive upset. As these upsets become more common, the child's general condition worsens. Eventually, he is wizened and emaciated. His legs and buttocks, in particular, show gross wasting. If the disease is allowed to progress, there may be complications, such as rickets and anaemia.

It is believed that coeliac children inherit some kind of sensitivity to a protein known as *gluten.* This substance is present in certain types of food, such as ordinary flour made from wheat. Studies in Great Britain and in Holland have shown that most children affected by coeliac disease show dramatic improvement when gluten is strictly excluded from the diet.

COFFEE is a drink obtained from the coffee plant, which grows throughout most of the tropics. Its most important ingredient, caffeine, is a mild stimulant which promotes wakefulness. If taken late at night, coffee can cause insomnia. As coffee also has a diuretic action, that is, it increases the flow of urine from the kidneys, it may be troublesome for those with urinary complaints.

COIL is a contraceptive device, often referred to as the I.U.D., or intra-uterine device. It is usually made of stainless steel or plastic and is about one inch across. The *loop* is very similar to the coil — it is merely of a different shape.

If a woman wishes to be fitted with a coil, her General Practitioner will usually refer her to a gynaecologist or to a family planning clinic and she is then examined carefully. The doctor inserts a device shaped like a drinking straw with a plunger at one end into the vagina. The tip of it is passed through the cervix (neck of the womb). Inside this instrument is the straightened out coil. Gentle pressure on the plunger puts the coil into place in the

womb. The entire procedure is painless. The insertion of the coil or any intra-uterine device is easier for women who have already given birth, and is easiest of all just after menstruation, when the opening of the womb is somewhat enlarged.

Immediately after the coil is introduced into the womb, there may be mild side effects, such as bleeding or discomfort, similar to that experienced during menstruation. Ordinarily, however, these symptoms soon disappear.

Few women, however, cannot tolerate the device. There is a slight risk that it may enter the abdomen, and it can also be expelled through the vagina.

It is not entirely clear why the coil is effective in preventing conception. But when properly fitted in position, it is very reliable. In underdeveloped countries, notably India, it is, after sterilization, the most widely used method of birth control.

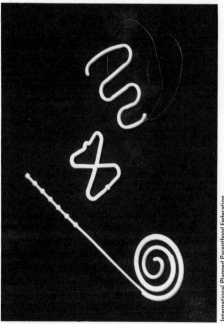

International Planned Parenthood Federation

Intra-uterine coils or loops are among the most effective contraceptive methods developed in the mid twentieth century.

COITUS is another name for sexual intercourse. (See **intercourse**.)

73

COLCHICINE is a drug, extracted from the autumn crocus. It is used to treat the severe pain of acute gout.

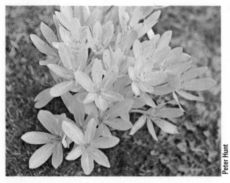

A drug to aid gout sufferers has its source in *Colchicum autumnale*, autumn crocus.

COLDS – see **chill**.

COLIC means a spasmodic gripping pain. The term does not designate a specific disease, as colicky pain can arise from such places as the intestine, the ureter (see **renal colic**), and from gall-stones (see **gall-stones**).

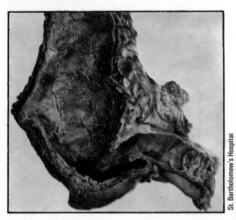

Ulcers on the inner lining of the colon may eat into its walls.

COLITIS means inflammation of the colon. (See **colon.**) It is now recognized that there is no single specific disease which constitutes the disorder. There are, however, a number of separate forms of
74

inflammation of the colon, the commonest and most important of which is ulcerative colitis (see **ulcerative colitis**).

COLLAGEN DISEASES are disorders of the body's connective tissue. In recent years it has been discovered that they are common afflictions. The types most frequently encountered are D.L.E. (see **D.L.E.**) and polyarteritis nodosa (see **polyarteritis nodosa**). All the collagen diseases seem to be closely related, and it is sometimes difficult to determine one from another. Steroids (see **steroids**) are commonly used for treating all the diseases of this group.

COLLARBONE, or clavicle, is the bone which joins the shoulder to the breast bone, or sternum. It is shaped like an elongated 'S' and forms a strut to support the shoulder girdle in front and provide an attachment for the pectoral muscles.

Fractures of the collarbone are common and are usually caused by falling on the shoulder or arm. As a rule, such injuries are not serious and normally heal in about six weeks. Depending on the degree of displacement of the broken bone, it may be necessary for the patient to wear strapping for two or three weeks. Occasionally, it is of value to wear a complex arrangement of slings to keep the fractured bone in place until it knits together.

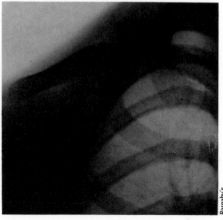

The jagged edge of the broken collar-bone shows up clearly on the X-ray.

COLLES' FRACTURE is fracture of the wrist which usually results from a fall on an outstretched hand. The lower end of the radius (one of the two long bones of the forearm) breaks and is pushed forward. The fracture is accompanied by intense pain in the wrist and marked by a bony lump over the area.

The process of 'reducing' (correcting the deformity of) this fracture is very painful, and it is therefore carried out under a general anaesthetic.

(For other kinds of wrist fracture, see **wrist**.)

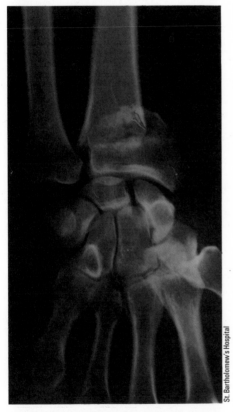

St. Bartholomew's Hospital

In Colles' fracture, the lower end of the radius close to the wrist is broken, resulting in a displacement of the hand.

COLON is the main part of the large intestine (see **alimentary canal**), four to six feet long, extending from the end of the small intestine to the rectum.

COLONIC LAVAGE is the process of washing out the bowel. Except where there is a specific medical indication for an enema, this practice is not justifiable.

COLOSTOMY is the process of making an opening in the colon (see **colon**). The operation is performed for various conditions including cancer of the colon and diverticular disease (see **diverticular disease**), in cases where the bowels are obstructed. A colostomy is not always permanent, and it may be possible to close it off after several months.

The edges of the opening are often stitched to the skin of the abdomen, so that the motions are passed through the incision into a receptacle such as a plastic bag.

COLOSTRUM is the thin fluid which is secreted from the breasts until about two days following childbirth when a mother begins to produce milk.

COLOUR BLINDNESS is the inability to distinguish colours accurately. It is often an inherited condition which is passed on to the male through a 'sex-linked' gene. Colour blindness does not mean, as many people believe, that those who suffer from it perceive everything as black or white. The commonest type of colour blindness, which occurs in eight per cent of the male population, is the inability to distinguish between red and green.

Many men who have this form of colour blindness are completely unaware of it. Entry examinations for the military services often reveal the defect for the first time. The subject is shown a book containing a series of coloured plates composed of dots. A person with normal colour perception would see a number, say five, on a plate, but the design is such that a colour-blind man would, perhaps, see the number three.

Colour is perceived by special structures called 'cones' in the retina, the screen at the back of the eye. It is probable that colour-blind persons have a deficiency in these cones.

The introduction of traffic light signals has made colour blindness a problem of obvious importance, yet driving tests do not include tests for colour-blindness.

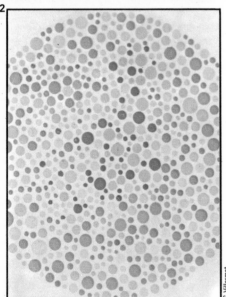

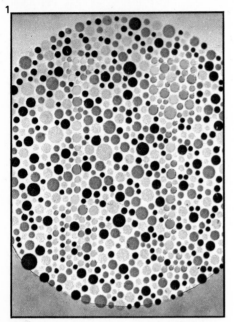

A colour blind person would fail to detect or misinterpret the objects in the arrangements of dots. 1 normal eyes see a spade and fork, pointing in opposite directions;

G. Villermet

defective eyes, see one or other. 2 In the circle, a child holding a ball sits on a chair. Defective eyes would not see the child, only the ball and chair.

COMA is deep unconsciousness and usually implies a state from which a person cannot be roused. The most common causes of coma are malaria, strokes, head injuries, and various types of poisoning, for instance, from barbiturate drugs. An insufficient amount of insulin may cause a diabetic to go into a **diabetic coma,** but, among diabetics, the most frequent form of coma is **hypoglycaemiá**, which results from an overdose of insulin. Excessive use of alcohol or drugs may also produce coma. Other causes include epilepsy, meningitis, cerebral tumour, and indeed, almost any disorder which affects the brain or the surrounding tissues.

Some types of mental illness, notably hysteria, may produce a condition difficult to distinguish from true coma. Hypnotism, too, can put a patient into a completely unrousable state, as do general anaesthetics. Any patient unconscious on an operating table, is, of course, in coma.

With modern medical and nursing techniques, death no longer invariably occurs if a coma persists longer than twenty-four hours. Some patients have remained in coma for periods of months or years. Few of these, however, ever recover normal brain function.

COMPLEXES are groups of symptoms. The term is particularly applied in psychological medicine, though less commonly than forty years ago. It is proposed that complexes are groups of emotionally charged ideas, desires, or concepts which are repressed in childhood at the conscious level, or 'ego', but are powerful, during adult life, in the unconscious mind, or 'id'. These include: the Oedipus or the Electra complex (unconscious sexual desire for the parent of the opposite sex), the castration complex (fear of castration as punishment for desire for the parent of the opposite sex), and the inferiority complex (frustration which results from striving, unsuccessfully, to overcome weaknesses and to achieve superiority).

COMPRESSED AIR is widely used in factories, garages, and in deep-sea diving. Misuse of it can cause a variety of accidental injuries. Caisson disease, also known as 'the bends' (see **bends**), develops in divers or tunnellers who, after breathing compressed air, return too quickly to air at normal pressure. In addition, divers who breathe compressed air at depths below 150 feet may suffer nitrogen narcosis – popularly called 'the narks'.

In factories, playing practical jokes with compressed air hoses has led to a number of deaths. Discharging a compressed air hose under a work-mate's buttocks may, if the jet enters his rectum, perforate his intestine. Discharging compressed air hoses near the ears can damage the ear drums and affect the hearing.

CONCEPTION is the union of a female egg, the ovum, and a male sperm which marks the beginning of the development of a foetus. It generally occurs between the 14th and 18th day of the menstrual cycle. The egg, released from the ovary during the process of ovulation, passes down the Fallopian tube. Millions of sperms ejaculated by the male into the vagina swim towards the egg, but only one sperm can fertilize it. A fertilized egg divides into two then four, and so on, as the embryo begins to develop. At the end of approximately 280 days, the baby is born.

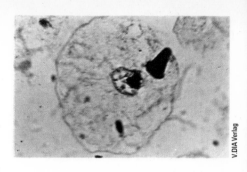

V. DIA Verlag

The sperm enters the outer membrane of the ovum and makes towards its nucleus.

CONCUSSION is an injury to the brain which results from a blow on the head. Brain injuries are generally considered under three categories – concussion, contusion, and laceration. Although contusion means 'bruising of the brain', and laceration means 'tearing of the brain', it is not usually possible to make a clear clinical distinction between the three conditions. They should be regarded as three stages in the same process. Anyone who has been knocked out has, at the very least had concussion. He should be kept quiet, given nothing by mouth (and, in particular no alcohol), and taken to hospital immediately for a skull X-ray and full examination of his central nervous system.

CONDOM or French letter, is a contraceptive sheath which fits over the penis, and prevents the emission of sperm into the vagina. Throughout the centuries, sheaths have been improvised from various materials, such as fish skin. Within the last 50 years condoms have been manufactured which consist of very thin rubber. Such condoms are reasonably safe means of birth control, but they tend to decrease sensitivity. Greater protection is afforded if a condom is used with a spermicide. (See **contraception**.)

CONGENITAL means originating before birth, for example, certain disorders which result either from abnormal foetal development or are transmitted through heredity.

CONGESTIVE CARDIAC FAILURE is a condition in which the activity of the

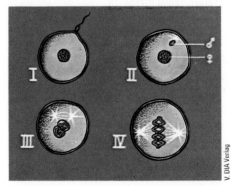

V. DIA Verlag

1 The sperm penetrates the ovum; 2 the sperm's pronucleus guides it towards the egg's pronucleus; 3 chromosomes are visible; 4 the pronuclei fuse; the chromosomes arrange themselves for division.

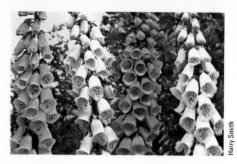

The flowers of foxglove produce digitalis, a drug used to treat cardiac failure.

heart is insufficient to meet the body's needs. Failure of the heart is classified as 'right-sided', 'left-sided', or as a combination of the two. Failure of the left side of the heart causes congestion of fluid in the lungs, with resulting breathlessness. The patient may find that he can only breathe comfortably when his head is elevated. At night, if he should fall into a flat position during sleep, he may suddenly become desperately breathless. Other symptoms of left-sided heart failure include wheezing, and coughing of pink, frothy sputum. In right-sided heart failure, the blood returning to the heart from the body is 'dammed back' so that the veins of the neck tend to stand out. Fluid may collect around the ankles and in the abdomen, and the liver may become congested and swollen.

Heart failure also seems to be associated with over-production of substances which promote the retention of salt and water in the body, so that the patient becomes 'waterlogged'. Some of these alterations are connected with over-production of the hormone aldosterone (see **aldosterone**).

The drug *digoxin*, or the closely related *digitalis*, is widely used in the treatment of heart failure. It has a highly beneficial effect on the contraction of heart muscle and enables the heart to pump the stagnant fluid more readily and to pass it out of the body as urine. *Salt restriction* also enables the body to retain less fluid. *Diuretics* are drugs which enable the kidneys to secrete more water. In severe cases of heart failure, *bed rest* may be

invaluable in helping the patient to recover. *Southey's tubes,* tubes with needles which drain the fluid out of waterlogged legs, over a period of several hours, are a less frequently used method of treatment.

CONJUNCTIVA is the thin membrane covering the front of the eye.

CONJUNCTIVITIS, commonly referred to as 'red eye', is inflammation of the conjunctiva. It is commonly caused by dust in the eye. The numerous vessels which spread over the conjunctival surface dilate and produce the characteristic redness. The condition usually clears up spontaneously, or with very simple treatment.

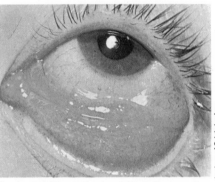

Conjunctivitis or 'red eye' is inflammation of the membrane covering the eye.

CONSTIPATION is failure to pass motions with customary regularity. Constipation rarely indicates a disorder and purgatives are seldom necessary. The use of aperients (especially regularly) can, under certain circumstances, even be harmful. The sudden appearance of constipation during and after middle age may, however, be dangerous, as it sometimes indicates a bowel growth. It should, therefore, be investigated fully.

CONTACT LENSES are lenses made of plastic which fit directly on to the eye and move with it. They are worn instead of spectacles. Large lenses (haptics) are used for sport, while small ones (micros), often tinted, are mainly used for cosmetic purposes. Except on close examination they are invisible.

CONTRACEPTION means prevention of fertilization. For thousands of years, various methods of contraceptive devices have been used, but, until relatively recently, with limited success. Now there are several effective forms available.

Vasectomy, or sterilization, is a method favoured in the East, particularly in India. It involves a minor operation, usually under local anaesthetic, to divide the vasa deferentia, the ducts which carry sperm, from the testes (see **vas deferens**). This procedure does not interfere in any way with the man's ability to have an erection or to perform sexual intercourse. Seminal fluid *is* emitted, but it does not contain sperm; therefore, the female egg cannot be fertilized.

A sterilizing operation can be performed on a woman. The fallopian tubes carrying ripe eggs from the ovary are cut and the ends tied. Sometimes the ovaries are removed for absolute certainty of sterility. Many women have it done in hospital when they are recovering from the birth of their last baby.

The oral contraceptive, or Pill, developed in the mid 1950s, is used by millions of women throughout the world. If the Pill is taken regularly according to instructions, there is almost no possibility of pregnancy. As there may be unwanted side-effects, this type of contraceptive should be prescribed by a doctor (see **Pill**).

The intra-uterine device, or I.U.D., also known as the coil or loop, is a piece of stainless steel, plastic, or nylon thread which is inserted into the womb through the vagina. There is only a small possibility of conceiving with this method (see **coil**).

The diaphragm, cervical cap, or Dutch cap, is basically a dome-shaped object which is inserted into the vagina and covers the cervix, the neck of the womb. It should be fitted by a doctor and used with a spermicidal cream to afford maximum protection. There is a larger failure rate with this device than with the pill or coil (see **Dutch cap**).

Condoms, or 'French letters', are rubber sheaths which cover the penis. When they are used with a chemical they are about as reliable as the combination of a cervical cap and a chemical. However, as they diminish sensitivity, they tend to reduce sexual enjoyment. (See **condom**.)

Coitus interruptus, or withdrawal of the penis from the vagina before the emission of sperm, is widely practised, but is not very safe. As there is some flow of sperm before emission, conception can occur despite withdrawal. Coitus interruptus as a regular practice is not recommended, since it may sexually frustrate the wife.

Foams, pessaries, and other chemicals which are spermicidal are relatively unreliable. When they are used with another device, the cap or condom, they afford greater protection.

The rhythm method is the only type of contraception authorized by the Roman Catholic Church. It regulates intercourse, according to the woman's menstrual cycle, to coincide with the infertile or 'safe' period when conception is unlikely. As this period is extremely difficult to determine, the method is unreliable (see **rhythm method**).

CONVULSIONS, or fits, are rapidly alternating contractions and relaxations of the muscles which result in spasmodic bodily movements. They are usually accompanied by unconsciousness. Apart from true epilepsy (see **epilepsy**) the majority of convulsive seizures occur in childhood. They are frequently caused by upper respiratory tract infection.

A sudden rise of temperature frequently caused by pneumonia or tonsillitis may produce a **febrile convulsion.** Convulsions of this sort are fairly common and not generally dangerous. When they occur, call the doctor at once, turn the child on his side and make sure that he can breathe. Put something between his teeth and be certain that no vomit is obstructing the airway. (See **epilepsy** and **fits**.)

CORNEA is the clear outer layer of the eyeball through which light passes to the pupil (see **eye**) the dark opening in the centre of the coloured iris. The cornea is subject to disease or to injury and the resulting opacity may well produce blindness. The grafting of corneas from deceased persons is now used to restore sight.

In cases where the cornea has been damaged by disease or accident, corneal graft is often successful.

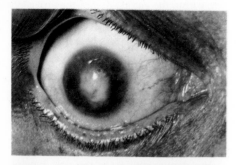
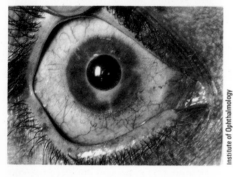

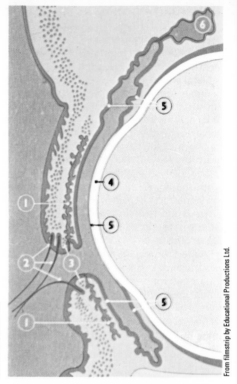

A damaged cornea, *top*, produces opacity. After a successful corneal graft, *above*, vision has been restored. A cornea removed within ten hours of death can be stored for twenty days before it is used.

A diagrammatic vertical section shows the position of the lids in relation to the front of the eye: 1 meibomian glands; 2 eyelashes; 3 muscles of eyelids; 4 cornea; 5 conjunctiva; 6 lachrymal glands.

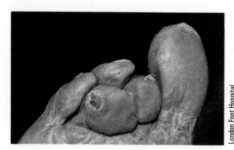

A corn has a cone-like shape; the point is directed inwards towards the 'eye'.

CORNS are localized thickened areas of skin caused by the pressure of tight or ill-fitting shoes. When they occur on the sole of the foot, they result from an unevenness of the surface. Because of the pressure, the skin grows more rapidly and becomes hardened by the pressure. Corns are best treated by chiropodists.

CORONARY THROMBOSIS is the lay term for myocardial infarction, the death of a section of the heart muscle due to a deficient supply of blood. When the coronary arteries which supply the heart muscle are constricted because of disease, the blood flow is slowed down and clots or thromboses may be formed. Intense pain in the chest, often collapse, and even death may result.

CORONER is an officer who holds inquests on deaths resulting from unnatural or unknown causes, for example, death resulting from violence.

COR PULMONALE, or pulmonary heart disease, is a disorder of the right side of the heart which is caused by lung disease. Blood is normally pumped into the lungs by the right side of the heart to receive a fresh supply of oxygen. A lung disorder may cause a strain on the right side of the heart and a subsequent malfunction. Various signs and symptoms of 'right heart failure' develop, notably, swelling of the ankles.

The most common cause of cor pulmonale is chronic bronchitis with emphysema (see **bronchitis** and **emphysema**).

CORPUSCLES are cells. The term usually refers to the red and white cells of the blood (see **blood**), about $\frac{1}{3000}$ of an inch in size, which carry oxygen, repair tissue and destroy bacteria.

CORTICOSTEROIDS are steroids, chemical compounds (see **steroids**), which are produced by the cortex of the adrenal glands (see **adrenal**).

CORTICOTROPHIN, also known as A.C.T.H. or adrenocorticotrophic hormone, is a chemical produced by the pituitary gland situated at the base of the brain.

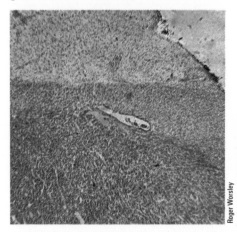

Roger Worsley

The pituitary gland, shown in section, secretes the hormone corticotrophin.

CORTISONE is a steroid hormone (see **steroids**), produced by the cortex of the adrenal glands (see **adrenal**). In the late 1940s, it was found that cortisone had a dramatic effect on certain cases of arthritis. Unfortunately it became clear within a few months that the effect was not permanent, and that a number of dangerous side effects had resulted. The hormone is now little used in medicine, as other steroids, such as prednisone and prednisolone, have proved more useful in treating conditions such as rheumatoid arthritis and asthma.

CORYZA is a rarely used name for the 'common cold'.

COSTAL means pertaining to the ribs.

COSTIVE means constipated (see **constipation**).

COUNTER-IRRITANTS are substances applied to the skin in an attempt to relieve an underlying disorder. They are employed on the principle that external irritation causes congestion of the tissues immediately below the skin, thereby acting upon the nerves which regulate the size of the capillaries. The congestion of internal organs is said to be subsequently relieved.

Until quite recently this method was widely practised: counter-irritants and even blistering of the skin was used to treat conditions such as bronchitis, pleurisy, and 'congestion of the stomach'. More accurate diagnosis and the development of specific drugs to treat specific diseases have caused therapy by counter-irritants to be largely abandoned.

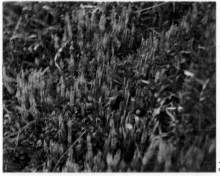

C. Jermy

Spores of the club-moss, lycopodium, are used as a mild counter-irritant.

COW-POX is a mild infectious disease which affects the udders of cows. It can be communicated to humans, and principally occurs among those who work with cattle. In the late 1700s a British surgeon, Edward Jenner, investigated the folk tradition that individuals who had suffered an attack of cow-pox never contracted the feared disease small-pox. The popular belief was confirmed by his observations and experiments. He soon developed the technique of vaccination with fluid from a cow-pox pustule as immunization against small-pox.

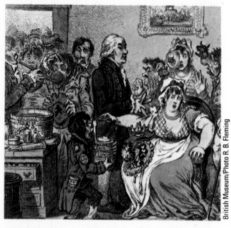

Dr. Jenner's cow-pox serum was treated with some scorn in the 1800s, *above*. The 'gun', *below*, has no needle and gives small-pox vaccine almost painlessly.

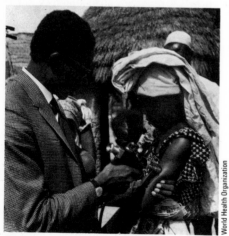

COXSACKIE VIRUSES are a group of disease-producing viruses, which was first isolated in Coxsackie, New York. These viruses can produce a number of feverish illnesses, including a rare type of meningitis and Bornholm disease (see **meningitis** and **Bornholm disease**).

CRABS is the common name for lice affecting pubic hair. They are often transmitted through sexual contact with an infected person. The first symptom of 'crabs' is intense itching around the pubic region. After approximately a week the tiny crab-lice are visible.

The condition generally will not disappear without medical treatment. A D.D.T. preparation is usually prescribed.

CRADLE-CAP is a scaly condition of the scalp which often appears in young babies. It usually responds to treatment with olive oil rubbed on the scalp several times a day for a period of one or two months. Combing afterwards usually dislodges the crusts. Soap and water should not be used on the scalp during the treatment.

CRAMP is a painful muscular spasm which most often occurs in the legs, but it may also affect other parts of the body. The causes of a cramp are little understood by medical science: but causes which have been suggested in the past include: salt depletion, excessive exercise (particularly after a heavy meal) and exposure to cold, for instance in swimming.

A cramp occurs suddenly. It often comes on during sleep and may result from a particular position which an arm or leg has taken during the night. In certain occupations which require the habitual use of certain muscle groups, a 'professional cramp' may develop. In 'writer's cramp', the attempt to write produces painful spasms in the muscles of the hand. A similar condition develops in bricklayer's and seamstress' cramp.

The most effective means of relieving a cramp is to rub the affected part with the hand. Stretching the muscle often causes the condition to disappear. A cramp is rarely symptomatic of a serious disorder, but if attacks recur, consult a doctor.

CRANIAL NERVES are the twelve pairs of nerves which emerge from the brain. They affect important bodily functions including the senses of smell, sight, and hearing, the movements of the eyes, sensation of the skin of the face, movement of the facial muscles and the tongue, and swallowing. Certain brain disorders may be localized by testing the functions which these nerves control.

CRETINISM is a disease caused by defective function of the thyroid gland. It can be recognized within a few months of birth: the baby is dull and listless, and his swollen protruding tongue is prominent. In former times, cretinous children invariably became mentally defective, but now the condition is curable once the diagnosis is made. Thyroid extract is given to counteract the deficiency.

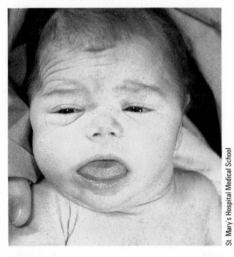

This baby was given treatment with thyroid hormone soon after birth and was completely cured.

CROHN'S DISEASE is a condition in which an area of the small intestine becomes inflamed. It commonly occurs where the small intestine joins the large bowel. Thickening of the intestinal wall produces a stenosis, or narrowing, of the calibre of the bowel. The cause of the disease is obscure. Treatment by drugs is usually preferred to surgical measures, but sometimes operation is necessary.

CROUP refers to any childhood condition in which obstruction of the larynx (or voice box) causes noisy breathing. It includes a number of disorders, for instance, laryngitis and laryngo-tracheo-bronchitis. As a child's air passages are extremely narrow an obstruction is dangerous and may be fatal. For this reason, a doctor should always be called.

CURARE is a poison derived from some trees belonging to the *Strychnos* family. South American Indians use it as an arrow poison and it may cause paralysis and indeed, death, if the respiratory muscles are affected. A derivative of the poison, **tubocurarine**, is a drug used in anaesthesia. An injection produces complete muscular relaxation. Although the respiratory muscles become paralysed, there is no danger of death, as the anaesthetist supplements the patient's breathing by pumping air into him – either by squeezing a rubber bag or by using a mechanical respirator.

CUSHING'S SYNDROME is a condition of glandular imbalance which occurs when the adrenal cortex over-secretes hormones (see **adrenal**), and marked changes take place in the body. These are obesity (with a rather unusual distribution of fat), tiredness, high blood pressure, abnormal growth of hair (notably on the face), absence of menstrual periods in women, and purple marks on the skin. Personality is also affected.

The condition may be caused by an adrenal disorder itself, or by an overgrowth of certain cells in the pituitary gland (see **pituitary**) located at the base of the brain.

The disorder was first described by an American brain surgeon, Dr. Harvey Cushing, in 1932.

CYANIDE is the highly poisonous salt of hydrocyanic or, prussic acid. It was once used widely in gaseous form in the United States to execute criminals. Inhalation is said to produce nearly instantaneous death. Taken by mouth, death is slower.

CYANOCOBALAMIN is vitamin B_{12} (see **vitamins**). Deficiency of this vitamin causes pernicious anaemia (see **anaemia**).

CYANOSIS (see **blueness**).

CYSTITIS is an inflammation of the bladder usually caused by bacterial infection in the urine (see **urinary infection**). It is a common condition particularly among women. In the female the urethra, the tube which runs from the bladder to the exterior, is short and germs can easily pass up through it into the bladder. The condition known as 'honeymoon cystitis' may be caused by the repeated mild injuries to the lower end of the urethra which are likely to occur during a woman's first sexual experiences and may be an inflammation of the urethra. The symptoms are pain passing water and frequency of urination which may also disturb sleep. All patients who have these should consult a doctor immediately. If cystitis is not treated promptly and thoroughly it may lead to serious complications at a later time. A urine specimen sent to the lab. will determine the germs which are present and the antibiotic which will eradicate them. At the end of about a fortnight's treatment with the antibiotic, a further specimen should be taken to see if the infection has cleared up. *Disappearance of the symptoms does not indicate that the infection has been eliminated.*

CYSTS are hollow tumours which may occur at various sites in the body. As a rule, surgeons can remove them easily, and they do not return. In structure, cysts have a definite wall and contain fluid, semi-fluid, or solid material. Some cysts are caused by a fault in the body's development; others by the blockage of a duct; others by a parasite.

Cysts in the breast may be caused by a blocked milk duct. In the ovary, cysts may reach a large size, taking many years to do so. 'Daughter' cysts may bud from the original cyst wall. Cysts on the skin — most commonly on the face or scalp — are called *wens*. They contain fatty material, and are caused by the blocking of a gland. They are unsightly, but not dangerous, and can often be removed under a local anaesthetic. Cysts which develop on the ovaries and kidney often grow to a large size over a period of many years.

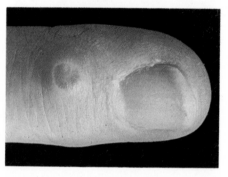

Two cysts, one on the finger and the other inside the mouth, look very similar. Most cysts can be removed surgically.

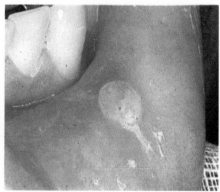

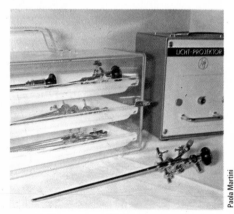

Through the *cystoscope*, the doctor can look into the inside of the bladder.

Paola Martini

84

D.D.T. is the common abbreviation for a chemical insecticide, officially known as dicophane, which came into widespread use during the 1940s. D.D.T. has a toxic action on lice, bedbugs, fleas, mosquitoes, and many other insects. Its lethal effect on lice is particularly valuable, as these insects are responsible for the spread of epidemic typhus — the commonest and most terrible of the group of typhus fevers (see **typhus**). This disease tends to occur whenever there is over-crowding and lack of proper facilities for washing — conditions which occur in prisoner-of-war camps, in refugee camps, and in armies on the march. At the end of the Second World War, conditions were suitable for typhus outbreaks all over Europe and the Far East. Because of the scientific application of D.D.T. few of these outbreaks occurred.

D.D.T. is poisonous to human beings and animals. It should, therefore, be used with great caution. Indiscriminate use has lead to the poisoning of vast areas of lakes and rivers making them largely uninhabitable for fish. Great numbers of insects which are actually valuable to Man, such as those which prey on pests, have been killed off. Because of its widespread application in agriculture, it has been suggested that the level of D.D.T. in human tissues is now approaching dangerous levels. It may therefore result in some kind of poisoning. This point, however, is much disputed.

D.F. 118, or dihydrocodeine bitartrate, is a useful pain-killing tablet. Chemically related to both codeine and morphine, it produces effective relief of pain without drowsiness or risk of addiction.

D.L.E. is the abbreviation for the disease *disseminated lupus erythematosus*. The alternative name is S.L.E. (*systemic lupus erythematosus*). D.L.E. is one of the collagen diseases (see **collagen diseases**) and, like the other members of this group, affects the connective tissue. It appears in various sites of the body, and it may produce a number of different symptoms, depending on the site which is most affected. In women, the first sign is often a 'butterfly rash' over the bridge of the nose.

Rashes may appear in other parts of the body; a malfunction of the kidneys may also develop. Arthritis can be produced by D.L.E., and the condition is often difficult to distinguish from rheumatoid arthritis. Treatment of D.L.E. usually involves the use of steroid drugs, which have an anti-inflammatory effect on the tissues involved.

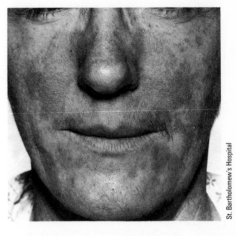

St. Bartholomew's Hospital

The butterfly rash over this woman's nose is one of the first signs of D.L.E.

D.T.'s (see **delirium tremens**).

DA COSTA'S SYNDROME, also known as D.A.H. (disorderly action of the heart), is a condition in which an individual, often a young person, particularly a young man, imagines he has disease of the heart. The condition was first clearly described in young men conscripted for military service, hence the alternative name 'soldier's heart'. The sufferer interprets normal slight palpitations and odd aches in the left lower chest as symptoms of heart trouble. His agitation makes the palpitations worse and sometimes his life is almost crippled because of the conviction that the heart may stop at any moment. A few people with this condition refuse to accept that they have no cardiac trouble, and spend the rest of their lives in a state of what is called 'cardiac neurosis'. Most patients, however, lose their symptoms rapidly once the nature of the condition has been explained to them and their anxiety is thereby eliminated.

85

DANDRUFF is a condition of scurf on the scalp: the epidermis, or outer layer of the skin, proliferates in the form of dry, white scales. The condition is extremely widespread, but remarkably little is known about it. Dandruff is not contagious as many people imagine, so that it cannot be passed on by sharing a comb. Nor does it inevitably lead to baldness — the other popular misconception. Mild cases can be treated by using a medicated lotion or shampoo, but more serious cases may require the attention of a dermatologist.

DEADLY NIGHTSHADE is the plant *Atropa belladonna*, which contains the drug atropine (see **Belladonna**).

DEAFNESS is the absolute or relative impairment of hearing.

There are two main categories of deafness: **conductive deafness** and **perceptive deafness**, depending on which part of the ear is affected. Conductive deafness, which affects the external and middle ear, is generally more amenable to treatment. The causes of this type of deafness include plugs of wax in the outer ear, which is readily cleared up by syringing, and otosclerosis, a disorder involving the tiny bones of the middle ear — the malleus, incus, and stapes. Until the 1960s little could be done to treat otosclerosis but now it is possible to operate on the middle ear and greatly improve hearing. (See **otosclerosis**.)

Perceptive deafness affects the inner ear or the auditory nerve (the nerve which carries impulses from the ear to the brain). It may be present from birth or be caused by such disorders as meningitis, but it is common in old people. Regrettably, at the present time, cure is not usually practicable, but modern hearing aids can help greatly.

Some elderly people exploit slight degrees of hardness of hearing, hearing only what they wish. This 'selective' deafness is an understandable reaction in one who encounters an environment with which he feels unable to cope.

The causes of deafness are numerous, and it is unfortunate that only a small proportion of cases can be completely cured

by surgical operation. However, an increasingly large number of deaf people are being helped through both surgical and non-surgical methods to achieve a useful degree of hearing. (See **ear**.)

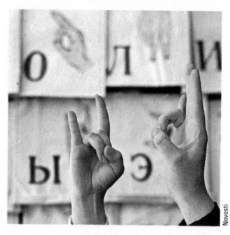

Deaf Russians learn a separate sign for each letter in their thirty-three letter alphabet.

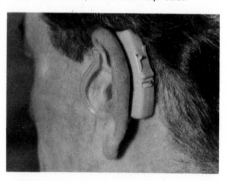

The small hearing aid worn behind the ear, *above*, has become more popular than the larger, more clumsy devices, *below*.

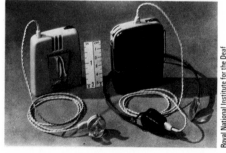

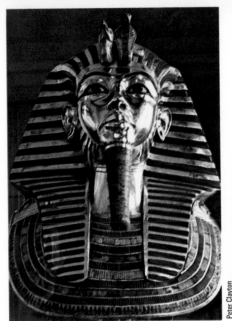

Peter Clayton

Death masks were placed on the mummified bodies of the Egyptian pharaohs.

DEATH is the cessation of life. The actual *moment of death* is difficult to distinguish. In past years, the stoppage of breathing was regarded as a satisfactory indication: a mirror was held in front of the person's lips, and if it did not become misted-up, death was pronounced. But the absence of breath is no guide to the absence of life; nor, as we have learnt since the 1950s is cessation of the heart beat.

It would be more accurate to say that an individual dies when his brain ceases to function. However, it is difficult to determine when this occurs. Brain activity can be recorded in the form of waves by means of an electro-encephalogram (see **E.E.G.**), but a 'flat' electro-encephalogram does not necessarily mean that the patient has no possibility of recovering.

Defining the moment of death has always been a difficult problem for doctors. Today it is a crucial one, largely because of the widespread introduction of transplant surgery. Organs which are transplanted, whether they are hearts, livers, or kidneys, must themselves be living when they are removed from the donor. At the same time, the donor himself must be dead — not only to meet the law's requirements, but to fulfil the doctor's moral obligation towards his patient. In such circumstances, current medical opinion recommends that the pronouncement of death should always be undertaken by someone who has no interest in the subsequent transplant operation which will make use of the organ.

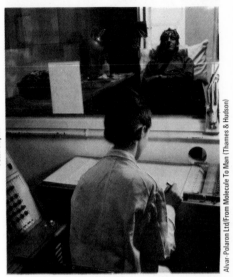

Alvar-Polaron Ltd/From Molecule To Man (Thames & Hudson)

Brain waves recorded on the E.E.G. are often used as proof of life or death.

The *causes of death* vary greatly from country to country. In underdeveloped lands, infectious diseases, such as malaria, sleeping sickness, typhoid, and T.B. are the prime killers. In these countries, there is also a high mortality rate among newborn babies, just as there once was in Western countries. In the West the main causes of death are 'degenerative' diseases of the heart and blood vessels (for instance, heart attacks and strokes), followed by cancer, and, in some countries (notably in England), by chronic respiratory diseases, such as emphysema and chronic bronchitis.

Fear of death is strong in most human beings. Many people think that it will be agonizing or terrifying. But, from repeated observation, most doctors would agree that the vast majority of people suffer very little, if at all, at the point of death.

Changes after death are quite rapid in their onset. Within a few minutes, the

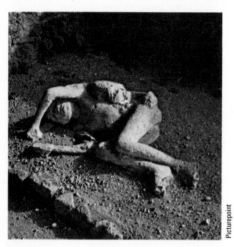

A child who died in the eruption of Vesuvius was petrified and preserved by lava.

pupils become dilated and staring, and the face muscles sag. Within an hour or two the skin usually acquires a rather waxen appearance. A few hours later, post mortem lividity, a bluish discoloration which resembles bruising, develops in those parts of the body which are nearest to the ground. The occurrence of this phenomenon indicates to forensic pathologists whether the body has been moved after death. For instance, if a body were found face downwards, but with lividity on the back, this would reveal that it had been turned over.

Rigor mortis, or stiffness, is variable in its onset. It is usually complete about 12 hours after death and passes off after about 48 hours, but these times can be influenced by many factors.

A much more accurate guide to the time when death actually occurs is the temperature of the body, which decreases at a uniform rate, depending on the surroundings.

Disposal after death generally takes the form of burial or cremation. Burial is undoubtedly the most widespread method and the one hallowed in Judaeo-Christian tradition. In most countries, it requires

88

only formal permission from an official registrar of deaths who will invariably give such permission if a death certificate, signed by a doctor, is submitted to him.

Cremation has also been practised for thousands of years in India and elsewhere, but it was not until late in the 1800s that it began to gain any respectability in the West. Because cremation is so final, in that the body can never be examined again, most countries require special cremation certificates to be signed by two doctors. (As a rule, such matters as the examination of the body after death are more strictly governed for cremation than for burial.) When all procedures have been duly carried out, the body is taken to a crematorium and incinerated over a furnace. Most of the substance is carried off as smoke, but a few pounds of ashes usually remain. Cremation is now approved by the Roman Catholic Church, which had for hundreds of years opposed it.

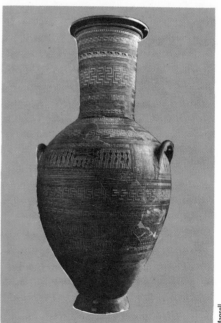

From ancient times, the ashes of cremated bodies have been placed in cinerary urns.

DEFAECATION, the evacuation of faeces, is the act of opening the bowels.

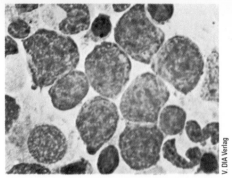

Iron deficiency distorts blood forming cells and produces anaemia.

DEFICIENCY DISEASES

DEFICIENCY DISEASES stem from the lack of an ingredient in the diet. Nutritional science can remedy these deficiencies but such diseases are still common in under-developed countries.

The most widespread deficiency disease is **iron-deficiency anaemia** (see **anaemia**). Women, in particular, need iron because menstruation, and the requirements of unborn babies during pregnancy can produce deficiency of iron. Anaemia is almost universal in pregnancy but it can be cured by iron tablets or injections.

Vitamin A deficiency *(Avitaminosis-A)* occurs in people whose diet lacks *carotenes* (carotenes, colouring matter in carrots and other vegetables are converted to vitamin A by the liver), or with intestinal troubles (such as tropical sprue) which make them difficult to absorb. Avitaminosis is most commonly found in children in the Orient. It causes night-blindness, and atrophy, degeneration, or even ulceration of the outer layer of the eyeball.

Of the B-group vitamins, the most important from the point of view of deficiency diseases are nicotinic acid, thiamine (aneurine) and riboflavin.

Nicotinic acid deficiency results in pellagra. Its most common symptoms are dermatitis, diarrhoea, and dementia (see **dementia**). It stems from a diet consisting largely of maize (corn) with little animal protein or green vegetables. Pellagra occurs in a great belt across the world, extending as far north as Italy, and as far south as Chile. Pellagra caused 7000 deaths in the southern states of the U.S.A. in 1928, but enriched bread, with vitamin additives, has almost eliminated it in recent years.

Thiamine deficiency causes beri-beri. The main sources of thiamine are whole cereals, liver and lean meat in general, peas and beans, and yeast or yeast products. Milled cereals, such as polished rice (which constitutes the staple diet in much of the East) contain practically no thiamine at all.

60 years ago Christian Eijbman and Gerrit, two Dutch physicians in Java, discovered that a continuous diet of milled cereals produces one or more types of beri-beri. The most important are 'dry' beri-beri, which produces neuritis, and 'wet' beri-beri, heart failure (see **beri-beri**). Both were common among inmates of Japanese prisoner-of-war camps during the second world war.

Riboflavin deficiency results in atrophy and cracking of the skin and of the tongue. It is often associated with pellagra, and occurs in the same areas of the world.

Vitamin C deficiency can produce scurvy. In children the main symptoms are severe pain, especially in the bones of the legs, swelling and bleeding of the gums and anaemia; in adults small cuts in the skin refuse to heal. Sailors on long voyages suffered from scurvy until the eighteenth century, when James Lynd, a British naval surgeon, gave them lemon juice (a rich source of vitamin C) to vary the constant diet of biscuits and salt pork. Children between the ages of six and eighteen months who have not been given diet supplements, such as orange juice, which contain vitamin C may contract scurvy. If untreated the consequences (especially to the development of the bones) may be serious.

Vitamin D deficiency, which causes rickets (see **rickets**), is uncommon as almost all dried milk preparations for infants are fortified with vitamin D. However, children require sunlight, and fresh air to assimilate sufficient quantities of vitamin D.

Proteins, which we get from meat, cheese, and to a lesser extent eggs, may be lacking in the diet. Normally they supply energy and are essential for growth. One extreme form of protein deficiency disease, *kwashiorkor* (see **kwashiorkor**) is widespread in children living in underdeveloped countries. It is characterized by mottled skin, reddish patchy hair and swollen abdomen. High protein foods have been developed to meet this condition.

DEFLORATION is breaking the *hymen*, a thin membrane partially covering the vagina. This occurs usually during sexual intercourse, or medical examination.

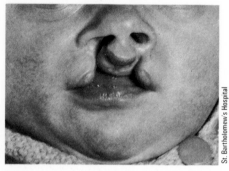

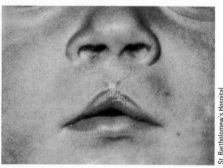

Above, embryonic tissue which fails to join can form a hare-lip. Below, plastic surgery soon after birth removes the disfiguration which has prevented the baby from sucking.

DEFORMITIES are abnormalities of structure of any part of the body. Some deformities are acquired, by injury, but the term is most often used to imply congenital abnormalities present at birth. Common examples include clubfoot and hare-lip, while less common ones include
90

malformations such as those caused by certain drugs taken during pregnancy.

DEGENERATION is deterioration of a tissue or organ. Degeneration, common in old age, coupled with excessive strain on an organ, such as toxins, for instance copper and alcohol, exert on the liver, or disease, such as arteriosclerosis exerts on the heart, can bring about failure.

DEHYDRATION may result from lack of drinking water, excessive loss of water in the urine or by sweating, or most commonly by intestinal disturbances. Severe gastro-enteritis in a child can rapidly deplete his small stores of water, by vomiting and diarrhoea, and may thus threaten his life.

The signs of dehydration include a dry skin which, when pinched, remains puckered for some seconds, sunken eyes, and, in babies, a sunken fontanelle (see **fontanelle**). When these signs appear, there is urgent need for treatment, usually in the form of a rapid 'drip' of fluid into a vein.

DELIRIUM is a temporary state of mental disorientation as opposed to the more permanent disorder of mental function, *dementia* (see **dementia**).

Feverish illness, alcoholism or a blow on the head can all cause delirium. A special case is the withdrawal symptoms exhibited by drug addicts if their supplies are abruptly stopped. The delirious patient is confused, restless and sometimes terrified. He may suffer frightening hallucinations, lose his sense of balance and become overexcited. He is completely disorientated as to where, or who, he is. He should not be left alone as frequently delirious patients attempt suicide.

DELIRIUM TREMENS (the D.T.s) results from the physical deterioration associated with chronic alcoholism. Delirium of this type does not usually persist for more than a few days. Like other abnormalities which occur in alcoholics it may be caused by interference with the absorption of B group vitamins, specifically nicotinic acid, and injections of these vitamins are often used to treat it.

DELIVERY (see **labour**).

DELOUSING is the removal or killing of lice on the body. It is usually effected with the application of D.D.T. to body and clothing.

DELUSIONS are irrational and mistaken beliefs. In psychiatric terminology, they denote beliefs held in spite of contrary evidence which would adequately convince a normal person of similar age, cultural, and religious background. Delusions are a feature of several types of mental disorder, such as schizophrenia, paranoia and senile dementia.

DEMAND FEEDING is the feeding of young babies whenever they want food, as opposed to feeding on a rigid three-hour or four-hour schedule. Both systems have received support among paediatricians, and neither method can be proposed as 'better'. A mother should try whichever method seems likely to be more convenient for her, and, if this does not work, change to the other.

DEMENTIA is a state of disordered brain function. The term normally implies a permanent state of mental confusion (as opposed to delirium, which describes temporary disturbances). The main features of dementia are irrationality, irritability, restlessness, and poor memory. The failure of memory is of a characteristic type, in that the sufferer can recall very clearly events which happened fifty, sixty or seventy years ago (and may think they occurred recently); he cannot, however, remember things which took place the previous day. The commonest type of dementia is **senile**, or **arteriosclerotic dementia**, which occurs in many old people. This is related to the degeneration of the brain cells and of the blood vessels supplying the brain which occur in advanced age. Other, rarer causes of dementia include syphilis, in the later stages, and a number of uncommon types of atrophy of the brain tissues.

    Dementia praecox is a form of mental disorder now more commonly known as schizophrenia (see **schizophrenia**).

DEMEROL is the American name for the valuable pain-killing drug pethidine (see **pethidine**).

DENDRITE is a fine, many-branched fibre which carries impulses to a nerve cell from other nerve cells and sensory areas of the body. There are usually several dendrites connected to each nerve cell.

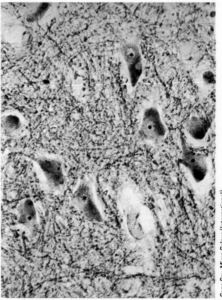

Gene Cox, Micro Colour (International)

Dendrites show up as a blue tracery among the red cells in a motor nerve. They are found in all sensory areas.

DENGUE (pronounced den-gee) is a viral illness transmitted by mosquitoes. It is also known as 'break-bone fever' because of the severe pain associated with it. The virus is transmitted by the *Aedes Aegypti*, the same species which is responsible for the spread of yellow fever (see **yellow fever**). Dengue is common in hot countries, particularly in the East, where it tends to occur in epidemics. About six days after being bitten by a mosquito carrying the virus, the victim will develop a fever, feel desperately weak, and have severe pain in the legs and the back. The fever tends to remit after a few days, and then come back again. Normally, recovery follows after several weeks. It is very rarely fatal.

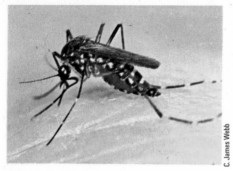

C. James Webb

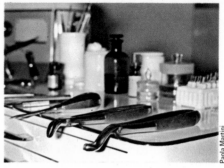

Paola Martini

Aedes Aegypti, the mosquito which carries dengue, feasts on a human finger.

In the dentist's armoury, forceps are among the most important weapons.

DENTINE, or dentin, is the dense white substance which composes the main part of the tooth and surrounds the pulp in the central hollow. When the thin layer of enamel which covers the dentine is eaten away or broken, the dentine is liable to decay and a cavity may then form beneath it. The sensitive pulp is thereby exposed.

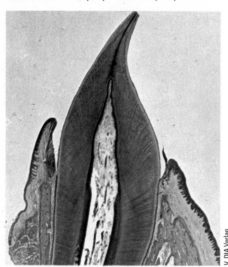

V. DIA Verlag

Dentine, dyed pink in the photograph, protects a tooth's sensitive nerve.

DENTIST is a practitioner of the branch of medicine which is concerned with the prevention, diagnosis, and treatment of diseases of the teeth and gums.

DENTURE is a term which is usually applied to any number of artificial teeth from one, to a complete set of 32.

DEODORANTS are substances used to destroy or disguise odours. Examples are aerosols to dispel unpleasant smells in rooms and the numerous preparations for use on the human body. The latter type includes mouth deodorants (toothpaste, mouth washes, and tablets) and body deodorants (sprays, creams, and liquids and certain kinds of soap).

Toothpaste, especially if 'flavoured' is undoubtedly an effective breath-sweetener, and the proprietary antiseptic mouthwashes also have some value. Chlorophyll tablets, which were popular in the early 1960s are quite useless. The best way of avoiding mouth odour is to visit the dentist regularly and to clean the teeth twice a day.

Frequent bathing is effective in eliminating perspiration secreted from the sweat glands located all over the body.

Perspiration odour from the axillary glands of the armpit can normally be countered by the use of deodorant preparations. Some of these contain antiperspirants which actually prevent the formation of sweat, as opposed to removing its smell. However, many people are allergic to body deodorants and antiperspirants, and they should be used with care, particularly if infection develops in the armpit (see **perspiration**).

DEPRESSION is a feeling of dejection and unhappiness. Such a state of mind is a normal occurrence at times, but, in its severe forms, depression amounts to a serious and often crippling mental illness. In psychological medicine, depression is divided into two types: **reactive** (in which depression appears because of some specific event, such as the death of a loved one), and **endogenous** (in which there is no obvious antecedent event). Distinction between the two types, however, is often difficult.

The main characteristics of depressive illness (as opposed to normal depression) are misery and self-reproach, often with unjustified feelings of guilt, slowness of thought, difficulty in making decision, and, often, loss of appetite and disturbance of sleep. There may be a marked variation of mood, so that the patient feels depressed every morning but improves every evening (or, sometimes, the other way round). This type of depression may entirely cripple the life of the sufferer.

A particularly severe form of the disorder, sometimes called *involutional melancholia*, occurs in people who are around the age of retirement. Suddenly, the individual feels that his whole life has been worthless, that he has never achieved anything, and that he has been a constant burden to his family. Suicide is a serious risk, and medical or psychiatric help should be arranged at once. These cases respond particularly well to electroconvulsive therapy (see **E.C.T.**), or to antidepressant drugs which, in a reasonable proportion of patients, produce considerable improvement after some weeks and change their attitudes dramatically.

DERMATITIS is inflammation of the skin. Normally, the term is only used to indicate a specific type of inflammation which is characterized by redness and flaking of the skin. Certain types of dermatitis are probably a form of eczema (see **eczema**). But the disorder has a variety of causes, including allergy and skin irritants like certain plants. Industrial dermatitis, for example, results from sensitivity to some substance the patient works with in a factory, or place of work.

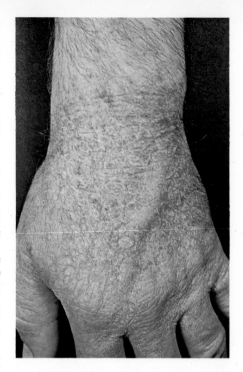
Dermatitis can result from handling chemicals, or even too strong a soap.

DERMATOLOGY is the study of disorders of the skin. Dermatologists, or specialists in this field of medicine, also have a general or specialized knowledge of internal medicine, as a great variety of internal illnesses can produce abnormalities of the skin.

DERMATOPHYTES are primitive fungal organisms which can invade the skin, the nails, or the hair follicles. They cause such skin diseases as ringworm and athlete's foot.

DESENSITIZATION means freeing a patient from some unwanted 'sensitivity'. The term is generally applied both to allergic reactions and mental disorder. A patient who is allergic to a foreign protein, such as pollen or dust, may be given a series of desensitization injections consisting of minute doses of the foreign protein. Gradually he becomes accustomed to the substance, so that eventually the allergy disappears.

In psychiatry, desensitization is used to describe a form of treatment for such disorders as phobias and anxiety states. A barbiturate drug (see **barbiturates**), may be injected intravenously to influence the patient who is asked to imagine the object or situation which terrifies him (for instance, travelling on a train). Each time he feels fear, he is given a little more barbiturate sedation. After a series of such sessions, many patients are completely desensitized, or 'deconditioned'. They can then approach the object or situation which previously terrified them without showing, or feeling fear.

DETERGENTS are chemicals which lower the surface tension of various substances, such as greasy dirt, allowing the dirt to be broken up into small particles which can be readily washed away. In the same way, however detergents can remove the natural oils from the skin and cause dry, chapped hands. Because detergents are chemicals, a small number of women develop violent allergies to them. These reactions can be quite severe, and anyone who develops a rash after using a particular detergent should discontinue its use immediately.

DEVELOPMENT IN CHILDREN can be assessed from certain 'targets', or 'milestones'. These are achievements which a child may be expected to reach at a given age based on surveys of those reached by other children of that age.

The following are usually considered to be among the significant 'milestones'. Babies normally begin to smile when they are about two months old. At about six months, they usually cut the first tooth (which is very often one of the lower incisors, or front teeth). Some normal babies however, do not teethe until several months later, while a small number of children are actually born with teeth.

At about eight months, the baby can usually remain in a sitting position unaided, though, initially, he will often topple over. By about nine months, he is usually crawling; and not long after this, he may drag himself into a standing position by using the bars of his play pen. At the age of

94

one year, he will probably be standing unsupported and may be walking. Many children do not walk until about eighteen months, but a paediatrician should be consulted if walking is delayed any further. Talking is extremely variable in onset, and no set age can be given for it. Many extremely intelligent children do not talk to any extent until they are well past their second birthday. By the age of two he may be dry during the day.

Children vary greatly in their rates of development. There is, for instance, considerable variation between races: coloured babies often walk very much earlier than white ones. Because many children are 'slow developers', it is essential that mothers should not be overly concerned if their child seems to be a little behind in some respect — in a few months' time, he will probably prove to be ahead in some other field. The 'milestones' of development are at the best only rough guides to a child's future progress.

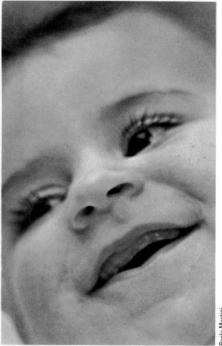

Paola Martini

This happy 7-month-old, with eight teeth through, is ahead of the average.

DEXEDRINE, a member of the amphetamine group, (see **amphetamines**), is a drug which stimulates the central nervous system. It was once used as an appetite-suppressant in the treatment of obesity (though as such it was of doubtful value); in cases of depression (see **depression**), it was used to produce elevation of mood. However, the risk of addiction to the drug is so great that it is now rarely prescribed.

DEXTRAN is a chemical substance composed of carbon, hydrogen and oxygen which may be infused into a vein in place of blood, for instance, in an emergency if blood is not available. It is, however, only a temporary substitute in cases where there has been relatively minor blood loss and can not be used in place of transfusion.

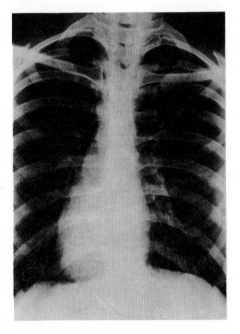

An X-ray photograph reveals dextrocardia, a 'wrong-sided' heart.

DEXTROCARDIA is a condition in which the heart is located on the right side of the chest cavity instead of the left. Although it is uncommon, the exact incidence is unknown, as some people may have the condition without being aware of it. In these cases, dextrocardia is not likely to involve any other abnormality. Other cases, however, may be associated with gross structural abnormalities of the heart and blood vessels.

When the heart is on the 'wrong' side, other organs, for instance, the liver and spleen, may be reversed as well, so that the internal arrangements are a 'mirror image' of what is normal.

DEXTROSE is a form of glucose (see **glucose**).

DIAPERS (see **nappies**).

DHOBIE'S ITCH is an irritation of the crutch area. It is usually caused by infection from a fungus, similar to that which causes athlete's foot (see **athlete's foot**). The condition is common in hot countries. It is made worse by the excessive sweating which tends to occur with non-natives and the subsequent urge to scratch the affected area. Antifungal ointment and careful hygiene will usually clear up this troublesome condition quite rapidly.

DIABETES INSIPIDUS, a relatively rare disease, is a disorder of the pituitary gland, a gland which grows out of the base of the brain (see **pituitary**).

ADH (anti-diuretic hormone), one of the hormones produced by this gland, normally prevents the kidneys from producing too much urine. If, however, the posterior part of the pituitary gland or the nerve connections supplying it are diseased, there may be reduced production of ADH and, consequently, an increased flow of urine, often as much as twenty pints a day. Treatment consists in administration of an extract of pituitary glands obtained from animals. This is administered by injection or nasal insufflation.

Diabetes insipidus is in no way related to the more common **diabetes mellitus**, which is the condition invariably meant by the term 'diabetes'. One of the few things the two disorders have in common is the passing of a large quantity of urine.

DIABETES MELLITUS, which is usually known simply as 'diabetes', is a disorder

95

in which the level of sugar in the blood tends to be higher than it should be.

Sugars and starches are broken down through the process of digestion into a simple sugar called glucose, the energy-giving fuel of the body. In order to 'burn' this fuel, the body requires insulin. This chemical is secreted into the bloodstream by the pancreas, a gland which lies in the upper part of the abdomen. In diabetes mellitus, the amount of insulin produced is insufficient to burn up the glucose. Characteristically, the urine which is then passed has a high sugar content.

Although the forms which diabetes may take vary considerably, particularly between the races, there are two main varieties. In the first type, the patient is usually under the age of 45 when the disease appears, and he may be slightly overweight. The onset is relatively sudden, often within the course of a few days. The patient begins to lose weight rapidly and feels generally unwell. He becomes very thirsty and passes large quantities of urine. Diagnosis can usually be made readily by testing the urine for sugar. If the diabetic does not seek treatment immediately, he may, within one or two days, pass into diabetic coma (see **diabetic coma**) which can prove fatal.

Under treatment, this type of patient usually requires daily injections of insulin for the rest of his life. This is combined with a strict diet — one which contains no sugar and certain, limited quantities of starchy foods, like bread and potatoes. However, if the prescribed amount of these carbohydrates is not received, his blood sugar will be so lowered by the insulin injection that he will suddenly become confused, and then unconscious. These 'insulin reactions', or hypoglycaemic attacks, are extremely common, in fact much more common than diabetic coma (in which the blood sugar is too high, rather than too low). In the event of hypoglycaemic attack, a patient who is still in the confused stage should be given oral doses of sugar; if he is unconscious, he should be taken to hospital immediately, where he will be given glucose into a vein.

The other main group of diabetics do not, as a rule, require insulin injections.

The patient is usually over 40 to 45 years old at the onset of the disease, which is much more gradual. Frequently, he is very overweight. Strict dieting is again necessary, often combined with tablets which lower the blood sugar. There is usually little risk of diabetic coma. The patient's health will, in general, be greatly benefited by a reduction in weight to the ideal figure indicated in life insurance companies' tables. It has been statistically shown that such weight loss will lengthen the patient's life.

Diabetes frequently affects different members of a family. Those who have diabetic relatives are well-advised to keep their weight down and have their urine checked occasionally for sugar.

For several hundred years diabetes has been a recognized condition and known to be associated with the passing of large quantities of sugary urine. Experiments in the late 1800s showed that this symptom was produced in animals from which the pancreas had been surgically removed. It was, however, not until 1921 that Frederick Banting and Charles Best, working in Canada, managed to extract insulin from the pancreatic glands of animals and demonstrated that it had a life saving effect on diabetic sufferers.

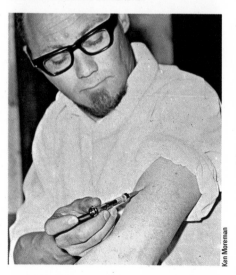

Ken Moreman

Insulin injections may be necessary for those suffering from diabetes mellitus.

DIABETIC COMA is a condition of unconsciousness which may occur in diabetes mellitus (see **diabetes mellitus**). It is associated with a very high level of sugar in the blood. It may occur in patients who have recently developed diabetes or in diabetics who have been taking no insulin or insufficient insulin for a period of several days. In this latter case, the diabetic may be suffering from some other illness, such as 'flu'. Not realizing that diabetics usually need *more* insulin when they have intercurrent infections, the patient may mistakenly cut down on his insulin.

Diabetic coma develops over a period of one or two days and is initially characterized by thirst and the passing of large quantities of urine. The patient vomits with increasing frequency; eventually he becomes drowsy and lapses into coma. A distinct smell of acetone is discernible on the breath. Immediate hospitalization is necessary. In hospital, the patient is given large quantities of intravenous fluids to combat the severe dehydration, and insulin, to reduce his blood sugar.

Diabetic coma is far less common than hypoglycaemic coma, or insulin reaction, which results when the blood sugar is too low (as opposed to too high). The onset of this condition is sudden, and follows a short period of mental confusion. In a reaction, the patient has invariably taken his last dose of insulin earlier in the day, whereas, in diabetic coma, he may have omitted it or reduced the dose.

All diabetics should test their urine daily for sugar, and keep a record of the result. A high sugar content in the urine normally precedes diabetic coma, whereas the urine is usually relatively free of sugar before an insulin reaction.

DIABINESE, or chlorpropamide, is a drug used in the treatment of diabetes (see **diabetes mellitus**) and has a valuable effect in lowering blood sugar. It is often administered to an older patient suffering from mild diabetes. Its use must be combined with the strict dietary rationing of starchy foods.

DIAGNOSIS is the process of determining the nature of an illness. The principal aid to diagnosis is usually the history given by the patient. Secondary to this are the findings of the doctor's examination which consists of inspection, palpation (feeling), percussion (tapping) and auscultation (listening), and possibly other methods.

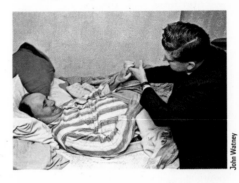

John Watney

A doctor diagnoses disease by careful questioning of a patient and thorough examination.

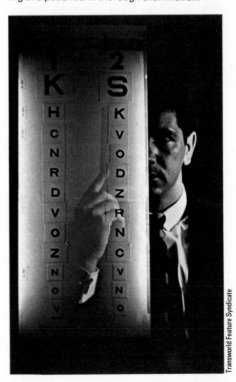

Transworld Feature Syndicate

Diagnosis of the future. Here the results of an eye test are recorded for a computer.

DIALYSIS refers to the process of 'purifying' a person's blood of poisons by means of an artificial kidney (see **kidney, artificial**).

DIANABOL is a chemical compound of the group known as 'anabolic steroids' (see **steroids**), which encourage the formation of muscle in the body. Dianabol has gained particular fame because of its use among athletes, as the taking of the drug increases muscle bulk and often enables the individual to gain three or four stones in weight. There is a corresponding increase in his performance. It is, however, possible that the side effects of these drugs may be highly dangerous.

DIAPHRAGM refers to any dividing membrane. In medicine, it has two distinct meanings.

The *muscular diaphragm* is the membrane which divides the contents of the chest from those of the abdomen. Through its three main apertures pass the gullet (which enters the stomach immediately below the level of the diaphragm), the aorta (the largest artery of the body, which carries blood away from the heart), and the inferior vena cava (the main vein which brings blood back from the lower part of the body to the heart).

It is possible for some of the contents of the abdomen to herniate, or bulge, through the apertures in the diaphragm. The stomach, in particular, may protrude through the hole which is traversed by the gullet. This common condition is called *hiatus hernia*.

The word diaphragm is also used to mean an *intravaginal contraceptive device* (see **contraception**).

DIARRHOEA means looseness of the bowels. In young babies, the condition may occur if the milk is too sweet — in such cases reducing the sugar content will help greatly. Some babies pass diarrhoeal stools shortly after being put to the breast — this is a natural reflex emptying of the bowel in response to feeding. The one dangerous cause of diarrhoea in babies is infectious gastro-enteritis. This may be caused by bacteria (see **bacteria**) or
98

viruses (see **virus**) and, in either case, the real danger is dehydration. Because infants have such minute reserves of fluid, a severe attack of diarrhoea and vomiting can have fatal consequences. Severe dehydration must be rapidly treated with replacement of fluid lost — usually by an intravenous drip (see **dehydration**).

For mild cases of infective diarrhoea in infants, it is often recommended that feeding be suspended for 24 to 48 hours, and fluid be replaced by mouth with boiled water containing a little salt and sugar.

In both children and adults, the common cause of diarrhoea is infection, particularly when people are living together under cramped and insanitary conditions. Clearly, the best defence against this is strict hygiene — careful washing of hands before eating or preparing food and, especially, after visiting the toilet. Dietary indiscretion may also give rise to diarrhoea.

Diarrhoea in adults can, of course, be caused by a variety of other bowel conditions. Any sudden change in bowel habit (either diarrhoea or constipation) which occurs for no apparent reason in a person over the age of 35 to 40 should be immediately investigated by a specialist.

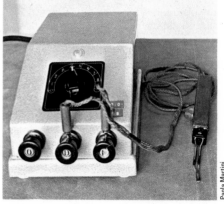

Paola Martini

Diathermy apparatus, much used during operations, to cut through tissues without bleeding.

DIATHERMY is the therapeutic use of heat. It is applied to two forms of therapy: short-wave diathermy, or heat treatment, which is used in painful conditions of muscles and joints, and the process of cauterization by heat. In the latter procedure, a hot electrode is used to burn away unwanted tissue, much as a scalpel would be used. Because the diathermy electrode coagulates blood which passes through the tissue being cut, it has the advantage of reducing haemorrhage.

DIET is the food regularly consumed in the course of normal living.

There are three types of energy-giving food: the carbohydrates, the proteins, and the fats. The carbohydrates (see **carbohydrate**), the sugars and starches, are contained in such foods as bread, potatoes, cakes, biscuits, milk and rice. At the present time it is generally felt that the overconsumption of carbohydrates is related to obesity. It has also been suggested that a high sugar content in the diet may increase an individual's liability to 'coronaries'.

Proteins, which are contained in lean meat and fish, cheese, milk, eggs, peas and beans, are the vital building blocks of the body and are essential for growth and development, particularly in children.

Fats are an important source of body fuel, but it has been suspected for some years that animal fats (as opposed to vegetable fats) may be related to the development of diseases of the heart and blood vessels.

Vitamins (see **vitamins**), the complex chemical substances which exist in most foods, are essential to a balanced diet. But any adult who eats vegetables and fruit is in no danger of vitamin deficiency and should not require the use of vitamin pills. In Western countries, vitamin deficiencies are almost entirely confined to infants, all of whom need vitamin supplements in some form, and impoverished elderly people who live on meagre rations and never eat vegetables nor vary their diet in any way.

Minerals like iron and calcium are essential in the diet. Calcium is particularly important for expectant and nursing mothers and growing children; if sufficient amounts of milk are consumed, calcium deficiency is not likely to occur. Iron-rich foods include the lean portions of all meats, spinach, and red wine. A lack of iron commonly leads to iron-deficiency

anaemia (see **anaemia**), especially in women.

Given a completely free choice, most people (including young children) will select a diet which is nutritionally balanced. However, because of economic reasons, not everyone has a completely free choice; and, in most countries of the world, people

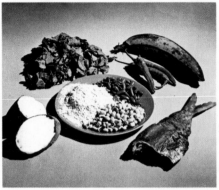

Contrasting diets. *Above,* average daily diet of a Ghanaian child aged 5. Carbohydrates predominate. *Below,* diet of a British child contains a greater proportion of proteins.

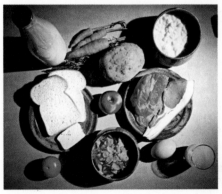

tend to consume cheap starchy and sugary foods.

Within the last thirty or forty years, there has been a significant tendency in the Western world to over-eat. There is evidence that this overindulgence, coupled with the increasingly sedentary nature of Western life, has been responsible for the marked rise in deaths from disorders of the heart. Regular exercise, and a careful

99

watch on diet and weight, can do much to avert damage to the heart and prevent coronary damage.

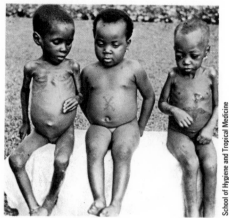

Left, a Kwashiorkor victim; *Centre*, a normal child; *Right*, sufferer from protein deficiency.

DIETING means adhering to a particular pattern of eating; in common speech, it usually refers to restricting eating with a view to losing weight. To be effective, a slimming diet generally must make the dieter feel hungry. After a week or so, the 'appestats' the body's hunger control centres, become readjusted, and hunger diminishes considerably. Trick diets and fad diets which promise a major weight loss without the feeling of hunger are not effective. In order to reduce, the daily intake of food must be decreased and *kept* decreased until the desired weight is actually lost.

Most doctors agree that the main types of food to be cut down or eliminated from the slimmer's diet are the carbohydrates (see **diet**). This includes all sugar, bread, potatoes, milk and other starchy and sugary foods. It is unnecessary and undesirable to reduce the intake of green vegetables, but all other foods should be eaten only in moderation.

For many years, people have tried to lose weight by taking 'slimming pills', and often these preparations have consisted of nothing more than chalk. In the period after the Second World War, many doctors prescribed drugs of the amphetamine group (see **amphetamines**) for overweight patients, as these were believed to reduce the desire for food. Such pills were not only completely ineffective, but frequently addictive. Young people who received the drugs in illicit ways often progressed to heroin or cocaine. As a result most doctors do not prescribe them.

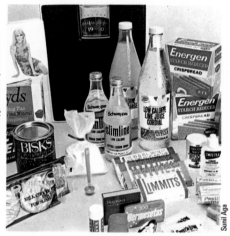

Numerous aids to slimming are available, with low carbohydrate content, yet still palatable.

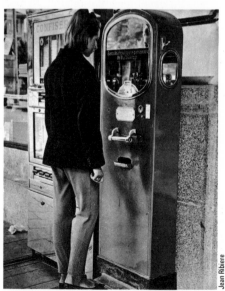

A regular check on one's weight enables dietary adjustment to maintain good health.

DIETITIANS are those specially trained in the science of dietetics, or nutrition. The dietitian is an expert on the chemical content of food, the constituents of a balanced diet and on the type of diet required for various types of illness. The attractive preparation of food for invalids is part of the training process. Normally, dietitians advise on the type of food which should be served in hospitals, schools, and other places where people eat.

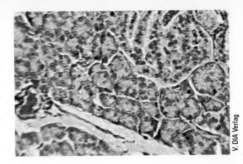

The pancreas secretes an enzyme-rich juice which is essential to digestion.

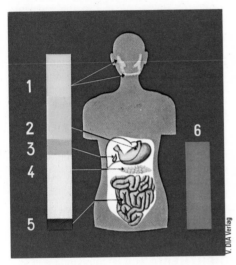

This key shows the digestive juice produced in 24 hours: 1 saliva, 2 stomach juice, 3 bile, 4 pancreatic juice, 5 intestinal juice. 6 is total blood volume.

DIGESTION is the process of breaking down food from its natural state into relatively simple chemicals so that it can be absorbed from the intestine into the bloodstream.

The cooking of food may be said to be a part of the digestive process, as it often alters the food's chemical nature. Raw meat, for example, would be largely indigestible to civilized man.

In the mouth, starchy foods, such as bread or potatoes, are mixed with an enzyme (see **enzyme**) called *ptyalin*, contained in the saliva. Pytalin reduces the starches to sugars, which are simpler chemical substances.

In the stomach, hydrochloric acid and the enzymes pepsin and renin carry on the process of digestion. The chemical action is facilitated by the movement of the stomach, which churns the mixture thoroughly.

When the food is ready to leave the stomach (which may be after about five minutes or as long as several hours, depending on the particular content of the food and the amount of fluid taken with it), it has been reduced to a freely flowing pulp known as *chyme*. At this time, however, no absorption has taken place. The only substance which can be directly absorbed from the stomach into the bloodstream is alcohol, which accounts for the rapidity of its effects.

From the stomach, the chyme enters the duodenum, the short C-shaped tube which forms the beginning of the small intestine. Into the duodenum lead the common bile duct, which carries *bile,* and the pancreatic duct, which carries *pancreatic juice.*

Bile is a golden yellow liquid which gives the intestinal contents their characteristic colour. By emulsifying the fats in foods, bile breaks down the large fat globules into smaller, uniformly distributed particles.

The juice from the pancreas contains several enzymes, including *lipase* (which splits fats), *amylase* (which splits carbohydrates), and *trypsin* (which splits proteins).

As a result of this chemical activity, all the large and complex molecules of chyme have been rendered into simple forms by the time it passes into the main part of the small intestine. The fats have been transformed into readily-absorbable chemicals, such as fatty acids; the proteins have been broken down into basic building blocks called amino-acids; and the carbohydrates have become simple sugars, such as glucose.

The simple chemicals which have been produced by the process of digestion are then absorbed through the wall of the small intestine into the blood.

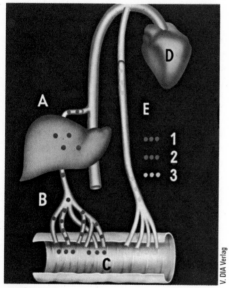

Carbohydrates and proteins, 2, 3, are absorbed in the intestine, C, and carried to the liver, A, by the portal vein, B. Fats diffuse into the lymph, E, and are emptied into the blood near the heart, D.

DIGITALIS is a valuable drug used in the treatment of heart failure. It is extracted from the leaves of the foxglove. The properties of this plant first became known to medicine in the late 1700s as a remedy for dropsy. It was later discovered that the drug exercised its effect by the help it gave to the failing heart. Digitalis has now been very largely replaced in medicine by the closely related compound digoxin (see **digoxin**).

DIGOXIN is a drug used in cases of heart failure. It slows the pulse, improves the
102

efficiency of the heart's contraction, and thus increases the flow of urine. It thereby rids the body of the excess fluid characteristic of heart failure.

Like digitalis, to which it is chemically related, digoxin is a dangerous drug which must be used with great care. Overdoses are very common, especially among old people. The principal symptoms of toxicity include loss of appetite, nausea, vomiting, a very slow pulse (or, sometimes, an extremely rapid one), and blurring of vision. Characteristically, in this blurring, the patient may see everything through a green haze.

DINDEVAN is an anticoagulant drug, that is, one which prevents the clotting of blood. It is often used in cases of coronary occlusion (or 'coronary thrombosis') to try to prevent the formation of clots in the arteries which supply the heart, or in the veins of the legs. Clots in either of these sites can, under certain circumstances, prove fatal. In the heart, clots may lead to the occlusion of the vital blood supply to the cardiac muscle; clots from the leg veins may circulate through the bloodstream and lodge in the lungs (see **pulmonary embolism**).

DIPHTHERIA is a highly dangerous infectious disease caused by a bacterium called *Corynebacterium diphtheriae*. The commonest site of infection is the back of the throat, where a pearly grey membrane appears. The victim, ordinarily a child, becomes ill within a few days. The usual symptoms are fever, loss of appetite, and, sometimes, difficulty in breathing. The latter indicates that the pearly membrane is blocking the air passages. In such cases, it may be necessary to perform an emergency tracheotomy, that is, to make an opening in the windpipe to prevent the patient's choking to death.

Before the Second World War, diphtheria was a common cause of death in babies, but, in countries where inoculation is given, it has become exceedingly rare. Even with modern treatment, however, the disease is often fatal. The 'Shick Test' has been devised to test an individual's susceptibility to diphtheria.

DIPSOMANIA is the old term for chronic alcoholism. This disorder is extremely common, and there is some evidence that it is becoming more prevalent. In three-quarters of all cases, the patient is already a heavy drinker before the age of twenty-five. Five, ten, or even fifteen years may pass, during which he is able to drink increasing amounts of alcohol without apparent serious ill effects. At this time, the dipsomaniac is completely dependent on alcohol and cannot refrain from it. His career and marriage may be wrecked, and he may become a total dissolute. Admission to mental hospitals, interspersed with nights in jail, and periods of sleeping in any available place, usually in the company of other alcoholics are the prelude to eventual death from general neglect and malnutrition or from alcoholic damage to the liver.

However, certainly not all alcoholics follow this pattern. Success in coping with the disorder depends in part on early recognition of the symptoms by the patient or his family. When a man starts drinking heavily in order to blur the edges of unpleasant reality, and, in particular, when he needs to drink in the mornings, even though he does not become drunk, it is time for help. It is probable that the disastrous complications of alcoholism could be substantially reduced if the family doctor were consulted by a member of the victim's family, and informed of the problem. Psychiatric help should be arranged as soon as possible, as there are invariably severe mental problems underlying chronic alcoholism. The Alcoholics Anonymous organization cannot be too highly recommended. Its method of frank, open discussion between alcoholics at regular meetings is remarkably effective. The mere fact of knowing that there are others who have gone through the same backslidings and social disasters is a considerable help to the alcoholic. Even more encouraging to him is the realization that many of the men and women he meets have managed, by sheer power of will to pick themselves up and save their family and their career.

Of course, the alcoholic who wants to help himself (and many do not) must give up alcohol completely. Even the smallest drink is almost certain to start off a wild bout of uncontrollable drinking.

There are several methods of treatment which help the victim to resist temptation. An alcoholic receiving hospital care may be given daily doses of a drug called *antabuse*. He is then given alcohol to drink. The combination of the two within the body produces an appalling physical reaction. If, after leaving hospital, antabuse is taken regularly, the alcoholic will have an additional reason to avoid drinking since he realizes the effect it will produce.

Other methods of therapy include *aversion*. In this procedure, the patient is usually taken to a treatment room which resembles a bar. Bottles are on the shelves and drinks are freely available to him, but, each time he drinks, he is given an injection of a drug called *apomorphine*, which makes him violently sick. The object of this treatment is to establish a conditioned reflex whereby the patient is revolted by bars, bottles of alcohol, and, indeed, everything to do with drinking.

DISEASE is a disordered condition of the body which is recognizable as a specific entity. Literally tens of thousands of different types of diseases have been described, some of which are very common, and others which have occurred in only two or three people. There are various ways of classifying disease. One convenient method is to consider them as **congenital** and **acquired**. Congenital diseases are those which are present from birth. Acquired diseases may originate from infection, inflammation, or injury, or may be associated with some degenerative or ageing process or with benign or malignant growths.

This classification may be applied to any organ. The various diseases which may affect the brain, for example, can be divided in this way. Brain diseases, then, may be congenital (as in certain cases of familial idiocy), or, if they are acquired, they may be infectious (for instance, meningitis), or related to trauma (as in cases of severe head injury), or degenerative (as in hardening of the arteries leading to the brain), or associated with growths (such as cerebral tumours).

DISINFECTANTS are chemicals which kill micro-organisms. They are widely used on such objects as bedclothes, drains, and lavatories, where bacteria are likely to grow and spread.

DISLOCATIONS are displacements of bones from their correct position in a joint. There is generally considerable pain, and this may be increased if the bone presses on a nerve. Common dislocations are those of the shoulder, the elbow, and the fingers. Correction of dislocations should not be attempted by any but medically qualified persons. There is a definite risk of nipping nerves and blood vessels, and harm may be done to the bones themselves. Dislocations should always be dealt with by a doctor, preferably in hospital, where X-ray facilities are available.

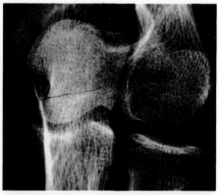

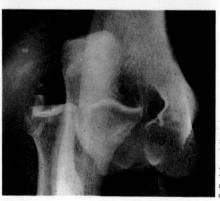

A fall down stairs can have shattering effects. Above, a normal elbow joint. Below, a fractured and dislocated one.

St. Bartholomew's Hospital

104

DISSEMINATED SCLEROSIS (D.S., multiple sclerosis, or M.S.) is one of the most common chronic disorders of the nervous system. It is characterized by symptoms such as transient numbness or weakness of a limb, or temporary interference with vision which occur at intervals over a period of years. The cause of the disease is not known.

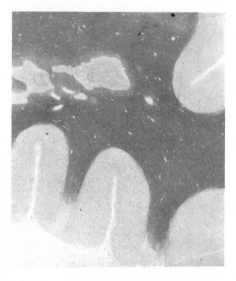

In DS, the sheaths insulating the brain's nerve-fibres (in blue) are destroyed (shown in white).

DIURETICS are drugs which increase the flow of urine, and thus rid the body of excess salt and fluid. The latter is characteristic of such disorders as heart failure and cirrhosis. Commonly used diuretics include the **thiazides** (which are taken in tablet form, usually each morning), **frusemide** and **ethacrynic acid** (two fast-acting drugs introduced in the early 1960s). All these drugs must be taken under careful supervision, because they have potentially dangerous side-effects, such as a tendency to deplete the body's vital stores of potassium and so cause progressive muscle weakness and heart damage. Many diuretics are, therefore, given with potassium supplements or together with one of the two diuretics which cause retention of potassium, **spironolactone** (an aldosterone antagonist – see **aldosterone**) and **triamterene.**

DIVERTICULAR DISEASE is a common condition affecting the large intestine, in which little pouches, or **diverticula,** bulge out from the intestinal wall. Although these can occur at almost any site in the small and large intestines, the vast majority develop in the large bowel just above the rectum. It is likely that between five and ten per cent of all people over the age of forty have diverticula at this site.

It seems that the recurring major changes of pressure which occur inside the large tube forming the colon gradually cause the inner lining of the bowel to bulge through the muscular wall. In many people, so many diverticula are formed in this way that the last part of the colon resembles a bunch of grapes.

When diverticula are present without the symptoms of pain in the abdomen, diarrhoea, blood in the motions, and sometimes obstruction of the bowels, the condition is referred to as **diverticulosis.** When the tiny sacs become inflamed, however, and the symptoms do develop as a result, the condition is then described as **diverticulitis.**

Diverticulitis is usually treated with antibiotics, bed-rest, and a special diet. However, the infection can proceed to the extent that a large abscess is formed which may completely obstruct the bowel. In such cases it may be necessary to perform a temporary colostomy (see **colostomy**) to relieve the obstruction.

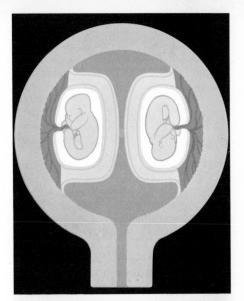

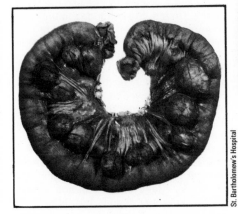

Diverticula are revealed on the jejunum, or upper part, of the small intestine.

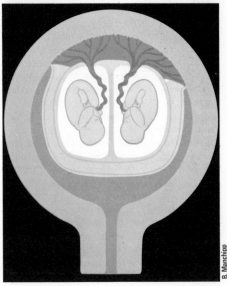

Dizygotic twins, *above*, come from two separate ova. Fertilized and nourished individually in the womb, they can be of mixed sexes. Contrast them with monozygotic, or 'identical', twins, *below*, which share one placenta and develop from one ovum which divides into two.

DIZYGOTIC TWINS, or binovular twins, are twins produced from two separate eggs. Two eggs instead of one are released

105

by the mother during ovulation, and each is fertilized by a different sperm. Each foetus is nourished in the womb by separate placentae. As dizygotic twins have a different genetic inheritance, they bear exactly the same relationship to each other as do ordinary brothers and sisters (hence their description as 'fraternal'); they may be of different sexes and unlike in every way. (See **monozygotic twins**.)

DIZZINESS is a feeling of unsteadiness or 'giddiness'. The term is used to describe two different conditions: feelings of faintness and being about to fall, and (much less commonly) feelings of true vertigo, in which the sufferer feels the room spinning round him.

In the first type, there is no sensation of spinning. The giddiness may result from many causes, the most common being what is called *postural hypotension*. This occurs in perfectly healthy people: they get out of bed quickly or stand up suddenly from a chair and, about six or seven seconds later, they suddenly feel weak, 'light-headed', and faint. Occasionally they may even pass out. The feeling lasts only a short time and is immediately relieved by sitting or lying down. The giddiness is caused by the sudden movement which disturbs the relaxed state of the body's blood vessels: the blood literally drains away from the head for a few seconds, depriving the brain of oxygen. Other causes of giddiness include various debilitating illnesses, and any disorder which affects the blood vessels leading to the brain — for instance, the common degenerative changes which affect the cerebral arteries of older people.

True vertigo is less common. It usually indicates some disturbance of the balance mechanisms inside the skull, and it may be accompanied by noises in the ears and vomiting. Among the possible causes are diseases of the cerebellum (see **cerebellum**), the part of the brain which is connected with the inner ear and controls balance, Menière's disease and acute labyrinthitis, both of which are disorders of the inner ear, and any disorder affecting the nerve which connects the ear to the brain. (See **ear**.)

106

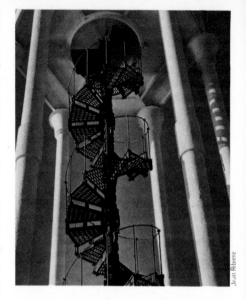

Jean Ribiere

Unaccustomed heights, here accentuated by the 'whirling' staircase, can cause an unpleasant sense of dizziness.

DOCTOR is a term applied to a medical practitioner. Strictly speaking, it is only a courtesy title, since only someone with a doctorate degree (such as a Ph.D) can officially be called doctor. By tradition, doctorates are only awarded to those who submit a learned thesis to an academic board. However, the term has now been extended by long usage to include those who have a licence to practise medicine. In the United States and a number of countries in which the influence of U.S. medicine is strong, the degree of M.D. (Doctor of Medicine) is given on qualifying; and, indeed, dentists and veterinary surgeons are addressed as 'doctor'. In the British Commonwealth, however, with the exception of Canada, the M.D. is still quite a rare and coveted award, given not on qualification but on submission and acceptance of a doctoral thesis.

The degree given by Commonwealth medical schools is the M.B. (Bachelor of Medicine). Many doctors do not, in fact, take a university degree, but, after completion of training, receive a diploma issued by such bodies as the Royal College of Physicians or the Society of Apothecaries.

DOG BITES, fortunately, are usually superficial, but any dog of moderate size can inflict fatal wounds – particularly on babies and children. No small child should ever be left completely alone with a large dog, especially if the animal has been out of sorts or the weather is hot. An irritable animal can easily be frightened, by a child's sudden movement, into a violent reaction – and, once he has tasted blood, may not stop until it is too late.

In countries where there is no rabies (see **rabies**), minor lacerations from dog bites require only careful cleaning, with a mild disinfectant, and a simple dressing. As with any cut in the skin (especially dirty ones), it is worth while ensuring that protection against tetanus is up to date.

In many countries, however, rabies (often known as *hydrophobia*) is endemic. Animals which are apparently in perfect health can infect human beings, and the results may be fatal.

Except in a small number of countries, Britain and Scandanavia for example, which have instituted strict quarantining of imported dogs, it is essential, after a dog bite, to take medical advice as to whether anti-rabies inoculation is necessary, as, once the manifestations of the disease appear, death is inevitable.

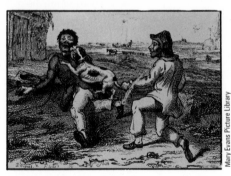

Before quarantine regulations were enforced any bite could cause rabies.

DONOR (see **blood donation**).

DORSAL means pertaining to the back. The **dorsal vertebrae** are the twelve bones of the spinal column between the neck and the loins.

DOSAGE is the amount of a particular drug taken by a patient. It is extremely important to keep to the correct dosage of any preparation whether prescribed by a doctor or bought over the counter; this applies even more forcibly to medicines given to children. As a general rule, there is an optimum dose of a drug; exceeding it will bring no benefit, and, in many instances, may be highly dangerous. Similarly, taking *less* than the prescribed dosage of a drug is also unwise, since it may have no effect at all on the illness; taking less than the prescribed dose of certain antibiotics may be highly dangerous. Similar considerations, of course, apply to the habit of discontinuing a drug before the prescribed course is complete.

All doses should be measured accurately. Doctors now usually prescribe in exact units, such as millilitres (m.l.), instead of teaspoons or dessertspoons. In Britain, all medicines which require it are now dispensed together with a 5 m.l. spoon.

Adults should never be tempted to give children adult medicines and attempt to work out the correct child's dosage for themselves. Although some books give formulas for working out children's dosage, this is a highly risky business; the formulas simply do not apply to all medicines. When treating children, use extreme care, and, if in doubt, consult your doctor.

DOUBLE VISION *(diplopia)* consists of seeing two images of an object at the same time. It may result from disease of the eyeball or failure of the eyeball's muscles. Injury to an eyeball or a blow on the head can both cause double vision.

DOUCHES are applications of water, or any other fluid, to the body. Usually, the word implies a stream of fluid intended to flush out a cavity. Nowadays, the term tends to be most used in connection with vaginal douches. These are still quite often employed in certain gynaecological disorders. Usually, the doctor prescribes a particular fluid, which is poured into a large douche can, attached to a rubber tube. The can is then raised above the level of the body, so that the fluid flows into the vagina. It then runs into a bidet or bedpan.

Mary Evans Picture Library

DRAIN means to draw fluid or pus from an abnormal accumulation in a body cavity or wound (see **dropsy**). A drain tube may be used to empty the bladder when the patient lacks control of his bladder after an injury to his spine.

DRAMAMINE *(dimenhydrinate)* is a useful anti-emetic — that is, a drug used against nausea and vomiting. It is often employed to ward off travel sickness. Those who take it for this purpose should remember that all drugs of this group have a marked sedative effect. Drivers should use such drugs cautiously; the prescribed dose should never be exceeded and, most important of all, alcohol should not be taken with them.

DRAW SHEET is a roll of muslin or small sheet used to provide an unsoiled bed for an incontinent patient. It can be changed quickly and prevents the patient lying in his own excrement.

DREAMS are images passing through the mind during sleep. In sleep, brain waves have a pattern quite different from those of wakefulness. For about an hour the waves are big and slow and the eyeballs remain motionless. Then there is a sudden change into a different kind of sleep with different kinds of brain waves. Most of the body's muscles go limp, and the brain becomes more active. The internal temperature of the brain rises, the blood flows through it faster, the heart beats with sudden quickenings, the eyeballs jerk rapidly. In the male, the penis may become erect.

It is at these times that if a sleeping man is wakened and asked if he has just been dreaming, he will nearly always answer 'Yes' and give a detailed account of a dream. These *'rapid eye movement'* or *'paradoxical'* periods of sleep recur every night. It is now realized that dreaming occurs at least five times nightly for a total of some two hours, and that it is broken up into periods of around 20 minutes each, separated by 60-90 minute intervals. Now research has made it plain that at probably no time during sleep is the mind totally blank.

Today most psychologists agree that dreams are symbolic — not prophetic, that they represent persons, places and things which are significant in the problems and emotional conflicts of waking life. Sigmund Freud (see **Freud**), the founder of psycho-analysis, thought that dreams could be symbols of unresolved conflicts in the individual mind, and tended to stress what he saw as strong sexual overtones. Freud's work on dreams was extremely important but it has since been challenged by many other researchers.

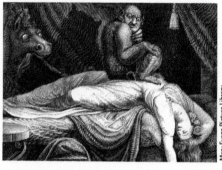

The problems of waking life are represented symbolically in dreams.

DRESSING is covering or protecting a wound or injury. For first-aid treatment a simple dressing of a clean cloth, held in place with a folded handkerchief, can be used. The person treating a wound must clean his own hands thoroughly before washing the skin around the wound and applying the dressing.

DRIP is the drop by drop injection of fluid into a vein, the rectum or (by a tube passed through the nose) the stomach. Glucose solution may be given as a nutrient; saline solution (salt and distilled water) replaces losses from dehydration.

DROPSY means an abnormal accumulation of fluid beneath the skin or in the cavities of the body (see **ascites** and **oedema**). It may result from heart disease, when the circulation is too sluggish to carry fluid away, or failure of the kidneys to remove waste products and excess water from the blood. The cause of dropsy must be found before it can be alleviated.

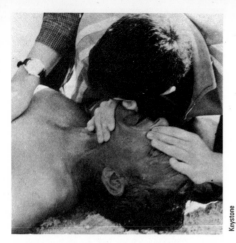

A victim of drowning is revived by artificial respiration, the 'kiss of life'.

DROWNING is death by inhalation of water into the air passages and lungs.

There are two different types of drowning — fresh water drowning and salt water drowning. In fresh water drowning, the victim inhales water into his lungs, and this is quickly absorbed into the bloodstream and destroys the red blood cells. These cells contain large quantities of potassium, which, when released into the bloodstream, stop the heart, and sudden death follows.

Drowning in sea water is a slightly slower process and holds a greater chance of survival. Salt water enters the lungs and, by the process of osmosis, draws large quantities of fluid out of the blood and into the lungs. In this situation, heart failure is more gradual.

In both types of drowning, death is likely to occur within about ten minutes of submergence. Where large quantities of water have been inhaled, the chance of survival is slim. However, the immediate application of artificial respiration may revive a victim even though he appears to be dead.

Life-saving. The head of the drowning person *must* be kept above the water. A simple method involves swimming on the back beside the drowning person and close against him. One arm holds his left elbow, and the other is thrown round his shoulders

so that his right elbow can be held.

First aid in drowning. It is absolutely essential to start resuscitation the moment the drowning person is dragged from the water. Lay the victim flat on his back. If he is on a sloping beach, ensure that his head is lower than his feet. Put a finger as far down his throat as possible and rapidly clear out any seaweed or sand. Then close off the victim's nose with your finger and thumb, place your mouth over his and inflate his chest with about 15 breaths per minute. (In the case of a child, the rescuer's mouth goes over both the nose and the mouth.) If there is another person present, get him to massage the heart by firm pressure on the lower end of the breastbone, about once every second. This has to be done very energetically and it is difficult to keep it up for more than five minutes at a time. The two rescuers should, therefore, change places every few minutes. It is absolutely essential to apply continuous artificial respiration until medical help arrives.

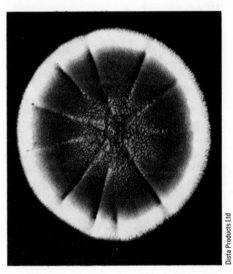

The antibiotic drug penicillin is derived from the mould *Penicillium chrysogenum*.

DRUGS are chemicals which have a specific effect on the metabolism of the human body. Any medicine, whether bought over the counter or prescribed by a doctor, is a drug.

109

The action of drugs on the body can be divided into two groups: *local* and *general* (or *systemic*).

When a drug is applied locally, or direct, to a tissue or organ, it usually affects only the immediate area and does not spread to the rest of the body. A drug of general or systemic action enters the blood stream by absorption from the intestines or lungs, or by direct injection. It affects organs or tissues which are not near the place of entry. Some drugs of this type are cumulative in their effect, because they are not immediately excreted from the system.

DRUG ADDICTION is a state of complete dependence on a drug. The word 'addiction' has slightly varying connotations. Some doctors use it in referring to the desire for tobacco felt by heavy smokers. Others use 'addiction' only when they feel that the patient's need for a specific drug is such that the body's cells require the drug in order to function.

The phrase 'drug addiction' usually means addiction to drugs of the heroin-morphine-opium group, to cocaine, to amphetamines (such as benzedrine), or to alcohol. The effects of drug addiction vary greatly, depending on the drug involved. However, addiction to all the above drugs will produce gross mental disturbance and, eventually, lead to severe physical illness as well.

The spread of drug addiction among teenagers is often caused by complete ignorance about the dangers of drug-taking — they often believe that addictive drugs can be taken a few times 'for kicks', and then stopped. Usually, the habit is impossible to break; even prolonged psychiatric treatment is often unsuccessful.

DUCTLESS GLANDS – see **endocrine glands.**

DUMBNESS – see **speech therapy.**

DUODENAL ULCER is an ulcer occurring in the duodenum, the first part of the small intestine. The mucous membrane of this structure breaks down. The main symptom of this condition is pain in the upper abdomen (see **peptic ulcers**).

110

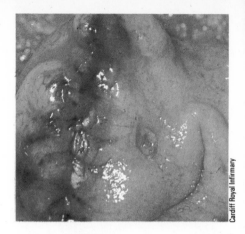

A duodenal ulcer, about half an inch across, is surrounded by swelling and redness.

DUODENUM is the first part of the small intestine. Food passes into it from the lower end of the stomach and is then passed into the rest of the small intestine. The duodenum is a vital section of the alimentary canal, because into it flow bile and pancreatic juice which play an important part in the process of digestion.

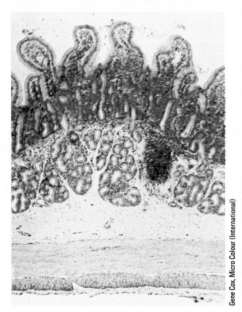

The duodenum, shown in section, is a C-shaped structure about 10 inches long.

DUOGASTRONE is a preparation used in the treatment of duodenal ulcers (see **duodenal ulcer**). It is supplied in the form of a special capsule designed to burst open as it leaves the stomach and enters the duodenum. Duogastrone contains carbonoxolone, a chemical derived from licorice, which is also valuable in the treatment of ulcers of the stomach (gastric ulcers). It has been shown to be the only substance which can help ulcers to heal.

DUPUYTREN'S CONTRACTURE is a common deformity of the fingers, usually of the ring, or the little finger, in which the digit becomes permanently flexed. The condition seems to be caused by a thickening of the tissues of the palm of the hand, thereby affecting the tendons which lead to the fingers. Early cases may be treated by regular, gentle stretching of the finger, but advanced ones require operation.

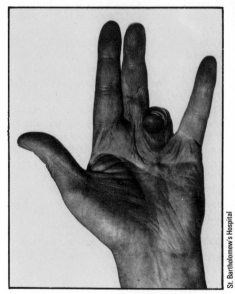

St. Bartholomew's Hospital

The ring finger, clearly affected by Dupuytren's contracture, may need an operation.

DURA MATER is the outermost and strongest of the three membranes covering the brain and spinal cord. The other two cerebral membranes are the arachnoid mater (the middle layer) and the pia mater (the innermost layer).

DUST is the fine debris which gathers on floors, in corners, in carpets, and, on all surfaces where it is allowed to settle. There are two reasons for its importance in medicine — firstly, because it may contain bacteria (which is why the floor of hospital wards are kept scrupulously clean), and secondly, because it induces attacks of

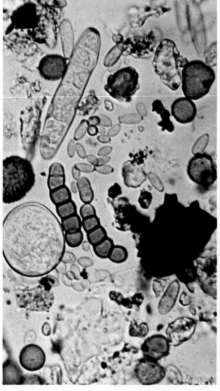

Allergy Dept. Wright Fleming Institute

Dust examined under the microscope shows a mass of microorganisms; some are potentially a risk to your health.

hay-fever and asthma in many people who suffer from allergies. As dust often contains microscopic organisms called mites, an allergic reaction may possibly result from the protein which is present in the bodies of such creatures.

DUTCH CAP, or diaphragm, is a commonly used type of intravaginal contraceptive device, so called because it was first developed in Holland (see **contraception**).

111

DWARFISM is the condition of under-development of the body. Its causes include hereditary disorders, malfunctions of the endrocrine glands (such as cretinism) deficiency diseases (such as rickets), kidney insufficiency, and diseases of the skeleton (such as achondroplasia). Because the incidence of some of the causative diseases has been substantially reduced by proper nutrition and others are rapidly treated, dwarfs are infrequently seen in Western countries.

Dwarfs do not necessarily suffer from any intellectual subnormality. This, however, depends on the specific cause of their condition (see **cretinism, rickets, achondroplasia**).

DYS – is a prefix meaning difficult or painful, such as dyslexia and dyspepsia.

DYSENTERY, which literally means 'difficulty with the bowels', applies to two distinct diseases, **amoebic dysentery** and **bacillary dysentery**.

Amoebic dysentery is an infection of the large bowel by a parasite known as *Entamoeba hystolytica*. This disease, which is widespread in many parts of the tropics, is characterized by diarrhoea and colicky pain in the abdomen. Like most infective bowel diseases, it is spread by faulty hygiene. An infected person may fail to wash his hands after using the toilet. If he then handles food, it may be contaminated by amoebic cysts from his fingers. Anyone who eats the food may later develop the characteristic pain, diarrhoea, and general ill-health. Resulting complications, particularly infection of the liver, may make the condition even more serious.

Bacillary dysentery is an infection of the bowel caused by a group of bacteria called *Shigella*. It is usually a much more acute illness than the amoebic type, with great abdominal pain, fever, and copious, bloody diarrhoea. Although it can occur almost anywhere in the world, it is considerably more common in the tropical countries. The infective organisms are passed out in the motions of diseased people and, if these motions contaminate drinking water or food, infection will spread and serious illness will develop

112

within a week. Careful observation, bed-rest, replacement of fluid loss, and the use

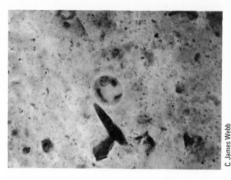

The cyst of the parasite which causes amoebic dysentery is usually found in faeces.

of antibiotics or sulphonamides are generally effective treatments. When victims are weak, starved, or suffering from other infections, however, the death rate may be high, particularly if the necessary medical care is not provided.

DYSLEXIA is difficulty in reading. This condition may be due to mental deficiency. However, many intelligent children suffer from 'word blindness', that is, a visual confusion in which, for instance, similarly shaped letters such as *o, e, c, a* and *p, b, h, d* are transposed. A word like 'god' might be seen 'dog'. Since the 1950s, the disorder has been recognized. With great care and patience, it is possible to teach many of these children (who would formerly have been labelled 'backward') to attain quite reasonable reading ability.

DYSPEPSIA is pain associated with digestion, and is more commonly known as 'indigestion'. Although it is a common affliction, the causes are not very well understood. Overeating, improper diet, and the taking of tablets which contain aspirin may sometimes provoke dyspepsia. Occasional mild dyspepsia can safely be treated with any of the bland antacid preparations available without prescription. Aspirin, or any of the many aspirin-containing pain killing tablets, should *not* be used for any pain in the abdomen. Dyspepsia can be a symptom of some other disorder.

EACA is epsilon-amino caproic acid, a relatively new drug used in the treatment of disorders of blood clotting.

ECG is the usual abbreviation for electrocardiogram, the recording instrument which enables doctors to study the electrical changes occurring in the heart. The ECG was invented by the scientist Eindthoven, who discovered that electrodes attached to the limbs and the chest picked up electrical impulses from the heart, and that it was possible to show on graph paper the passage through the heart muscle of the electrical impulses accompanying each heart beat.

Eindthoven found that in healthy people a wave of characteristic shape was produced on the moving graph paper. Increases in the height of the waves usually indicated an overdevelopment of one or other particular part of the heart wall. A widening of the waves indicated slowing of conduction inside the heart, while distorted or extra waves indicated the development of abnormal rhythms in the heart's action. Certain other typical changes from a normal pattern showed damage of heart muscle due to angina pectoris or 'coronary thrombosis'.

The electrocardiogram has probably contributed more to the study of the heart than any device since the stethoscope, and today ECG tracings greatly augment the cardiologist's diagnostic ability. Although his clinical skill in interpreting the signs and symptoms of the different types of heart disease remains the cardiologist's greatest asset, the ECG enables him to understand far more about the condition of the heart muscle, and quickly reach an accurate diagnosis. In combination with specialized X-rays, cardiac catheterization (see **catheterization**), and such sophisticated techniques as ballistocardiography, the ECG has enabled the diagnosis of almost all types of heart disease to be made with reasonable certainty.

ECHO is a name applied to a group of viruses (see **viruses**). Their full name is Enteric Cytopathogenic Human Orphan viruses. They commonly occur in the digestive tract, usually without producing any disorder there. However, if they spread to other parts of the body, such as the brain or spinal cord, they may produce very serious illnesses, for instance, meningitis, and encephalitis (see **meningitis**, and **encephalitis**), particularly among young children. These illnesses may occur in epidemics.

As with most germs which are basically bowel-dwellers, ECHO viruses are passed on by the 'faecal-oral route' — that is to say, lack of elementary hygienic precautions, such as washing the hands after visiting the toilet, eventually leads to the viruses reaching someone else's mouth and infecting them.

ECT is the abbreviation for electro-convulsive therapy, a form of psychiatric treatment used with remarkable success in certain depressive illnesses (see **depression**). Its value is all the more remarkable in that no-one knows how it works — its original introduction into medicine was based on a belief since shown to be false.

The word 'convulsive' is probably responsible for the many horror stories which circulate about the use of ECT. It is not painful, and certainly not a form of torture (as ill-informed persons · have claimed). Often the depressed patient, who is frequently seen on an out-patient basis these days, attends hospital one afternoon a week for treatment. To allay nervousness he is given a 'pre-med' injection, and sits in a waiting room for half an hour or so. He is then asked to lie on a couch, and given a general anaesthetic (normally by means of a simple injection in the arm) which renders him completely unconscious. At the same time, he is given a relaxant drug, which reduces muscle movements and reduces the risk of him injuring himself.

Once he is asleep, and completely unable to feel anything, electrodes are placed on either side of his head, and an electric current is passed briefly between them. As a rule, this produces only a very minor convulsion, in which the hands and feet merely tremble for a few seconds.

A few minutes later, the patient comes round. Within an hour or so, he is usually able to go home with a relative. The effect of a course of ECT in relieving some types of mental depression, particularly in older patients, is often very good indeed.

EEG is the abbreviation for electroencephalogram, a method of recording the electrical changes which accompany activity in the brain – the 'brain-waves'. Numerous small electrodes are attached to the scalp, and the variations in electrical potential which they pick up are traced on a moving strip, as a complicated wave pattern. From distortions of the normal pattern it is possible to diagnose certain brain disorders, such as epilepsy and cerebral tumours, and pinpoint local damage to brain tissue. Several sorts of wave are recognized, the *alpha* waves being the most marked, with a frequency of about ten per second. *Beta* waves are much more rapid, *delta* waves are slower. *Theta* waves are rare.

EARS are the organs of hearing. The ear does not just consist of the external flap of skin and gristle, on each side of the head. In fact it is an extremely complex structure, most of which lies deep inside the head, within the bony skull.

The external ear of man is the vestigial remnant of the long ear of animals. In the hare or rabbit, for instance, the external ear flap can be moved around and seems ideally designed for capturing sounds, and identifying their direction. Man, however, has practically lost the ability to move his ears, and it is doubtful if the external ear serves as anything more than a useful prop for spectacles.

A narrow tube leads from the exterior to the middle ear – in fact, it is so narrow that it very readily becomes blocked with wax. At the end of the tube is the eardrum – a roughly circular membrane which, as the name suggests is like the skin of a drum. Sound waves make this diaphragm vibrate, and it transmits the vibrations to three tiny bones, called the malleus (hammer), incus (anvil) and stapes (stirrup-bone). They carry the vibrations on to a structure known as the labyrinth, where, in a snail-shell-like helix called the cochlea, they are translated into nervous impulses. These pass up the auditory nerve to the brain, which registers them as

114

either meaningless or meaningful sounds.

Exactly how the vibrations reaching the cochlea are turned into nerve impulses representing different sounds is still a matter of controversy. In one theory, each of the fine hairs in the spiral canal corresponds to a particular sound wavelength, but other scientists disagree.

Also a part of the labyrinth are the semicircular canals — three fluid filled tubes which provide information about balance. It is the movement of the fluid in these tubes that gives an indication of which way the body is turning or falling. When the fluid in the semi-circular canals is made to spin continuously in one particular direction (for instance, by turning rapidly in a circle), it causes a sensation of giddiness, which continues until the fluid comes to rest. Disease can also cause giddiness.

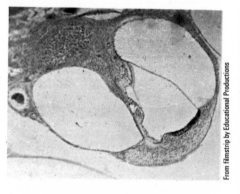

A highly-magnified cross-section of the cochlea, responsible for distinguishing sounds.

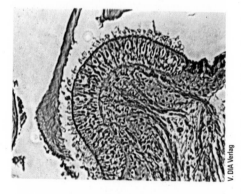

A section of the delicate organ of balance in the inner ear, which detects all head movements.

EAR DISORDERS are among the most common conditions seen in a doctor's surgery. *Earache* is particularly common among young children. The commonest cause is otitis media, which is an infection of the middle ear by germs. The child is miserable and usually feverish. If he is not old enough to complain of earache, he may hold his ear. Sometimes there is a little discharge.

Before antibiotics were discovered, little could be done for this common condition. Many children with it suffered subsequent mastoid infections and severe ear damage. Nowadays, however, as soon as a doctor has looked at the ear-drum (with a special instrument called an auriscope), and established that it is inflamed, he can put the child on a week's course of antibiotics — usually given by mouth, but sometimes by injection to start with.

Discharge from the ear always calls for medical advice. It can be due to an eczematous condition of the skin of the ear, to the presence of a foreign body, or to infection, acute or chronic. Lay people often imagine that this type of discharge is of no importance; they either neglect it or, worse still, plug up their ears with cotton wool. If infection is present, blocking the ears will only make things worse. It is essential that a doctor examines any discharging ear with his auriscope.

Deafness (see **deafness**) may be

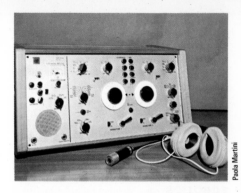

The audiometer is an instrument used to investigate different forms of hearing defect.

either perceptive or conductive. In perceptive deafness, it is the nervous connections between the ear and the brain which are affected. This type of deafness (which is common in old age) is not amenable to surgery, but can often be helped by the use of a hearing aid.

Conductive deafness, on the other hand, is caused by disorders of the middle ear. One of the most common of these is otosclerosis, which can produce a severe and rapidly advancing deafness in people as young as 30. Fortunately, delicate surgical techniques have been developed since the mid-1950s which have enabled ear, nose and throat (ENT) specialists to improve the hearing of patients afflicted with this condition beyond all measure (see **otosclerosis**). One of the other common causes of conductive deafness is, of course, wax in the ear. It is astonishing how many middle aged or elderly people accept increasing deafness over a period of years when, in fact, a brief examination by their doctor would disclose that all that is needed is to syringe the ear out with warm water.

Noises in the ear (tinnitus) characteristically take the form of whistling, ringing, hissing or throbbing. The latter type of noise is usually in time with the pulse, and the patient may be troubled by it as he falls off to sleep at night. It is usually of little significance, and a slight change in posture will abolish it. Other types of noise are usually associated with some type of middle-ear disorder — for instance,

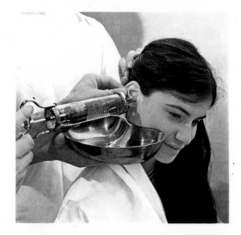

Syringing the ears to remove wax may sometimes be all that is needed to restore hearing.

115

catarrh in the eustachian tubes (see **eustachian tubes**), or inflammation of the labyrinth (labyrinthitis), or Menière's disease (see **Menière's disease**). Because the mechanisms of hearing (see **ear**) are so closely bound up with those of balance, any disorder of the labyrinthine region which produces noises in the ear is also liable to produce vertigo.

Fortunately today surgery is progressing to the stage where many such disorders, even of the inner ear, can be corrected.

ECBOLICS are drugs taken with the intention of producing an abortion. In fact, although disreputable people have made a good deal of money in the past by selling supposed ecbolic drugs, it is now considered highly doubtful whether any drug really can have this effect without seriously threatening the life of the expectant mother.

ECDYSIS means the shedding of outer coverings. The word is applied to the process whereby insects throw off their outer skin, and to the sloughing of the top layers of skin which occurs in certain forms of dermatitis.

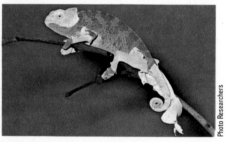

When a chameleon outgrows its skin, it simply grows a new one, sloughing off the old.

ECHINOCOCCUS is a type of tapeworm. The commonest species is Echinococcus granulosus, which infests dogs. The eggs of the tapeworm are passed out in the dog's motions. It is extremely easy for anyone who handles such a dog to get these eggs on his hands, and thus carry them to his mouth. (Similarly, sheep and other animals can become infected by grazing on grass where an infested dog has defaecated.)

116

Once the tapeworm eggs are ingested by a human being, they release tiny embryos which burrow their way through the walls of the intestines, and eventually find their way to the liver or the lungs, where they form cysts. The commonest symptoms are general ill-health, jaundice, anaphylactic shock (see **anaphylactic shock**), and, if cysts form in the brain, epileptic fits. Fortunately, this last occurrence is rare.

Not surprisingly, this type of tapeworm infection tends to occur in areas of the world where man works closely with dogs. In the United Kingdom, for instance, it is generally recognized that the likely candidate for the disease is the Welsh sheep-farmer, who works with collies. Other areas in which infection is found include the sheep and cattle rearing plains of South America and Australia.

Surgical removal of cysts offers the only prospect of cure. However, prevention of the disease is possible, wherever people are willing to observe sensibly hygienic precautions. In Iceland, for instance, where the disease was once widespread, the incidence has been greatly reduced. Firstly, dogs are not allowed to eat the carcases of infected sheep, from which they themselves could become infested. Secondly, shepherds and other people who own dogs are educated to realize that these animals are potential sources of disease, and that it is necessary to wash one's hands after handling them, especially before touching food.

ECLAMPSIA is a condition occurring in toxaemia of pregnancy (see **toxaemia of pregnancy**). It is characterized by fits, which usually occur shortly before the end of pregnancy, but may also come on during labour or even shortly after delivery. The blood pressure of the patient increases, and may greatly exceed the normal. Fortunately, if a mother has proper antenatal care, the signs and symptoms of toxaemia will often give adequate warning of the imminence of this very serious condition. Treatment consists in skilled nursing under heavy sedation in a quiet, darkened room.

ECTOPIC PREGNANCIES are those in which the fertilized egg becomes attached to some part of the mother other than its correct position inside the womb. When an unfertilized egg is released from a woman's ovary at the time of ovulation, it has to traverse a short distance within the abdominal cavity before it enters the Fallopian tube, which is the tube attached to the uterus, one on each side, and extends sideways, with fingerlike projections, out to the ovary. Normally, fertilization occurs inside the tube (when a sperm meets the egg), and the fertilized egg then passes on into the womb and becomes attached to its lining.

Very rarely, an egg may become fertilized within the abdominal cavity; it may attach itself to the ovary, or to the lining of the cavity itself (the peritoneum). Surgical removal is necessary in such cases.

Much more commonly, however, the ectopic pregnancy occurs in the tube. The fertilized ovum burrows its way into the wall of the tube, which can only accommodate it for a limited length of time – usually about eight weeks or so. If the condition has not already been diagnosed by then, and the pregnancy terminated, the sac containing the embryo will probably rupture. The features of an ectopic pregnancy are therefore usually as follows: One or two periods are missed, and the patient realizes she is pregnant. She then begins to feel pain low down in the abdomen, usually on the side of the affected tube. This pain is usually of gradual onset, but occasionally it may be very sudden and severe, so that she may collapse. As a rule, a certain amount of vaginal bleeding follows the onset of the pain, often a few hours later. This depends, however, on the direction in which the sac has ruptured – if it has burst into the abdominal cavity, then vaginal bleeding may well be absent.

In any case, the patient must be taken to hospital at once. If the gynaecologist there decides that she definitely has an ectopic pregnancy, and not some condition producing similar symptoms, such as a miscarriage (abortion) or salpingitis (inflammation of the tubes), then she will be operated on.

It is usually necessary to remove the affected Fallopian tube with the embryo. This does *not*, however, mean that it is impossible to have another pregnancy. Provided the tube on the other side is healthy, there should be no obstacle to a further, successful, pregnancy.

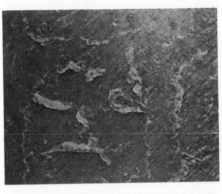

In severe eczema the outer layers of the skin are often dry and scaly.

ECZEMA is a skin disorder which is characterized by patchy eruptions of red, scaly skin. There may be crust formation, itching and sometimes oozing of liquid from the affected areas.

Eczema is part of what is often called 'the eczema – dermatitis group' of disorders, which probably make up about 50 per cent of all skin conditions seen by doctors. Eczema is not one single disease, and individual cases vary greatly from each other. We do not know why one person develops eczema, and another does not. However, infantile eczema in particular does seem to run in families. Frequently one or other parent of a child with eczema has a history either of the disorder itself, or of asthma or hayfever. The child may sometimes, as he grows out of infancy, lose his eczema, and develop asthma instead. These findings have led doctors to suppose that there is a marked allergic factor involved in the production of eczema. In addition, psychological factors undoubtedly play a part in some patients – as with asthma, an episode of mental stress (such as an exam.) may trigger off an attack. Infection of an affected area of the skin may also make things worse. Nowadays, doctors have a

117

wide variety of treatments which have greatly improved the outlook for the patient with eczema, including antibiotics (where infection is present) and steroid applications. It is also worth bearing in mind that a considerable proportion of patients (particularly children) with eczema undergo spontaneous cure for no apparent reason.

EDEMA is the American way of spelling oedema (see **oedema**).

EFFORT SYNDROME is a condition almost identical with Da Costa's syndrome (see **Da Costa's syndrome**), except that the symptoms (mainly palpitations and pains in the lower left chest) tend to be brought on by exercise. It is of psychological origin, and usually clears up readily as soon as the patient understands this fact.

EFFUSIONS are outpourings of fluid into any cavity of the body for instance, the cavities of joints, or the thoracic cavity. Effusions into joints are usually due to injury. The joint becomes swollen and painful; although the swelling will usually disappear after a few days' rest, it is occasionally necessary to aspirate (suck out) the fluid with a needle.

Effusions in other parts of the body are usually aspirated if they interfere with the body's function — for instance, fluid collecting in the chest as a result of pleurisy is frequently tapped off, as it may interfere with breathing by compressing the lung.

EGGS are the oval structures in which the embryos of birds and many reptiles develop. By extension, the term 'egg' is widely applied to the ovum (Latin **an egg**) of human beings, which is a very similar structure to that found in birds and reptiles, the most obvious difference being that the ovum of human beings (and almost all other mammals) does not need protection for existence outside the mother's body; therefore it has no hard shell. The organ responsible for the production of the ova (plural of ovum) is usually known as the ovary.

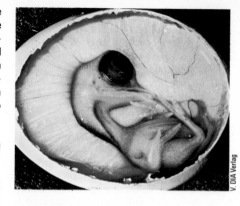

V. DIA Verlag

Above After only two weeks the main body features of a bird can be discerned. *Below* An ostrich hatches.

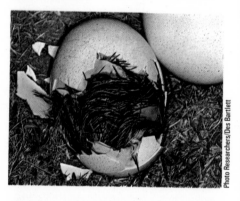

Photo Researchers/Des Bartlett

EGO is a Latin word meaning 'I'. Freud, the founder of psychoanalysis introduced the term into medicine. Basically, he suggested that there were three main divisions of the human mind — the id, the ego, and the super-ego. The id represents man's basic self-preservative and completely selfish nature — the part of his mind that satisfies his basic needs. The ego represents the conscious, 'day-to-day' part of his mind, while the super-ego is the highest intellectual component — the portion which is responsible for man's finest thoughts and actions. In a sense the super-ego keeps the id in check, by preventing our baser urges from ruling our lives, while the ego concerns itself with running the routine affairs of our existence. Subsequent work has somewhat modified the way that psychologists regard Freud's original views.

EJACULATION is the word applied to the process whereby drops of seminal fluid are forcibly squirted from the penis at the male climax (see **climax**) during sexual intercourse, and so reach the region of the cervix, or neck of the womb. Spermatozoa in the ejaculated fluid are thus able to enter the uterus, if all conditions are favourable. Failure of ejaculation is sometimes found in patients treated with certain drugs to reduce high blood pressure, but stopping the drug restores normal function. For premature ejaculation see **premature climax.**

ELBOW is the joint formed between the single bone called the humerus in the upper arm and the two in the forearm called the radius and ulna. It is an extremely complicated joint, but, since it does not bear weight (as does the knee joint), it is fortunately not particularly prone to strains and injuries. However, dislocation of the elbow is quite common in children, and fractures around the joint also occur quite frequently. Because of the presence of important nerves and blood vessels close to the elbow joint, such injuries must be treated with considerable care to avoid further damage.

TENNIS ELBOW is a rather mysterious ailment in which there is considerable pain immediately above the joint. Its cause has never been clear, but it is probably related to recurrent minor strains on muscle fibres attached to the humerus.

ELECTRIC SHOCK causes a considerable number of deaths every year — mostly from such causes as handling faulty electrical apparatus, or touching such apparatus with wet hands. In addition, a very small number of deaths are caused by electric shock from lightning.

Minor electric shocks produce only a painful sensation and a local contraction of the muscles. However, more severe shocks may cause serious burns. High voltage shocks, at whatever current, usually cause immediate unconsciousness, and the heart may stop beating. Unless prompt action is taken to start the heart beating and keep respiration going,

death will follow.

FIRST AID IN SEVERE ELECTRIC SHOCK: If the unconscious victim is still in contact with the source of the shock, do not touch him. If there is a nearby switch, turn off the current. Otherwise drag the victim away by using any non-conductor (e.g. a rope, a stick, or best of all, rubber gloves). If there is no pulse, start immediate cardiac massage by chest compression as described under 'drowning'. Get someone else to carry out mouth to mouth respiration. Keep this up without cease for at least an hour, or until medical aid arrives.

ELECTRICITY is used in medicine for many purposes. Direct application of electricity is mainly employed by specialists in physical medicine, and by physiotherapists, for the relief of painful conditions and the improvement of the tone of wasted muscles.

ELECTROCARDIOGRAM – see **ECG.**

ELECTROCAUTERY is an electrically heated device used to burn away diseased tissue.

ELECTROENCEPHALOGRAM – see **EEG.**

ELEPHANTIASIS means gross swelling of any part of the body (literally, to elephantine proportions). Invariably, the cause of this phenomenon is blockage of the tiny lymph vessels, which drain fluid away from the tissues. In temperate countries, the commonest factor involved in the production of such a blockage is radiotherapy. Frequently, radiotherapy has to be given in doses which produce a certain amount of unwanted tissue damage, and unfortunately sometimes the result is gross swelling of a leg, for instance.

In many areas of the tropics, however, elephantiasis is quite common. Here, the condition is due to blockage of the lymph vessels by multitudes of tiny worms called filaria. The larvae of these worms enter the body when a man is bitten by an infected mosquito. Filariasis (as infection with these worms is called) is endemic in areas of most countries between the latitudes of 40°N. and 30°S.

ELIXIR means a medicinal extract, usually containing sweetening and aromatic ingredients, to give a pleasant taste. The 'elixir of life' was sought throughout the middle ages, by alchemists, who thought it would give them eternal life.

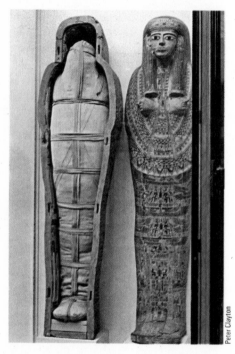

In ancient Egypt the bodies of important people were embalmed and turned into 'mummies'.

EMBALMING is the preservation of dead bodies from decay. In ancient Egypt it was extremely popular, the favoured method being the removal of certain internal organs shortly after death, followed by the wrapping of the entire corpse in bandages impregnated with preserving solutions. This process is called 'mummification'. Modern embalmers use more sophisticated techniques, such as injecting preservative materials into the blood vessels within a few days of death. This technique is used for scientific purposes — e.g. where it is essential that a body be preserved intact for examination over

120

some period of time. Undertakers also practise it, however, at the request of relatives of the dead person, or to honour his own wishes.

This custom is particularly widespread in the United States, where it is frequently combined with post-mortem cosmetic techniques which enable the relatives to visit the departed over a period of weeks if they so wish.

EMBOLISM is a word which literally means 'a plug'. It is used in medicine to describe any condition in which matter passes along a blood vessel to another part of the body, where it blocks up the blood vessel and cuts off the blood supply or otherwise damages the tissues. An embolus (as the matter which causes the embolism is called) may be a clot, a piece of tumour, a fragment of infected tissue, or an air bubble, among other things.

PULMONARY EMBOLISM is a condition in which a clot passes up the veins which return blood from the legs and lower trunk, passes through the right side of the heart and lodges in the pulmonary artery (the blood vessel which carries blood from the right side of the heart to the lungs), or one of its branches. The result may be fatal if the clot is very big. The embolus may, however, only cause sudden failure of the right side of the heart, which may respond to treatment. Smaller clots will cause the condition known as pulmonary infarction, which is characterized by sudden pain in the chest, and often coughing with blood-stained sputum.

CEREBRAL EMBOLISM is a condition in which a clot (or other matter) passes up an artery leading to the brain, and cuts off the blood supply. Normally, this happening manifests itself as a 'stroke' (see **stroke**).

AIR EMBOLISM occurs when air bubbles get into a blood vessel. Common causes include the accidental opening of a vein carrying blood from the brain (e.g. during surgery), and accidents while aqualung diving. In the latter instance, pressurized air forms bubbles in the blood if a diver ascends too rapidly without using proper breathing techniques. This is the cause of the extremely painful divers' condition known as 'the bends'.

EMBROCATIONS, or liniments, are oily aromatic preparations rubbed into the skin to relieve the pain and stiffness of muscle strains and similar ailments. Any effect they have is often due mainly to the massage which is used in applying them, since intensive rubbing increases blood flow through the affected part and produces a warm feeling. They are not absorbed to significant degree through the skin, although in some, mildly irritant substances cause a reddening of the surface.

EMBRYO is a word applied to the unborn child in the very early part of its existence. As a rule, embryonic life is considered as starting at the time when the fertilized egg first loses its round shape and becomes discernibly lengthened. The foetus is referred to as an embryo until about eight weeks of the pregnancy have passed, at which stage all the basic organs of the body have been formed. Embryology is the study of the formation of these organs.

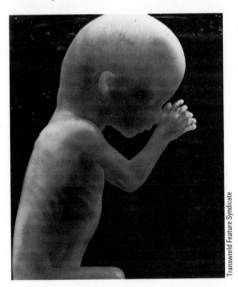

A human foetus at about four and a half months. Blood vessels can easily be seen.

EMETICS are substances which bring about vomiting. Common examples are salt-water and mustard-and-water, both of which are useful to induce vomiting as immediate treatment when a poison has been swallowed. (N.B. when a corrosive poison, such as a strong acid or alkali is involved, the use of emetics is highly dangerous.) This type of emetic acts by irritation of the stomach, though the unpleasant taste undoubtedly adds to the nausea. Certain drugs, such as morphine, have an *indirect* emetic effect, by passing into the bloodstream and acting on the 'vomiting centre' in the brain.

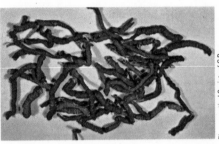

Emetine is extracted from the roots of the Brazilian shrub called Cephaelis ipecacuanha.

EMETINE is a useful drug employed in the treatment of amoebic dysentery (see **dysentery**). It is extracted from the root of the Brazilian shrub Ipecacuanha.

EMISSIONS are discharges of any sort from the body. Usually, however, the word is applied to nocturnal emissions. These are the discharges of seminal fluid during sleep which occur in most males from the age of puberty onwards. As a rule, they are accompanied by erotic dreams (usually called 'wet dreams'), though there may be no recollection of these in the morning. It is a natural physiological phenomenon, and it is a fallacy that nocturnal emissions are in any way bad for the health.

EMPHYSEMA means the abnormal presence of air. The word is used in two principal senses. Firstly, it indicates the relatively uncommon condition of *surgical emphysema*, in which air gets under the skin or into the body tissues. It does occasionally follow surgical operations but more frequently as a result of injury (for instance, a fractured rib). The air under

121

the skin can then be detected by a characteristic crackling noise and feeling whenever the skin is touched.

The second sense in which the word is used is to describe the common condition of *emphysema of the lungs*, of which there are several varieties.

The disorder is frequently associated with chronic bronchitis (see **bronchitis**). It is characterized by distension and breakdown of the alveoli — the tiny air sacs that form the lung. Although the cause of emphysema is unknown, it seems likely that, very often, the inflammatory processes of chronic bronchitis start the lung changes. However, some patients with emphysema have no history of chronic bronchitis.

The emphysematous man tends to be a barrel-chested individual. In his forties or fifties he usually first consults his doctor, complaining of breathlessness on exertion, and probably of the main symptom of chronic bronchitis, which is a long-standing cough. He is frequently a heavy smoker.

After some time, the patient begins to experience breathlessness at rest, as well as on exertion. What is happening now is that the disruption of the tiny air sacs has led to a reduction in the surface area of the lung which is available for transport of oxygen into the body. The blood vessels which supply the lungs degenerate, and this, in turn, tends to lead to failure of the right side of the heart, and the characteristic symptoms of swollen ankles and fluid in the abdominal cavity. When the doctor examines the emphysematous patient, he notes that the lungs are over-distended with air, and that the patient has difficulty in breathing out. There is often blueness of the face (cyanosis), and wheezing may be a feature.

However, emphysema is a disease which progresses very slowly indeed, if the patient has proper medical care, and looks after himself. If he is a smoker, he should give it up immediately, since inflammation of the lungs will only accelerate the progress of the disorder. All chest infections must be treated promptly — here the advent of the antibiotics has greatly improved the outlook for the emphysematous patient. If heart failure occurs, the

doctor will treat it accordingly. Breathing exercises will be found to be of very considerable value. Finally, if the patient is at all overweight, he should reduce.

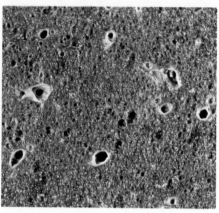

Contrast the size of the air-spaces in a normal lung and in emphysema.

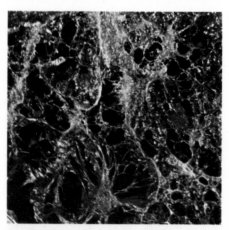

EMPYEMA is a collection of pus (an abscess) within the cavity of the chest, between the lung and the chest wall itself. It occurs following infection in some nearby structure, usually the lung itself, perhaps pneumonia or tuberculosis; however, infection can spread inwards — for instance through a stab wound in the chest wall. The pus must be removed as soon as possible (this may necessitate tapping with a needle, or a surgical operation), and antibiotics are then used to eliminate the infection.

EMULSIONS are liquids in which various kinds of oil or fat are contained in the form of very small globules. An every-day example is milk. A pint of milk contains, on average, about 20 grams of fat (varying according to the species of cow) dispersed throughout the liquid in tiny invisible globules.

There are many other examples of emulsions in medicine. When food passes through the small intestine, the fats in it are converted into minute globules by the action of bile salts. The resulting emulsion is easier for the body to absorb. The same principle is used in prescribing emulsions, such as cod-liver oil, in medical practice — the process of emulsification makes such preparations easier to digest, because the droplets are so small.

ENAMEL is the thin hard protective layer of the teeth. It is quite difficult to damage enamel, but its brittle nature is such that cracks, once made, are likely to be extensive. For this reason, children should be discouraged from such practices as opening bottles with their teeth. Cracks formed in the enamel may lead to subsequent destruction of the underlying dentine (see **dentine**). The enamel is the hardest tissue in the body, and is composed of the same material as is found in bone. The salts are in the form of six-sided prisms arranged on the dentine.

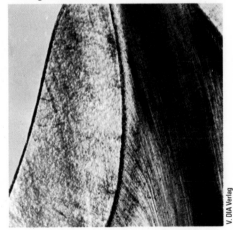

Structure of the tooth, showing the outer layer of enamel, protecting the dentine within.

ENCEPHALITIS means inflammation of the brain. In the majority of cases it is due to infection by viruses (see **viruses**). There are various ways in which such infection can penetrate the brain tissue, and it is not always clear how the organisms responsible entered the body. Probably the majority enter the body via the nose, lodge in the upper air passages and thence make their way to the brain. The viruses which are commonly involved in encephalitis include those of mumps, measles, chickenpox and influenza. Rarer causes are glandular fever, rabies and equine encephalitis (a disease transmitted by horses, which occurs in scattered outbreaks in North America).

Encephalitis may also rarely follow vaccination against smallpox or measles, or occur a fortnight or so after the diseases. In such cases, the brain inflammation is probably not due to infection but to some form of allergy to the virus. The main features of encephalitis are as follows: The patient becomes ill over a period of a day or two. He is feverish, and his temperature may be over 106°F. Initially he is lethargic and irritable but he may well soon become unconscious. Most patients complain of headache and vomiting. Pain tends to occur down the back of the head and neck, and is made worse by bending the head forward so that the chin is on the chest. This sign is called *meningism* because it is characteristic of inflammation of the meninges, or membranes of the brain and spinal cord. In fact, meningitis and encephalitis are often associated, and the combination of the two is called meningoencephalitis.

Encephalitis lethargica is a special form of the disorder which was extremely widespread in many parts of the world during the period 1918–1930. It is believed that one of the many influenza-like illnesses which swept around the world at that time was responsible. The great significance of encephalitis lethargica is that it is believed that, many years later, hundreds of thousands of those who originally acquired the viral illness developed a form of Parkinsonism (see **Parkinsonism**). This is 'the palsy', the shaking disease which affects many elderly people.

123

In the management of encephalitis, the important thing is to be sure that the patient does not, in fact, have meningitis (see **meningitis**), which is usually, though not always, a bacterial, and not a viral illness, and is therefore likely to be amenable to treatment with antibiotics. The difference between the two disorders can, as a rule, be determined by lumbar puncture – putting a needle into the lower part of the back and tapping off some spinal fluid. Once the diagnosis is made the treatment of encephalitis consists largely in skilled nursing care and sometimes steroid drugs are used to try to reduce inflammation.

ENCEPHALOPATHY is any generalized brain disease. Examples include encephalitis (see **encephalitis**), and poisoning due to such toxins as lead (lead encephalopathy). *Hypertensive encephalopathy* is a rare complication of high blood pressure. It is characterized by headache, visual disturbances and mental confusion.

ENDEMIC means existing continuously in a particular locality. It is applied to diseases to indicate their geographical distribution – yellow fever, for instance, is endemic in certain areas of South America.

ENDOCARDITIS means inflammation of the inner lining of the heart, the endocardium. The endocardium is particularly liable to become inflamed where it covers the heart valves. Here, the blood is subjected to extreme turbulence, which apparently renders the endocardium more liable to injury.

Almost invariably, endocarditis is due to infection by bacteria which have entered the blood stream (blood-poisoning or *septicaemia*) in one of many ways. For instance a mother's blood stream may become infected if bacteria enter her womb shortly after delivery. Particularly if the heart is deformed in any way, bacteria can produce an acute and very severe inflammation of the endocardium, with consequent destruction and distortion of the tissue of the heart valves.

More commonly, however, bacteria enter the blood stream via tooth sockets,

following dental extraction. In a patient whose heart valves are healthy, this occurrence is not likely to be serious, but a patient who already has valvular heart disease is very likely to develop *sub-acute bacterial endocarditis* (SBE). This is a most serious disorder, which, before the antibiotic era, was invariably fatal, since it was characterized by the slow and inexorable destruction of the victims' heart valves. Nowadays, provided the diagnosis is made early enough, sub-acute bacterial endocarditis can be successfully treated with antibiotics. 90 per cent of patients with bacterial endocarditis can be cured if treated within six weeks of the onset of the disease.

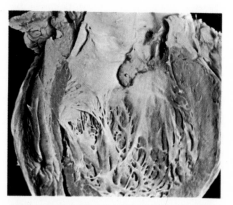

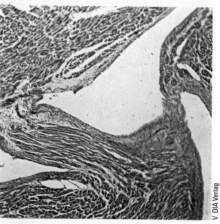

V. DIA Verlag

Endocarditis may so distort the normal structure of the heart valves that they become useless. *Above* Aortic valve almost completely destroyed. *Below* As seen through microscope.

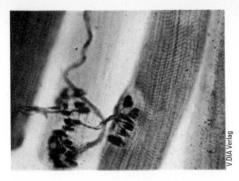

The end-plate is a minute plate at the end of a nerve, where it joins the fibre of a muscle.

END-PLATE is the term for the minute structure found at the endings of nerve fibres, where they pass on their electrical messages to the muscle cells, so causing them to contract.

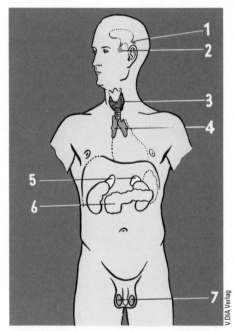

The main endocrine glands. *1* The pineal gland *2* The pituitary *3* The thyroid and parathyroids *4* The thymus *5* The adrenals *6* The pancreas *7* The testes. In women the gonads are ovaries.

ENDOCRINE GLANDS are the glands of the body which pour their secretions containing the chemical messengers called *hormones* (see **hormones**), directly into the blood stream. They were once known as *ductless glands.* The important endocrine glands are the pituitary (see **pituitary gland**), the thyroid (see **thyroid gland**), the parathyroids (see **parathyroids**), the pancreas (see **pancreas**), the adrenals (see **adrenal**) and the gonads, or sexual glands.

The pituitary gland has been called the 'leader of the endocrine orchestra', which aptly describes how it seems to regulate the working of the other endocrine glands. Pituitary hormones stimulate the other glands to release their own particular hormones, and there is in most cases a sort of 'feed-back' control system to keep the concentration of each hormone in the blood at the right level. Thus, for example, the thyrotropic hormone from the pituitary stimulates the thyroid gland, in the neck, to secrete the hormone thyroxine. Thyroxine is essential for normal growth, and also speeds up the body metabolism and production of energy. A person with too much thyroxine in the blood would eventually lose weight, develop a very rapid heart-rate and become nervous and 'jittery'. To avoid this overproduction, above a certain level, thyroxine itself acts as a brake on the system, and stops the pituitary from producing more thyrotropic hormone. When the blood-level of thyroxine drops, the pituitary again starts to release thyrotropic hormone; thus a balance is achieved.

Similar feed-back mechanisms regulate the production of the important steroid hormones by the adrenal glands, of sex hormones by the testicles and the ovaries, and in a rather more complex and less well understood way, of insulin by the pancreas. Diabetic patients produce too little insulin (see **diabetes**).

The remaining important endocrine gland not yet mentioned is the placenta, or afterbirth, which although it is only a temporary structure present in the mother's womb for the last six months or so of pregnancy, is nonetheless a rich source of hormones. These it pours into the blood stream, creating conditions which enable the pregnancy to continue, and promoting changes throughout the mother's body which prepare her for motherhood.

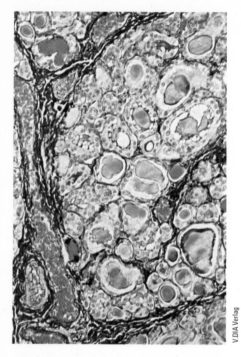

A highly-magnified cross-section of the thyroid gland, as it appears under the microscope.

ENDOMETRIOSIS is a relatively common condition in women; it is characterized by the occurrence in abnormal sites of tissue which should properly constitute the lining of the womb. Endometrial tissue, as it is called, may occur in the muscular wall of the womb, in the tubes, in the ovaries, or anywhere in the pelvis. More rarely, it may occur in the navel, in operation scars, or in the appendix.

Why this curious misplacement of tissue should occur is not clear — some doctors think it is a developmental abnormality, during the formation of the human body but others do not.

In any case, the problem is that the misplaced tissue responds to the sex hormones from the ovary just as correctly placed uterine lining would. Therefore, at the time of the menstrual periods, the scattered particles of tissue swell, become painful and may bleed. To take an example

126

a piece of endometrial tissue in the appendix may cause symptoms which mimic those of appendicitis at each period. Fortunately, such an occurrence is rare. Cure of endometriosis is usually by surgery. However, in certain circumstances it may be possible to help the patient by altering the hormone drive from the ovaries — e.g. by giving hormones by mouth, or by irradiating the ovaries and inducing an artificial menopause.

ENDOMETRITIS means inflammation of the lining of the womb (the endometrium). Usually this is due to infection, which may enter following abortion or child-birth. Infection can also be due to gonorrhoea or tuberculosis. In elderly women, resistance to other germs is lessened, because the vagina becomes less acid, and hence less hostile to germs, as the years go by. Women who have gynaecological operations involving the womb, or who suffer from prolapse (see **prolapse**) are also more likely to suffer from endometritis.

The patient usually complains of pain, fever and discharge. Antibiotics are indicated with, if necessary, local treatment of the womb to clear up the infection.

ENDOMETRIUM is the lining of the womb.

ENDOSCOPE is any instrument used to look into the inside of the body.

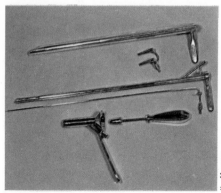

Endoscopes. *From above* oesophagoscope, bronchoscope and proctoscope.

ENEMA means an instillation of fluid into the bowel via the anus. Enemas are used for various purposes. In small children or delirious persons, they provide a convenient way of administering a sedative drug without disturbing the patient. In surgical wards, enemas are widely used to empty the bowel of motions prior to an operation, while in obstetric units, an enema is a standard method of trying to bring on labour. Enemas containing drugs (for instance, steroids) are administered to patients with certain diseases of the bowel, with the object of bringing the drug into direct contact with the diseased area. Enemas containing radio-opaque barium are used for X-raying the bowel.

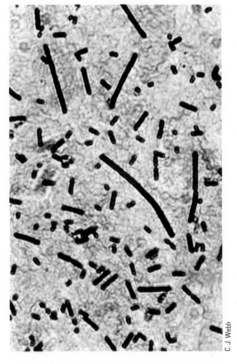

The organisms which are responsible for the extremely dangerous disease typhoid.

ENTERIC FEVERS are infections of the typhoid and paratyphoid group. Enteric literally means 'pertaining to the gut' and these disorders do, in fact, affect principally the gastro-intestinal tract. Like most infectious intestinal diseases, the enteric fevers are likely to be passed on where hygiene is inadequate. In practically all such conditions, the germs are passed out in the motions of infected people; it is remarkably easy for the organisms eventually to enter other peoples' bodies (via their mouths) if precautions are not strict. In the case of typhoid and paratyphoid fevers, the bacteria may get into water supplies and rapidly spread infection.

The basic features of enteric fevers are severe diarrhoea, with some abdominal pain and a high temperature. The diarrhoea may be profuse enough to threaten the life of a patient through dehydration (see **dehydration**), but, where death supervenes, it is more commonly the result of ulceration of the intestinal wall by the disease process. Treatment, if instituted early enough, is usually curative nowadays, although the patient may become a symptomless 'carrier' of the disease. The two antibiotics most commonly used are chloramphenicol and ampicillin. (see also **typhoid,** and **paratyphoid**).

ENTERITIS means inflammation of the gut or intestine, usually due to infection. Very frequently, the stomach is involved as well as the intestine, and it is then customary to refer to the illness as gastroenteritis. The characteristic features of enteritis are diarrhoea and abdominal pain. Where there is gastro-enteritis, there is also vomiting. The mode of infection, is, as with so many other intestinal diseases, the 'faecal-oral' route, that is to say germs are conveyed from one person's motions to another person's mouth because of inadequate hygiene.

A typical example is that of infantile enteritis, or gastro-enteritis. This may be caused by a variety of germs – for instance viruses of many types and 'wild' strains of E. coli, the germ which is a normal inhabitant of the bowel. 'Summer diarrhoea' as it used to be called, was epidemic in many countries before the First World War, when it caused the death of thousands of babies. Isolated, and often disastrous outbreaks of infantile enteritis still occur, and there were quite a number of deaths in England in the early part of 1969 as a result of such occurrences. It may be that the character of the germs is changing, possibly under the influence of Man's widespread use of antibiotics. However, in countries where hygiene is less strict, the death rate from infantile enteritis is very much higher. Mexico for example, has nearly 600 deaths per 100,000 of population a year. The prevention of infantile enteritis is mainly a question of strict hygiene.

ENURESIS means involuntary passing of urine. Normally, the word is used in the term *nocturnal enuresis*, which means bed-wetting. This is a relatively common disorder. *Primary enuresis* is said to occur when children simply take a long time to stay dry at night. Children vary greatly in this respect, but if a child goes on wetting the bed regularly after the fourth birthday, it is advisable to consult a doctor, particularly as a certain percentage of such children have either urinary infections or structural abnormalities of the urinary tract which can only be shown up on X-ray.

Secondary enuresis occurs when a child who has regularly been dry at night for some considerable time suddenly starts bed-wetting again — for instance at the age of five or six. Such an occurrence is almost invariably due to some form of psychological upset, which should not be too difficult to find. On no account should the child be scolded for bed-wetting; this may make things worse. Avoidance of drinks during the last two hours before bed-time may help, as may a frank discussion with the child, to find if a problem is worrying him. If these measures fail, the doctor should be consulted.

ENZYMES are chemicals which are produced by living cells, and which have the property of being able to break down tissue. They were once known as 'ferments'. Enzymes are present in the digestive fluid (see **digestion**), their function here being to break down the food into readily absorbable chemicals. Enzymes began to be used commercially in detergents during the late 1960s, because of their value in breaking down the organic matter in 'biological' stains, such as blood. They are destroyed by high temperatures.

128

EOSINOPHIL is a type of cell with granules which stain easily with the dye eosin. In certain diseases the number of eosinophils in the blood increases sharply, for example in asthma, hay-fever, and some parasitic diseases. Their exact function in the human body is not known.

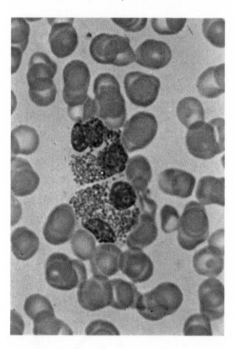

Eosinophil cells, seen in the centre of the microphotograph surrounded by red blood cells.

EPICANTHIC FOLD is the fold of skin which is found above the upper eyelid in the Mongolian races, giving the eyes a characteristic appearance. It may occur as a congenital disorder in Western races (see **Mongolism**).

EPICONDYLE is the term for a bony prominence sticking out near a joint; muscles which move the joint are often attached to it by means of tendons.

EPHEDRINE is a drug related to adrenaline. It is used in nose drops and sprays to relieve congestion, and also in tablets. It has been widely used as a treatment for asthma although it is now being superseded by other drugs.

EPIDEMIC means occurring in large numbers of people over a short period of time. The word is usually contrasted with the term 'endemic' (see **endemic**), which implies that a disease is always present to a greater or lesser extent in the country or area in question.

There have been many great epidemics in history. The diseases which tend to produce epidemics include typhoid, cholera, influenza, yellow fever, typhus and plague. Certainly the worst epidemic in recorded history is the great wave of plague (the Black Death) which swept across Europe in the years 1348–50; at least a quarter of the population of Europe was wiped out in these years. Although it was not realized at the time, the organism causing the disease, Pasteurella pestis, was transmitted to Man by fleas from black rats. In modern times, the most severe epidemic was the 'Spanish Flu' of 1918, which claimed over twenty million lives.

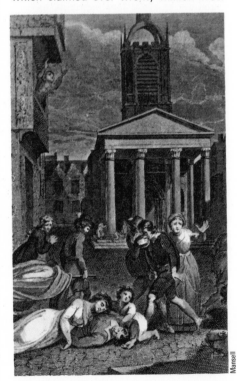
Terror and despair in the streets of London during the Great Plague outbreak of 1665.

EPIDIDYMITIS is inflammation of the epididymis – the coiled tube which lies on top of the testicle. Epididymitis is characterized by pain, often associated with mild fever. The commonest cause is gonorrhoea (see **gonorrhoea**), but tuberculosis was at one time quite frequently responsible.

EPIGLOTTIS is a structure which forms a lid to the voice-box, or larynx. It is constituted mainly of cartilage, and is situated immediately behind and below the root of the tongue. In many people the hard epiglottis can be felt in the throat with a finger, and in some it can actually be seen if the mouth is opened widely. The main function of the epiglottis is to stop food or drink going down the wrong way. During swallowing, it shuts off the entrance to the wind-pipe.

EPILEPSY is an intermittent disorder of brain function associated with disturbance of consciousness. It is not one disease, but many. Although the commonest type of epilepsy (major epilepsy) is associated with fits, these do not occur in other types.

Major epilepsy, or grand mal, is fairly common. It is characterized by recurrent episodes of generalized convulsions, in which the whole body shakes in a series of short jerks. It should be emphasized, however, that all convulsions are not epileptic in nature. In young children particularly, convulsions may occur without any evidence of epilepsy in later life (see **convulsions**), due to the effect of illness (for instance, a high temperature due to tonsillitis) on a baby's immature nervous system.

Major epileptic fits follow a set pattern. In about half the cases, the patient has a distinct warning that a fit is going to take place. This is called the aura. It may take the form of an odd sense of discomfort, a peculiar smell, or an impression of flashing lights. After a few seconds, the patient falls unconscious. There is a short tonic phase, in which all the muscles go into spasm; the patient does not breathe, and thus may go blue. This is followed by the clonic phase, in which characteristic short jerking movements of the limbs

129

occur. During this stage, the patient may bite his tongue; to prevent this it is a standard first-aid procedure to push a firm object between the teeth. Nothing else is necessary, apart from turning the patient on his side and making sure he can breathe. In the vast majority of cases, the convulsions will cease after a minute or so, and there usually follows a period of sleep. If, however, the convulsions persist for more than a few minutes, it becomes necessary to get the patient to hospital.

Minor epilepsy (petit mal) is also common, especially among children. It is an almost momentary impairment of consciousness — the child simply stops whatever he is doing and stands very still, with a vacant expression on his face.

Rarer types of epilepsy include Jacksonian attacks, in which the twitching starts in one part of the body before spreading to involve the whole body.

Where the diagnosis of epilepsy is not immediately clear from the history the patient gives to the doctor, it can frequently be confirmed by an electro-encephalogram test (see **EEG**).

Today, it is possible to control most forms of epilepsy and prevent attacks with suitable drugs, taken regularly. The vast majority of epileptics are now able to lead virtually normal lives. There are, however, certain classes of occupation, and hazardous pastimes, which it is clearly better for them to avoid unless the epilepsy is satisfactorily controlled.

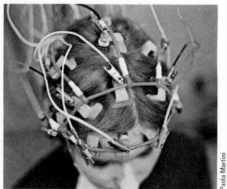

Paola Martini

Recording the brain's activity by EEG to find the exact location of an epileptic focus.

130

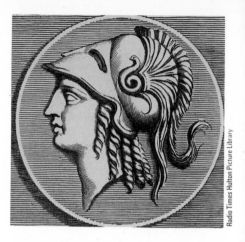

Radio Times Hulton Picture Library

Alexander the Great, one of the best-known historical figures to suffer from epilepsy. This complaint obviously did not hamper his activities in the field of military exploits.

EPISIOTOMY is the incision which is frequently made a few moments before delivery to widen the birth passage and make it easier for the baby's head to be born. An increasingly high proportion of births today are helped by episiotomy. The incision is made after injection of local anaesthetic, so there should be practically no pain. Although stitches are required afterwards, the clean surgical incision heals very much better than would a tear in the tissues. Within a fortnight, healing should be complete.

EPISTAXIS means a nose-bleed. Minor nose-bleeds happen occasionally to everyone, and it is only when they recur very frequently, or when large quantities of blood are lost, that medical attention is needed. The basic rule in dealing with nose-bleeds is not to interfere with the inside of the nose. All that is necessary is to press a finger firmly along the outside of the nose, so that the nostril is compressed, for about five minutes. The nose should not be blown or anything poked inside. However, if there is a really severe haemorrhage, a large plug of cotton wool should be left in the entrance to the nostril. It should *not* be removed frequently for inspection — this only restarts the bleeding. Most nose-bleeds stop in a few minutes.

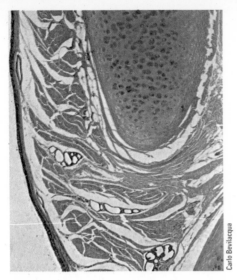

The epithelium of the trachea, *above,* is the dark layer on the left. In the duodenum the epithelium is of the secretory, columnar type.

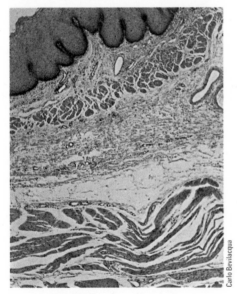

EPITHELIUM means the layer, one or more cells deep, which forms the outer covering of the body — the cuticle of the skin — and the lining of the digestive tract, the hollow organs of the body, and their ducts. The structure of the epithelium is different in the different regions of the body. That of the skin is composed of several layers of cells which are more or less flattened and parallel to the surface (see **skin**), while the bowels are lined with 'columnar' epithelium, which has long narrow cells. The air passages have a lining of special 'ciliated' epithelium, each cell of which is provided with minute 'cilia', or lashes, which are in constant motion. The movement of the lashes gradually propels the fluid covering the surface towards the throat. In the bladder the cells of the epithelium are intermediate in shape between those of the skin and those of the bowel.

EPIZOOTIC is the term which should be used for an epidemic occurring in animals other than Man, (Greek derivations *demos* 'the people', and *zoion,* 'animal'). Thus myxomatosis in rabbits should strictly be called an epizootic, not an epidemic. Sometimes epidemics and epizootics may go together — for instance, an epidemic of plague in Man follows or accompanies an epizootic in rats (see **plague**).

EPSOM SALTS is the name applied to a popular purgative. Its chemical name is magnesium sulphate, and it was first discovered at Epsom, England — hence its name. The dose is one to two teaspoonfuls of the salts, or half to one ounce of the mixture. Magnesium sulphate appears to attract water into the bowel and retain it, by a process called osmosis. The presence of this bulk of fluid produces a bowel movement within a few hours. As with all purges, the use of Epsom salts should not be abused.

Magnesium sulphate also has other uses in medicine. Injections and enemas of Epsom salts are said to be of benefit to certain cases of convulsions, while a paste made from the chemical is very commonly applied to boils and carbuncles. The object here is to attract fluids (again, by osmosis), but it is rather doubtful if such a process really occurs.

ERECTION is the term applied to the process by which certain structures in the body composed of 'erectile' tissue, lose their normal flaccid state and become

131

distended and rigid. The underlying mechanism is an increase in the amount of blood in the tissue, which causes expansion and stiffening.

In men the most important erectile structure is the penis; in women the nipples and the clitoris (see **clitoris**). Erection of the penis is necessary to make possible its introduction into the vagina during sexual intercourse, but erection may occur for other reasons than sexual arousal. In children particularly, erection may occur reflexly when the bladder is full, or following irritation of the penis. When for some reason erection is regularly found impossible in the adult, this is termed impotence (see **impotence**).

In women, erection of the clitoris, which has a structure very similar to the penis, also accompanies sexual arousal.

Erection of the nipples occurs to its greatest extent when a mother is breast-feeding her child, as the breasts are most developed at this stage, but also follows sexual stimulation.

ERGOMETRINE is a drug derived from ergot (see **ergot**). It induces the womb to contract, and is therefore of value in treating bleeding following labour or miscarriage. It is also widely employed in illegal attempts to procure abortion, but it is doubtful if it has any effect whatever in this respect.

ERGOT is a fungus which grows on rye. It contains a number of drugs which are of importance in medicine – notably ergometrine (see **ergometrine**) and ergotamine (see **ergotamine**). Ergot has been responsible for one of the most extraordinary illnesses in history – *ergotism*. When bread made from rye contaminated with the fungus is eaten, the results are extremely bizarre. The victim may become temporarily insane, be subject to all sorts of strange delusions, and want to dance until he is exhausted. In addition, constituents of ergot such as ergotamine may produce severe spasm of the blood vessels and hence gangrene, with subsequent loss of fingers or toes. Throughout recorded history, but most especially in the middle ages, there have been terrible outbreaks of

ergotism in countries where rye bread is eaten. At Aachen, in Germany, in 1374, for instance, hundreds of men and women went completely berserk, and danced in the streets until the majority had either collapsed exhausted or been trampled under-foot. Similar episodes recurred throughout the years; they were referred to as 'St Anthony's Fire', though this term has caused some confusion, as it is also used to refer to erysipelas (see **erysipelas**). The last recorded outbreak of ergotism was probably in Languedoc, France, in 1951, when the exact pattern of Aachen six hundred years before was repeated. People screamed like animals as they danced; one man leapt from a window and broke both his legs, but continued to try to dance down the streets on his shattered limbs. Since that time, stringent public health measures seem to have kept ergotism in check.

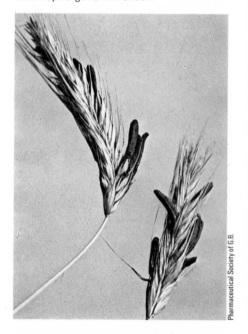

Pharmaceutical Society of G.B.

Ergot of rye is a black fungus which grows on the ear of the grain. In Man it causes ergotism.

ERGOTAMINE is an extract of ergot (see **ergot**). It constricts blood vessels, and has been found useful to treat attacks of migraine (see **migraine**).

EROGENOUS ZONES are the areas of the body which are most responsive to sexual stimulation, and which take a part in love-play. The psychological importance of these areas has often been exaggerated, and at one time it was even widely believed that stimulation of a particular erogenous zone, especially during infancy, could lead to perversion of the sexual instincts. The only proven fact seems to be, however, that human beings derive a pleasurable sensation from being touched on certain areas including the genitals and the lips; in women touching the breasts also produces a pleasant sensation. There is an extremely wide variation from person to person in the areas which can be truly termed the erogenous zones.

EROSION means a 'wearing away' of any tissue of the body. Thus an aneurysm (see **aneurysm**) of an artery may by pressure cause erosion of a nearby bone, or too much acidity in the stomach may cause an erosion or small ulcer of the stomach lining. Cervical erosions, found at the cervix, or neck of the womb, are quite common. They are bright red velvety areas which can be seen by the doctor with a speculum (a small metal device which aids inspection of the vagina and cervix). Erosions are often secondary to some mild cervical infection. Others occur after delivery and are noted at the postnatal examination — these usually clear up readily without treatment. A few occur in virgins; the cause of this type is not understood, but they may be due to some hormonal imbalance.

Erosions of the cervix may bleed slightly — for instance, after intercourse — but they are not, of course, malignant. However, it should be understood clearly that bleeding between the periods or bleeding after intercourse is not necessarily due to an erosion. Such symptoms need *immediate* full medical investigation.

Treatment of erosions is very simple. Small ones (particularly those occurring after delivery) can often be left to heal by themselves. Large erosions can be cauterized within a few minutes, a trivial and completely painless procedure, and will then cease to give trouble.

EROTIC means pertaining to love or sex. The term may be applied to almost anything — art, literature, music or even perfume — which has an arousing effect on human beings. For hundreds of years, Western morality heaped opprobrium on all forms of eroticism, though artists like Rubens, Titian, and, later, Manet, Renoir and Rodin somehow or other managed to keep the traditions of classical times going. In the East, however, particularly in India, erotic art has a long and honourable history, and in Japan eroticism (particularly in the form of 'pillow-books') was considered to play an important part in love-play (see **love-play**). In general it is widely recognized nowadays that eroticism is a perfectly acceptable and healthy part of an individual's sexual development.

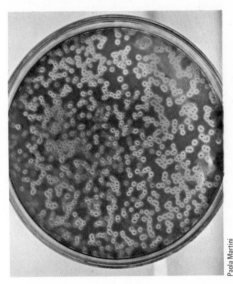

Paola Martini

The organism which causes erysipelas can be grown on a special gelatine plate for study.

ERYSIPELAS is a skin condition caused by infection with the common germ called the Streptococcus. The condition itself is, however, quite rare nowadays. It is characterized by areas of reddened skin which have a sharply defined margin. The infected skin feels hard to the touch. Very often the cheek is affected. Laboratory tests will usually demonstrate the presence of the Streptococcus. The infection

133

is sometimes liable to spread to other parts of the body if it is not treated promptly. Antibiotics, such as penicillin, should produce a complete cure.

Erysipelas was for many years known as 'St Anthony's Fire', but this term has caused some confusion, since it is also applied to poisoning by ergot (see **ergot**).

ERYTHEMA is any redness of the skin.

ERYTHEMA AB IGNE is the mottled net-like rash which develops very frequently on the lower legs of people who sit next to the fire a lot. The condition is extremely common in women in cooler countries such as the United Kingdom.

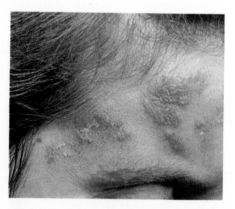

The unsightly reddened and nodular lumps which are characteristic of erythema nodosum.

ERYTHEMA NODOSUM is a condition in which the skin becomes reddened and 'nodular', or lumpy, over certain areas — particularly the front of the leg, over the shin bone. Erythema nodosum is particularly common in children. It may be caused by any infection with the streptoccus germ (such as a sore throat), or by rheumatic fever (which itself is believed to be an unusual reaction to this type of infection). More rarely, erythema nodosum is caused by tuberculous infection. It may also be related to an unusual disease called sarcoidosis, or to recent treatment with particular drugs. In all these cases, the eruption seems to constitute some form of hypersensitivity reaction, triggered off by the stimulus of infection or drug

134

therapy. It is characteristic of such reactions that they occur after a delay of about 9–14 days from the original stimulus. Thus, a fairly typical story would be that a child has a sore throat, starts getting better, and then, about 10 days after the original infection, an eruption appears on his shins. Although it may last for a week or two it will invariably clear up.

ERYTHROBLASTOSIS FOETALIS is the condition produced by the severest form of Rhesus incompatibility (see **rhesus factor**). Fortunately the condition is uncommon thanks to modern obstetrical techniques, and in particular, early delivery of babies who seem likely to be badly affected if the pregnancy were allowed to go to term. However, at one time many babies died shortly after birth from erythroblastosis foetalis, or were stillborn. They were usually jaundiced and their bodies were grossly swollen. Milder forms of disorder due to Rhesus incompatibility do still occur very frequently, taking the form of anaemia and jaundice (haemolytic disease of the newborn). There is, however, hope that even this condition will soon claim fewer babies' lives, in view of new techniques being developed (see **rhesus factor**).

ERYTHROCYTE means a red blood cell. There are literally thousands of millions of these tiny cells in the bloodstream; a cubic millilitre of blood contains about five million. Each cell is shaped like a minute biconcave disc, and, although it is so small, it is capable of a quite fantastic amount of work in keeping the body's vital chemistry working. Its most important function is to carry oxygen to the tissues — and on this function depends life itself. Erythrocytes passing through the blood vessels of the lungs pick up oxygen from the inhaled air, and it becomes temporarily attached to the oxygen-carrying pigment haemoglobin. Each red cell in the oxygenated blood travels in the blood stream to the tissue and releases its oxygen, before returning in the now deoxygenated blood through the veins and the heart, to the lungs for 'recharging'. Each erythrocyte has a life of about 115 days.

ERYTHROMYCIN is a very important antibiotic which was developed during the latter half of the 1950s. It attacks much the same range of germs as does penicillin (see **penicillin**), but its great value is that it can be used to treat infections which are resistant to other antibiotics. For this reason, doctors tend to keep it 'in reserve' for use in resistant infections. Unlike some other antibiotics, it is relatively free from side-effects.

ESSENTIAL HYPERTENSION means high blood pressure for which no definite reason can be found. The term unfortunately covers the majority of cases of raised blood pressure, since in only a few instances can a precise and specific cause be found, such as disease of the kidney, or a tumour of the adrenal gland. In all other cases, the doctor can only say that certain factors seem to have played a part in causing the illness. Among these factors is heredity − the child of a patient with essential hypertension has roughly a one in three chance of having it himself, while if both parents are hypertensive, the chances are one in two.

Obesity is also an important contributing factor. Those who are very fat are far more liable to high blood pressure than those who are thin, and reduction of a stone or two in weight by a fat man with high blood pressure will usually bring down his blood pressure considerably. Restriction of salt in the diet may also help.

The mechanism of this very common disorder appears basically to be an increased resistance to the blood flow in the tissues of the body, caused by intermittent muscular contraction of the arterioles − the smallest branches of the arteries. In time, the arterioles may become permanently narrowed, and affected by the degenerative or 'hardening' process called arteriolosclerosis.

However, whether the hardening is caused by the high blood pressure or vice versa is not clear. In addition, some authorities believe that all these changes are due to a process noted to go on in the kidneys in cases of high blood pressure; while still others think that the kidney changes are secondary to the hypertension.

What is certain, however, is that essential hypertension is becoming increasingly common in the population as a whole. It causes about 20 per cent of all deaths over the age of 50. However, drugs are now available which, used regularly, have the effect of lowering the blood pressure in patients with hypertension, and reducing its harmful effects on the organs of the body. It is to be hoped that further research into this baffling disease will eventually reveal its mysteries. Early diagnosis of the condition is very important, because steps can be taken to slow down its progress in young patients, and so add years of extra life to people who might otherwise die before their time.

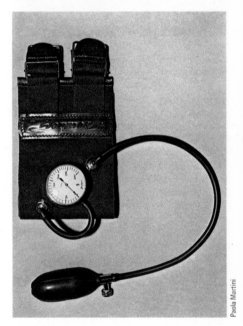

Paola Martini

The sphygmomanometer is an instrument to detect blood pressure changes.

ETHACRYNIC ACID is an extremely useful and powerful diuretic (see **diuretics**) − a drug which helps people to get rid of excess fluid from the body. First developed in the early 1960s, its great advantage is its remarkable speed of action; an injection of Ethacrynic acid into a vein will produce a dramatic increase in urine flow in less than a minute.

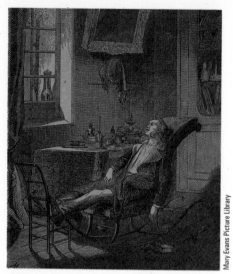

An early experimenter with ether tries out its properties for himself.

ETHER is an anaesthetic, a solvent, and a cleansing agent. There are in fact a number of chemical compounds called ethers, but, in medical terminology, the word 'ether' always means *ethyl* ether. It is a volatile liquid which rapidly becomes converted into gaseous form at higher room temperatures. As a solvent, it is still widely used in medicine to dissolve drugs, and as a cleansing agent for the skin.

As an anaesthetic, ether was used in the early experiments in America, around 1840. It continued to be used with considerable success for 100 years after that time. Ether and chloroform were so much the mainstay of anaesthesis for many years, that all hospitals developed the same characteristic smell. Until well into the 1920s and 1930s, the technique of administering ether was by the 'open drop' method. Many middle-aged and elderly people will recall having a mask (shaped like a metal basket, with a piece of gauze in it) placed over their mouths prior to operation. The anaesthetist then opened a bottle of ether, and carefully counted out a set number of drops on the gauze every minute. This method was known as 'rag-and-bottle' administration, since, in the old days, the ether was simply poured on a

136

clean rag, or the surgeon's glove. New methods came in, however; more scientific ways of giving ether were developed, and, eventually, after the Second World War, new anaesthetic gases were introduced. These gases, and injectable anaesthetics, such as pentothal, gradually replaced ether (and, indeed, chloroform) in the majority of the world's major hospitals.

ETHOSUXIMIDE is a valuable drug in the treatment of children with petit mal — the attacks of transient loss of awareness of the environment which are a common form of childhood epilepsy (see **epilepsy**).

ETHYL CHLORIDE is a clear colourless liquid with a characteristic smell, and very easily vaporized by slight heat. When sprayed on the warm skin it evaporates rapidly and has a freezing effect. It is therefore used to produce local anaesthesia for minor operations such as ear-piercing and the removal of warts. It is sometimes also used as a general anaesthetic for brief operations such as the removal of tonsils or teeth.

ETIOLOGY (aetiology) is a term for the group of causes which are known to underlie any disease.

EUPHORIA means a feeling of well-being or elation. Such a feeling may be produced by certain drugs which have for many years been used to counteract mild mental depression, and also the more powerful drugs of addiction.

EUGENICS is the study of the means whereby the human race may be improved. Eugenicists are particularly interested in improving the conditions of conception, gestation and birth of human beings, with the object of producing a human race which is morally, intellectually and physically superior to that of today. Unfortunately, experiments to this end have not, so far, been very successful.

From time to time, groups of people have attempted experiments, which, in theory, would lead to the production of children likely to grow up into adults possessing several physical and mental advantages.

EUSTACHIAN TUBES are the two narrow passages, one on either side of the head, which form a direct connection between the throat and the ear. Each is rather less than two inches long. The diameter of the Eustachian tube varies considerably, but the entrance may be wide enough to admit the tip of a finger.

The ear is a complex structure (see **ear**) which contains a thin membrane — the eardrum. Relatively minor changes in pressure — for instance, those caused by going up a hill (or ascending in an aeroplane) or by diving only a few feet down into water — will cause bulging of this delicate membrane. So that the eardrum will not burst, it is necessary to have a pressure-equalization system, and this is provided by the Eustachian tube, which allows air to move between the throat and the middle ear. Most of the time this process of equalization is not noticed, although going up or down a very steep hill rapidly in a car may cause the ears to 'pop', as the pressure on the drum is relieved. Rapid ascent in an aircraft (particularly one that is badly pressurized) will bring on mild earache and deafness in most people. The well-known methods of avoiding these symptoms (swallowing and yawning) are simply means of stretching the muscles of the throat, and thus opening more widely the orifices of the Eustachian tubes. When air at the same pressure as that outside the eardrum enters the middle ear from the throat, the symptoms stop immediately.

The same thing happens in reverse when an unpressurized plane descends rapidly — the eardrum bulges inwards as a result of the sudden increase in pressure outside. An absolutely identical phenomenon occurs when a swimmer dives to thirty or forty feet (depths which are very easily attained in skin diving). The weight of water is such, however, that the change in pressure is very marked; severe damage to the ears could ensue if the swimmer were not able to 'clear' them. For this reason, skin divers learn a special technique of ear-clearing by manipulation of the muscles of the throat.

The Eustachian tubes very readily become blocked with catarrh during colds. Under normal conditions, this is merely uncomfortable but, of course, it could be dangerous to the ears if one were to undergo any violent changes of pressure.

EUTHANASIA means, literally, a gentle or happy death. It has come to mean the bringing about of a person's death in order to save him from unnecessary suffering. The religious and moral principles involved have made euthanasia an extremely controversial topic throughout history.

EXANTHEM is another term for a 'rash', or eruption of the skin, accompanied by inflammation, which occurs in diseases such as measles, chickenpox and many others.

EXCRETION is the elimination of waste matter from the body. Although commonly taken to include the expulsion of waste from the bowel, it is more correctly applied to the processes by which unwanted material is removed from the bloodstream. The main routes of excretion are through the kidneys (water, urea, uric acid, creatine and other nitrogen-containing compounds, mineral salts), through the lungs (carbon dioxide and water vapour) and the skin (water, salt, and small quantities of urea).

EXERCISE carried out regularly is one of the most important factors in maintaining the health of the human body. This has always been a widely-held view, but its truth has become abundantly clear in the last decade or so. During this period, it has been evident that a virtual epidemic of coronary heart disease threatens western man. In the U.S.A. particularly, more and more men are dying in their forties, and even their thirties, from this cause. The reasons which lie behind the development of this disease are not yet very clear. One thing that does seem fairly certain, however, is that lack of exercise greatly predisposes to death from coronary disease. A typical story might be that a man leads an active life physically until he is thirty. He then settles down, takes no exercise whatever and drives everywhere by car, where once he would have walked. At the age of forty, he drops dead of a heart attack. Man simply was not designed for the sedentary life that many people live in the West today. Certainly, one of the most valuable precautions one can take against heart attacks is regular daily exercise. This need not be (and should not be) violent exercise. A walk to the station in the morning (instead of a car ride), a short stroll after lunch, and another walk, or a spot of gardening, in the evening are sufficient. A game of golf, or half an hour's tennis, once a week is *not* adequate, though such intermittent activities may be a useful adjunct to regular daily exercise of the type described above.

Home exercises of the PT type, if carried out daily, are also useful. It makes no particular difference what exercises are used, as long as they provide the body with mild exertion over a reasonable period of time each day. However, *isometric exercises* are not of value in this respect. These exercises have become extremely popular in recent years, particularly in America. They involve tensing opposing muscle groups against each other during a short period of intense effort lasting a matter of seconds. There is no actual movement of the body involved. For this reason, although isometric exercises are very helpful for those interested in muscle building, and will undeniably lead to the development of a powerful physique in a relatively short time, they appear to be of no real use in regard to warding off heart disease, as other forms of graded exercise may.

For this purpose, the body needs the benefit of regular daily sustained exercising. Primitive man was a hunter and a cultivator, and it is not without significance that men who work all their lives in the fields live longer than desk-bound city dwellers. There is no need for the ordinary person to go to great lengths to develop his physique, or to go in for strenuous daily routines which leave him exhausted. Exhaustion is not a sign that the exercise is 'working', and in fact may indicate that the exercise being taken is excessive. The point is that the exercise should be regular.

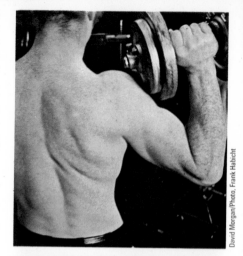

David Morgan/Photo. Frank Habicht

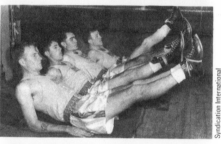

Syndication International

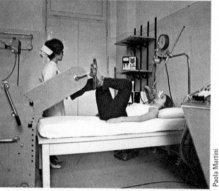

Paola Martini

Exercise with weights is a favourite means of developing particular groups of muscles, whether the aim is to simply improve the physique, or to increase physical strength. Leg-raising exercises tone up abdominal muscles, essential to protect boxers from injury. To determine how much energy is expended during exercise, the oxygen used is measured with an 'ergometer'.

EXOMPHALOS is a fortunately uncommon condition in new-born babies; there is a gap in the abdominal wall at the umbilical region. The bowel and other contents of the abdomen may come through this aperture. Minor degrees of exomphalos can readily be dealt with surgically, but in some cases there is practically no abdominal wall present, and the outlook is not so good. The cause of this developmental abnormality is unknown.

EXOPHTHALMOS means protrusion of the eyes. There are a number of possible causes for this symptom, but much the most common is *exophthalmic goitre.* Known as Graves' disease (after the Irish physician who first described it), exophthalmic goitre is a condition of the thyroid gland. The patient has a marked swelling (or goitre) at the front of the neck, and grossly staring eyes. One or both eyes may be affected. In addition, the patient (who, four times out of five is a female) usually has the other symptoms of overactivity of the thyroid gland (thyrotoxicosis). These include marked weight loss, despite a voracious appetite. The patient is jumpy, irritable and nervous. She constantly finds herself feeling too hot, and greatly prefers colder weather. She may also suffer from palpitations, and her pulse is likely to be very fast.

If the diagnosis is not obvious, it can be confirmed by laboratory tests of thyroid function. The patient can then be treated in three ways.

Anti-thyroid drugs can be given to damp down the gland's activity. These may need to be taken for life.

The patient can also be treated with radioactive materials, which have the effect of damping down the thyroid. However, this method is rarely used in women of child-bearing age, because of the possible damaging effects of radioactivity on the ovaries.

Finally, the thyroid gland may be removed surgically. (In fact, a small portion of it is always left behind – the object being to remove about nine-tenths).

All these methods of treatment will clear up all the other symptoms, but, unfortunately, they do not always relieve the protrusion of the eyeballs, and in rare cases may even make the protrusion worse. This is because the complex balance between the thyroid and the pituitary gland is upset. In this case other treatment with hormones may be effective, or the use of special eye drops. Surgical treatment is necessary in some cases.

EXPECTORANTS are medicines given with the object of helping the patient to bring up phlegm or sputum. Their use has been hallowed by tradition for hundreds of years. Unfortunately, it is becoming increasingly apparent that few, if any, of the preparations held to be 'expectorants' in the past have any such function, and that any benefit they produce is largely psychological, and dependent on their impressive colour, and unpleasant taste and smell.

EXTRASYSTOLES are extra beats of the heart, 'thrown-in' among the normal rhythm of its action. Many healthy people have extrasystoles quite frequently (usually without noticing them). These extrasystoles may become particularly frequent during severe exercise.

Where a person notices extrasystoles (perhaps by feeling his own pulse), he may become alarmed, but a doctor will be able to reassure him, though it may be necessary to check the diagnosis by means of an electrocardiograph (see **ECG**).

EYES are the organs of sight. Each is a globular structure, about two inches in diameter. Basically, the eye works like a camera. There is an aperture to admit light (the pupil), the size of which is controlled by the iris – which is the coloured part of the eye surrounding the pupil.

Immediately behind these structures is the lens – a biconvex (or converging) lens which is so constituted that its shape can be varied greatly according to need. Behind the lens is a 'screen', or retina, on which the pictures the eye receives are thrown.

Of course, the eye is infinitely more complicated than any camera, though its principles may be the same. It is capable

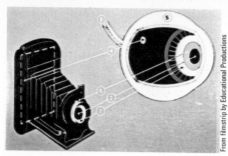

From filmstrip by Educational Productions

1 Lens of camera and lens of eye. 2 Diaphragm of camera and pupil of eye. 3 Diaphragm control and iris. 4 Sensitized film and retina. 5 The sclerotic layer of the eyeball. 6 The optic nerve connecting eye to brain.

of the most astonishing feats of definition of objects at varying distances, and of adapting itself to all sorts of conditions from dazzling brilliance to near pitch darkness.

The light which enters the eye passes first through what is, in effect, an additional lens, the cornea, or outer covering of the eyeball. It is believed that the major part of the refraction (bending) of light takes place here, while the lens itself probably only acts as an adjusting lens, varying its shape according to whether the object being viewed is near or far away.

Having traversed the lens, the light crosses the vitreous humour (the fluid which fills the back compartment of the eye), and is brought to a focus on the retina.

The retina is composed of many tiny nerve cells called 'rods' and 'cones'. The cones, which are concerned with colour vision, are densest in the middle part of the retina, while the rods, which are concerned with black and white vision, are more evenly spread out. At the edges of the retina, there are many rods and practically no cones. This explains why colour is seen very poorly towards the edge of the field of vision, and why, in the black-and-white viewing conditions of night-time, it is often easier to see something by looking sideways at it.

All the cells of the retina are connected to the optic nerve, which leaves the retina

at the 'blind spot' (see **blind spot**). From there, the optic nerve relays all the information regarding the picture received to the brain. The area of the retina which is most sensitive to light under normal viewing conditions is called the fovea. This takes the form of a small depression lying at the very back of the eye, on the axis of the lens. In birds the fovea is a deep pit; this enables them to detect the movement of other animals at great distances.

The eye is one of the most delicate structures of the whole human body, and is extremely easily damaged by blows or penetrating injuries. Many other disorders affect it — (see **blepharitis, blindness, cataract, conjunctivitis, keratitis** and **stye**). Fortunately, many can be cured.

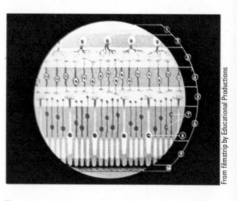

From filmstrip by Educational Productions

The layers of the retina. 1 Nerve fibres forming the optic nerve. 2 Multipolar nerve cells. 3 Inner dendrite layer. 4 Bipolar layer. 5 Outer dendrite layer. 6 Outer nuclei of rods and cones. 7 Nuclei of the rod cells. 8 Nucleus of a cone cell. Light reaches all layers.

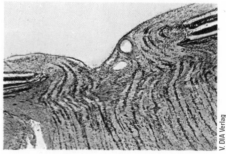

V. DIA Verlag

Section of the region where the optic nerve leaves the retina on its way to the brain.

FACE is the front part of the head. The basic structure of the head is the same in all human beings but there are racial variations in the proportions of the bones which make up the skull, and several skull 'types' are recognized — such as the Caucasoid, Mongoloid and Negroid — which have characteristic facial proportions. Even within one race, however, there are wide variations in the detailed structure of the face, and no two people have exactly the same appearance; on close scrutiny the most identical twins are distinguishable because of differences in skin pigmentation and texture, and the development of the muscles under the skin.

One of the main muscles which make up the face is the orbicularis oculi, which surrounds the eye and is responsible for closing the eyelids. Similarly the orbicularis oris muscle encircles the mouth and moves the lips. A complex group of smaller muscles enables the corners of the mouth to be turned up or down at will to give a smile, a grimace or a pout.

Little movement of the nose is possible, beyond dilating or twitching the nostrils, because it is mainly cartilage, with few muscles. The cheeks, however, have the important masseter and temporal muscles, which aid chewing movements.

The external ears consist almost entirely of cartilage and skin, and Man, unlike many animals, is incapable of significant movement of the ears, apart from slight twitching, achieved by contracting nearby scalp muscles.

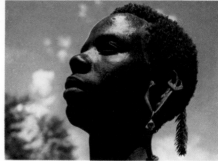

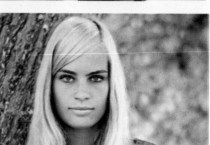

Paf International

Picturepoint

The Negroid type of face, *top*, with rather flattened nose and large lips, contrasted with a typical Caucasoid face, *below*. To one race, the members of another may all look alike, but small differences spell beauty or ugliness.

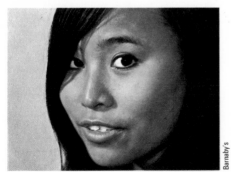

Barnaby's

The Mongoloid type of face. Perhaps the most outstanding feature is the shape of the eye.

FAECES are the stools or motions passed from the bowel. The process of elimination of faeces is known as 'defaecation'. Faeces are composed of the indigestible residue of food, together with countless millions of mainly dead bacteria from the bowel, and bile pigments (see **bile**). The latter are responsible for the characteristic brown colour of faeces. If the faeces are putty-coloured instead of their normal shade, this often indicates a blockage of the bile, a condition which is usually accompanied by jaundice. Medical aid should be sought without delay.

Similarly, faeces which are black and tarry may be a sign of ill-health. The black colour could be due to bleeding into the bowel; a medical opinion should be sought. Darkening of the faeces, but without any medical significance, can also be due to a diet very rich in meat, or to taking iron tablets.

FAINTING, or syncope, is a temporary loss of consciousness, due to insufficient blood reaching the brain. In normal circumstances the heart is perfectly capable of maintaining the circulation, in whatever position the body may be, but sometimes factors combine to cause 'pooling' of the blood in the vessels of the legs, so that there is not enough to meet the needs of the brain. Hot weather causes the blood vessels to dilate, and standing still aggravates the situation, because movement of the leg muscles normally assists the blood to return to the heart against the force of gravity. Emotion can also cause dilatation of the blood vessels, and sluggishness in the return of blood to the heart.

Falling into a horizontal position quickly restores the blood flow to the brain and consciousness is regained. In this respect fainting acts as safety valve. A person who has fainted should *not* be immediately dragged into an upright or sitting position.

Another situation in which a healthy person may feel faint is getting out of bed quickly in the morning, or rising suddenly from a chair. This is termed *postural hypotension.* Certain drugs may make it worse. All that happens is that the blood vessels have been dilated and relaxed while sitting or lying down, and rising suddenly causes pooling of blood in the lower extremities. After about 7–10 seconds, there is a feeling of weakness and dizziness. The remedy is to sit or lie down again for half a minute until the circulation has adapted itself. In the treatment of this or any other type of fainting, brandy or any other kind of alcohol should not be given. Lying flat for a short while is all that is needed.

FALLOPIAN TUBES are the two tubes, one on each side, which lead from the ovaries to the uterus (womb). Each is about four inches in length. The end of each tube near the ovary is wide, so that it acts as a funnel to collect the ova (eggs) released from the ovary at ovulation. The other end of the tube, at the point of entry into the womb, is very narrow, and can thus be easily blocked by TB or gonorrhoea, hence leading to infertility.

It is believed that fertilization of the egg by the sperm usually takes place in the

Fallopian tube, and that the fertilized egg then passes on into the womb, where it embeds itself. Sometimes, the fertilized egg becomes lodged in the Fallopian tube instead, and in this situation it is impossible for it to develop (see **ectopic pregnancies**). The affected tube has then to be removed surgically together with the embryo. However, this does not affect the ability to have children, since eggs may still reach the womb via the other tube.

FALSE MEMBRANE is the deposit that forms on the walls of the air passages in cases of diphtheria. A yellowish deposit, it either sticks to the mucous membrane or is incorporated in its damaged surface. If removed, it leaves a raw, bleeding area on which a new false membrane forms.

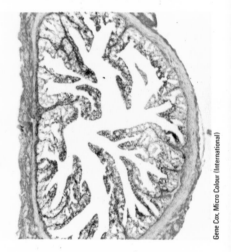

Gene Cox, Micro Colour (International)

The intricate structure of the inside of the Fallopian tube, as seen under the microscope.

FARMER'S LUNG is a disorder whose symptoms are rather similar to those of asthma. It occurs in men who are exposed to dusts from hay or grain. It seems that the dusts contain various fungi, but these do not actually infect the lung. The disorder is in fact an allergy to fungi, and it is this allergic reaction which produces the characteristic wheezing, breathlessness and cough. The symptoms occur, at certain seasons of the year, in farmers and stableworkers. Removal from exposure to dust usually relieves the symptoms.

FATS are one of the three types of energy-giving foods in the diet (see **diet**) the other two being carbohydrates (see **carbohydrates**) and proteins (see **proteins**). Fat is a very rich source of energy, providing more than twice as many calories per gram as do carbohydrates or proteins.

Fatty foods include, of course, butter, milk and fatty meats. Western Man has tended recently to eat more and more of this type of fat (called *saturated* fat). The alarming rise in death rate from coronary disease in recent years has led doctors to speculate that such disease might be related to consumption of saturated fats in the diet. There is some evidence to support this theory. It is possible to show that people whose diets are rich in butter, milk, and meats such as beef or pork have higher blood levels of certain blood chemicals, including cholesterol (see **cholesterol**) and triglycerides. The levels of these chemicals are also increased in many people with coronary heart disease. People who live in economically deprived areas of the world and who eat very little saturated fats (which are essentially 'rich men's food') tend to have low blood levels of these chemicals, and a low incidence of these types of heart disease. If the economic conditions in a country improve over the years, so that the population can afford butter and other saturated fats, the incidence of coronary disease tends to increase. This does not prove, however, that saturated fats are responsible for the virtual epidemic of heart disease threatening Western Man; there are other factors which could well be responsible – for instance, the increasing tendency to a sedentary life, or the ever-growing consumption of sugar. Nevertheless, a considerable number of physicians (particularly in America) now suggest to likely subjects of heart disease that they give up butter and other sources of saturated fat as far as possible. Instead of these foods (which are, in fact, largely animal fats) such patients can eat unsaturated (mainly vegetable) fats such as margarine, corn oil and cotton-seed oil. Drugs can also be given to lower the levels of cholesterol and triglycerides in the blood.

FAVUS is a disease of the skin, uncommon in Great Britain, caused by a fungus. It is also known as honeycomb ringworm.

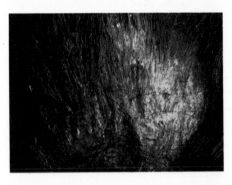

The typical appearance of the scalp affected by the fungus which causes honeycomb ringworm.

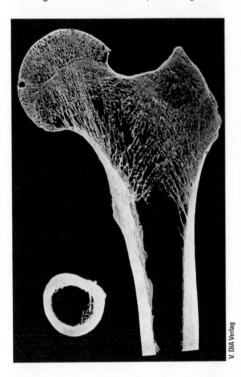

V. DIA Verlag

A cross-section of the upper end of the femur shows its complicated internal bony structure.

FEMUR is the thigh bone. Extending from hip to the knee, it is the longest bone in the human body, to which the most powerful muscles of the body are attached.

143

Fractures of the femur are usually serious. In young, healthy people such breaks are rare except in the type of severe injury seen after car accidents. In old people, however, fractures of the upper end of the bone ('hip' fractures) are more common and the complications which may follow are sometimes fatal. As a rule, treatment is directed to getting the patient mobile again as soon as possible, since the incidence of complications increases with the length of the time spent in bed. The orthopaedic surgeon therefore usually attempts to repair the fracture surgically. This can often be done by pinning the broken femur with a steel nail or blade.

FETISHISM is a form of sexual perversion in which a particular object or material comes to have a sexual significance for the person. Probably the most frequently encountered form of fetishism is that which involves an unnatural interest in clothing of rubber, leather or plastic, and there are a number of men (and some women) who cannot enjoy a satisfactory sexual relationship unless their partner is wearing some garment made of these materials. Some psychoanalysts believe that this affliction is due to an error in the development of the sex drive during infancy.

FEVER means any elevation of body temperature above normal. There are many possible causes of fever, but the most common is infection. Almost any kind of infection can cause fever. In children, it is sometimes difficult to be certain of the site of the infection and of the nature of the infecting organism. The commonest infections causing fever in children, however, are colds and other upper respiratory tract viral infections (see **chills**), tonsillitis (see **tonsillitis**), ear infections (otitis media; see **ear disorders**) and chest infections (see **bronchitis,** and **bronchiolitis**). Other fairly common causes include appendicitis, urinary infections (such as pyelitis) and meningitis. In addition, the common infectious fevers of childhood — measles, German measles, chickenpox and mumps, all produce an elevation of temperature. In general, it is

144

reasonable for a parent to assume that any child with a fever probably has an infection. Crying and emotional upsets can produce minor elevations in temperature but it is not always safe to assume as parents often do, that fevers of 101F. or upwards are due to teething.

FIBRILLATION means rapid contraction of muscle fibres (fibrils). The term is used in a number of senses but is applied in particular in connection with an abnormal heart rhythm called atrial (auricular) fibrillation. This is one of the most frequently encountered causes of heart failure (see **congestive heart failure**). It is characterized by a completely irregular pulse at the wrist. The two upper chambers of the heart (the atria) do not contract rhythmically. Instead, the muscle contracts very rapidly and pumps ineffectively. The lower chambers (the ventricles), which under normal conditions beat synchronously with the atria, are thrown out of gear, and themselves contract fast and irregularly, thus producing the characteristic pulse.

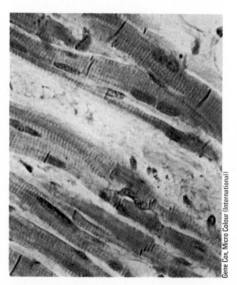

Gene Cox, Micro Colour (International)

Microscopic view of heart muscle fibres. In fibrillation they contract in an erratic way.

FIBRIN is a protein in the blood which forms a mesh-like structure, the basis of blood clots which plug bleeding vessels.

FIBROBLASTS are special cells which help to lay down connective tissue. They appear in large numbers wherever a tissue is damaged, and are involved in the healing process of wounds.

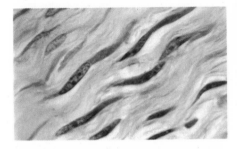

Fibroblasts are cells responsible for laying down new fibrous tissue when scars form.

FIBROCYSTIC DISEASE is a serious disorder of childhood. Various mucus-secreting tissues of the body are affected — notably the pancreas (see **pancreas**) and the lungs. Absence of digestive pancreatic enzymes makes it difficult for food to be absorbed from the digestive tract, and frequent diarrhoea results. More important, infants fail to gain weight, and become grossly wasted. The lung disorder leads to recurrent chest infection.

FIBROIDS are non-malignant tumours (lumps) which occur in the wall of the womb. They are common in middle-aged women, especially those who have not borne children. Occasionally, fibroids may attain great size, and it is sometimes necessary to remove them, or the entire womb. (See **hysterectomy**.)

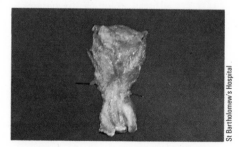

Fibroids are a common cause of bleeding from the womb, and abnormally heavy periods.

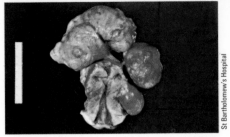

Fibroids removed from the uterus. Although not malignant, they may attain great size.

FIBROSIS means the formation of fibrous tissue, usually in response to inflammation. Pulmonary fibrosis is an example of this process occurring in the lungs; it may be caused by tuberculosis (see **tuberculosis**), pneumoconiosis (see **pneumoconiosis**), sarcoidosis (see **sarcoidosis**) and a number of other lung conditions.

FIBROSITIS means inflammation of fibrous tissue. The word is used loosely to describe various minor aches and pains — in particular those associated with muscle strains and arthritis. There is, however, no medical condition called fibrositis.

FIBULA is the smaller of the two bones which make up the lower leg.

FILARIASIS means infestation with filarial worms. These are minute parasites found in tropical regions. Among the serious disorders they can cause is a form of elephantiasis — the condition in which a part of the body (for instance the leg) becomes swollen to elephantine proportions. The worms (of a species called Wurcheria bancrofti) block the lymph channels which normally drain the affected part. The disease is transmitted by mosquitoes, but in other types of filariasis worms may be passed on by other insects, such as gnats.

FINGERS are the digits of the hand. Despite their delicacy and relatively slim structure, the fingers are very strong, the muscles which control them being principally situated in the forearm and in the palm of the hand. The fingers themselves consist of little more than skin, nails, tendons running from the muscles of the forearm, and bones. Each finger contains three bones (or phalanges) except the thumb, with only two.

FIRST AID is attention given in an emergency, before the arrival of medical assistance or transport to hospital. Knowledge of some of the basic principles of first aid is well worth while. Perhaps the most important rule of first aid is – do not interfere unnecessarily. A doctor called to a person injured in an accident will interfere with him as little as possible, but many lay people regrettably regard the sight of an injured man as an invitation to start sitting him up, forcing his head down, pouring liquid down his throat and so on. A good example is the treatment of fainting (see **fainting**) – a person who faints should be allowed to lie flat until he recovers – not dragged upright.

The second important rule of first aid is to ensure the patient is able to breathe. Many unconscious people die after accidents simply because their 'airway' (the passage from the nose and mouth to the lungs) is blocked. The mouth should be cleared of blood or vomit with a finger and dentures removed; then with the patient lying on one side, the jaw should be brought forward and supported. If the patient does not start to breathe, artificial respiration by the mouth-to-mouth method should be started at once. (This technique is described under drowning.) **First aid in common emergencies.** *Burns and scalds:* there is nothing to put on the skin to help; if the affected area needs medical attention, simply cover it with a clean cloth (e.g. a freshly laundered handkerchief) and get the patient to hospital. *Drowning:* clear the airway and start immediate mouth-to-mouth respiration (see **drowning**). *Electric shock:* give immediate mouth-to-mouth respiration if the patient is not breathing, and, if possible, cardiac massage as well (described under drowning). *Fits:* put a firm object between the patients teeth and turn him on his side (see **epilepsy**). *Fractures and dislocations:* try to immobilize the part if possible; do not attempt any

manipulation yourself; get the patient to hospital (see **fractures**). *Gassing:* drag the patient into the open air, and give immediate mouth-to-mouth respiration (see **carbon monoxide**). *Haemorrhage* (bleeding): maintain firm continuous pressure on the bleeding point with a pad (e.g. a clean handkerchief); do not apply a tourniquet (see **bleeding**). *Head injuries:* if the patient is unconscious, ensure he can breathe without obstruction, as outlined above. Any patient who has been knocked out must go to hospital; disregard of this rule may have fatal consequences. *Poisoning or drug overdose:* except in the case of corrosive poisons (acids and alkalies), make the patient vomit at once, and then rush him to hospital. *Unconsciousness:* ensure the patient can breathe, as outlined above; do not try to give alcohol or any other fluid.

The last point applies to all persons who are injured in any way whatsoever; give no fluids, and indeed, nothing by mouth at all until the patient has been seen by a doctor.

FISSURE means a narrow ulcer or crack in skin or mucous membrane. Examples include the fissures at the corner of the mouth which most people get at one time or another, and fissure-in-ano. The latter is an extremely common and painful condition of the back passage.

FISTULA literally means 'a pipe'. In medicine it means any abnormal channel leading from one body cavity to another, or from a body cavity to the skin.

FITS are attacks in which the patient is overcome by a convulsion, with characteristic rapid alternate contraction and relaxation of muscle groups, so that parts of the body twitch.

Fits have many possible causes. In early childhood, they are usually related simply to the immaturity of the child's central nervous system, and may be provoked by such factors as a rise in temperature, due to infection (see **convulsions**). Such fits are rarely indicative of epilepsy. Epilepsy is, however, the commonest cause of fits in adult life. (See **epilepsy**.)

FLAGELLATION means whipping. In previous times many religious orders indulged in flagellation, as a means of punishing 'the sins of the flesh'. Today in medical terms, it is a variety of sado-masochistic perversion (see **sadism, masochism, perversion**). The sufferer can achieve sexual satisfaction only while whipping (or, more often, being whipped by) his partner. Flagellation is often associated with other perversions – in particular leather fetishism (see **fetishism**).

FLAT FOOT is a deformity in which there is an absence of the normal 'arch' of the foot, so that the entire sole rests flat on the ground. This can be demonstrated very clearly by looking at the patient's footprints. A normal footprint is extremely narrow at the middle part of the foot, since only the outer edge of the sole should be in contact with the ground here. The footprint of a person with flat foot is very much wider.

Flat foot is a very considerable disability. It more or less rules out any serious athletic activity, and makes certain occupations involving walking unsuitable for the patient. The origin of flat foot is problematical. It certainly occurs in some people who have to stand or walk a lot (e.g. policemen). However, degrees of flat foot also occur in quite young children. In any case, the actual loss of the arch of the foot is due to laxness of the muscles, tendons and ligaments which should maintain the normal posture. The condition can therefore be considerably ameliorated by improving the tone of the muscles and tendons, and this can be done by careful exercises. These should be prescribed by an orthopaedic surgeon, who will also advise if any other form of treatment is necessary.

FLATULENCE means gas ('wind'), in the stomach or intestines. Except in one quite rare condition, gas does not actually form in the stomach, and it can be shown by X-ray studies that gas which is brought up by belching has almost invariably been swallowed by the patient who is suffering from flatulence. He is unaware, as a rule, that he is doing this, and shortly after belching he swallows more air, and so perpetuates the process. All that is required is a conscious effort to stop swallowing air. Taking remedies like bicarbonate of soda will not help. Bicarbonate has a considerable reputation for 'helping to get the wind up', but in fact all it does is to release carbon dioxide gas into the stomach. Naturally, this gas is itself belched up within a few minutes, and the patient imagines that the bicarbonate has therefore done him some good.

The main exception to the rule that gas which is belched is merely swallowed air occurs when there is an obstruction to the exit from the stomach. Occasionally, a gastric ulcer may cause such a narrowing. Under these circumstances, food may be retained for long periods in the stomach and may actually break down with the formation of gaseous products. It sometimes happens that the gaseous mixture is explosive, and there have been occasional reports of violent (but fortunately harmless) detonations when a patient has belched while smoking a cigarette.

Although gas does not normally form in the stomach, a considerable quantity is produced in the intestines, through the breakdown of food by the digestive processes. Almost everyone occasionally experiences colicky pain due to pockets of gas becoming trapped for a few minutes. No treatment is effective, or, indeed, required for such occasional episodes. It is possible that reduction in the quantity of starchy foods, such as bread and potatoes, in the diet will help to prevent the development of such flatulence.

FLATUS is the medical name for wind passed from the back passage.

FLEAS are minute parasitic insects. The common flea which lives on Man's body and feeds on his blood is called Pulex irritans. It is found throughout the world, being, of course, much more common where hygiene is lax. As a rule, the insect is merely a source of irritation to Man, but, under certain circumstances, fleas can carry infection. For instance, plague (Black Death) is passed on by fleas which have bitten infected rats. Fortunately, such

147

insecticides as DDT are extremely effective against fleas. The best protection, of course, is scrupulous hygiene — especially in regard to washing, and to laundering of clothes and bed clothes.

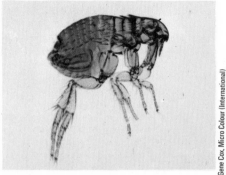

This dog flea will make your dog scratch, but it will not live on a human body.

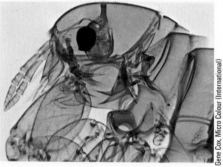

The human flea injects a chemical through its mouthparts that stops the blood from clotting.

FLIES of various kinds are important in relation to disease. The common house fly is one of the most widespread of all pests. It lays its eggs in manure or other rotting matter, and tends to settle and feed on all kinds of filth. Material containing germs is thus carried on its legs and around its mouth. When it alights on human food, bacteria are scattered from its legs. In addition, it both vomits material from its crop onto the food and also leaves its droppings. It is therefore one of the filthiest of insects, and no effort should be spared to eradicate it from kitchens and anywhere where food is stored, prepared or eaten. Although many house flies are now resistant to DDT, newer preparations

148

including some in aerosol form, are very effective in ridding a house of the insects. Other measures which should be taken against them include the careful covering of dustbins, hygienic sewage disposal, and the prompt incineration of material on rubbish tips; all these are sites which are favoured by flies for settling, feeding and breeding.

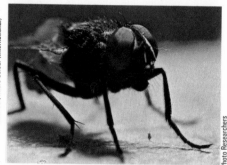

The house fly settles on all kinds of filth then scatters bacteria on human food.

FLOODING is the lay term for heavy vaginal bleeding. *Bleeding during pregnancy* needs immediate medical attention; among the common causes are miscarriage (in early pregnancy) and antipartum haemorrhage (in late pregnancy).

Flooding occurring at the menopause (change of life) is always an abnormal symptom. Many women do not realize this fact. In a normal change of life, the periods should not be unduly heavy — they should either gradually dwindle in amount, or occur at greater and greater intervals of time, or merely stop suddenly and never return. Anything else is abnormal and merits a full gynaecological examination.

Flooding occurring at the periods also needs investigation. Sometimes hormone treatment is helpful. Not infrequently, a sudden episode of flooding may not be due to a period at all, but to an unnoticed miscarriage (a *missed abortion*). This condition should be suspected if a woman has always had normal periods and then, perhaps after missing one or even two, develops severe flooding. The minor operation of dilatation and curettage ('*D and C*'), in which the womb is scraped, will clear up the condition.

FLUKES are minute parasitic worms which infect both Man and animals. Examples include the liver fluke, the lung fluke and the schistosome. The last is the parasite responsible for schistosomiasis (Bilharzia), the disease which ravages many tropical countries, (see **Bilharzia**).

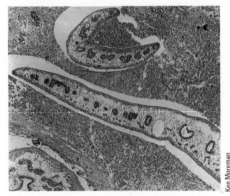

Flukes in the liver, as seen under the microscope. They may remain undetected for years.

FLUORIDE means any compound of a chemical base with fluorine, a gas closely related to chlorine. Fluorides have been used in the past to treat certain bone diseases — notably osteoporosis, a generalized loss in density of the bones which occurs in elderly people. Their use has now been abandoned in such conditions, however, because of the danger of toxic effects — notably blindness. Fluorides in very small doses (about one to two parts per million) are used in the fluoridation of water (see **fluoridation**).

FLUORIDATION is the addition of fluoride to mains water. Children who drink water containing about one part fluorine per million have a lessened incidence of dental decay. The weight of medical and dental opinion has to date been in favour of fluoridation of water. However, despite the fact that much of the opposition to fluoridation has been wildly irrational (there being, for instance a school of thought in America which holds that the process is part of a Communist plot to sap the virility of Western Man), nonetheless it is worth bearing in mind that doctors and scientists are occasionally very wrong.

FOETOR means an offensive smell on the breath (see **breath**).

FOETUS is the name applied to the unborn child in the womb (uterus). The fertilized egg enters the uterus via the Fallopian tube (see **Fallopian tube**), and embeds itself in the uterine lining. Before long, the spherical ovum has developed a more elongated appearance, and from this stage until about the eighth week of intra-uterine life, the foetus referred to as the embryo (see **embryo**). By the eighth week, all the organs are fully formed, and from then onwards the foetus simply grows in size. Although it can move its limbs at this stage, it is not until about the eighteenth week of pregnancy (later in women who are pregnant for the first time) that the mother feels the foetus move inside her. At about the twenty-sixth to twenty-eighth week of pregnancy, the foetus is just about capable of separate existence from the mother, but only under very favourable conditions. Such very premature babies weigh about two pounds, and even with modern medical techniques, few of them survive. Under normal circumstances, however, a foetus will remain in the mother's womb until fully mature, at about the fortieth week of pregnancy.

FOLIC ACID is one of the B group of vitamins. It is found in many green vegetables. Deficiency of folic acid leads to a form of anaemia very similar to pernicious anaemia (see **anaemia**). In temperate climates, such a deficiency is not uncommon in pregnant women, due to the demands of the foetus. Doctors frequently give expectant mothers routine folic acid, as well as iron, to guard against anaemia. Folic acid treatment carries one particular danger — if the patient actually has pernicious anaemia (which is due to vitamin B12 deficiency) then folic acid will make things very much worse, and also make the condition harder to diagnose. For this reason many doctors feel that proprietary 'tonics' containing folic acid should be banned.

FONTANELLE is a word applied to the gaps between the growing bones in a

149

baby's skull, which form 'soft' areas. There are two main fontanelles – the anterior and posterior. The posterior is only present for a very short time after birth as a small triangular area towards the back of the skull, in the mid-line, and rapidly closes as the bones around it develop.

The anterior fontanelle, on the other hand, is present for about 18 months after birth. It is a four-sided aperture, readily felt under the skin, about an inch above the hair-line of the forehead. Doctors frequently examine this fontanelle, since its condition provides some help in the evaluation of certain disorders. For instance, the skin over the fontanelle bulges in cases of raised intracranial pressure (e.g. meningitis), but is sunken where a child is badly dehydrated as in severe gastro-enteritis).

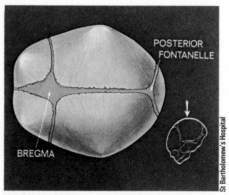

POSTERIOR FONTANELLE

BREGMA

St Bartholomew's Hospital

The fontanelles are the gaps between the developing bones of a baby's skull.

FOOD see **diet**.

FOOD POISONING is a general term which covers accidental poisoning through eating contaminated food. The contamination may be by chemical poisons, by the toxins of certain germs, or by the germs themselves.

An example of the first type of food poisoning would be contamination of (say) a mushroom omelette by poisonous fungi. More commonly, however, the term 'food poisoning' implies poisoning through the agency of bacteria (see **bacteria**). The commonest type of bacteria which produce a toxin (poison) are Staphylococci (see **staphylococcus**).

150

The Staphylococcus is present in the noses of a high proportion of the population, and also in boils and infected cuts. It is a matter of the greatest ease for such germs to get into food during preparation, if those responsible do not take care, such as thorough washing of the hands. The foods which tend to be affected are those containing cream and cream products – for instance, many types of cake. Once in the food, the germs produce their toxin, and from this stage onwards *no amount of heating will provide protection against food poisoning*. Cooking will kill the germs, but will not destroy the toxin.

Bacteria which themselves cause food poisoning, without producing any toxin, include the Salmonellae. These germs are harboured by many animals, and Man may be infected by eating contaminated meat from such animals (particularly processed or tinned meat). Ducks also harbour Salmonellae, and duck eggs are liable to contain the germs. For this reason, they should be boiled for at least 15 minutes. Humans may be 'carriers' of germs in their alimentary tracts, and readily infect others.

There are many other organisms which may cause food poisoning. In most cases, however, the symptoms are the same – abdominal pain, diarrhoea and vomiting. If the symptoms are severe, call a doctor.

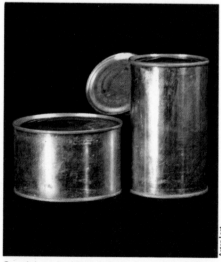

Anton Last

Suspicious-looking bulges in cans of food. They may indicate the presence of bacteria.

FOOT is the part of the leg below the ankle. In many ways, its bony structure is similar to that of the hand; there are five digits (the toes); four of these contain three bones each and the fifth (the big or great toe) contains two bones. The bones of the middle part of the foot are arranged in an arch; loss of this arch structure leads to the condition known as *flat foot* (see **flat foot**).

FORESKIN or prepuce is the fold of skin which covers the glans penis completely in young boys (and incompletely in adults). Many doctors believe it has a valuable protective function, and circumcision (see **circumcision**), the removal of the foreskin, is recommended less frequently today than it used to be, except in the United States. Many paediatricians hold that it is unwise of mothers to stretch the baby's foreskin and break the delicate adhesions which bind it down by pulling it back, as many do. Some of the adhesions, around the base of the glans penis, may not normally part until adolescence. However, boys should be taught, at about the age of 3 or 4 to wash the foreskin carefully each day. This prevents irritation and inflammation (see **balanitis**), which are quite common but should not be allowed to develop. Chronic inflammation over a period of many years may lead to cancer of the penis in later life.

The condition called *paraphimosis* occurs when the foreskin becomes tightly constricted around the penis at the base of the glans. This condition is extremely painful, and may sometimes necessitate a minor operation to relieve it.

FORGETFULNESS affects most people at one time or another, particularly in later life. Patients quite frequently consult their doctors because they cannot recall facts (e.g. for an exam) but there is little or nothing that can be done medically in such cases, except in the case of a serious psychological disturbance. In a healthy person, a tendency to forget important facts can often be combated by employing mnemonics or similar tricks of association. All commercial memory-improving courses are based on such schemes. To take a simple example, a person may not be able to recall the name of an important client, say, Mr Green, but be able to fix it in his mind by associating the person with the colour green.

FRACTURES are breaks in bones. There is no difference whatever in meaning between the words 'break' and 'fracture', as many people imagine.

Fractures are generally divided into two types – *compound* and *simple*. A compound fracture is one in which the skin is broken, though the bone may not necessarily be protruding. The significance of this is considerable, because it greatly increases the chance of infection of the broken bone. Antibiotics have lessened the danger from such infection considerably. Simple fractures are those in which the skin is not broken – the majority of all fractures. *Comminuted* fractures are those in which the bone is shattered into many fragments.

Except where there is only a very minor crack, fractured bones are frequently immobilized at the joints above and below the break to give the bony tissues the best

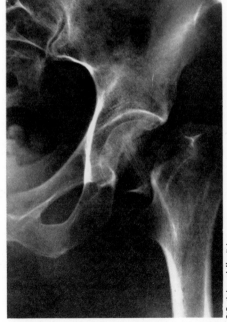

St Bartholomew's Hospital

Fractures can be seen in X-ray pictures. Here the head of the thigh-bone is fractured.

151

chance of rapid healing. In young, healthy people, most bones of the body take about 6 weeks to mend after an uncomplicated fracture. The rate of healing can, however, be slowed by numerous factors.

FRATERNAL TWINS (see **dizygotic twins**).

FRECKLES are brown spots which appear on the skin, particularly on the face, after exposure to the sun. They are particularly common in children, especially those with fair skins. The spots are due to the dark pigment melanin. Nothing can be done to make freckles go away. Girls may not like them, but they can be attractive.

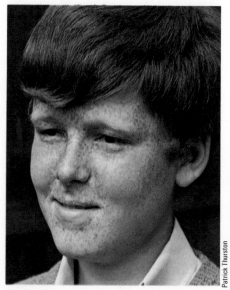
Patrick Thurston

Freckles are caused by small concentrated specks of the pigment melanin in the skin.

FRENCH LETTERS are condoms, or sheaths worn over the penis to prevent pregnancy. They form a moderately effective type of contraception, but considerably diminish sensitivity during intercourse. The thinner types of sheath (with which sensitivity is less impaired) are more likely to fail. Sheaths provide only incomplete protection against venereal disease.

FREUD, SIGMUND, was the great Austrian neuropsychiatrist who founded

152

psychoanalysis. His contribution to the study of mental health has probably been unequalled. Although some of his theories have been considerably modified by his successors, his place in the history of medicine is assured.

Freud conceived of the human mind as being in three parts – the id, the superego and the ego (see **ego**). He pointed out the great importance of the subconscious – that vast portion of the mind of which we are never aware, but which may come to the surface during dreams. Some of Freud's most important work was done on the significance of dreams and the part they play in helping us to act out unconscious desires. Freud suggested that most, if not all, dreams represented a 'safety-valve', but that unconscious desires might make their appearance in dreams in an altered and therefore more acceptable form because of the existence of what he called the 'dream censor'. The classic instance of the dream censor in operation is the example of a sexually frustrated woman dreaming of a church steeple (which represented the male organ).

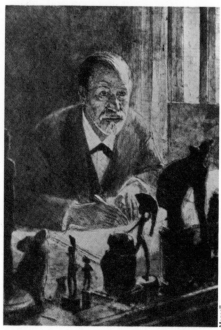
Mansell

Sigmund Freud, founder of psychoanalysis, caused a revolution in psychological ideas.

FROSTBITE is injury to the body through exposure to cold. Commonly, frostbite affects the fingers and toes, because the temperature at the extremities is rather lower than that elsewhere in the body, and because the blood supply to these parts can very easily be cut off. In addition, because people have to use their hands even in cold climates, they tend to wear insufficient protection on them.

In a typical case of frostbite, after exposure to severe cold, the fingers become white, cold, powerless and numb. If immediate counter-measures are not taken the consequences are likely to be gangrene, and the eventual loss of the fingers. Rapid re-warming of the hand, however, is dangerous, since it may lead to further damage to the delicate tissues of the blood vessels. Excess warmth will usually make the fingers flush a bright red and become very painful. What is required is gentle warming over a prolonged period. The traditional Eskimo method is to place the frozen part for several hours against someone else's body. There is a widespread belief that frostbite can be treated by rubbing handfuls of snow on the affected part. This is untrue and dangerous since it may damage the tissues further.

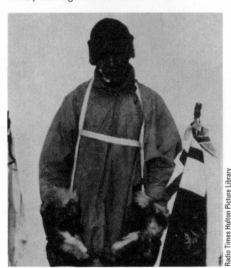

Frostbite is a grave hazard to polar explorers. Oates, who went to the South Pole with Captain Scott, left his companions and died because he had frostbite.

FROZEN SHOULDER is a painful condition occurring in the middle-aged and elderly, characterised by stiffness and limitation of movement in the joint. Treatment involves physiotherapy.

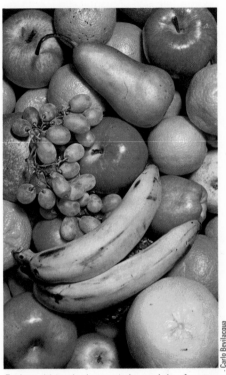

Fruits, although they consist mainly of water, are valuable for their vitamin C.

FRUITS are useful sources of vitamin C, and constitute an important part of the diet. Most fruits consist mainly of water, with a moderate amount of carbohydrate (see **carbohydrate**). An average sized orange contains some 10 grams of carbohydrate, or the equivalent of two heaped teaspoonfuls of sugar. Apart from the vitamin C content, fruits such as apples may help to clean teeth and remove other food debris. Many dentists believe that for this reason there is considerable justification for giving a child 'an apple a day'.

FUGUE is a type of hysterical state (see **hysteria**) in which a patient tends to wander off by himself, often for several days at a time, and usually returns without

153

any clear idea of what has happened. This condition occurs quite commonly among teenagers, particularly girls, unable to cope with some particularly difficult situation or problem. There is no conscious decision to go into this kind of mental state, or to 'go missing' and the loss of memory is perfectly genuine. Such episodes should not be dismissed as mere wilfulness or treated as minor emotional upsets — the patient needs expert psychiatric help (see also **hysteria**).

FUNGI are members of a very large group of living things related more closely to the plant than to the animal kingdom. (Some biologists actually classify all fungi as plants, while others place them in a category by themselves). A large number of fungi are either parasitic (living off other living things) or saprophytic (living off dead plants or animals). Among the latter are many of the largest fungi, such as those found on rotton trees or dead vegetation.

The fungi of main medical interest are the edible and poisonous ones and those which actually live on the human body.

The commonest fungus which is eaten is the mushroom *(Psalliota campestris)*. This fungus is completely harmless, even if it has little nutritive value. Its skin is white, its gills are brown, and the base of its stem is clubbed. There is also a small downward pointing 'collar' round the stem, just below the gills, and there is *no* volva, or upward pointing ring, round the base of the stem — a feature which characterises the highly poisonous 'Death Cap' mushroom *(Amanita phalloides)*. Otherwise, the latter may look very like the edible mushroom, though its gills tend to be whiter and its skin more discoloured and often yellowish.

Other poisonous fungi, such as Fly Agaric *(Amanita muscaria)* which has a red cap with white spots on it, are so striking in appearance that they are unlikely to be eaten, except possibly by small children, left unattended.

The main danger is the Death Cap fungus, which contains certain alkaloids, notably muscarine, which cause vomiting, diarrhoea, and abdominal pain. Once in the bloodstream, muscarine may stop the

most vital pumping action of the heart.

Treatment of this type of poisoning consists in encouraging the patient to vomit, and giving him atropine injections, which block the effect of the muscarine. Very few people actually die from fungus poisoning.

Certain fungi found in South and Central America may produce hallucinations if eaten. Some of these contain a chemical similar in chemical structure to LSD.

The fungi which live on the human body are usually microscopic. They include the dermatophytes (see **dermatophytes**) which cause athlete's foot (see **athlete's foot**) and the fungus called *Candida albicans* or *Monilia* which is responsible for thrush in babies, a type of vaginal discharge in women, and a chronic disorder of the finger nails.

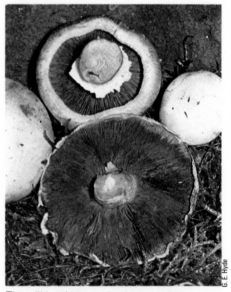

The edible mushroom is a harmless fungus, but some other kinds are poisonous.

FURUNCLE means a boil (see **boil**).

FUSIDIC ACID is a relatively new antibiotic, introduced during the 1960s, chemically related to the new semi-synthetic penicillins. It is usually kept in reserve for hospital use against penicillin-resistant germs, in particular various staphylococci (see **staphylococci**).

GALL BLADDER is a pear-shaped sac which lies on the under surface of the liver. It is about 4 inches long and has a capacity of about an ounce and a half in the undistended state. The only opening in the gall bladder is at the apex, where a narrow duct (the cystic duct) leads out to join the main biliary passage from the liver (the common hepatic duct), and form the common bile duct, through which bile flows into the first part of the intestine, or duodenum.

The function of bile is to aid the digestion of fat (see **bile**). About a pint is produced by the liver each day. The flow is not continuous, however, occurring mainly when a fatty meal is eaten. The gall bladder acts as a reservoir in which bile is stored until required; whenever anything fatty is eaten the organ contracts and pours bile into the duodenum. In addition, the gall bladder is capable of concentrating the bile considerably — when produced by the liver it is too dilute to be wholly effective as a digestive agent. There are a number of conditions which affect the gall bladder, including cholelithiasis, or gall stones (see **gall stones**), and cholecystitis (see **cholecystitis**). Cancer occasionally occurs in the gall bladder; it is more common in patients over the age of 60 than in younger people.

Gall bladder disease can be investigated by means of the procedure called *cholecystography*, in which a special radio-opaque dye is used to outline the gall bladder on X-rays. The dye is given by mouth the night before the X-rays. Next morning, the resultant concentration of bile should show up on the X-ray screen and, after a fatty meal, becomes smaller as the gall bladder contracts and empties. A similar dye can also be given by injection.

Removal of the gall bladder (cholecystectomy) may be necessary when it is seriously diseased.

GALL STONES are stones which form in the gall bladder (see **gall bladder**). They are made up of various chemicals, including cholesterol (see **cholesterol**) and calcium. Those which contain much calcium are easily seen on an ordinary X-ray of the upper abdomen, but pure

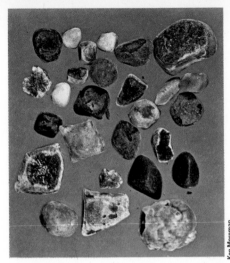

Gall stones vary in size, and may derive from calcium salts or cholesterol.

Ken Moreman

cholesterol stones do not show up. Special X-rays of the gall bladder and biliary passages (see **gall bladder**), are used if gall stones are suspected. Traditionally, gall stones are said to be commonest in women who are 'fair, fat, fertile and forty to fifty'. The stones may be very large (the size of a pigeon's egg) or very small indeed, and they may be single or multiple. Some gall bladders are found at operation to have hundreds of tiny stones within them.

Smaller stones are liable to pass out of the gall bladder into the cystic duct or common bile duct. Larger stones are unlikely to leave the gall bladder. Probably about one in ten of the population have at least one stone in the gall bladder after the age of fifty. They may cause little harm, but many doctors believe that their presence can cause dyspepsia, and perhaps predispose to cholecystitis (see **cholecystitis**). There is also a very small but definite risk of perforation of the gall bladder, and even cancerous change.

It is when gall stones move out of the gall bladder and lodge in the cystic duct, effectively blocking off the flow of bile, that trouble starts. The dammed-back bile in the gall bladder is likely to become infected, and cause acute cholecystitis. If the stone passes further on and jams in the

155

common bile duct, it obstructs outflow from the liver as well. (Stones sometimes actually form in the common bile duct itself). The obstruction leads to intense muscular contractions of the bile duct walls in an effort to expel the stone. The great pain which may result is known as 'biliary colic'.

Continued obstruction leads to 'obstructive jaundice' in which the motions become very pale, through absence of bile pigment reaching the intestines, and the urine very dark because the excess pigment passes instead into the blood and so to the kidneys. The treatment of gall stones is usually surgical.

GANGLION has two medical meanings. It is a term for a collection of nerve cells forming a swelling in the course of a nerve, and also for a swelling, filled with jelly-like material, which sometimes appears in the sheaths of tendons. The back of the wrist is a common site for the latter. A ganglion sometimes disperses if pressure is applied, but may require surgery.

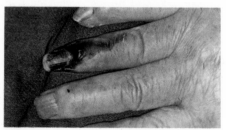

Gangrene occurs when the blood supply to the tissues is stopped and they die.

GANGRENE means the death of tissue, combined with putrefaction. There are two main types, *dry* and *moist*. Dry gangrene occurs when there has been a gradual impairment of the blood supply to a part of the body – for instance where arterial disease in elderly diabetics leads to gangrene of the toes. Moist gangrene occurs when an artery is *suddenly* blocked, crushed or cut across, and in certain conditions where veins draining a part (as well as arteries supplying blood to it) are blocked. In such cases, the tissues become swollen and infection usually follows. In either case, gangrenous parts of the body 156

cannot be brought back to life, and amputation is necessary. If this is not carried out, infection may spread.

GAS For poisoning by household gas (see **carbon monoxide**).

GASTRECTOMY means removal of the stomach by operation. Nowadays the word usually implies partial (as opposed to total) gastrectomy, in which roughly a third of the stomach is left. The operation has been performed on thousands of ulcer sufferers throughout the world since its introduction in Vienna in the late 1800s.

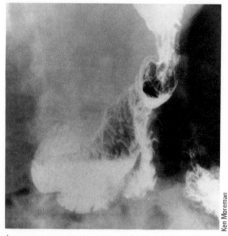

In gastrectomy, part of the stomach is removed. X-ray pictures show the stomach before *(above)* and after *(below)*.

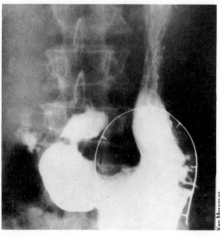

GASTRIC means of the stomach.

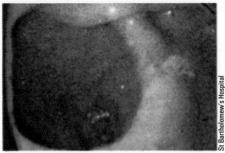

A gastric ulcer, in which there is a hole in the stomach lining, causes intense pain.

GASTRIC ULCERS are gaps in the lining, or epithelium, of the stomach wall which allow the acid gastric juice to attack the underlying tissues, and gradually erode them. There is normally a layer of mucus which protects the stomach from this digestive action; until the epithelium can heal, and re-establish its mucus layer, an ulcer will persist. The cause of gastric ulceration is unknown, but it does tend to run in families.

The chief symptom of gastric ulcer is usually pain in the upper abdomen, in the mid-line, often occurring when the stomach is empty. The pain may be relieved by taking food or alkalis, and worsened by certain substances such as aspirin. There may also be flatulence and nausea. Less common but more severe symptoms include the vomiting of blood, and the passing of altered blood in the stools (see **black motions**). Perforation of an ulcer occurs if the ulcer erodes its way completely through the stomach wall, thus allowing the acid stomach contents to escape into the abdominal cavity, causing peritonitis (see **peritonitis**). There is sudden severe abdominal pain and usually collapse. Hospital treatment — often surgical — is necessary.

For the uncomplicated case of gastric ulcer, however, treatment can be on an outpatient basis. Pain can be prevented and relieved by alkalis (antacids), and avoided by simple dietary measures; eating usually relieves pain for an hour or two, and the usual object of diet should be to try to keep the stomach full. Eating 'little and often' is therefore the rule. Many doctors nowadays believe that it does not greatly matter what actual food is eaten, though others still prefer to prescribe a diet consisting only of 'bland' foods — such as steamed fish and milk puddings. The only methods of treatment which seem to actually promote healing, as well as relieve symptoms, are bed rest, use of the drug carbenoxolone (see **carbenoxolone**) and stopping smoking. The only other curative treatment is by operation (see **gastrectomy; vagotomy;** also **peptic ulcers**).

GASTRITIS means inflammation of the stomach. There is no one condition called 'gastritis', since a variety of irritant agents may produce such inflammation. Perhaps the commonest of these is alcohol: concentrated alcohol in sufficient doses will produce symptoms of gastritis in almost anyone. These symptoms are pain of the 'indigestion' type, nausea, retching and (if the irritation is severe enough) even vomiting of blood.

GASTRO-ENTERITIS means inflammation of both stomach and intestines. The symptoms and causes are the same as those of enteritis (see **enteritis**), except that, since the stomach is involved as well as the intestines, there may be vomiting, in addition to diarrhoea, abdominal pain, and sometimes fever.

GASTROSCOPE is an instrument designed for looking at the interior of the stomach. At its simplest, a gastroscope is a long tube, with an eyepiece, and a light at the lower end, to enable inspection of the nature and progress of ulcers and other stomach conditions. A camera can be fitted to the gastroscope to preserve a permanent record of the patient's progress.

To reduce the discomfort of the examination the patient usually has pre-medication (see **pre-med**) to calm him down, and a local anaesthetic is sprayed on the back of the throat to make it easier to tolerate the gastroscope. Nonetheless, with this older type of gastroscope, he is virtually being asked to do what a sword-swallower does — allow a straight and rigid rod to be passed down into his stomach.

A newer type of gastroscope has been developed which is flexible, and much more comfortable for the patient. Called the *fibrescope* — it consists of a thick bundle of tiny glass rods, which will still transmit a good image of the interior of the stomach when bent. It was hoped at one stage that the tip of the fibrescope could be passed right through the stomach, and into the first part of the small intestine (the duodenum) where it could be used to inspect duodenal ulcers. This has not proved so, but the instrument is easier to use, and will get much farther round the stomach curve than the old rigid gastroscope.

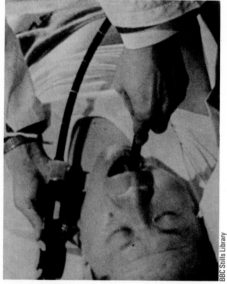

A gastroscope, with camera attached, enables a doctor to photograph a patient's stomach.

GPI is the commonly used abbreviation for *general paralysis of the insane*, one of the late manifestations of syphilis (see **syphilis**); paralysis and insanity are caused by the effect of the syphilis bacteria on the central nervous system. GPI is fortunately rare nowadays in most countries, but until the introduction of salvarsan as a treatment for syphilis in the early 1900s it was quite common. Many lives were ruined by it, and hospitals were full of people with this and other manifestations of late syphilis. The careers of many famous men, including Lord Randolph Churchill, one of

158

the most brilliant politicians of Victorian England, were ruined by it.

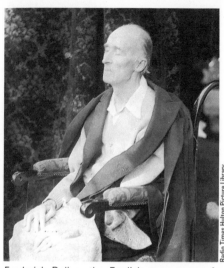

Frederick Delius, the English composer, suffered from general paralysis of the insane.

GENES are the minute carriers of our hereditary traits, whose existence was first postulated by Mendel, the founder of the science of genetics (see **genetics**). They are arranged in lines along the chromosomes, the tiny strands of genetic material found in 23 pairs in the nuclei of all body cells. During fertilization, 23 *single* chromosomes are contributed by the father (in a sperm cell) and 23 by the mother (in the ovum), so that the new individual has 23 *pairs*, with sets of genes from both parents. The child will thus grow up with characteristics inherited from both mother and father.

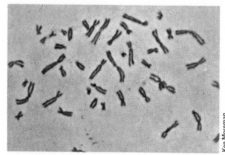

Chromosomes, seen here through a powerful microscope, carry the genes.

GENETICS is the science of heredity. Although it has long been realized that children inherit their parents' (and, to a less marked extent, their grandparents') characteristics, it was not until the 1860s that the study of inheritance was first put on a scientific basis by the abbot Gregor Mendel, who lived at Brno in what is now called Czechoslovakia. From his classic experiments with plants it became clear (after an interval of many years, during which his work was forgotten) that his conclusions applied, in general, to all living things.

Mendel's experiments showed that when two plants with a particular type of inheritance were cross-pollinated, there were simple laws that governed the likely nature of the new plants which were produced. These statistical laws were subsequently tested in such easily studied creatures as laboratory mice and fruit-flies and in due course, geneticists who studied patterns of inherited disease and of unusual characteristics found that the same rules applied to Man.

The applications of these discoveries are varied. For instance, knowledge of the inheritance of blood groups supplies valuable information in cases of disputed paternity. In another field, geneticists are being called in more and more to counsel people who have hereditary disorders in the family; in many such cases, it is possible to tell someone who is contemplating marriage or having children just exactly what the chances will be of transmitting the illness to future generations.

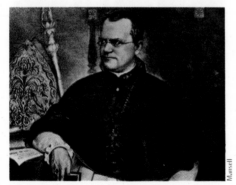

The Abbé Gregor Mendel, founder of the science of genetics and human heredity.

GERIATRICS is the speciality of medicine which deals with care of the aged. As Man lives longer, so the average age of the population becomes steadily more advanced. It is conceivable that children now alive will know a time when a third of the world's population is over sixty years of age.

Prolonging the lifespan of Man has inevitably created new problems. In all Western societies, there are now many old people who simply cannot look after themselves — even though many of them are not 'ill' in the usual sense of the word. In addition, family links have tended to break down in Western civilization — the aged Chinese peasant is likely to be looked after and revered by his children and grandchildren and great-grandchildren, but his counterpart in the West may find himself sent off to the old people's home or the geriatric ward.

Doctors who specialize in geriatrics (geriatricians) have a formidable task. Much of their work is concerned with social problems — for instance, putting old people in touch with the social services, so that they can be properly fed, clothed and housed. Much of the geriatrician's time is also devoted to 'remedial medicine' — for instance, helping people to learn to walk and feed themselves again after a stroke.

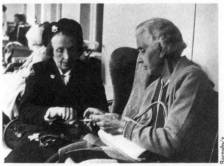

The elderly have problems all of their own. A WVS worker may help a doctor considerably.

GERMAN MEASLES or rubella, is an infectious virus illness spread by means of infection through the nose and mouth. The virus is carried in the tiny invisible droplets which are formed and released during breathing, laughing, coughing and sneezing. It is more common in childhood.

The infected child becomes mildly 'off-colour' about twelve to fourteen days later. Usually he has catarrh, slightly red eyes, and, most characteristically, enlarged lymph glands (see **glands**) in the neck. As a rule, a rash appears on the second day of the illness consisting of small, pink spots which usually appear first on the head, and then spread to the body, arms and legs. The child recovers within a couple of days, and complications are almost unknown. No special treatment is required. One attack probably gives lifelong immunity from re-infection, but it is so easy to mistake the disorder for several others (notably mild cases of measles) that no pregnant woman who thinks she has had the disease should ever assume she is immune and run the risk of infection. Rubella caught during early pregnancy is serious; where infection occurs in the first two to three months, the baby is likely to be born with one or more of a variety of defects, including blindness due to cataracts, heart and ear deformities and mental defects. Giving the mother an injection of human gamma-globulin may protect the child. Where, however, an expectant mother has definitely had an attack of German measles in the first two to three months of pregnancy, many doctors favour immediate abortion as the best course.

Little girls should certainly be encouraged to catch German measles (e.g. at 'German measles parties') but their parents must ensure that they do not come into contact with anyone who is pregnant.

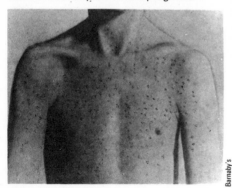

The fully-developed rash of German measles. It rarely lasts for more than a day or so.

GERMS are micro-organisms. Usually the word is used of both bacteria (which are, basically, large germs) and viruses (which are very much smaller germs), but it can be used to describe other types of microscopic living things as well (see **bacteriology; bacteria; viruses**).

GESTATION means pregnancy. The commonly-used phrase *period of gestation* means 'length of pregnancy'. The longest period of gestation in the animal world is that of the elephant, which is roughly two years. In humans, the average period of gestation is about 40 weeks (280 days), but much longer periods, in the region of 330 days, are occasionally accepted by courts, trying legitimacy cases.

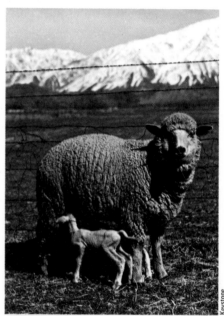

In general the larger the animal, the longer the gestation; for a sheep it is five months.

GIDDINESS (see **dizziness**).

GIN is an alcoholic drink flavoured with juniper. It has no particular medical value, and, like all forms of alcohol, should not be given to sick people, or as a form of first-aid, except with a doctor's consent. Its reputation for producing abortions is due to mere wishful thinking.

GLANDS are organs of the body which produce secretions. In the widest sense, the word gland could be applied to many organs including, for instance, the liver, which secretes bile. By convention, however, the term is restricted to certain groups of organs: the exocrine glands, the endocrine glands, and the lymph glands.

Exocrine glands, or glands of external secretion, are those which have a *duct.* These do not release their secretions into the blood-stream, but via the duct, or channel. Examples of exocrine glands include the sweat glands of the skin, each of which releases its sweat down a minute duct which leads to the skin. Other exocrine glands include the mammaries (breasts), which have ducts opening at the nipple.

Endocrine glands, or 'glands of internal secretion', are ductless. These secrete chemicals directly into the blood-stream. Such released chemicals are called 'hormones', a term meaning 'chemical messengers'. Examples of endocrine glands include the pituitary, thyroid and adrenal glands (see **endocrine glands**).

Some glands of the body are both exocrine and endocrine in nature, since they produce more than one secretion. The pancreas, for example (see **pancreas**) produces an exocrine secretion which passes down the pancreatic duct into the intestine, where it aids digestion. However, the gland also produces certain hormones, released directly into the blood-stream. The most well-known of these is insulin.

The lymph, or lymphatic, glands (see **lymph glands**) are small aggregations of tissue occurring in various parts of the body — notably the neck, armpits, and groins. It is these glands which enlarge when there is infection or inflammation in the area which they drain — for instance, the neck glands if the throat is sore.

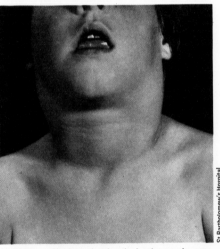
St Bartholomew's Hospital

In illness, the lymph glands in the neck, armpit and groin are likely to swell up.

GLANDULAR FEVER or infectious mononucleosis, is an infectious disease which is almost certainly due to a virus. However, efforts to isolate such an organism have not so far been successful. It is commonest in young adults and adolescents; this may not be entirely unrelated to the fact that many doctors believe it can be passed on by kissing, a theory which is fairly credible.

The symptoms vary, but usually include fever and enlargement of the glands at the sides and back of the neck. Other features may include sore throat, generalized aches and pains, a rash and a feeling of prostration. The diagnosis is made by means of blood tests. These show at some stage in

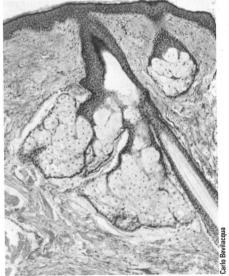
Carlo Bevilacqua

Sebaceous glands release oil which lubricates the skin and keeps it in good condition.

161

the disease a characteristic increase in the number of one kind of white blood cell; in addition, they usually show a positive reaction to a laboratory procedure called the Paul Bunnell test. There is no specific treatment, but recovery is the rule.

GLAUCOMA is a condition characterized by increase of pressure within the eye. There are many types of glaucoma, but untreated, all are liable to lead to blindness. In one common type, the patient has occasional attacks of dimness of vision, in which he sees haloes round lights. Eventually, he develops a severe attack, in which there is marked impairment of vision, associated with severe pain in the eye. The pain is frequently so bad that the patient vomits repeatedly. Acute glaucoma of this type is an emergency, and must be treated in hospital without delay. Fortunately, surgical and medical treatment, including the administration of special eyedrops, have considerably improved the outlook for most cases of glaucoma.

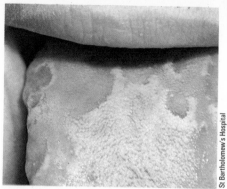

Inflammation of the tongue signals glossitis, often the result of deficiency diseases.

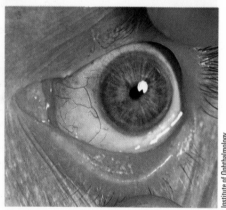

Glaucoma produces high pressure within the eyeball which leads to dimness of vision.

GLEET is a term for the discharge which occurs in gonorrhoea (see **gonorrhoea**).

GLOMERULONEPHRITIS is a type of inflammation of the kidney (see **nephritis**).

GLOSSITIS means inflammation of the tongue. This may occur in many conditions – for instance, certain types of vitamin deficiency and anaemia.

162

GLUCOSE is a form of sugar, and therefore a carbohydrate (see **carbohydrate**). It is found in honey, and in many fruits. All carbohydrate foods are eventually broken down into glucose during digestion, and glucose is normally the only form in which sugar is present in the blood. A patient's 'blood sugar' level means the amount of glucose in the blood.

Normally, the blood sugar level remains between certain limits. Too little causes weakness and hunger, and the body takes steps to put matters right by mobilizing more glucose from the stores of another carbohydrate (called glycogen) in the liver. If, on the other hand, the blood glucose is too high, insulin (see **insulin**) which is produced by the pancreas, helps to bring it down to normal levels.

In diabetes mellitus (see **diabetes**), the normal mechanism for preventing glucose levels from rising too high fails to operate properly; the patient therefore has to go on a diet with a much reduced carbohydrate content in order to lower the blood glucose level. He may well have to take tablets for the same purpose, or inject himself daily with insulin.

GLUTEN is a protein (see **protein**) found in wheat and wheat products. Its particular importance from a medical point of view lies in the fact that certain children ('coeliac children') and adults develop chronic diarrhoea and malabsorption of nutriment if it is not excluded completely from their diet (see **'coeliac children'**).

St Bartholomew's Hospital

Institute of Ophthalmology

GOITRE means a swelling of the front part of the neck, due to enlargement of the thyroid gland (see **thyroid gland**). Slight fullness of this gland is common and quite normal in some women at puberty, in pregnancy, and whenever a period is due. However, larger, persistent goitres may be due to thyrotoxicosis (see **thyrotoxicosis**), which is over-activity of the thyroid, or to certain rarer conditions of the gland (see **thyroid**).

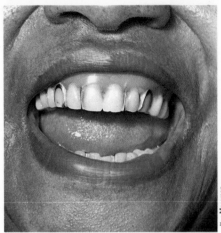

Gold is used extensively in dentistry to repair damaged teeth and prevent further decay.

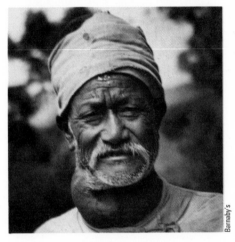

Typical appearance of the neck in goitre, due to gross enlargement of the thyroid gland.

GOLD is not only a precious metal; it is also of some value in medicine. Its toughness makes it particularly useful as a filling for teeth affected by decay; such fillings last many years longer than the amalgam type, but are expensive.

The administration of various forms of gold has been used as a treatment for several diseases. However, by beginning of the twentieth century, the use of gold salts was restricted to the treatment of tuberculosis and rheumatoid arthritis, and they now find only occasional use in patients with rheumatoid arthritis. Some patients with rheumatoid arthritis do seem to benefit from injections of gold salts, although their mode of action is not well understood. There are sometimes side effects such as skin rashes, kidney damage and blood disorders. Radioactive gold is used to treat certain tumours.

GOLDEN EYE OINTMENT is an ointment containing a compound of mercury, which gives it a yellow colour. It has been used in such conditions as styes and mild inflammation of the eyelids (blepharitis).

GONADS are the sex glands, i.e. the ovaries in women (see **ovaries**) and the testicles (see **testicles**) in men. The gonads in both sexes are formed from a ridge of tissue which develops inside the abdominal cavity of the embryo (see **embryo**) within a few weeks of fertilization of the egg. In female embryos, the tissue remains within the abdomen and eventually becomes the ovary, while in males the gonad on each side is slowly drawn down, out of the abdominal cavity into the scrotum. In a small proportion of boys, this process is not complete, and one gonad fails to descend into the scrotum. An operation may be necessary to draw it down.

GONADOTROPHINS or gonadotrophic hormones, are hormones which control the activity of the gonads. The pituitary gland produces three different gonadotrophins, and another, called chorionic gonadotrophin is produced by the placenta during pregnancy. In the male they control the production of spermatozoa, and in the female, of the ova.

163

GONOCOCCI are the germs responsible for gonorrhoea (see **gonorrhoea**).

GONORRHOEA is probably the most common venereal disease. It is caused by infection with bacteria (see **bacteria**) called gonococci, and transmitted by sexual intercourse, other forms of sexual contact and occasionally by contact with infected clothing, towels, etc. There is evidence that the incidence of gonorrhoea (which dropped dramatically after the introduction of penicillin) is now rising again. The apparent rise is possibly due in part to the fact that the germs themselves have, in many instances, become resistant to penicillin therapy.

In men, the initial symptoms of gonorrhoea (or 'clap' as lay people often call it) occur, on average, about 5 days after infection. (Possibly as soon as 2 days or as late as 30 days afterwards.)

The commonest symptoms are burning pain on passing urine and discharge (usually yellowish) from the penis. These symptoms demand immediate investigation and treatment.

In men, the late complications of untreated gonorrhoea may be severe. Stricture (constriction) of the urinary passages, formation of abscesses in the penis, inflammation of the prostate gland and of the passage leading from the testicles, sterility, eye disease and arthritis — all these are a high price to pay for not attending a clinic immediately.

One final aspect of gonorrhoea in men which should be noted is that (contrary to widespread belief) it may occur in homosexuals, who get pain and discharge not only in the genitals, but in the back passage.

In women, the symptoms of gonorrhoea are unfortunately vaguer than they are in men, and some women undoubtedly have the disease for a very long time without recognizable symptoms.

However, many women with the disease notice an unusual amount of vaginal discharge, often yellow and offensive a few days after infection. Pain on passing urine is also common, and it is easy for it to be dismissed as 'cystitis'. Pus may cause a swelling of the glands of Bartholin, which lie in the lower part of the labia (lips) of the female genital tract.

Since the late complications (including sterility, chronic infection of the neck of the womb, and chronic inflammation of all the pelvic tissues) are also very serious in women, it is extremely important to seek advice at the slightest suspicion of infection. Most large hospitals have clinics for the diagnosis and treatment of venereal disease, run by sympathetic and helpful medical and nursing staff; names are not used, and few patients who have been treated at these clinics (or even simply reassured there that they have not contracted venereal disease) feel in the least embarrassed — in the main, they only feel grateful.

In all countries, prostitutes are likely to form a reservoir of infection. One survey of London prostitutes showed that as many as half of them had gonorrhoea. This suggests that any man who has intercourse with a London prostitute may well have a fifty-fifty chance of catching the disease. Condoms (French letters) are *not* a fully adequate protection.

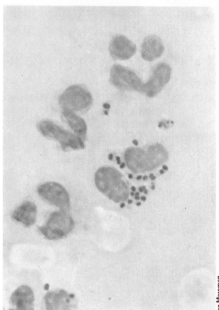

Ken Moreman

The organisms responsible for causing gonorrhoea, seen together with larger cells in pus.

GOUT is a disorder in which various joints of the body (most notably that at the base of the big toe) become inflamed and painful from time to time. It is due to an inborn error in the body's chemical processes, and an increase in the level of a substance called uric acid in the blood.

Gout has been recognized as an illness for over two thousand years — it was well known to the ancient Greeks and Romans, who believed it to be associated with high living and debauchery. When the first really clear description of the disorder was written by the English physician Thomas Sydenham in the 1600s it was generally believed that gout would not attack a man until he had had his first experience of both wine and women. This belief in the slightly disreputable nature of the origin of gout has persisted among lay people to this day. However, the condition is simply a defect in body chemistry, though it is possible that attacks may be precipitated by over-indulgence in alcohol.

Apart from the severe joint pain which gout produces, it may produce considerable destruction of the bone around the joint. There may also be kidney complications after many years.

Fortunately, a number of drugs have been developed which are extremely useful in the treatment of gout. Some of these, such as colchicine (see **colchicine**) are principally of use in relieving the pain of the acute attack, while others are taken long-term to keep the level of uric acid down, and so ward off complications.

GRAFT means any tissue removed from one site and placed on another. Grafts may be taken from one area of a person and transplanted elsewhere on his body — for instance, where skin is removed from the thigh to cover a burnt area elsewhere. Grafts may also be from one person to another, or, indeed, from animals to human beings (though this type of graft is rarely successful). The subject is more fully discussed under the heading **transplants.**

GRAM'S STAIN is one of the most important methods of distinguishing between different types of bacteria. When a thin film of the bacteria to be identified is treated with the stain, if the bacteria are Gram-positive the dye is 'fixed', and cannot afterwards be washed out; Gram-negative bacteria, however, readily lose the blue dye. Under the microscope the difference can readily be seen.

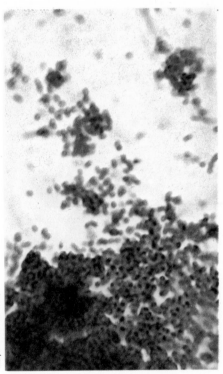

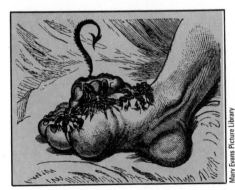

The intense pain of an attack of gout, as seen by an imaginative eighteenth century artist.

Gram-positive bacteria retain the blue colour of the dye, unlike these Gram-negative bacteria.

165

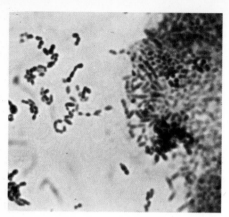

Typical appearance of Gram-positive bacteria. These are a species of streptococcus.

GRAND MAL is a term applied to what is probably the commonest form of epilepsy (see **epilepsy**), in which the patient's attacks are characterized by unconsciousness and generalized convulsions.

GREENSTICK FRACTURE is a type of fracture occurring in children. Just as a green stick, when bent, does not snap across, but splits incompletely, so, frequently do the long bones of children. The bones which are commonly affected are the upper and lower bones of the arm and leg. It is usually necessary to give the child a general anaesthetic, straighten the bone, and encase the limb in a plaster of paris splint for several weeks.

GREY POWDERS were once widely used for the treatment of intestinal upsets. They were popular 'home remedies' and were often given by parents with no idea of the correct dosage. The powders contained mercury, and it was eventually realized that an unpleasant and highly dangerous illness of young babies called 'pink disease' was actually caused by the mercury in these and similar preparations.

For this reason, the use of such powders was completely discontinued. Any parent who still has such a preparation in the medicine cupboard should destroy it.

GRIPPE is a word which used to be much used by lay people to describe transient feverish illnesses which were characterized by aches and pains – for instance, influenza (see **influenza**) and Bornholm disease (see **Bornholm disease**). There is no medical entity called 'grippe', but to be able to say that one had such an illness (instead of 'flu or a cold) became immensely fashionable in Europe, particularly Paris, during the late nineteenth and early twentieth century. Nowadays, the word is dropping out of use in favour of such terms as 'virus infection'.

GROWING PAINS are pains supposedly associated with growth in children.

For many years, doctors held that the process of development of children's bones was likely to cause them pain, and that this was an entirely natural phenomenon. In the 1930s and 1940s, however, this view came to be questioned. Many doctors suspected that the pains of rheumatic fever (see **rheumatic fever**) could well have been mistaken for 'growing pains' in the past. The consequences of such a mistake could be extremely serious.

The present state of medical opinion on this subject is undecided. Most doctors agree that 'growing pains' do not exist. Any child who complains of persistent pains in the limbs (particularly in the joints) should have a full medical investigation. This may well fail to reveal the presence of any disease, but it is nonetheless an essential precaution.

GROWTH is a word which is used in two senses in medicine – to describe the process of growing in children, and to describe tumours, both benign and malignant (see **cancer; tumours**). In the second sense, the word 'growth' does *not*, therefore, necessarily imply cancer. The subject is more fully discussed under the heading **tumours.**

Growth, in the sense of increase in height and weight, is usually a good index of a child's healthy development. (See also **development in children**). A few general guides can be given as to how fast a child should grow. It must be stressed, however, that children vary considerably: differences from the figures given (see tables at end) are not important.

GRUEL is a mixture of oatmeal and milk or water. At one time it enjoyed a considerable reputation as an invalid food.

GRUTUM are small pink and white patches on the skin of the face and scrotum.

GUANETHIDINE is a drug used principally in the treatment of high blood pressure (hypertension), though in the form of eye-drops it is also of use in the treatment of glaucoma (see **glaucoma**) and of over-activity of the thyroid associated with staring eyes (see **exophthalmos**).

In cases of high blood pressure, the action of the drug is to block nerve impulses from the 'sympathetic' nervous system, which maintain a certain tone in the blood vessels. When the impulses are blocked, the vessels relax and widen, and the pressure in them drops.

Guanethidine is one of the most useful drugs to have been developed, but it has certain predictable side-effects — notably diarrhoea, faintness on standing up (for reasons which are explained under the heading **fainting**) and failure of ejaculation (see **ejaculation**). Fortunately, these unwanted effects are harmless and disappear when dosage is reduced.

GUANOCLOR is a drug used in the treatment of high blood pressure (hypertension). It was introduced during the 1960s, and is quite widely employed in some countries. It lowers the blood pressure effectively, and has much the same side-effects as guanethidine (see above).

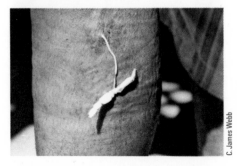

Extracting a Guinea worm by winding it slowly round a stick. The process takes many days.

GUINEA WORM is a parasitic worm found in India, Arabia, Persia, parts of Africa, Brazil and the Caribbean. It burrows through the tissues, but may not cause any trouble for as long as a year, when it nears the surface of the body and causes a painful swelling.

GULLET is the oesophagus (American spelling esophagus), the pipe which carries food from the throat to the stomach. It is a muscular structure about ten inches in length, running behind the trachea (windpipe) in its upper part, and then between the heart and the spinal column, before piercing the diaphragm (see **diaphragm**) and entering the stomach. The muscles which principally make up its wall have the ability to contract and 'squeeze' food or drink down into the stomach. It is thus possible to swallow even when lying flat or standing on one's head.

There are a number of conditions which may affect or involve the oesophagus. Among these are hiatus hernia (see **hiatus hernia**), diverticula or pouches, growths and ulcers. Oesophagitis, which is inflammation of the gullet, is quite a common form of indigestion. Very often, it is associated with the above-mentioned condition of hiatus hernia. Achalasia of the gullet, also known as cardiospasm, is a relatively unusual condition characterized by persistent regurgitation of food; this is due to the existence of a gross sac-like dilatation of the gullet above a narrow 'neck' where the organ joins the stomach.

In new-born babies, the gullet is sometimes malformed. This condition (oesophageal atresia) is said to be as common as cleft palate. In all cases, there exists no complete communication between the throat and the stomach — obviously a most serious state of affairs, as the baby cannot feed. Things are made worse in the majority of cases by the fact that an abnormal communication, or fistula (see **fistula**) exists between the gullet and the windpipe. Fortunately, if the condition is diagnosed within a few hours of birth, a surgical operation is possible which can correct the abnormality, and save the lives of babies who might otherwise die.

167

GUMBOIL is an abscess arising near a decayed tooth. Usually, the treatment consists in opening the abscess, letting out the pus, and dealing with the diseased tooth.

GUMMA is a deposit characteristic of the later stages of syphilis (see **syphilis**). These deposits are usually hard masses of tissue which may form in many organs of the body — for instance, the liver, skull or brain. Anti-syphilitic treatment (which is almost invariably penicillin nowadays) will cause considerable shrinking and even disappearance of gummas, though the tissue they have destroyed may never regenerate.

GUMS are ridges of dense fibrous tissue covered with pink mucous membrane. They overlie the bones of the upper and lower jaws. Disorders of the gums, such as gingivitis, are dealt with almost entirely by the dental surgeon. Such disorders, if left untreated, can very readily lead to loss of teeth. In the event of any soreness, inflammation, ulcer or swelling of the gums which persists more than a few days, it is essential to obtain the prompt advice of a dentist.

GUNSTOCK DEFORMITY is the name for a deformity in which the long axis of the extended forearm is turned outwardly from the upper arm. It is caused by a fracture of the elbow.

GUSTATION meant tasting; four classes of taste are generally recognized — sweet, salt, bitter and acid, distinguished by the taste-buds of the tongue.

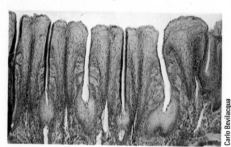

The taste-buds, responsible for gustation, are specialized cells in the tongue epithelium.

GUT is another name for the intestine. In man it is about 28 to 30 feet long. It plays the major role in digestion.

GYNAECOLOGY is the branch of surgery and medicine dealing with disorders of the female genital organs. A gynaecologist is a specialist in such diseases. As a rule (though not invariably), he practises in obstetrics (midwifery) as well.

All gynaecologists, however, have a training in both gynaecology and obstetrics, and, indeed, surgery as well. As a rule, the doctor who decides to be a gynaecologist will start his career by taking posts in both general medicine and general surgery, as well as obstetrics and gynaecology. The training to become proficient in gynaecology is long and arduous, as befits one of the most varied specialities in the whole of medical science.

GYNAECOMASTIA is a condition in which the male breast increases in size — often to female proportions. Usually, it is due to a hormone disturbance, but may be a side-effect of one of a number of drugs, including digoxin, digitalis and stilboestrol. Reduction in drug dosage usually helps the condition.

GYRUS is a term for one of the many ridges of the surface of the brain; each 'valley' on either side of a gyrus is called a sulcus (see **sulcus**).

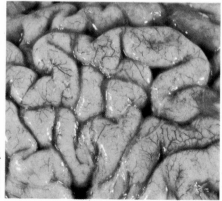

Carlo Bevilacqua

The tortuous folds of the surface layers of the brain, with sulci separating the gyri.

HAEM- is a prefix meaning 'blood'. It occurs frequently in medical words, as will be seen from the following entries.

HAEMATEMESIS means the vomiting of blood. When such vomiting occurs, it is essential that full investigations are carried out to determine the source of the bleeding. Common causes include ulcers; gastritis (inflammation of the stomach) often due to alcohol or aspirin; hiatus hernia (see **hiatus hernia**); varices (varicose veins) at the lower end of the gullet due to cirrhosis of the liver; and malignant diseases of the stomach.

Vomiting of blood is sometimes confused with *coughing* of blood (haemoptysis) by the patient. It is usually fairly easy to tell the difference, since coughed up blood is likely to be bright red, while vomited blood will probably have been turned a dark colour (perhaps even black) by the gastric juice.

HAEMATOLOGY is the study of the blood and its disorders. A haematologist is a specialist in these disorders.

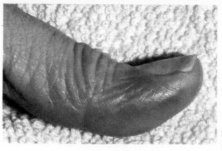
Bruises are accumulations of blood in areas of tissue where the blood vessels are damaged.

HAEMATURIA is the passing of blood in the urine. This always demands full investigation to determine the cause, which may be relatively easy to treat (for instance, a urinary infection). On the other hand, haematuria may be due to any of a wide range of disorders of the urinary tract – i.e. the kidneys, ureters, bladder and urethra. Extensive investigation, involving special X-rays and examination by means of a cystoscope (see **cystoscope**), may be necessary to discover which of these structures is involved, and what disease process is causing the bleeding.

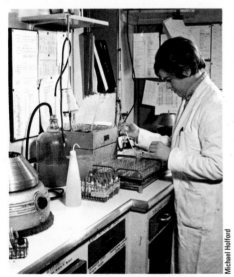
A haematologist working with samples of blood to determine to which groups they belong.

HAEMATOMA is a collection of blood forming a swelling. The commonest example is a bruise.

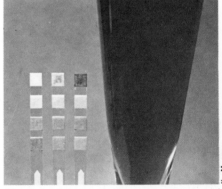
'Smoky' urine may indicate the presence of blood. A blue colour in this test is confirmation.

HAEMOCHROMATOSIS is a disease in which an excessive deposition of iron in the body occurs. This excess iron is deposited in the skin (where it causes a grey or brown discoloration), in the pancreas (where it can cause diabetes – see **diabetes mellitus**), and in the liver (where it causes a disorder akin to cirrhosis). It is

169

thought that haemochromatosis (or 'bronzed diabetes') occurs because too much iron is absorbed from the intestines. Occasionally, however, patients develop the disease because they have received too much iron during repeated blood transfusions.

HAEMOGLOBIN is an iron-containing pigment in the red corpuscles (or erythrocytes) of the blood (see **blood**). It has a remarkable ability to take up oxygen, forming a compound called oxyhaemoglobin. When air enters the lungs, oxygen diffuses into the bloodstream and immediately combines with haemoglobin. The red cells carry the bright red oxyhaemoglobin round the body in the arteries to the tissues, which remove the oxygen for their own use, leaving the blood deoxygenated, with a bluish colour. The veins carrying deoxygenated blood therefore appear darker than the arteries.

People from certain areas of the world (notably the Mediterranean and Africa) occasionally inherit disorders in which the haemoglobin in the blood is of an abnormal type, conditions called 'haemoglobinopathies'. The symptoms of these diseases are related to the fact that the abnormal haemoglobin may not carry oxygen efficiently (see **sickle cell anaemia**, and **thalassaemia**).

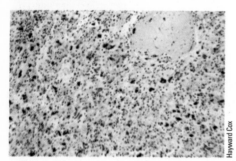

Iron-containing compounds in the tissues are shown as blue patches by dye techniques.

HAEMOLYTIC ANAEMIAS (see **anaemias**) are those in which anaemia is due to breaking-up (lysis) of red blood cells. Normally, a red corpuscle has a life of about 4 months, but in these disorders the red cell breaks up very much earlier than this.

170

Common types of haemolytic anaemias include the anaemia found in Rhesus babies (see **haemolytic disease of the newborn**), and those associated with sickle cell disease **sickle cell anaemia**) and thalassaemia (see **thalassaemia**). Haemolytic anaemia can also occur as a complicating factor in leukaemia and other conditions.

HAEMOLYTIC DISEASE OF THE NEWBORN is a type of anaemia occurring in Rhesus babies. (See **Rhesus factor**). About 85 per cent of the population are *Rhesus positive*, and the remaining 15 per cent are *Rhesus negative*. When a Rhesus negative woman marries a Rhesus positive man and becomes pregnant, it is possible that the child she bears may 'sensitize' her to produce antibodies against future Rhesus positive babies. Fortunately, this is not a common eventuality.

However, if sensitization *does* occur, then the second Rhesus positive baby may be affected by the mother's antibodies to a varying degree. A large dose of antibody, occurring early in pregnancy, causes the condition called *hydrops foetalis*, in which the child usually dies in the womb. If the child is less severely affected, however, as is usually the case, he or she will suffer haemolysis (break-up of the red blood cells) at or about the time of birth. The resulting anaemia is accompanied by jaundice, since bilirubin, the yellow pigment which causes jaundice, is released when the red cells break down (see **jaundice**, and **bilirubin**).

Nowadays, severe manifestations of Rhesus incompatibility are uncommon, because doctors are able to measure antibody levels in an expectant mother and, if necessary, bring on labour early (or even perform a Caesarean operation) if these antibody levels seem to be dangerously high. New techniques to prevent a mother ever becoming sensitized at all are coming into use. Finally, when a Rhesus baby is born, and it becomes apparent by its increasing jaundice and anaemia that a dangerous amount of destruction of its red cells is taking place, then it is possible to perform an 'exchange transfusion'. This involves exchanging all the blood in its body for fresh blood.

HAEMOPHILIA is a hereditary disorder which is characterized by an abnormal tendency to bleed. Except in rare circumstances, it occurs only in males. It is, however, passed on to sons by their mothers. Men do not pass it on to their sons, but all the daughters of a haemophiliac male will be healthy 'carriers' and liable to transmit the disease to roughly half of any boy children born to them.

Perhaps the most famous family to be affected by the disease was that of the Czars of Russia. What is not generally realized is that the gene of haemophilia appeared throughout many branches of the family tree of the descendants of Queen Victoria. At the present time, there are believed to be no affected males living, among the royal families of Europe, but it is possible that one or two female descendants of Queen Victoria who are now living may be carriers. It may be many years before we know.

The early symptoms of haemophilia are persistent bleeding after minor cuts. There is, contrary to popular belief, no serious danger of bleeding to death from such minor injuries. Before very long, the affected person develops a symptom which is very much more troublesome — namely, painful bleeding into joints such as the knee. These episodes occur at the least provocation, and they make it almost impossible for the boy to play football or do anything which entails the slightest risk of twisting a joint, even very slightly.

Unfortunately, the collections of blood in joint cavities (haemarthroses) may soon cause the affected joints to become completely stiff, so that the child is crippled. He may also have unexpected haemorrhages into muscles, and such episodes are again extremely painful.

The cause of haemophilia is a deficiency of a factor in the blood called AHG (or anti-haemophilic globulin). Normal people have adequate quantities of this chemical, which is essential for proper clotting of the blood to take place.

The basis of treatment is to give anti-haemophilic globulin. However, AHG keeps for only a short time, so it is usual to treat any severe haemorrhage, whether it is a haemarthrosis or a troublesome bleeding tooth socket, with either a transfusion of *fresh* blood, or one of fresh plasma. These measures have a dramatic effect, and, if applied in time, they will prevent the miseries and the crippling deformities so common in the past.

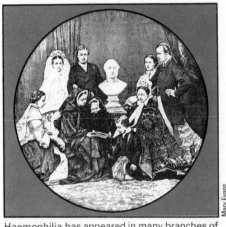

Haemophilia has appeared in many branches of the family tree of Queen Victoria's descendants.

HAEMOPTYSIS means the coughing or spitting up of blood. It is often confused by the patient with *vomiting* of blood which has accumulated in the stomach (haematemesis). However, vomited blood is usually dark red or even black, because of the action of the gastric juices, while blood which is coughed up is almost

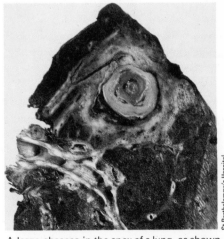

A large abscess in the apex of a lung, as shown here, may cause haemoptysis if vessels burst.

always bright red, or perhaps pink if it is mixed with sputum.

Causes of blood-spitting are many. *All, however, demand examination by a doctor, and, at the very least, a chest X-ray.*

The vast majority of cases of haemoptysis are related to disorders of the lungs and respiratory passages. Ordinary chest infections sometimes cause this symptom, but much more serious causes cannot be ruled out without the aid of an X-ray. Tuberculosis, lung cancer, bronchiectasis (see **bronchiectasis**), lung abscess and pneumonia are among the commoner of the lung conditions which may be implicated.

Certain heart conditions, notably *mitral stenosis* (narrowing of the mitral valve) may also result in blood being coughed up.

HAEMORRHAGE means bleeding (see **bleeding**). There is no verb 'to haemorrhage', despite the frequent use of this expression on television programmes about hospitals. The correct expression is 'to bleed'.

HAEMORRHAGIC DISORDERS, or bleeding disorders, are those in which the patient has an abnormal tendency to bleed, internally or externally.

There are many chemical and other factors in the bloodstream which react together to form a clot whenever blood vessels are damaged, so that bleeding stops quite rapidly. If any of these factors is deficient, then a haemorrhagic disorder results. Deficiencies of most of these factors have been described, and the common ones are as follows: haemophilia (see **haemophilia**) is due to lack of anti-haemophilic globulin (AHG); Christmas disease, which is called after a patient named Christmas, is due to deficiency of Christmas factor; hypoprothrombinaemia is due to lack of prothrombin in the blood; hypofibraogenaenia is due to deficiency of fibrin; thrombocytopaenic purpura, characterized by bleeding into the skin, is due to lack of blood platelets.

Many other disorders, such as various forms of purpura, and scurvy cause bleeding by rather different mechanisms. Usually, a number of varied blood tests are required to determine the cause of any type of bleeding disorder.

HAEMORRHOIDS are piles. It is usual to say that these are varicose veins of the back passage, but, in fact, this is by no means always the case. Internal piles are indeed varicose veins, but external ones may be composed simply of skin tags around the anus, though there can be varicose veins present under this layer of skin.

Haemorrhoids are among the most common afflictions of mankind — an astonishingly high proportion of men have them, and not a few women, especially during pregnancy.

The initial symptom is usually bleeding (which is very slight), often associated with discomfort and some itching. It is absolutely essential to have a full rectal examination at this stage, because, even if piles are present, the doctor has to be sure that it is not a cancer of the rectum higher up which is causing bleeding.

At this stage, piles can be treated very adequately by suppositories or soothing creams. If complications (such as prolapse) develop, however, operation may be necessary. There are a number of possible operations which can be carried out. While all of them mean that there will be a few days' discomfort, the results are very good indeed.

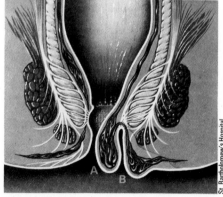

St. Bartholomew's Hospital

Diagram showing the formation of the two sorts of haemorrhoid, *A*, internal, and *B*, external, as the lining of the anal canal bulges.

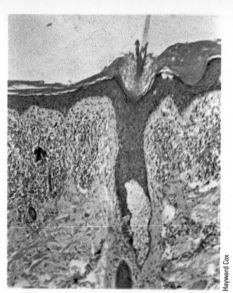

A section through the skin, showing a hair follicle, from which the hair grows upwards.

crime.

Hair on the head usually grows at a rate of about 6 inches a year. There are roughly 100,000 hairs on an average person's head — though this number varies greatly from one person to another. At any given moment, about eighty-five per cent of these hairs are actually growing, while the remainder are 'resting'. 'Resting' hairs eventually either fall out or are forced out by fresh hairs pushing up from underneath. In bald people, no fresh hairs develop to replace the 'resting ones'. It should be understood that the hair shaft itself is *not* living tissue, and nothing put on it or rubbed into it will make it grow. This is why there is at the present time, regrettably, no cure for the ordinary type of male baldness (see **baldness**), despite many claims to the contrary.

HAIRS are actually small horny tubes which grow out from the skin. The shaft of each hair grows upwards from a bulb, set in a recess in the skin termed the hair *follicle.* Sebaceous glands pour their secretions into these follicles, so that all hairs (particularly, of course, those of the head) are slightly oily — though the actual amount of oil varies from person to person. Hair colour also varies, of course, and this is due to the fact that people have different amounts of pigment in their hair. Depending on genetic inheritance, some people have curly hair, while others have wavy or straight hair. These are characteristics which cannot be altered, though it is, of course, possible to curl or straighten hair artificially for a time.

Hairs in various parts of the body differ considerably in their physical characteristics. Pubic and body hair, for instance, usually look different from head hair. Looked at under the microscope, the variations are much more marked. The hair of people of different races also varies appreciably in microscopic appearance. Even among people of the same race, differences in hair structure are often so marked as to be of considerable importance — for instance, to a pathologist investigating a

HALIBUT LIVER OIL is a vitamin supplement made from fish liver. It is rich in both vitamin A and vitamin D. Since it is particularly important that babies get sufficient amounts of the latter vitamin, which prevents rickets, either halibut liver oil or cod liver oil are often given routinely during the first two years of life. Halibut oil is a more concentrated source of vitamin D, and it is only necessary to give about 10 drops a day to a child. The dose should *not* be exceeded, as there are considerable dangers associated with an excessive intake of vitamin D. Most dried milk preparations now contain vitamin D, so a mother should usually discuss with her doctor whether it is wise to put her baby on halibut liver oil (see **vitamins,** and **deficiency diseases**).

HALITOSIS is bad breath (see **breath**).

HALLUCINATIONS are imaginary sensations. People may experience them through any senses: vision, hearing, touch, smell, or taste. In visual hallucinations, a patient may see all kinds of strange creatures which have no existence in reality. Such occurrences are characteristic of several types of mental illness — notably chronic alcoholism (see **dipsomania**). Visual hallucinations are also a feature of certain types of drug intoxica-

173

tion — a potent chemical in inducing this type of experience is LSD. 'Trips' with this drug are accompanied by bizarre visual hallucinations of colour and light; these are said usually to be pleasurable, but are sometimes terrifying.

Hallucinations of hearing are characteristic of certain types of schizophrenia. The patient usually reports that he hears voices, which may give him instructions. He may also hear music. Some medical historians have theorized that Joan of Arc might have suffered from such hallucinations, in common with other people who have claimed divine 'visions'.

HALLUCINOGENS are drugs which produce hallucinations (see **hallucinations**). These include LSD, mescaline and a number of so far unidentified chemicals which are found in certain Central American mushrooms. These hallucinogenic mushrooms have been used by Mexican Indians for many hundreds of years in connection with religious ceremonials.

HALLUX is the correct medical name for the big toe.

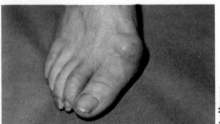

A bunion develops where pressure from a tight shoe causes inflammation over a deformed joint.

HALLUX VALGUS is an extremely common and troublesome deformity of the big toe which often develops in middle or later life. The toe becomes displaced outwards, towards the other toes, and the joint at its base becomes swollen. Often, a collection of fluid called a 'bursa' develops over this joint. Pressure of the shoe causes the bursa to become inflamed; the condition is then known as a bunion.

Very mild cases can be halted in their progress by avoiding wearing shoes with pointed toes, but the majority of patients

require surgical treatment to correct the distortion of the bones.

HAMMER TOE is a deformity which develops particularly frequently in people who wear over-tight shoes. It is commonest in the second toe, especially when this is subjected to additional pressure by a deformed big toe — e.g. where hallux valgus (see **hallux valgus**) is present. Instead of lying flat, the second toe is bent, so that one 'knuckle' is permanently in contact with the shoe. This leads to the development of severe corns on the 'knuckle'. Treatment consists initially in wearing shoes with plenty of room for the toes, although surgical correction may be needed.

HAMSTRINGS are the powerful muscles and tendons which lie at the back of the thigh. The tendons are attached to the bone immediately below the knee (the tibia), and the main function of the hamstrings is to bend this joint. Since they are subjected to so much stress in athletics and other sports, the hamstrings are very frequently injured. Fortunately, with rest, such injuries (which usually consist of a minor tearing of muscle fibres) usually heal completely. Problems arise if, as frequently happens, a sportsman will not, or cannot, rest the injured hamstring, and the damage becomes progressively worse, until permanent injury results.

HAND is the part of the arm below the wrist joint. It is one of the most complex structures in the body, and its ability to carry out the most delicate tasks with astonishing accuracy has been in no small measure responsible for Man's emergence at the top of the evolutionary tree.

The hand is made up of fourteen small bones in the fingers (see **fingers**), five metacarpal bones, in the palm of the hand (one at the base of each finger), and eight small bones which make up the 'carpus', or area immediately below the wrist joint.

The fleshy part of the hand consists of small muscles, but most of the power of the hand comes from the large muscles of the forearm, connected to the hand by long tendons (see also **fingers**).

HANGING is suspension by the neck with the object of producing death. In fact, there are two entirely different types – hanging by strangulation, and judicial hanging.

Judicial hanging was widely carried out in many European countries from the Middle Ages up to the mid-twentieth century, at which period it became used less and less frequently. Until only about 100 years ago, hanging was carried out in public, and seems to have been an extremely popular spectacle. Hundreds of morbid sightseers regularly attended such executions in England; public hanging was brought to an end after the execution of Michael Barrett, an Irish rebel, outside Newgate Jail in 1868.

By this time, the method of judicial hanging had become fairly standardized. A man who was to be hanged had a rope noose placed about his head, and a trapdoor was opened under him. The object was not to strangle him but to break his neck by means of the jerk. Occasionally, this method was not successful – in late Victorian times, a man was reprieved after the hangman had three times failed to execute him.

This type of death, caused by fracture of the upper vertebrae of the neck, is not instantaneous, although unconsciousness should be immediate.

Hanging by strangulation with a ligature is an entirely different matter. This is what occurs where there is no 'drop'; most suicidal hangings are of this type. Here, death is due to the rope or cord pressing on the blood vessels of the neck and cutting off the blood supply to the brain. Unconsciousness supervenes in about 7–10 seconds, and it is probable that the victim feels sensations very similar to those of a faint. Death is rapid; this fact is worth stressing, since it quite often happens that children at play put a rope round their necks. Such 'hanging games' may prove fatal. Sexual perverts may also accidentally hang themselves while taking part in bizarre antics involving putting a rope round the neck.

First aid for persons found hanging: cut the victim down at once, loosen the ligature from his neck and start artificial respiration (as described under the heading **drowning**) at once.

HANGNAIL is a tag of skin which forms at the side of the finger nail. It tends to catch on clothing, so that the split in the skin is readily lengthened. If germs enter this split, a whitlow may result. The best treatment for a hangnail is usually to cover the area with a dressing or with plastic skin. After a few days, the area rapidly heals over.

HARE LIP is a congenital deformity in which the upper lip is 'split', much like that of a hare's, but with the division to one side or the other, and not in the mid-line.

The cause of this deformity is an error in the development of the structure of the face during the first few weeks of life in the womb. The nose, upper lip and upper jaw are formed by three processes which grow downwards and together. If either of the outer processes fail to fuse properly with the centre one, a hare lip will result.

Because the palate is formed from the same three processes, failure of fusion can also lead to *cleft palate*, and the two conditions are very often associated. Fortunately, both hare lip and cleft palate are usually amenable to surgical treatment nowadays. Although both conditions may make it very difficult for a new born baby to suck, it is usually best to postpone operation until the child's lip, jaw and palate are larger, and easier for the plastic surgeon to deal with. In later life it is often difficult to detect any sign of the earlier surgical correction.

HASHIMOTO'S DISEASE is a condition of the thyroid gland, which lies in the front of the neck. When it was first described, it was thought to be very rare, but it is now recognized increasingly commonly. The cause is unknown. The condition is characterized by the occurrence of a firm, rubbery swelling (or goitre) of the thyroid gland, which has a characteristic appearance under the microscope. The patient may also suffer from myxoedema (see **myxoedema**) or underactivity of the thyroid gland. The presence in the blood of antibodies to one of the products of the gland suggests that this may be one of the autoimmune diseases, in which the body actually rejects its own tissues.

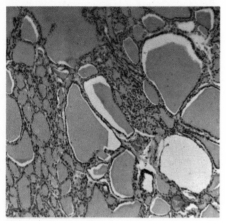

The normal thyroid gland, seen through the microscope, contains pools of colloid secretion, and little fibrous tissue. In Hashimoto's disease, below, the gland becomes very fibrous.

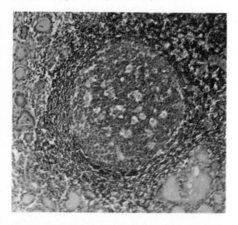

HAY FEVER is an allergic condition of the nose characterized by paroxysmal bouts of sneezing, coupled with copious nasal discharge. The eyes and throat are also involved as a rule, so that the mucous membranes of each may become inflamed and reddened. Very frequently the occurrence of the condition is seasonal — in Britain, for instance, attacks most commonly occur during the Summer, when there is most pollen in the atmosphere. Undoubtedly, allergy to such pollens is the cause of many attacks, though some patients may develop the distressing

176

symptoms of the condition after exposure to other *allergens* — for instance, dust.

The most effective way of dealing with hay fever is to avoid the allergen. For this reason, patients who have managed to establish whether it is grass pollen, tree pollen or dust that precipitates their attacks, often change their jobs, or even move house, to ensure that they are not exposed excessively. In addition, antihistamine drugs are of value in damping down the symptoms of hay fever. These drugs have to be used with considerable caution, however, since they very readily produce drowsiness; they are therefore not usually advisable for people who are driving, or operating machinery, and neither should they be taken with alcohol.

However, several new compounds have recently been discovered which have the effect of protecting an individual against allergic reactions. One of these has proved of considerable use in protection against asthma, and there are hopes that in the future it will be possible to help people with hay fever in the same way.

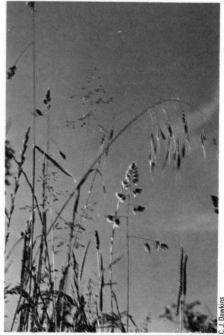

Hay fever is very often caused by the pollen of Cocksfoot, Ryegrass and Fescue, shown here.

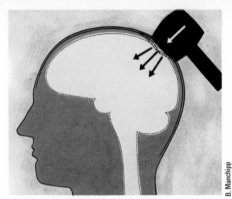

A blow on the head may be sufficient to break the skull; this absorbs much of the force, but any fragments which enter the brain tissue can cause damage which only comes to light much later, damage which is very often permanent.

HEAD INJURIES are among the most potentially serious types of accident. Any person who has had a head injury (other than slight knocks) should always be taken to hospital for a check-up and a skull X-ray. Disregard of this rule leads to many deaths every year. Particularly at risk are young men who sustain blows to the head during some sporting activity such as football or boxing. Even if such a blow knocks a sportsman out, he may feel that it is 'cissy' to go to hospital. *Nothing could be further from the truth.*

So important is it to ensure that a blow to the head has not produced internal injuries that hospitals make a practice of admitting for a night's observation anyone who has been knocked out — even if the period of unconsciousness has only been momentary. Patients often find this difficult to understand, since they may feel perfectly well in themselves. The great danger, however, is that internal bleeding may be taking place within the skull. If this is happening, the victim may feel in the best of health for hours after the original head injury. Meantime, the bleeding is slowly compressing his brain. All too frequently, he simply feels drowsy, goes to bed, and is found dead next morning.

Most doctors have seen tragedies of this type occur to young men in the prime of life. They can only be prevented if people realize that blows to the head are *not* the

trivial matters they are made out to be in many films and TV programmes — they are potentially very serious, especially if there has been an episode of unconsciousness following the blow. *The fact that the patient feels well is no guide* — he *must* have a medical examination, a skull X-ray, and if the doctor feels it is necessary, a period of observation in hospital. (See also **concussion**.)

HEADACHE is one of the commonest symptoms experienced by all of us at some time or another. Occasional headaches are of no significance whatever — little is known about their cause, but they may be related to occasional episodes in which the blood vessels in the brain become overstretched. The widespread belief that headaches are commonly due to constipation is completely without foundation.

Persistent, very severe, or recurrent headaches are a different matter, however, and all require medical advice.

Headaches that recur frequently and persist for many hours may be due to migraine, or occasionally to serious conditions inside the brain. A very sudden and severe headache, like a blow on the back of the skull, accompanied by weakness or unconsciousness, may be due to a particular form of cerebral haemorrhage known as sub-arachnoid haemorrhage. This is one of the very few serious causes of headache in young people.

Although severe or persistent headaches should be fully investigated, most such investigations prove negative. A great many patients who have this symptom are afraid that they may be suffering from a tumour of the brain, but, in the vast majority of cases, their fears prove groundless.

HEARING is the act of perceiving sound by means of the ears (see **ears**).

HEART is the powerful muscular pump, situated in the chest, which drives blood round our circulatory system.

To understand how the heart works, we must appreciate that it has to pump blood round two different circuits. The first of these is the system of blood vessels which

177

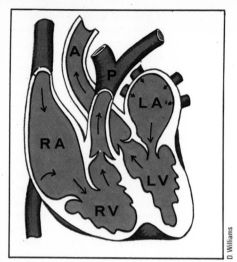

The heart with the front removed, showing the direction of blood flow in the four chambers. A indicates the aorta, P the pulmonary artery, RA and LA the right and left atria, RV and LV the right and left ventricles. Blood in the left chambers has been freshly reoxygenated.

D. Williams

supplies blood to the tissues and then returns it to the heart. The second is the smaller loop which carries the stale blood to the lungs to be enriched with oxygen before coming back to the heart.

In order to send blood round these two circuits, the heart has four muscular chambers — two atria and two ventricles. The right and left atria are basically receiving chambers to which blood returns; blood from the tissues flows into the right atrium, while blood from the lungs flows into the left atrium.

There is no connection between the right side and the left side of the heart, but each atrium is connected with the ventricle immediately below it. The ventricles are the pumping chambers; blood from the *right* ventricle is pumped to the lungs, while blood from the *left* goes to the tissues.

The entire sequence, therefore, is as follows. Blood returns from the tissues, enters the right atrium, and then flows into the right ventricle. This pumps it into the lung circuit, where it receives a fresh oxygen supply. Returning from the lungs, it enters the left atrium, and then flows into the left ventricle, which pumps it

around the tissues of the body.

There are valves between the chambers of the heart and at the points where blood leaves the heart; these valves may be malformed at birth, or affected later in life by disease (see **heart disorders**).

HEART ATTACKS are episodes in which parts of the heart muscle die because their blood supply is cut off. Laymen frequently refer to such attacks by the old term 'coronary thrombosis', which doctors have now abandoned in favour of the expression 'myocardial infarction' (because, in many cases, there is no actual thrombosis, or clot formation). See also **infarction,** and **coronary thrombosis.**

HEART DISORDERS are of many types. *Congenital disorders* are those which are present from birth. The structure of the heart is described under the heading **heart**; it can be seen that it is a most complex organ, and it is very easy for errors to occur during the early weeks of life in the womb when the heart is being formed. Such congenital defects include holes in the heart (forming an abnormal connection between the chambers on the right and left sides), and valve deformities.

Rheumatic heart disease is still common in most countries. Rheumatic fever, usually occurring in childhood, deforms the valves of the heart, and impairs its efficiency.

Heart disease due to syphilis is very much less common in Western countries than it used to be in the pre-penicillin era. The germ usually destroyed the valve leading from the left ventricle into the largest artery of the body, the aorta.

Heart disease due to other bacterial infections is also much less common since the introduction of penicillin (see **endocarditis**).

Heart disease due to various degenerative processes is increasingly common in Western civilization. Included in this group are 'heart attacks' (see **heart attacks**), which claim many lives yearly.

Other types of heart disorder include the cardiomyopathies — diseases of the heart muscle which were only first recognized in the late 1950s, but are now known to be quite common.

HEART FAILURE is inability of the heart to carry out its normal work. It does not, as many people imagine, mean either a heart attack or a stoppage of the heart causing death. The symptoms of heart failure are discussed under the heading **congestive cardiac failure.**

HEARTBURN is pain occurring in the abdomen and lower chest and related to digestive troubles (see **indigestion**).

HEAT STROKE is illness caused by exposure to great heat. Very frequently, it is associated with sun stroke. The early symptoms are faintness, thirst and confusion. Late symptoms include convulsions, extreme fever and even death.

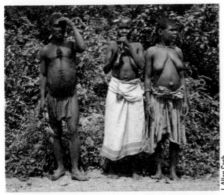

The pygmies of the Congo, above, contrasted in height with the Watutsi tribe, relatively huge.

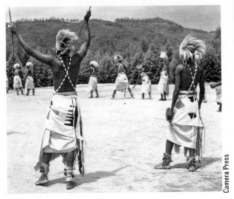

HEIGHT varies greatly from person to person and among different nations and races of humanity. For instance, the Watutsi (or Watusi) of Central Africa are believed to be the tallest people in the world — no accurate figures have been compiled, but their men are believed to average around six feet in height, as compared with the five feet seven or eight inches which is the mean for Englishmen. On the other hand, there are several tribes of pygmies in remote parts of the world (including one group living in the same area as the Watutsi) whose males average less than four feet six inches.

It is almost impossible to say who were the tallest and shortest men who ever lived. There are a few genuine instances of men whose height was between eight and nine feet. As regards midgets, the limit in height is roughly that of a new-born baby — i.e. about 22 to 24 inches.

Height in children is dealt with under the heading **development in children,** and tables are provided at the end of the dictionary.

Height and weight in adults are also dealt with in the tables at the end of the dictionary.

HELMINTHS are a group of parasitic worms. They include the threadworm (or pinworm) and the tapeworm.

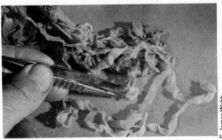

A tapeworm removed from the intestine of a patient who had eaten fish not properly cooked.

HEMIPLEGIA means paralysis of one side of the body. This condition is usually due to a stroke. The reason why only one side of the body is affected is that the brain is divided into two halves — the left half controls the right side of the body, and vice versa. If a stroke (for instance, in the form of a cerebral haemorrhage or cerebral thrombosis) occurs in one half of the brain, the other half of the body may be tem-

179

porarily or permanently paralysed.

HEMLOCK is a poisonous plant. Its properties have been known for thousands of years, and it was used as a poison by the ancient Greeks; Socrates was forced to commit suicide by drinking an extract of its leaves.

HEPARIN is an anticoagulant — that is, a drug which prevents blood from clotting. It is used in the treatment of disorders where there is abnormal clot formation — for instance, pulmonary embolism (see **pulmonary embolism**). Heparin is given by injection; the anticoagulant drugs which can be given by mouth do not take effect for about 48 hours, after which time heparin can be discontinued. Overdosage of heparin can occur quite readily and will produce severe bleeding; however, if the condition is recognized in time, it is relatively easy to treat it by giving protamine sulphate.

HEPATITIS literally means inflammation of the liver. These are many types of hepatitis, and doctors differ on terminology of this complicated group of disorders. *Infective hepatitis* is the common form of infectious jaundice. It is caused by a virus, and has an incubation period of about 40 days.

Its normal course is as follows: the patient feels ill for 3 or 4 days, and usually develops a slight fever. He loses his appetite and may feel nauseated; he then becomes jaundiced, and may remain so for anything from a few days to a few weeks. As a rule, despite the jaundice, he starts to feel better after only 48 hours. Nearly always, he makes a complete recovery. The only treatment recommended is rest and a nourishing diet. The patient should stay in his bedroom, but need not, as a rule, go into hospital. *All alcohol should be forbidden for six months.*

HERMAPHRODITE is a word derived from the names of the Greek god Hermes (Mercury) and the goddess Aphrodite (Venus). The term is properly applied to people who have the sex glands (testicles and ovaries) of both sexes; this condition is

very rare indeed. By extension, people in whom there is difficulty in determining their sex are sometimes described as hermaphrodite.

HERNIA means the protrusion of any body structure through the walls which are intended to contain it. Examples include hiatus hernia (see **hiatus hernia**). Commonly, the word is used to describe the several types of hernia, or rupture (see **rupture**) which occur around the region of the groin.

HEROIN, or diamorphine, is a potent and highly dangerous drug of addiction. Closely related to morphine, it is used in medicine to relieve intractable pain. However, much larger quantities than are used medicinally are employed by drug addicts. Heroin ('horse' or 'H' as it is called by addicts) is perhaps the most dangerous of all 'hard' drugs — unless an addict is rapidly weaned off it through pyschiatric treatment, this road to death is inevitable.

HERPES SIMPLEX is an infectious disease in which groups of blebs develop on the skin — commonly on the upper lip. It occurs particularly commonly in patients who have a severe illness such as pneumonia.

HERPES ZOSTER, or shingles, is a virus infection. The virus is believed to be the same one which causes chickenpox. The disorder is characterized by an eruption of small fluid-filled vesicles on the body or face. This eruption occurs over the area of skin supplied by one or other particular nerve, so that it occurs in great bands round one half of the body. It is thought that the herpes virus actually infects the nerves themselves, and it seems to have a predilection for particular nerves — notably the trigeminal, which supplies the skin of the face.

There is usually pain before an attack of herpes, but, as soon as the eruption comes out, the diagnosis is clear. In most cases, the rash eventually passes away, and the patient is cured, but some people, particularly the elderly, are prone to severe neuralgia after an attack.

180

HIATUS HERNIA is a protrusion of the stomach through the diaphragm (see **diaphragm**). This means that part of the organ, instead of lying in its correct place in the upper abdomen, finds its way through the hole by which the gullet passes from the chest to the abdomen.

Hiatus hernia is a fairly common condition. It occurs most often among middle aged people, particularly those who are overweight. The symptoms are pain in the upper abdomen or lower chest, in the midline, characteristically brought on (or made worse) by a change in posture — such as lying down or bending forward. Sometimes the patient may have persistent flatulence, or may complain of passing stools which are black and tarry due to the presence of blood (see **black motions**).

The diagnosis is confirmed by means of a barium X-ray. Treatment with antacids and correction of any obesity are often helpful, but surgery may be necessary.

HICCUP means a reflex contraction of the diaphragm (see **diaphragm**). It is usually due to irritation of that organ — often as a result of overdistension of the stomach. Orthodox medicine now has new remedies to improve on the traditional methods of treatment — such as drinking from the wrong side of a glass. Rarely, hiccups may occur persistently in the late stages of disease of the kidneys and liver.

HIP is the ball-and-socket joint between the femur, or thigh-bone, and the pelvis. A 'fractured hip' means a fracture of the upper part of the femur — a contingency which may be very serious in the elderly and debilitated (see **femur**).

HIRSCHSPRUNG'S DISEASE is a rare condition of the colon, or large intestine, which becomes grossly ballooned out. This occurrence is due to a deficiency of nerve connections at one point in the wall of the intestine. Megacolon, as the condition is also called, usually presents itself when a child is quite young — though occasionally it remains undiagnosed till later life. The features are bouts of diarrhoea alternating with constipation. There may be incontinence of faeces and abdominal pain. The diagnosis is established by means of a barium enema X-ray, which shows the abnormally distended intestine above the area deficient in nerves (the *aganglionic* segment). Operations are available nowadays, all of which give good results.

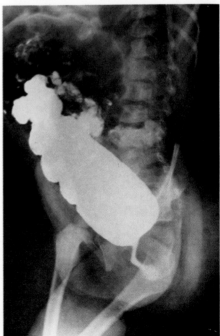

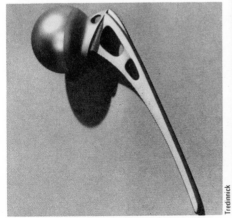

A badly diseased hip joint may be repaired using an artificial prosthesis of inert metal.

X-ray following a barium enema, showing the colon in Hirschprung's disease.

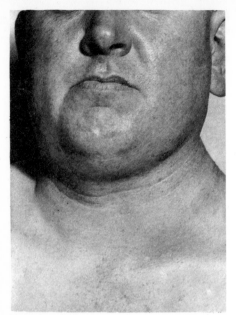

Typical appearance of the neck in a patient suffering from Hodgkin's disease.

HODGKIN'S DISEASE is a condition in which there is an overgrowth of lymph glands (see **glands**). It may occur at any age. The cause is completely unknown. The most common symptom is the occurrence of firm, painless, rubbery lymph nodes at the sides of the neck.

The outlook was bleak in Hodgkin's disease until only a few years ago. Nowadays, however, there is no doubt that cures have been effected in certain cases; there are many other patients alive today who have survived over 10 years with this condition, and hopes are high that a good proportion of them will also be eventually pronounced cured.

HOMEOPATHY, or homoeopathy, is a system of treatment not recognized by orthodox medical practitioners (though a few doctors do hold to its tenets). Basically, its theory is that to cure a disease, one should give a drug which produces similar symptoms to that disease, but in the most minute quantities. A 'homeopathic dose' is a phrase doctors use to describe a quantity of medicine literally thousands of times too small to have any effect on the human body.

HOMOSEXUALITY is sexual attraction between members of the same sex. The word does not derive, as many people imagine from the Latin word meaning 'man', but from the Greek word meaning 'the same'. Hence, both male and female homosexuality (lesbianism) are covered by the term. Nonetheless, most lay people use the word 'homosexual' to refer to male homosexuals, and hence female homosexuality is dealt with elsewhere in the dictionary, under the heading **lesbianism.**

Male homosexuality seems to be very much more widespread than was suspected 30, 20 or even 10 years ago. The exact incidence is completely unknown, if only because psychologists recognize that we are none of us entirely male, or entirely female. As regards *practising* homosexuals, figures are easier to obtain, and these suggest that about five or ten per cent of the male population may fall into this category. Dr Alfred Kinsey found that a much higher proportion of American men had had homosexual experiences, but it is likely that these were mainly adolescent escapades. The increased proportion of homosexuals in certain groups — the theatre and male nursing, for example — is well known.

What causes homosexuality? We simply do not know, though endless theories have been advanced. Some psychiatrists believe that the overpowerful influence of a mother who regards sex and all connection with women as 'dirty' can be a factor. In the present state of our knowledge, it is impossible to say. One elementary precaution which parents may take is to ensure that their sons are not exposed at puberty to the influence of persons who may be themselves homosexual.

Cure of homosexuality is only possible in the rare cases where the homosexual *wants* to be cured himself. In such instances, a psychiatrist may be successful in swinging the patient's sexual orientation from homosexuality to heterosexuality (attraction to persons of the opposite sex). To do this, he may use techniques such as aversion therapy (described under the heading **dipsomania**) and systematic desensitization (see **desensitization**) by several modern methods.

HOOKWORMS are parasitic worms which occur mainly in tropical countries. There are two important species – ankylostoma duodenale, and Necator americanus, both of which have roughly similar habits. Only the life cycle of the former type will be described. Ankylostoma duodenale lives in the duodenum (the uppermost part of the small intestine, which leads out of the stomach). It latches itself onto the wall of this part of the intestine by means of the tiny hooks at its head. From then on, it lives by sucking blood from the intestinal wall. The effect of this is to make the sufferer anaemic, and, in fact, hookworm is among the commonest causes of anaemia in tropical countries. There may also be abdominal pain and intestinal upsets. The hookworm's eggs are passed out in the stools. Where hygiene is poor, such infected stools may come into contact with the bare feet of children. The hookworms then penetrate the child's skin, and find their way round his body until they lodge in his intestines.

HORMONES are 'chemical messengers' produced by the endocrine glands (see **glands**).

HORNET STINGS are seldom serious. Some people recommend putting mild acids (such as vinegar) on them, but this is very rarely necessary.

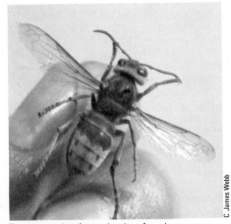

The hornet is often mistaken for a bee or wasp; its sting is painful but rarely dangerous.

HOUSEMAID'S KNEE is an inflammation of a sac of fluid (or bursa) in front of the knee. The medical term for the condition is pre-patellar bursitis. It is associated with constant kneeling, and rest or the use of kneeling-pad usually relieves the condition in a short time.

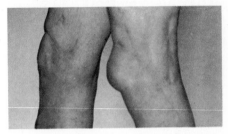

Swelling of the bursa at the front of the knee in 'housemaid's knee' – both unsightly and painful.

HUMERUS is the upper bone of the arm, which stretches from the shoulder joint to the elbow. It is known as the 'funny-bone', firstly because of an old pun on the word humorous, and secondly because of the fact that a nerve which runs over the bone at its lower end is liable to violent jarring, producing painful tingling.

HYALINE MEMBRANE DISEASE is a condition occurring in newly born babies, which is characterized by severe respiratory distress. This is due to the formation of a membrane in the lungs, which forms an obstruction to the breathing.

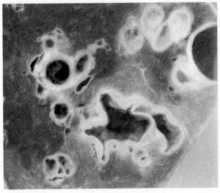

A section of a sheep's liver, showing the large cysts which form in hydatid disease.

HYDATID CYST is a type of parasitic

cyst common in people who live in sheep-rearing countries, who work with dogs. It occurs mainly in the liver of affected persons. The cyst is due to a parasite known as the Echinococcus (see **Echinococcus**).

HYDATIDIFORM MOLE is a serious condition which occurs in a very small number of pregnancies. Instead of developing normally, the contents of the womb degenerate into a collection of hundreds of tiny cysts, so that the appearance is that of a bunch of small grapes.

The characteristic symptoms are as follows. The woman becomes pregnant, and all goes well for the first three months or so. At this stage, vaginal bleeding commences; the blood may be brownish or bright red in colour. The woman normally goes to her doctor, who finds that the womb is about twice the size it should be at that stage of the pregnancy. The expectant mother may now be feeling ill, and have the symptoms of toxaemia (see **toxaemia of pregnancy**). By doing a special type of pregnancy test, the doctor can confirm the diagnosis. It is then necessary to terminate the pregnancy, which is of course, very upsetting for the mother but does not mean that she will never be able to have another baby.

A most important point is that any patient who has had this condition must be observed carefully, and have repeated pregnancy tests, over a period of at least eighteen months. This is because there is an appreciable risk (about 5 cases in a hundred) of a particular type of cancer developing in the womb during this time.

HYDRAMNIOS is a condition occurring commonly in pregnancy, in which there is too much fluid present in the womb. The unborn baby is normally surrounded by a quantity of fluid (the 'waters'), but, under certain circumstances, the volume of this fluid may become so great during the latter part of pregnancy as to be a serious embarrassment to the mother. Often, there is no evident cause for the occurrence of hydramnios, but sometimes the condition is associated with twins being present in the womb. Certain abnormalities of the foetus are occasionally found when the mother has this condition.

Hydramnios is liable to lead to problems with labour and delivery. Treatment is directed toward avoiding these complications. Bed rest and very careful observation during the last stages of pregnancy are essential.

HYDROCELE is a common condition occurring in men, in which fluid collects around the testicle. In fact, the fluid forms between the layers of the tissues which cover and protect the sex glands. Hydrocele appears, as a rule, in middle age; very often, the patient wrongly assumes that he has a hernia, or rupture. It is also important to distinguish this condition from another, called a *spermatocele*, which is a cyst-like swelling of the testicle itself.

A hydrocele can readily be tapped by a doctor, and the fluid drained off in a few minutes. Almost inevitably, however, the fluid will soon reaccumulate, and it is usually better to treat the condition by means of a simple operation.

HYDROCEPHALUS, or 'water on the brain' is a condition in which there is an excessive accumulation of fluid inside the skull. The characteristic feature is a great increase in size of the head – often, unfortunately, with a corresponding deleterious effect on the brain.

Hydrocephalus is due either to inflammatory disease, such as meningitis, or, more commonly, to some form of obstruction to the flow of cerebro-spinal fluid (CSF). Such obstruction is likely to be due to congenital deformity.

The outlook in this condition was generally very poor, but has been considerably improved in recent years by the development of valves which enable the excess fluid to be drawn off. The original valve was actually invented by an engineer with a hydrocephalic child.

HYDROCORTISONE is a corticosteroid (see **corticosteroids**) related to cortisone (see **cortisone**). It is often given by injection in certain inflammatory disorders.

HYDROPHOBIA means fear of water. The term is used to describe the disease also known as rabies, since one of the features of this terrible condition is that patients develop hideous spasms whenever they try to drink (or, in some cases, even look at) a glass of water.

Hydrophobia is a virus infection of the nervous system. It is normally caught from dogs, though occasionally other animals, such as bats, may be the cause. An infected dog, contrary to popular belief, may well not appear 'mad'; it may seem perfectly healthy, but its saliva contains the virus, and the slightest scratch from its teeth or even a lick will cause infection. Anything between 20 and 60 days later, the person bitten becomes ill. There is no treatment, and the condition is fatal, unless the person has acquired some immunity (see **immunity**) by being given injections against rabies. For this reason, countries such as the UK maintain a six months' quarantine period for imported dogs; as a result, cases of hydrophobia simply do not occur except in quarantine kennels (where they are usually mild, since the kennel attendants are immunized). In countries which do not have such measures, many children and adults die every year from the disease.

HYMEN, or virgin's veil, is a membrane which partly closes off the vagina. It does not, of course, close it off entirely, since it is important that the menstrual flow of blood escapes.

As a rule, the hymen is broken readily when defloration (see **defloration**) occurs; occasionally a very tough hymen may have to be broken by a doctor, but this is most unusual, and, as a rule the process is easy and painless.

HYPERTENSION means high blood pressure. (*Hypo*tension is low blood pressure.) There are many varieties of this condition, but by far the commonest is so-called 'essential' hypertension (see **essential hypertension**), in which there is no definite underlying cause.

However, in a small group of patients, there *is* an underlying reason – in some cases, a potentially curable one. Causes include various types of kidney disease, phaeochromocytoma (a relatively uncommon benign tumour of the adrenaline-producing tissue of the adrenal gland), certain other types of adrenal tumour, hyperthryroidism (see **hyperthyroidism**), coarctation (see **coarctation**) of the aorta (the large artery carrying blood from the heart) and toxaemia of pregnancy. (See **toxaemia of pregnancy**.)

While these causes are most unlikely in a person of advanced years, they should be considered in any young or middle-aged person who proves to have high blood pressure, and such a person should have full hospital investigation.

There are few actual symptoms of high blood pressure, although sometimes headaches may be associated with really severe elevations of pressure. In general, therefore, patients discover that their pressure is raised when they have a routine medical examination, or a check-up for some other condition.

Once hypertension has been discovered, it is essential that the patient should be under regular observation by the doctor, having his blood pressure checked at intervals. Not too much attention should be paid to individual readings as it is the pattern over many months which is important. It has been clearly established that treatment of high blood pressure lengthens life very considerably, Such treatment should not just consist of pills, but of weight-loss where the patient is even mildly obese (which is very often the case), and regular exercise to prevent the development of arterial disease (see **exercise**).

The drugs which are currently available for the treatment of high blood pressure are many and varied. They include reserpine, guanethidine (see **guanethidine**), bethanidine, guanoclor (see **guanoclor**), methyldopa (see **methyldopa**) and numerous others. Often, however, such powerful drugs, with potentially troublesome side-effects, are not required, and many patients benefit greatly from weight reduction alone.

HYPERTHYROIDISM is overactivity of the thyroid gland which lies at the front of the neck. (*Hypo*thyroidism is *under*activity of the thyroid). The symptoms include goitre (see **goitre**), anxiety, nervousness, a rapid pulse rate, tremor of the hands, excessive sweating, dislike of hot weather, and increased appetite despite a marked loss in weight. Finally, the patient often also has exophthalmos (see **exophthalmos**), or protrusion of the eyeballs.

In the vast majority of cases, all these symptoms (except, sometimes the staring eyes) can be cured by one of three methods of treatment. These are (a) radiotherapy, (b) anti-thyroid drugs and (c) removal of

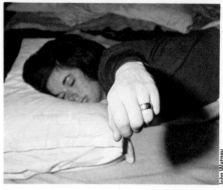

Hypnosis has been widely used to ease the process of childbirth. Hypnotized patients are insensible to pain, but still able to cooperate with the doctor and midwife during the delivery. Doing without pain-killing drugs at this time increases the safety of the birth.

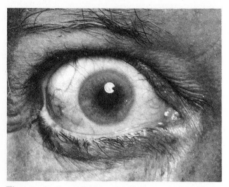

The typical appearance of the eye in hyperthyroidism, with white visible above the pupil.

the thyroid gland by surgical operation.

HYPNOSIS is a technique of putting a person into a state of trance by means of suggestion. People vary greatly in their suggestibility, but it is probable that between 30 and 50 per cent of the population are susceptible to hypnosis. Hypnosis is still used comparatively rarely – mainly in anaesthesia and psychiatry.

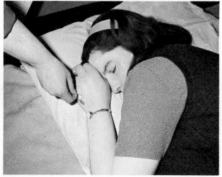

HYSTERECTOMY is removal of the womb by surgical operation. This is one of the most commonly performed of all surgical procedures, being usually carried out for such conditions as fibroids of the womb. A *sub-total* hysterectomy is one in which the cervix is not removed. A *total* hysterectomy involves the removal of the cervix as well. If the ovaries are removed at the same time, the 'artificial menopause' may cause quite unpleasant symptoms, such as hot flushes. More extensive types of hysterectomy operation, in which part of the vagina is removed, are employed for growths. However, in the vast majority of hysterectomies the vagina is left intact; therefore, marital life is unaffected.

HYSTERIA is a common condition. It is an illness (and a perfectly genuine one) in which the patient produces the symptoms or signs of some physical illness because of dissociation of normal mental processes, and to obtain relief from intolerable stress. The hysterical person is *not* a conscious malingerer, since he is totally unaware that the symptoms are not those of physical illness. Typical examples include transient periods of 'unconsciousness', or paralysis of an arm or leg. Psychiatric treatment is directed towards solving the deep seated problems which have produced the hysterical reaction.

IATROGENIC means literally 'caused by a doctor'. It is an expression applied to disorders such as unwanted side-effects of drugs, which have occurred as a result of medical treatment.

ILEITIS means inflammation of the ileum (see **ileum**), the last part of the small intestine. Symptoms include abdominal pain, diarrhoea and sometimes bleeding. The commonest cause is *regional ileitis,* or Crohn's disease (see **Crohn's disease**). This form of ileitis is called regional because it tends to be confined to small areas, notably the part of the ileum which leads directly into the large bowel.

ILEOSTOMY literally means making a hole in the ileum (see **ileum**), the last part of the small intestine. Very frequently, the edges of such an incision are stitched to the skin of the abdomen, so that material from the intestine can be passed through it into a receptacle such as a plastic bag. The operation is therefore very similar to that of colostomy (see **colostomy**), except that it is the small intestine and not the large intestine which is being opened by the surgeon. Usually, the object of such an operation is to 'rest' the large intestine, or perhaps permit its complete removal. The procedure is often of very great benefit to the patient in cases of ulcerative colitis. (See **ulcerative colitis**.)

ILEUM is the lower part of the small intestine, which connects the jejunum to the large intestine. (See also **alimentary canal**.)

IMMUNITY is the condition of being resistant to infection by a particular disease. It may be natural or artificial.

Natural immunity is acquired after infection by the germs producing the disease. To take a simple example, if a child has an attack of Rubella (german measles), it is likely that he or she will be immune from it for life. This is because the infection leads to the formation of antibodies (see **antibodies**), which remain present in the individual for the rest of his or her life, and which would effectively combat any attempts to re-infection by the same germ. Most of the infectious fevers of childhood provoke the formation of this type of antibody, and it is thus impossible to have these infections more than once. Furthermore, a mother who has antibodies against a specific disease will normally pass them on to her babies. These maternal antibodies remain effective for only about the first six months of a baby's life – but it is at this period that a baby is most vulnerable to death from infection, so that they perform a most useful function. It is therefore clear why babies under the age of six months are almost never infected by potentially serious diseases such as measles.

Artificial immunity was first introduced to medicine when vaccination against

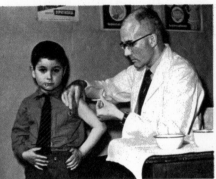

Receiving a booster immunization against both diphtheria and tetanus, to prolong immunity.

smallpox was developed. It may be of two types – active and passive.

Passive artificial immunity is a short term method of protection against disease. The basic principle is to give a patient antibodies against a specific infection, either from a human who has had the disease or from another animal, e.g. a horse. Serum from such an animal is injected into the patient to give him immediate, but short-lived, protection. In addition to the fact that the 'life' of the antibodies is short, there is another disadvantage of this method in that animal serum may provoke serious side-effects in human beings.

Active artificial immunity is therefore much preferable as a rule. This immunity

187

is obtained by stimulating the patient to produce his *own* antibodies. This can be done by giving him weakened or dead germs (which will not produce disease), or by injecting toxoids; these are chemically-treated, and therefore harmless, toxins produced by the germs in question.

If we give a patient active immunization then, he will produce his own antibodies against the disease, and these antibodies will last for many years. The only disadvantage is that it takes several weeks for the antibodies to be formed.

To take an example of the use of both active and passive immunization, let us imagine a patient with suspected tetanus (lockjaw). It is essential to provide him with some antibodies against the disease at once, so he is passively immunized by being given horse serum containing such antibodies. He will, however, need long-term protection, and to this end he is actively immunized by being given a course of injections of tetanus toxoid, which will stimulate him to produce his own antibodies.

IMPETIGO is a contagious skin eruption, often occurring on the face. The germ involved is usually the Staphylococcus (see **Staphylococci**), an organism very commonly present on skin, in people's noses, infected cuts, and boils.

IMPOTENCE is inability to achieve erection. Such occurrences happen occasionally to almost all men, but persistent impotence requires medical help. In the vast majority of instances, the origin of the trouble is psychological, and associated with guilt feelings about sex. It is therefore not surprising that husbands who attempt illicit liaisons sometimes find themselves impotent, while they are not so with their wives. Of course, the reverse may be the case if the wife's attitude to sexual relations is one of disgust while that of the mistress is enthusiastic.

Mild cases of impotence can be entirely cured with the help of a frank talk with the family doctor, and with the aid of a sympathetic wife. Unfortunately, what so often happens is that the husband finds

he is impotent and is afraid to tell his wife, who assumes that he no longer desires her and becomes hostile to him. A vicious circle thus develops. If, however, the husband is frank with his wife and she treats him with sympathy and understanding (using, perhaps, some of the techniques mentioned under the heading **love play** to help him with his difficulty), tragedy can be averted.

Quite commonly, impotence requires psychiatric help. The psychiatrist is nowadays able, by means of techniques such as desensitization (see **desensitization**), to cure many patients with this very widespread condition.

It should be mentioned that a small number of cases of impotence are due to a side-effect of certain drugs — notably those for high blood pressure. Stopping or changing the drug quickly produces cure.

INCONTINENCE is inability to control the emptying of the bowels or bladder.

INCUBATION PERIOD is the time an infectious disease takes to manifest itself. The incubation periods of the common infectious diseases are shown in a table at the end of the dictionary.

INDIAN HEMP is another name for cannabis (see **cannabis**).

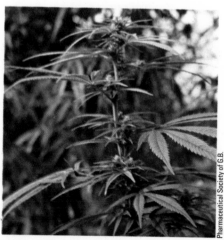

Indian Hemp, or *Cannabis indica,* the plant from which the drug 'pot' is derived.

INDIGESTION literally means 'inability to digest food properly'. It is not a medical term but to the layman it usually implies pain after eating food, and sometimes also a tendency to belching or flatulence.

All people, at some time or another, experience pain of the indigestion type. It occurs very commonly among children, who often get tummy-ache when 'the eyes are bigger than the stomach'. The cause of pain here is almost certainly a simple question of over-distention of the stomach and intestines by too much food.

In other types of indigestion, the cause of pain or flatulence is often obscure. Alcohol, foods to which a person is unaccustomed (for instance, curries and spices) and perhaps most important of all, aspirin (or, indeed, any of the proprietary pain-killing tablets – most of which actually contain aspirin as the principal ingredient) are important factors. Few people realize the danger in taking aspirin, and, in fact, patients often mistakenly try to treat indigestion with aspirin or aspirin-containing pills. As a rule, the best treatment for indigestion is an antacid, such as bicarbonate of soda.

If, on the other hand, pain of the indigestion type occurs frequently, it is essential to consult a doctor. A possible cause of such recurrent pain is an ulcer – either gastric or duodenal. An ulcer is particularly likely if the pain is in the middle part of the upper abdomen, occurs one or two hours after meals, and is relieved by having something to eat or drinking a glass of milk. In addition, the patient may notice that his motions are black, due to the presence of altered blood in them.

Other causes of recurrent indigestion pain include hiatus hernia (see **hiatus hernia**), the condition in which part of the stomach tends to slip through the diaphragm into the chest. The most characteristic feature of this condition is that pain comes on when the patient changes his or her posture – for instance, on lying down or bending forward.

All cases of recurrent indigestion need full investigation and, at the very least, a barium meal X-ray (see **barium meal**). This is particularly important because of the risk of such symptoms being due to

cancer of the stomach.

INFANT FEEDING is a complex subject, and one that poses problems for almost every mother. The basic principles of infant feeding are *cleanliness, choosing the right milk* for the baby, and giving him *the right quantity*.

These problems can usually be overcome if a mother chooses breast-feeding. Feeding from the breast provides absolutely ideal conditions of hygiene, in that it is practically impossible for germs to enter the milk. The situation with bottle-feeding is very different in this respect – it is only too easy for contamination to occur. A recent survey showed that few mothers who bottle-feed their babies managed to do so under conditions of proper sterility; the result of such a breakdown of hygiene may be infectious enteritis (see **enteritis**).

Breast milk is also undoubtedly the best *type* of food for the vast majority of babies (and, perhaps, all babies). No matter how cow's milk is treated to make it suitable for babies, it cannot provide an entirely adequate replacement for mother's milk. It is universally recognized that the health of breast-fed babies is in general superior to that of bottle-fed babies.

Problems of giving the baby the right *quantity* of milk are often considerably eased with breast-feeding. However, both underfeeding and (less commonly) overfeeding may occur in either breast-fed or bottle-fed infants.

Underfeeding is surprisingly widespread. In breast-fed babies, it sometimes occurs if the breasts do not contain much milk, though this is not common. In bottle-fed infants, it may be due to such mechanical problems as having too small a hole in the teat of the bottle. The symptoms of underfeeding are failure to gain weight, coupled with persistent crying between feeds.

Overfeeding is less frequently a problem; it may result from too large a feed being given, or from the fact that the mother has made the mixture up too richly. The main symptom is persistent regurgitation of food; the baby also has frequent loose stools, and perhaps experiences attacks of colic as well.

These and all similar severe digestive disturbances should be referred to the doctor or infant welfare clinic for advice. The doctor will also advise on the addition of vitamins to the diet. Many doctors recommend orange juice or some similar source of vitamin C from the second month onward. In addition, cod-liver oil may be given to ensure an adequate supply of vitamin D.

human 10 % **cow**

5

C

F

P

C

F

P

A comparison of the composition of human breast milk and cow's milk. C is carbohydrate content, F is total fat, and P is total protein. Dilution cannot make good the difference.

INFANT MORTALITY RATE is the annual number of deaths in the first year of life per thousand live births. In most countries, the rate has shown a steep fall over the last hundred years, and in several parts of Europe (for instance, the UK) there are now less than 20 deaths per 1000 live

births each year. Very much higher figures are unfortunately still recorded in the poorer countries of the world.

INFANTILE PARALYSIS – see **poliomyelitis.**

INFARCTION (or infarct) means death of tissue when its blood supply is cut off. Examples include myocardial infarction ('coronary thrombosis', see **heart attack**) and pulmonary infarction (see **pulmonary embolism**).

The former condition occurs when a branch of the coronary arteries (which supply blood to the muscle of the heart) become blocked – through atheroma, a fatty degeneration of the lining, or sometimes because of the formation of a thrombus (blood clot).

Pulmonary infarction, on the other hand, is always due to blockage of a branch of the pulmonary artery (which carries blood from the heart to the lungs) by an *embolism,* or piece of matter in the blood-stream. Usually this embolism consists of a thrombus (blood clot) which has formed in the leg veins and become detached from the walls of the blood vessels.

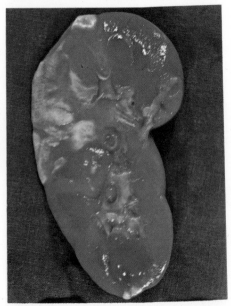

D. Williams

The effects of an infarct of the kidney, as seen in an autopsy specimen, recently removed.

INFECTION is the communication of disease caused by living organisms. Such organisms may be of many types — for instance, viruses (see **viruses**), bacteria (see **bacteria**), fungi (see **fungi**), tiny animals called protozoa (see **protozoa**), and larger animals such as tapeworms and hookworms. As a rule, viruses, bacteria and certain other infectious organisms of a similar size are referred to as 'germs'.

Until relatively recently, few people believed the 'germ theory' of disease, though it was vaguely understood that one person sometimes developed an illness after contact with someone else with the same disease. Even when men first saw germs through a microscope, they did not associate them with the idea of infection.

The first great step towards understanding of the nature of infection came in the middle of the 1800s, when the Viennese obstetrician Semmelweiss tried to reduce the incidence of deadly fever in his maternity wards. By introducing scrupulous cleanliness into nursing and surgical procedures, he was soon able greatly to reduce the death rate from this fever. Incredibly, few people were interested, and Semmelweiss died in comparative obscurity. One man who *was* interested was the Frenchman Louis Pasteur, who, although not a doctor, made perhaps one of the most outstanding individual contributions to medicine.

Despite abuse and ridicule from the scientists and medical men of his day, Pasteur pursued a series of experiments which demonstrated to all but the bigoted that many common diseases were acquired by a process of infection. The success of the surgeon Lord Lister in combating such infections made clear to most people the truth of the 'germ theory'.

The most common routes by which infection enters the body are: *The respiratory route.* Many infections, ranging from the common cold to measles, enter the body via the nose or mouth. Often the germs are carried in droplets sprayed out by other people when coughing, talking or even just breathing. It is to this route of infection that the phrase 'coughs and sneezes spread diseases' refers. *The gastro-intestinal route.* The great majority of intestinal infections enter by the mouth, in food or water contaminated by germs from the excreta of infected people. The infected excreta of a person with typhoid fever readily contaminates food or water, if hygienic measures are poor, and once the germ-carrying material is swallowed by other human beings, a typhoid epidemic is likely to result. *Infection through breaches in the skin.* It has been said that any cracks or cuts in the skin could be signposted 'germs — this way in'. Tissues provide an excellent breeding ground for organisms — once the protective barrier of the skin is broken. This is why cuts, grazes and burns so readily become septic. *Direct infection into mucous membranes.* Certain areas of the body, such as the mouth and genital areas, are covered, not in skin, but in mucous membranes. These are less effective in keeping out germs, such as those which cause venereal disease, and hence may be directly infected by contact.

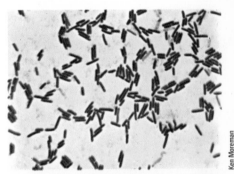

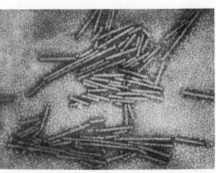

Bacteria such as Bacillus subtilis, *top*, may be seen through an ordinary microscope. Viruses need much greater magnification; the tobacco mosaic virus, *below*, is enlarged 125,000 times.

INFECTIOUS MONONUCLEOSIS is the medical name for glandular fever (see **glandular fever**). It is called mononucleosis because there is a characteristic increase in numbers of the type of blood cell, known as the mononuclear cell, found on microscopic examination.

INFLAMMATION is the process by which human or animal tissues react to injury, whether due to a blow, to infection, to a burn or to anything else. The cardinal signs of inflammation are swelling, warmth, pain, and redness, although all these signs may not be present in every kind of inflammation. Other signs which may be associated with inflammation include a raised body temperature and a raised pulse rate.

The signs of inflammation vary slightly, but the underlying mechanism is similar. Because of the injury to the tissues, the supplying blood vessels become dilated, and blood flow increases. Meanwhile, the defensive white cells of the body are mobilized. They pass through the walls of the blood vessels and into the tissues. At the same time there is a considerable outpouring of fluid into the inflamed regions. All these changes are directed towards making it easier for the body to combat the cause of the inflammation, and begin restorative work.

INFLUENZA, or 'flu, is one of the commonest afflictions of Mankind, even though many episodes of illness which are labelled as 'flu are probably not, in fact, due to influenza viruses. There are three types of these — A, B and C. Major epidemics are usually due to variants of type A; they occur every few years. Occasionally, as in 1918, 1957 and 1968, a particularly virulent strain causes many deaths, particularly among old people, across the whole world. The 1918 pandemic killed more people than did the First World War.

There is no *cure* for influenza, and antibiotics are of little use. However, in the vast majority of people, a few days in bed suffice.

INOCULATION (see **vaccination**).

192

INSULIN is a hormone produced by the pancreas. Its function is to regulate the level of sugar in the blood. A proportion of diabetic patients need insulin injections in order to live; for patients of this type, there was no hope at all until the year 1921, when Banting and Best in Canada succeeded in isolating the chemical from the pancreatic glands of animals (see **diabetes mellitus**).

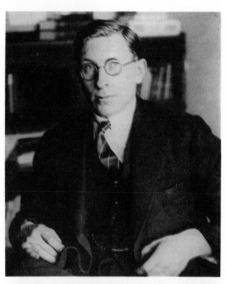

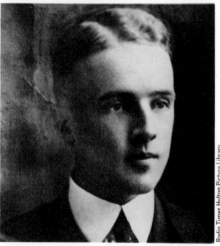

Above Dr Frederick Banting, who, with Dr Charles Best, *below*, discovered the relationship between the disease diabetes mellitus and the hormone insulin secreted by the pancreas.

INTERCOURSE is the sexual union of one person with another. As a rule, of course, the word 'intercourse' implies the act of love (genital union) between a man and a woman; strictly speaking, however, the word is used in medical terminology to describe other forms of sexual union as well – for instance, fellatio (see **love-play**) and also homosexual intercourse (see **homosexuality**).

Sexual intercourse between man and woman has been practised since our species began – yet ignorance about the act of love remains incredibly widespread. There is no doubt that the legacy of this state of affairs is the occurrence of sexual frustration and neurosis in quite a high percentage of the population. It is probable that few of the many people with sexual problems ever pluck up the courage to go to a doctor and talk about them; yet those who do often betray the most pitiable ignorance of sex. One example which suffices to demonstrate this is as follows: of young couples who consult gynaecologists because of infertility, a surprising number are found *never to have had true intercourse at all,* although they thought they had been doing so.

Fortunately, however, the Victorian attitude that intercourse was something bestial, and not to be talked about, is now gone. The work of Dr Alfred Kinsey in the 1940s and 1950s, and of Masters and Johnson in the 1960s, has put the study of the problems of intercourse on a scientific basis – and it is undeniable that there *are* problems. The technique of sexual intercourse is not something that can be learned overnight – which is why many wedding nights are something of a disaster. Particularly for a husband, who plays the more active part, the technique takes years, rather than months, to perfect.

For those whose sexual education is lacking, and who do not feel inclined to talk such matters over with their doctor (who will, in any case, not have the time for prolonged instruction in this complex subject), very helpful marriage manuals are obtainable at most bookshops. It is not too much to say that instruction of this type may well save a marriage, or greatly increase its happiness.

However, intercourse was not meant to be performed with a book in one hand, and both husband and wife will find that perhaps the most valuable thing to remember about intercourse is to retain a sense of humour, patience and kindness, which are more use in bed than all the marriage manuals in the world. In this connection also, the preparatory techniques described under the heading 'love play' will be found particularly valuable. Probably the greatest single mistake men make in bed is to devote insufficient time and effort to *preparing* their wives for intercourse. Furthermore, all too many men make little effort to *prolong* the act of love. If a husband tries to do these things, he will satisfy his wife; yet very often wives complain to doctors about their husbands that 'all he wants to do is get it over with in two minutes and go to sleep'. Husbands should remember that most women need to experience at least one climax (and probably considerably more than one) when they have intercourse (see **climax**). There is, however, no particular need for any such climax to be simultaneous with that of the husband. After some years of marriage, couples often feel that there is a sense of staleness and sameness about the act of love. It is usually easy to solve this problem. Firstly, both husband and wife should make every effort to make themselves as attractive as possible before love making. Intercourse between a wife with no make-up and her hair in curlers and a husband who hasn't shaved and who smells of beer is not likely to be over-successful. Secondly, a husband can readily make intercourse much more enjoyable for his wife by paying her compliments, taking her out to dinner and making love to her afterwards, and generally trying to recreate the atmosphere of their courting days. Thirdly, a good basic rule is 'try something new': help in this direction may be found in the section on **love play**; in addition, most couples find it stimulating to attempt intercourse in new and varied positions – an imaginative husband and wife will be able to work out literally dozens of such positions.

Painful intercourse usually needs investigation by a gynaecologist. *Bleeding from the vagina after intercourse* invariably does so.

INTERFERON is a chemical which interferes with the growth of viruses. Since most antibiotics, such as penicillin, have no effect at all on viruses, the isolation of interferon offers some hope that virus illnesses may be treated with a similar compound at some time in the future.

INTERMITTENT CLAUDICATION is a common symptom among elderly people with disease of the arteries supplying the legs. The patient finds that, after walking a short distance, he gets cramp or pain in the calves and has to stop. After resting for a few minutes, he finds that he can continue. In some cases a surgical operation can relieve the blockage of the arteries.

INTESTINE is that part of the alimentary canal (see **alimentary canal**) which runs as a continuous tube from the stomach to the anus. The narrow part (or small intestine) is about 20 feet long, and the broad portion (or large intestine) is usually about 6 or 7 feet long. The intestine is lined with special epithelium, containing numerous cells which secrete the digestive juices.

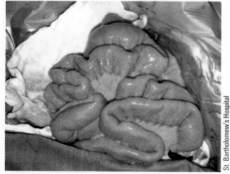

The glistening surface of the intestine as it appears to a surgeon operating on the abdomen.

INTUSSUSCEPTION is a condition of the intestine. One section of the tube which forms this organ actually enters the next segment, so that a blockage results.

194

The condition is particularly common in babies at around the time of weaning. The symptoms are spasms of pain, and screaming, usually with the passage of a small amount of bright red blood from the rectum. Treatment is usually by operation.

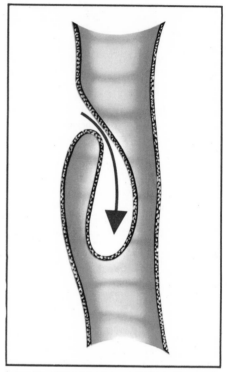

A portion of the intestine, pulled into the canal, may cause complete intestinal obstruction.

IODINE is an element essential to normal health. Lack of it in the diet can lead to thyroid disease (see **thyroid**). It is also used as an antiseptic.

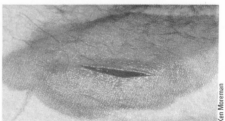

'Tincture of Iodine' is a solution of iodine in alcohol, for use as a surface antiseptic.

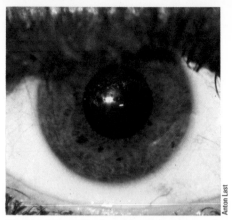

The iris of the eye is the coloured ring surrounding the pupil, acting like a camera diaphragm.

IRIS is the visible coloured part of the eye. It surrounds the pupil (which is itself just a round hole in the iris), and by expanding and contracting it varies the size of the latter, and regulates the amount of light which enters the eye. The colour of the iris depends on the amount of the pigment melanin which is present; in fair-skinned, blonde-haired people, there is likely to be little pigment present, and the iris then appears blue. This is the 'natural' colour of the eye in the unpigmented state — babies' eyes are blue because pigment does not appear in their eyes till they are several months old. The amount of pigment present in the iris regulates whether the eyes appear brown, hazel, green or other shades.

IRON is a metal which has been used by Man for thousands of years. It is only relatively recently, however, that it has been realized how important this mineral is to maintain life. Many people do not take in enough iron, despite the fact that only twelve to fifteen *milligrams* of the metal are needed every day in the diet. Iron-rich foods include meat (particularly liver), eggs and red wine. Among men, deficiency of iron is rare, save in those who are either poor, on a restricted, perhaps vegetarian diet, and eat meat rarely or not at all, and those who are suffering repeated loss of iron in the blood, through bleeding of any sort.

Among women, the situation is rather different. The average woman loses about 12 milligrams of iron at each period: some women however, may lose as much as 100 milligrams. This may not seem very much, but it should be remembered that the average adult only has about three or four grams of iron in the body, which *is equivalent to the weight of one small iron nail.*

The woman who has heavy periods may therefore lose about one fiftieth of her entire body store of iron at each menses. Furthermore, if she becomes pregnant, she will not only sustain blood losses at labour, but will also have to supply her unborn baby with enough iron to get him through not only nine months in her womb, but also the first six months of life outside it. Nearly all pregnant women tend to become anaemic unless they receive extra iron, and many other women have a degree of iron deficiency anaemia (see **anaemia,** and **iron deficiency anaemia**).

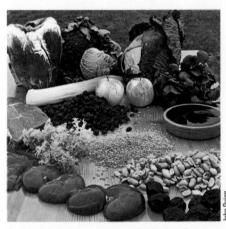

Foods rich in iron are essential in the diet, particularly for pregnant women.

IRON DEFICIENCY ANAEMIA is anaemia due to lack of iron (see **iron**). Although there are many types of anaemia (see **anaemia**), this is the most common variety, especially among women (see **iron**). The early symptoms of the disorder are tiredness, breathlessness on exertion, and sometimes dizziness. Pallor of the skin is usually present but may be masked in people who are sun-tanned or dark-skinned. It is almost always detectable to

195

the trained eye in the red margin which is exposed by turning down the lower eyelid: a doctor can usually make an estimate of the degree of anaemia by looking at this area.

When iron deficiency is more severe, further symptoms develop. These include a curious smooth, glossy appearance of the tongue, and characteristic changes in the nails of the fingers and (to a lesser extent) the toes, which become flattened and brittle. Later, they may even become concave or spoon-like. This condition is known as koilonychia: when it is severe, the patient can actually carry the contents of a small tea-spoon of salt in the concavity of the fingernail.

Today, iron deficiency anaemia is usually treated by means of tablets. Severe cases receive injections, while an occasional patient may need a blood transfusion. The condition is always curable.

ISCHAEMIA means impairment of the blood supply to any part of the body. Cardiac ischaemia, for instance, is characterized by an inadequate blood supply to the heart. If ischaemia is severe, it may lead to the condition known as infarction (see **infarction**).

ISONIAZID or **INAH** is isonicotinic acid hydrazide. This is one of the three drugs which defeated pulmonary tuberculosis. It was after the Second World War that research workers found chemicals which were effective against the bacillus responsible, and in the early 1950s isoniazid was used for this purpose. To begin with, it appeared that the tuberculosis organisms rapidly developed resistance to the drug, but it was found that by using isoniazid together with the antibiotic streptomycin and with another drug called P A S (para-amino-salicylic acid), the combination was nearly always successful. This discovery was one of the great advances in medicine.

ISOTOPES are elements which are identical chemically, but which have a slightly different atomic structure. They are used in medicine in two ways — as a source of radiation to treat growths and as a means of 'labelling' certain chemicals and making

it easy to follow their passage through the body.

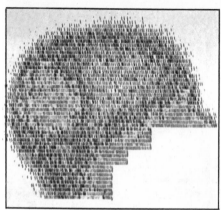

Radioactive isotopes can be used to outline tumours, such as this one within the skull.

ITCHING is a symptom of many conditions, including scabies (see **scabies**), obstructive jaundice (see **jaundice**), eczema, and fungal infections such as athlete's foot. Persistent itching is a symptom which requires medical advice.

-ITIS is a very common ending to medical words. It simply means 'inflammation'. For instance, appenticitis means inflammation of the appendix, tonsillitis, inflammation of the tonsils.

IVORY is the hard material which forms both the tusks of elephants and much of the bulk of human teeth. It is also known as dentine (see **dentine**).

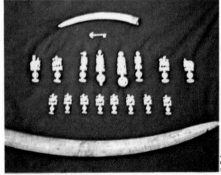

The texture of natural ivory makes it a favourite medium for the craftsman and artist.

196

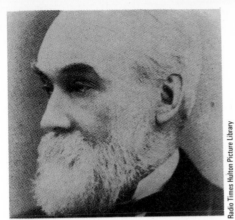
Doctor John Hughlings Jackson, who described the form of epilepsy now called after him.

Radio Times Hulton Picture Library

JACKSONIAN EPILEPSY

JACKSONIAN EPILEPSY is one of the less common forms of epilepsy (see **epilepsy**). Its characteristic feature is that attacks start in one particular part of the body, instead of being generalized, as is the case in most other types of the disorder.

A typical sequence of events is that the patient experiences a series of twitches in the fingers or toes, or at the corner of the mouth. These twitches may rapidly spread to involve a larger area (e.g. the arm or leg), and the patient may then go on to have an ordinary generalized epileptic attack, with complete loss of consciousness. On the other hand, the twitching may simply remain localized.

In another type of Jacksonian epilepsy, the patient experiences disturbances of sensation — for instance, pins and needles — in the affected part of the body, instead of twitches.

The occurrence of 'fits' of the Jacksonian type is usually an indication of some form of local, rather than generalized, brain disorder. For example, the small area of brain which sends messages to the hand and arm may be affected by a cerebral tumour, by an abscess, by damage caused through a blow to the head, or (quite commonly) by a stroke. Full investigation is necessary including an EEG (electro-encephalogram) test, skull X-rays and probably other special X-rays. Once the site of the disorder in the brain has been pin-pointed, it may be possible to deal with it surgically to prevent attacks.

JALAP is a very strong purgative which produces its effect through powerful irritation of the bowel. As with most strong purges, it is rarely prescribed nowadays.

JAUNDICE means yellowness of the skin, due to the presence in the blood and tissues of an excessive amount of bilirubin, a bile pigment (see **bile**).

There are many possible causes of jaundice, and, in order to follow the ways in which the condition may be produced, it is essential to understand the workings of the liver and the bile passages.

The liver produces about a pint of bile each day. This fluid passes down the hepatic duct and is concentrated in the gall bladder. From there, it is discharged at intervals into the duodenum (the part of the small intestine which leads out of the stomach). Once it is in the intestine, bile is of considerable value in aiding the processes of digestion.

If, however, the flow of bile is blocked at any point before it actually reaches the intestine, the damming-back will cause an accumulation of the pigment bilirubin in the bloodstream. This type of jaundice is known as *obstructive jaundice.*

Its characteristic features are as follows: there is usually some itching of the skin, due to the deposition of bile salts and pigment; the motions become pale and putty coloured, because there is no bile reaching the intestine to turn them brown and the urine becomes dark in colour, because of the accumulation of pigment in the blood.

There are a variety of causes of this type of jaundice, since the flow of bile can be obstructed at literally any point in the biliary passages, from beginning to end. For instance, the biliary passages within the liver may be obstructed during one phase of the common disorder known as *infectious jaundice* or *infective hepatitis.* Lower down, the hepatic duct and common bile duct can readily be blocked by gall-stones (see **gall-stones**), or by cancerous growths. Finally, the lower end of the common bile duct (just before it enters the intestine) may be blocked — sometimes by cancer of the pancreas, since the com-

197

mon bile duct passes through the tissue of this gland. However, it should be stressed that ordinary infective hepatitis, and *not* cancer, is the commonest cause of obstructive jaundice.

The second main group of causes of jaundice is that in which there is actual *liver disease* — for instance, cirrhosis of the liver. In this group, the destruction of liver tissue is responsible for the retention of bile pigment in the body.

Finally, jaundice may occur where there is excessive breakdown (*haemolysis*) of the red blood cells for some reason. In this type of *haemolytic jaundice*, pigment is actually released from the fragmented red corpuscles. This type of jaundice is seen, for example, in new-born babies affected by the Rhesus factor.

Jaundice is a symptom that invariably requires investigation, and, though the cause may not be serious, it is essential to consult a doctor as soon as possible.

JAW means the upper or lower teeth-bearing bone of the mouth region. The word is more usually employed to indicate the lower jaw or mandible.

The body of the mandible is horseshoe-shaped in front (in the region called 'the point of the jaw'); posteriorly it has a broad *ramus* on each side, running up to the joint at which the bone articulates with the rest of the skull. This ramus is very small during babyhood, but becomes much broader during childhood. At the same time, the horseshoe-shaped body of the jaw elongates to accommodate the full adult number of teeth. In old age, the body becomes much narrower as teeth are lost. These changes are of considerable interest to specialists in forensic medicine, since it is possible by examining the lower jaw-bone alone to determine fairly accurately the age of a skeleton, and this knowledge may be of value where an unidentified body is found.

Fractures of the mandible ('broken jaw') are quite common, especially among boxers. They may also occur during dental extractions. In the most frequently encountered type of break (fracture of the body of the mandible), the patient finds that he has intense pain and difficulty in speaking, after a blow to the chin; the teeth are noted to be out of line, and the saliva is blood-stained. As an immediate measure, the patient's jaw is supported by a 'barrel bandage'. As soon as possible the dental surgeon applies a rigid splint (usually consisting of steel wires) to the teeth adjacent to the fracture.

The upper jaw bone is known as the maxilla. It too can sometimes be fractured as a result of a direct blow or during a dental extraction. Such injuries are complicated by the fact that the bone contains on each side one of the sinuses, or air-cavities, of the skull. These sinuses communicate directly with the nose. Hence it is easy for a fractured maxilla to become infected, which delays healing.

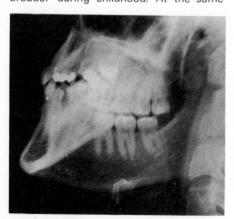

X-ray of a normal jaw, showing how the teeth have deep roots reaching down into the bone.

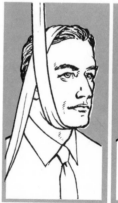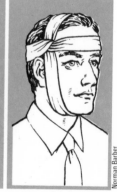

Norman Barber

Application of a 'barrel bandage', designed to support a fractured mandible, or lower jaw.

JEJUNUM is the anatomical name for the middle section of the small intestine. The first ten inches of the intestine are taken up by the duodenum, while the last part, joining the colon, is called the ileum. Between lies the jejunum, which is about two inches in diameter and some eight feet long. Its main function is to absorb nutriment from the food which has passed into it, and by alternate contraction and relaxation (peristalsis), to churn up the food and move it onwards to the ileum. (See also **alimentary canal**.)

JOINTS are points of junction or articulation between bones. In the case of the long bones of the body, such as the thigh bone (femur) and the shin bone (tibia), it is the ends of the bones which form the joints, but in flat bones, such as the bones of the skull, it is the edges.

Fibrous joints are articulations between bones, such as the flat bones of the skull, which are firmly linked together by fibrous tissue, so that practically no movement is possible.

Cartilaginous joints are those in which the bones are connected to each other by cartilage (gristle), so that some degree of movement is often possible. Examples include the joints between the vertebrae of the spine.

Synovial joints are what most people mean when they speak of 'joints' – for instance, the large joints of the limbs (the knee and elbow), and the small joints of the hands and feet. Synovial joints have much greater mobility than any other type, since the bones are not joined together. Instead, the articulating bony surfaces are each covered by a layer of cartilage (gristle). The joint as a whole is contained in a sac called the synovial membrane, inside which is a small amount of lubricating fluid called synovial fluid.

Any inflammation of a joint is called 'arthritis' – this is, therefore, a word which covers many different joint conditions producing inflammation. Arthritis is not a single disease in itself, as many people imagine.

The commonest type of arthritis is *osteoarthritis*, or degenerative joint disease. This is essentially a disintegration of the main weight-bearing joints of the body

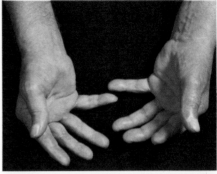
The distortion of the joints of the fingers and hand in a person with rheumatoid arthritis.

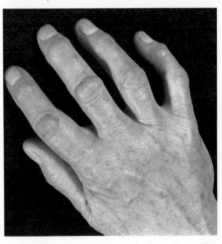
The swellings, called Heberden's nodes, which often appear in osteoarthritic subjects.

– the knee, leg, ankle and spine. The hands are not usually severely affected, but there are often small nodules, called Heberden's nodes, on the fingers. A very high proportion of all people over the age of 40 have at least some degree of osteoarthritis.

Rheumatoid arthritis, however, affects less than 5 per cent of the population, but may occur much earlier in life than osteoarthritis does and 'burn itself out'. It affects principally the small joints of the body – in particular, those of the hands and fingers, producing a characteristic type of deformity in which the fingers become 'spindle-shaped'.

Other types of arthritis include *ankylosing spondylitis*, or 'poker back', a condition which is quite common in youngish

199

men. *Gout* is also quite common; it affects principally the big toes, but may involve other joints as well. Various fevers, including *rheumatic fever,* may be associated with joint inflammation, as may a whole host of uncommon systemic disorders. However, it should be remembered that far and away the commonest of all joint disorders is osteoarthritis of the larger, weight-bearing joints of the body.

JUGULAR means pertaining to the neck. In particular, the word is applied to the large and often prominent veins (see **veins**) which carry blood from the brain, head and neck back to the heart.

KALA-AZAR is an infectious tropical disease, caused by a parasite known as Leishmania donovani. This parasite is transmitted to man by the bite of a sandfly. Any infection by a parasite of the Leishmania group is known as 'Leishmaniasis'; Kala-azar, however, is the special form of this disorder produced by Leishmania donovani. It occurs in the Mediterranean region, the Sudan, the Middle East, East Africa and also Russia and China. Very often, the 'reservoirs' of infection are dogs, foxes or jackals. They are bitten by the sand-flies, which then pass the disease on to human beings.

The symptoms, which may commence some months after infection are fever, weakness, pallor and weight loss. Internally, there is often gross swelling of the liver and spleen. Treatment consists in giving antimony compounds (which kill the parasite) and correcting the severe anaemia which is usually present by means of iron administration or blood transfusions. (See also **leishmaniasis**.)

KAOLIN is a white aluminium-containing powder. In the form of a mixture, it is used to treat mild cases of diarrhoea, either alone or with the addition of a small quantity of morphine. Because it retains heat, kaolin was also much used in the past in the form of poultices for application to the skin.

KELOID is an abnormal type of scar, in which the tissues, instead of healing in the
200

normal way, become grossly heaped-up and swollen along the scar line. The condition is particularly common in negroes. Often, keloids can be removed by plastic surgery, but there is always a slight risk that in some people the incisions made at the operation may in turn lead to fresh keloid formation.

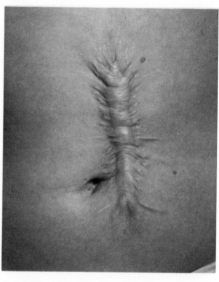

A keloid scar which has developed along the line of incision for a surgical operation.

KERATIN is a hard substance found in the horns of animals and in the hard, horny layers of human skin such as are found on the soles of the feet.

KERATITIS means inflammation of the cornea – the thin membrane in front of the eyeball, through which light passes to enter the eye itself. There are numerous possible causes of keratitis. For instance, if the eyelid cannot close for any reason, 'exposure keratitis' develops because of the fact that the cornea is not being protected adequately; another type of keratitis, 'interstitial keratitis', may be a manifestation of congenital syphilis.

KERATOMALACIA is softening of the cornea of the eye sometimes due to a lack of vitamin A in the diet. In advanced cases, there may even be ulceration of the eye. (See also **deficiency diseases**.)

KERNICTERUS is a type of brain damage in infants, caused by the deposition of bile pigment in areas called the basal nuclei. It follows the severe jaundice which occurs when large numbers of the child's red blood cells are destroyed *(haemolysed)* for some reason. The most common cause is the destruction of the blood cells by antibodies of the anti-Rh type (see **Rhesus factor**) passing into the bloodstream from the mother's circulation during pregnancy. If a Rh-negative mother, married to a Rh-positive father, is pregnant with a Rh-positive baby, she becomes sensitized to the Rh factor, and develops antibodies to it. These may not affect the first child seriously, but later Rh-positive babies are at hazard, and liable to become anaemic and severely jaundiced. The bile pigment damages the brain tissue and causes physical disability, in particular, the child may suffer from *athetosis*, a condition characterized by writhing movements.

Fortunately, kernicterus is much less commonly seen today than formerly. In newborn babies who are observed to have rapidly increasing jaundice, it is possible to tell very rapidly by blood tests whether the level of bile pigment is likely to reach a dangerous concentration. If so, the paediatrician will perform an exchange transfusion of the baby's blood, thus restoring the concentration of bile pigment to safe levels (see also **Rhesus factor**).

KETONES are a group of chemicals – the most well-known of which is acetone. The major importance of ketones in medicine is that they are produced from fats in the body under certain abnormal conditions – for instance, in starvation. In diabetes too (see **diabetes mellitus**), ketones are produced when the disease gets out of control (*diabetic coma* or *pre-coma*). A diabetic who is going into coma is almost certain to have ketones in his urine, and these can be detected by a very simple but valuable test; at the same time, his breath may well smell strongly of acetone.

KIDNEY – ARTIFICIAL The artificial kidney is one of the most remarkable medical inventions of all time. The kidneys (see **kidneys**) are essentially filters, which purify the blood and carry away all the poisonous waste products to be excreted in the urine. In quite an appreciable percentage of the population, disease eventually attacks these organs and impairs this function, so that dangerous concentrations of waste products build up in the blood. Tragically, severe kidney disease sometimes attacks quite young people. Until quite recent years, people who were so affected faced a very bleak outlook indeed.

In the 1940s, however, the first primitive artificial kidneys were developed. Many difficulties were encountered, however, and it was not until the 1960s that long term treatment of patients with kidney failure became a practical possibility.

As a typical case history, a young man with chronic kidney failure might become so ill that his life is in danger. His doctors then decide that he should either have a kidney transplant (if a suitable one is available) or be put on long-term *dialysis* (as artificial kidney treatment is called).

For long term dialysis, a plastic tube (called a 'shunt') is inserted into an artery and a vein of one limb, to connect them via a special filter which purifies the blood of toxic waste products. All the blood in the body has to be purified, and the process naturally takes many hours. In addition, waste products reaccumulate so quickly that it may be necessary to dialyse the patient two or three times a week; artificial kidney treatment is, therefore, a time-consuming business.

For this reason, techniques have been developed, in Britain and the United States, which enable a patient to have his own artificial kidney at home, and undergo dialysis at night whilst he is sleeping in his own bed.

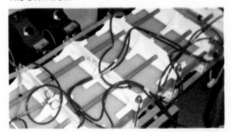

Part of the complicated tubing of an artificial kidney unit, used for dialysis.

KIDNEYS are two organs which filter impurities from the blood for excretion in the urine. Excretion is one of the most vital processes in the human body, and, if the kidneys are not working, treatment (dialysis) with an artificial kidney (see **kidney–artificial**), must be undertaken; or a kidney transplantation performed.

Each kidney, about four inches long and two and a half inches wide, lies at the back of the abdominal cavity, underneath the lowest ribs on each side. (It is for this reason that blows to this region may have such crippling effect, and are banned in boxing.)

Blood reaches the kidney via the renal artery. The smallest branches of this artery (the arterioles) lead into the capillaries, which are the tiniest blood vessels of all. The capillaries of each kidney are arranged in something like a million 'tufts'. Each tuft is surrounded by a membrane, through which fluid filtered from the blood under pressure passes into the narrow, coiled kidney tubules.

As the extracted fluid passes along the tubules, the cells of the walls absorb and pass back to the blood those constituents of the fluid which are needed by the body, and reject those which are not. To carry out this process requires an extremely complex series of chemical reactions in the walls of the tubule. In the healthy person, these reactions are so adjusted that the chemical constitution of the blood remains constant, and precisely the right amounts of waste product are removed.

Eventually, the tubules join together and deliver the excreted fluid, which by now is known as urine, into the region known as the pelvis of the kidney. From there, the urine leaves the kidney via the slim tube known as the ureter. The right and left ureters empty into the bladder, which is a reservoir from which urine is discharged through the urethra.

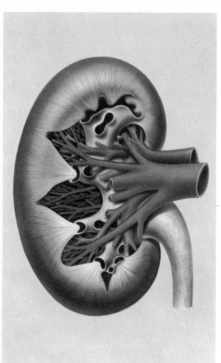

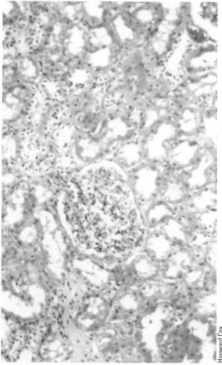

The structure of the kidney, showing the renal artery (red) and vein (blue), and the ureter (grey). The ureter leads down to the bladder.

Microscopic structure of the outer layer of the kidney (cortex), with the capsule of one of the nephrons seen in cross section.

Hayward Cox

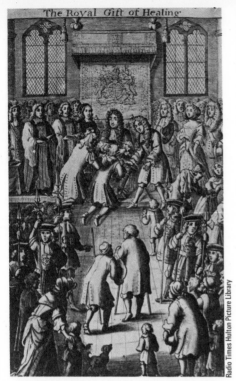

The Royal Gift of Healing

King Charles II touching his subjects to cure them of the skin disease called 'King's Evil'.

KING'S EVIL, or scrofula, is the old term for tuberculosis of the lymph glands of the neck — a condition which is nowadays very rare, but which was very frequently encountered in the Middle Ages, and, indeed, up till about the beginning of this century. The name 'King's evil' is due to the fact that people believed that the touch of the ruling monarch could lead to cure.

KLEPTOMANIA is a term which was once commonly used to indicate a supposed compulsion to steal objects, for instance from shops. There is, in fact, no single condition called kleptomania, but in a number of psychological disorders, patients do steal articles for no apparent reason. Some times this behaviour occurs because a person has deep inner conflicts which he or she cannot resolve except by carrying out some antisocial action. Again, guilt feelings may lead a person to steal in the hope of being caught and punished. In the type of personality defect known as psychopathy the person has, in effect, no 'conscience', and sees not the slightest reason why he should not steal to gain his own ends.

Persistent stealing also occurs in many disturbed children and adolescents. When this happens, psychiatric help should be sought and the child's parents should not hesitate to ask their doctor to refer the disturbed boy or girl to a child guidance clinic.

KNEE is the joint between the thigh-bone (the *femur*) and the shin bone (the *tibia*). Because so many different movements are required of it, its structure is quite complex, and because of the many strains which are placed upon it, it is very liable to injury.

The lower end of the femur in effect hinges on the upper end of the tibia, but between them is a cavity bounded by a structure called a joint-capsule, which is lined by a type of membrane peculiar to joints and known as the *synovial membrane.* In front of this cavity is the small bone called the *patella*, or knee-cap. Inside the cavity are strong ligaments and two half-moon shaped cartilages. It is these ligaments and cartilages which are so frequently damaged in the common sports injury which doctors call 'internal derangement of the knee joint'. In games like football or rugby, violent strains, in directions in which the knee is not equipped to bend, readily tear these structures. The symptoms are severe pain in the knee, often accompanied by swelling (as the joint cavity fills with fluid). Frequently, the patient suffers recurrent episodes in which the unstable knee seems to suddenly 'slip', and then becomes painfully 'locked' for a while. Attempts to manipulate such a locked knee are dangerous. Anyone who suspects he may have such a knee injury should be fully investigated at once, since the longer treatment is delayed, the greater is the risk of osteoarthritis setting in. Where a cartilage injury has been diagnosed, many orthopaedic surgeons recommend operation within a week if possible. This usually produces a complete disappearance of the symptoms.

Radio Times Hulton Picture Library

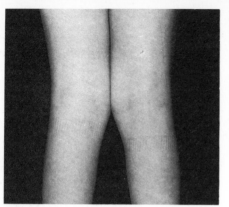

Photograph of a child with a fairly severe degree of genu valgum or 'knock-knees'.

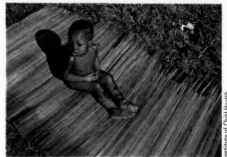

A child suffering from the protein deficiency disease called kwashiorkor, often rapidly fatal.

KNOCK-KNEE (or genu valgum) is a deformity in which the lower leg is displaced outwards so that the knees literally knock together while the patient is walking. In the past, it was very commonly due to rickets, but this is now very rare indeed in Western countries. Many healthy children have a very mild degree of knock-knee for no apparent reason, and these mild cases often correct themselves, though the parents of a child with the condition should, of course, always seek medical advice. If treatment is required, it may only be necessary to provide a special shoe which elevates the inner edge of the child's foot by a small amount. Children with slightly more severe deformity may need to wear leg splints at night. In addition, the parents are usually taught the technique of gentle manipulation of the legs in order to encourage the knee joint to 'grow straight'.

KOPLIK'S SPOTS are spots which appear inside the mouth early during an attack of measles (see **measles**). They are about the size of a pinhead and white or bluish-white in colour. As a rule, they are most readily found on the insides of the cheeks. Their importance is that (a) they confirm the diagnosis of measles, where this is in doubt, and (b) since they usually appear *before* the skin rash does, they often enable the doctor to make the diagnosis earlier than would otherwise be possible.

204

KWASHIORKOR is a form of starvation found very widely in children living in tropical countries. It is probably commonest of all in West Africa. It occurs when the child's diet is deficient in protein — the essential group of foods present in meat, fish, cheese, milk and eggs. The child may get more than adequate amounts of other foods — for instance, carbohydrates such as bread, rice, potatoes or sugar — and he may therefore be quite plump-looking. However, the gross deficiency of protein leads to chronic ill-health. The child's hair falls out, and what remains acquires a curious reddish discoloration, even in negro children. The skin becomes dry and flabby. As the condition progresses, the liver may increase in size and fluid (dropsy or oedema) may accumulate in the body, so that the starving child's abdomen actually appears swollen. Because the antibodies which help fight infection are formed from proteins, the child becomes an easy prey to any infectious disease. Death is certain, unless protein-rich foods are supplied. In the long run, kwashiorkor will not be wiped out while we have all over the world the situation that carbohydrate foods are very cheap and protein foods very dear.

KYPHOSIS is a curvature of the spine in a backward direction (as opposed to lordosis, which is a curvature in a forward direction). Such curvatures are very common, and most people are unaware that they have them. Severe kyphoses, however, need the attention of an orthopaedic surgeon.

LABIA is a Latin word meaning 'lips'. Although anatomists use the word to refer to any kind of lips (including, for instance, those of the mouth), the term is generally understood to mean the lips of the external female genitalia, or vulva.

The female organ is in fact, equipped with two pairs of lips – the labia majora, and the labia minora. The labia majora are the two external folds of tissue, one on either side of the vulva, running vertically from the region of the perineum (the area between the genitals and the anus) to the region of the mons veneris (the slight mound of tissue which lies in front of the pubic bone). The outer surfaces of the labia majora are pigmented and covered with pubic hair, while the inner surfaces are pink and relatively hairless.

The labia majora together form the homologue of the scrotum in the male – that is to say, they are formed from the same tissue in the embryo. In fact, in some patients whose sex is wrongly recorded as female at birth, the problem is that the scrotum is divided in the mid-line and contains no testicles (these being retained within the abdomen) – it therefore bears a strong resemblance to a pair of labia. If, in addition, the baby's penis is so small as to look like a clitoris, then the external resemblance to a female is complete.

The clitoris lies just below the mons-veneris, in front of the pubic bone, and between the upper ends of the two labia minora.

These smaller lips are situated within the labia majora. They run in a vertical direction, about $1\frac{1}{2}$–2 inches downwards from the area of the clitoris; they lie immediately external to the vestibule of the vagina. In the virgin, the lower ends of the labia minora are usually joined by the frenulum, a thin fold of skin. This is *not* the same structure as the hymen, or 'virgin's veil', which lies just inside the smaller pair of labia in the vestibule of the vagina. Also in the vestibule is the orifice of the urethra, or urinary passage; one of the most important functions of the two sets of labia is to protect this passage from contamination by germs.

Women are particularly susceptible to urinary infections, largely because it is so easy for germs from the rectum to make their way up the urethra into the bladder. This is particularly so in infants, in whom the nappy area is regularly contaminated by faeces. The labia majora and minora provide a double covering which gives considerable protection against the entry of bowel germs.

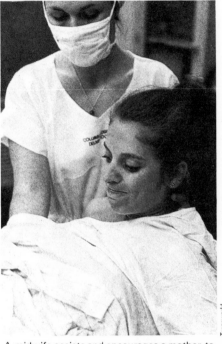

A midwife assists and encourages a mother-to-be, as the contractions of labour increase.

LABOUR is the process of repeated contractions of the womb which culminates in childbirth.

The *first stage of labour* is usually heralded by the onset of strong and regular contractions which produce some pain. (Contractions which occur in the weeks before labour are irregular and usually painless). When labour pains begin, they last only a short time – perhaps half a minute, and they may occur 20 or more minutes apart. Gradually, however, they become more and more frequent, and more painful, until really strong contractions are felt every few minutes.

The first stage of labour can also start, incidentally, with a 'show' of blood and

205

mucus, or with the breaking of the waters.

The *second stage of labour* should be reached well within 24 hours in the case of a woman who is having her first baby, and within 12 hours if she has given birth before. It starts when the cervix (or neck of the womb) is fully dilated. This precise moment can only be determined with absolute certainty by internal examination, but a fairly reliable indication that the second stage is imminent is the feeling which the mother has of wanting to 'bear down'. She should not try to 'push' with her pains before this, as straining downwards before the cervix is fully dilated is thought to be bad for the pelvic organs and lead to prolapse later in life.

The second stage is very short compared with the first one. It should not last more than 2 hours in a woman having her first child, and in a woman who has given birth before, it should not exceed one hour. Delay in the second stage is a common reason for the obstetrician to intervene and assist the baby's birth with forceps.

The *third stage of labour* begins when the baby is actually born, and ends when the mother is delivered of the placenta, or afterbirth. Usually it is a relatively pain-free and trouble-free period for the mother after what has gone before. Sometimes, however, she is unable to expel the placenta, and then the doctor has to remove it manually from the interior of the womb.

LACTATION is the process of producing milk from the breasts. When a woman is only a month or so pregnant, she notices a prickling sensation in the bosom. Shortly afterwards, the breasts become larger, and remain so during pregnancy and the period when the mother is nursing.

By about the third or fourth month of pregnancy, the nipples start to darken; soon afterwards, a thin fluid called 'colostrum' can be expressed from the breasts. This liquid is secreted until a few days after delivery, when certain hormonal changes taking place in the mother's body (as a result of the placenta no longer being in the womb) greatly increase the volume of the fluid and alter its composition to

206

that of milk (see **milk**). Milk usually continues to be produced by the breasts for as long as the mother wishes to feed: it is principally the stimulus of the baby sucking on the nipple which encourages its production.

All authorities agree that breast feeding is undoubtedly the best for almost all children — not only from a purely physiological but from an emotional point of view. It is only rarely that a mother absolutely cannot feed her baby, but regrettably quite a number of mothers are opposed to the idea these days, on such grounds as 'wanting to preserve their figures'. In fact, there is no real evidence that refraining from breast feeding has any such effect.

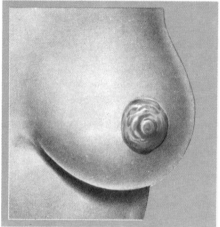

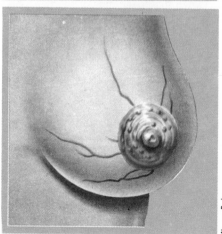

Norman Barber

The visible changes in the breast as pregnancy advances, in preparation for lactation.

LANOLIN is a fatty substance which is obtained from sheep's wool. It is used extensively in ointments, since it is a good solvent and does not become rancid like many other animal products. However, its function is only as a base in these applications; it does not itself have any curative properties. It has a limited use, because of its greasy nature, in soothing dry and chapped skin. For this reason, some mothers use it to apply to the nappy area to reduce chafing.

LAPAROTOMY means opening the abdomen by means of a surgical operation. The term is derived from two Greek words meaning 'cutting the flank'.

An 'exploratory laparotomy' does not just mean any abdominal operation, but one in which the diagnosis is in doubt. Very frequently, it is evident that a patient has some sort of trouble inside the abdominal cavity, but its nature may not be clear from examining him externally. For instance, it is relatively easy to confuse acute appendicitis, which usually produces pain in the lower right hand side of the abdomen, with salpingitis (inflammation of one of the Fallopian tubes), with an ectopic pregnancy on the right side, or with several other intra-abdominal conditions. Similarly, it is very often impossible without opening the abdomen to decide the cause of an obstruction of the bowel, which may be due to a growth, to adhesions (scar tissue) from a previous operation, to diverticulitis, or to some other cause. Very commonly too, a patient develops obstructive jaundice which is clearly due to something preventing bile from flowing down the common bile duct and into the intestine, and tests fail to reveal whether the obstruction is due to a gall-stone, to a growth of some sort, or to any other cause.

In all these circumstances, therefore, the surgeon will probably decide to undertake a laparotomy. Usually, as soon as he has opened the abdomen, the diagnosis will become clear, and he can take the appropriate action.

LARYNGITIS means inflammation of the larynx, the 'voice-box' which lies behind the Adam's apple at the top of the wind-pipe (trachea). It may be either acute or chronic.

Acute laryngitis is very common. It often follows an upper respiratory tract infection – for instance a head cold – when infection may spread downwards to the throat. Occasionally, infection starts in the chest (e.g. as bronchitis) and then spreads upwards until the larynx is involved. In these instances, the inflammation of the larynx is caused by infection by germs; sometimes, however, the inflammation has a 'mechanical' cause. This type of laryngitis occurs when a person indulges in loud and unaccustomed use of the voice. A common example is that of the football fan, who shouts himself hoarse during the first match of the season, and practically loses his voice for several days thereafter. The symptoms of acute laryngitis are familiar –

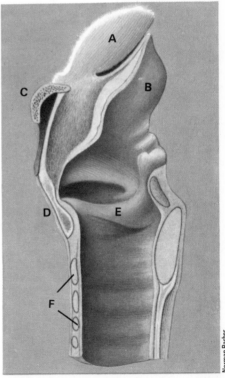

Norman Barber

Section of the larynx, showing *A* the tongue, *B* epiglottis, *C* hyoid bone, *D* thyroid cartilage, *E* vocal fold, *F* cartilages of the trachea. Laryngitis is inflammation of the tissues which form the lining of the larynx.

hoarseness, pain and dryness in the throat region, and some loss of voice. There may be a dry, painful cough.

Where acute laryngitis is due to infection, the treatment usually consists of antibiotics and the use of soothing warm gargles. In fact, gargles cannot reach the larynx itself, but they can soothe the tissues immediately above it.

Chronic laryngitis is much less common, and mainly occurs in those who persistently overstrain their voices — for instance, sergeant-majors and opera-singers. Essentially, what happens is that a series of episodes of acute laryngitis, occurring over many months or years, leads to a chronic thickening of the mucous membrane covering the interior of the larynx. The main symptom is huskiness and pain, which may be made worse on swallowing. In some cases, the condition progresses so far that small nodules develop on the vocal cords. Quite a number of well-known singers have had to have such nodules

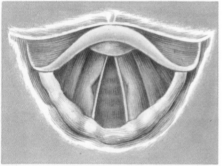

The vocal cords, as seen when a laryngoscope is used. During normal breathing the cords are wide apart, *above*, and are brought together during speech, to vibrate and produce sounds.

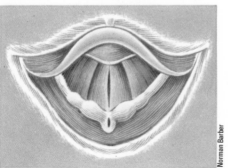

removed surgically.

The essence of treatment of chronic laryngitis is resting the voice. The ear, nose and throat surgeon, having inspected the larynx by means of his laryngoscope, may also prescribe sprays or soothing applications to the inflamed tissue.

Tuberculosis laryngitis is now fortunately rare. It was invariably due to spread of tuberculosis organisms from the lungs to the larynx.

Laryngo-tracheo-bronchitis is seen in young children. There is severe inflammation not only of the larynx but of the windpipe (trachea) and of the lower air passages (bronchi) as well. It is potentially an extremely serious condition, since the air passages of infants are so narrow that they may easily become blocked at the level of the larynx. The child is breathless and his respiration is extremely noisy (stridor). If his face becomes blue and congested, and it is evident that his larynx is obstructed, it may be necessary to perform a tracheotomy — that is, to open the windpipe in the lower part of the throat, below the obstructed larynx.

Diphtheritic laryngitis is now fortunately rare, since immunization against this terrible disease has become widespread. What happens is that the 'false membrane' characteristic of diphtheria blocks off the child's narrow larynx, and may literally choke him to death unless urgent measures are taken. Immediate tracheotomy is again indicated.

LARYNGOSCOPE means an instrument for examining the larynx. There are two basic types.

The first is the laryngoscopic mirror, which essentially consists of a tiny mirror, at the end of a long handle. The mirror is held at the back of the patient's throat, and the doctor illuminates the larynx by bouncing a light off this mirror. The light is often attached to a headband worn by the doctor.

In the other type of laryngoscope, which is mainly used by anaesthetists on unconscious patients, a curved blade with a light attached is slipped over the back of the tongue. This gives the observer a clear direct view of the larynx.

Norman Barber

LARYNX is the voice-box. It lies behind the prominence which is called the 'Adam's apple', and at the top of the trachea, or windpipe.

At the back of the throat, there are two passages – one for food and one for air. The one for food is the gullet, or oesophagus, and immediately in front of it lies the trachea, or windpipe. The opening of the trachea is guarded by a 'lid' called the epiglottis, and immediately below this lies the larynx.

The organ is about an inch and a half long, and slightly less in diameter. Its framework is made up of a number of cartilages. There are nine in all, including that which forms the lid-like epiglottis, and they are so joined together as to make up something very like a box. The largest of these cartilages is the thyroid cartilage, which actually forms the prominence of the Adam's apple in men. The cartilages are linked together by ligaments, and the interior of the whole structure is lined by mucous membrane.

There are two pairs of folds, one above the other, in the interior of the larynx. The upper pair are known as the false vocal cords, and the lower pair as the true vocal cords.

These true vocal cords normally lie rather slackly, like curtains drawn back, towards the sides of the larynx, but during speech, they tauten, and approach each other in the midline. Although the tongue, lips and palate do much to modify the sounds of speech, the voice is actually produced by the passage of air between the vocal cords. They also act in much the same way as the reed of a musical instrument, in that they are responsible for the actual notes produced. Depending on the tautness or slackness of the cords as they vibrate in the rush of air passing through the larynx, so a high or a low note emerges.

It can therefore be seen how a person who has lost his larynx due to cancer is no longer able to speak or sing. Such persons can, however, with practice learn to speak again by mastering the technique of swallowing air, and then regurgitating it back through the mouth.

Cancer of the larynx is fairly common. Until recent years, it was very frequently fatal. Nowadays, however, the operation of laryngectomy, or total removal of the larynx, gives remarkably good results, largely because this type of cancer does not usually tend to spread all over the body as so many others do. It is, however, essential to obtain treatment very early on in the course of the disease. *Any person over the age of 40 who has an episode of hoarseness persisting more than a week or so should consult his general practitioner at once.* If the condition does not clear up after a few days' treatment, the doctor will recommend an immediate examination by an ENT (ear, nose and throat) surgeon. Speed is essential, since early diagnosis and treatment can make all the difference between life and death.

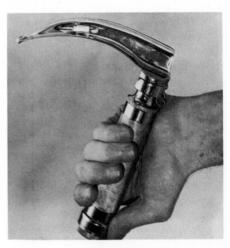

A laryngoscope of the sort commonly used by anaesthetists. The handle contains a battery.

LASER is a term which has been coined from the initials of the words 'light amplification by stimulated emission of radiation'. In recent years, it has been found possible to produce beams of light of such intensity and penetrative power that they can, for instance, be beamed all the way to the moon, and bounced back by means of a mirror.

Such powerful laser beams are also finding applications in medicine. Some types of beam can be used to cut through tissue just as a surgeon's knife would, for instance. However, the main medical

209

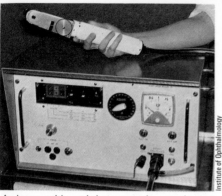

A laser with ophthalmoscopic attachment, used to attach the retina back in its position.

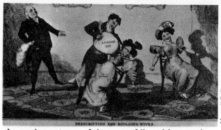

An early cartoon of the use of 'laughing gas'.

importance of the laser so far has been in treatment of the condition known as detached retina. In this disorder, the retina (the screen at the back of the eye) breaks loose from its attachment to the inside of the eyeball. One of the most difficult tasks of the ophthalmic surgeon is to re-attach the retina and so restore full sight to the patient. It has proved possible to do this in certain instances by 'welding' the retina to the eyeball by means of a laser beam. It seems likely that many other medical applications will be found for this remarkable invention.

LASSAR'S PASTE is a name commonly applied to a preparation of zinc oxide and salicylic acid with starch in white paraffin. It is one of the group of dermatological preparations described as *keratolytics*; these soften the horny layer of the skin and so reduce its thickness. It is widely used in the treatment of eczema.

LAUDANUM is tincture of opium. Although this medicine was once widely employed by doctors, it has largely fallen out of use since the development of other derivatives of opium, and also other pain-killing drugs with less dangerous side effects and no risk of addiction.

LAUGHING GAS is nitrous oxide, the gas usually employed for dental extractions, and, very often, for producing *twilight sleep* during labour. It is also used by anaesthetists for surgical operations,

210

but with the addition of some other anaesthetic. (See also **anaesthesia**.)

It was first suggested by Sir Humphry Davy about 150 years ago that nitrous oxide (or N_2O, to give it its chemical name) could be used to produce unconsciousness, and hence avoid the pain of surgical operations. Surprisingly, little attention was paid to his experiments, and he did not pursue them. About 40 years later, however, several Americans began to use both ether and laughing gas to produce unconsciousness — principally for the extraction of teeth. The gas was called *laughing gas* because it produced wild excitement in those who inhaled it, just before they became unconscious. In fact, it was used for this purpose at fairgrounds, where people paid a few cents to be rendered hysterical with laughter by the 'laughing gas man'.

In fact, nitrous oxide is felt nowadays to be suitable for use by itself as a general anaesthetic only where the period of unconsciousness is to be very short (as in tooth-extractions), since, in order to produce unconsciousness, it is necessary to reduce the amount of oxygen in the gas mixture being breathed to dangerously low levels.

LAXATIVES are drugs given to induce the bowels to act. For hundreds of years they were used very extensively by the medical profession largely because the intestinal tract was almost the only system of the body readily affected by medicines. Apart from laxatives, most of the 'draughts' given by doctors had no effect whatsoever. As a result, doctors and lay people generally came more and more to believe that 'purging' had a beneficial effect on all kinds of illnesses. This belief was, of course, totally unjustified, and it is now clear that in many conditions the administration of laxatives is positively dangerous.

Nonetheless, even today many members of the public (especially older people) firmly believe in the value of taking these preparations regularly, especially if they do not have a bowel action every single morning. In fact, although a *sudden* change in bowel habit (e.g. sudden constipation) in middle or later life is a serious symptom demanding immediate full investigation, most healthy children and adults need never worry about the regularity of their bowels. It is a significant fact that few doctors nowadays keep laxatives in their own family medicine cupboards.

However, there are specific circumstances in which it is necessary to prescribe laxatives. These drugs can be divided into various types.

Saline laxatives, such as magnesium sulphate, act by virtue of the fact that they attract water into the bowel through a process known as osmosis. This increases the bulk of the bowel contents; in response to this extra bulk, the intestinal wall contracts forcibly. This results in a bowel movement within two or three hours of taking the aperient.

Lubricants, such as liquid paraffin, simply make the bowel contents more 'slippery'; hence they speed their passage along the intestine.

Irritants, such as cascara, as the name implies, irritate the wall of the large bowel, so that it contracts violently. They usually take less than eight hours to produce an effect.

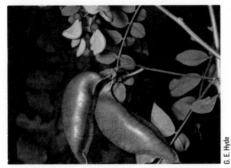

The Bladder Senna plant, whose pods were used to make an infusion with laxative action.

G. E. Hyde

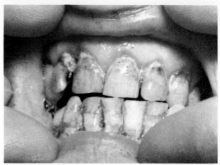

The 'lead line' which appears as a characteristic symptom of chronic lead-poisoning.

LEAD is a heavy metal which is a relatively common cause of accidental poisoning in both adults and children.

Among adults, poisoning by lead tends to occur in painters working with lead paint, plumbers, and people working in the production and smelting of the metal. It also occurs in people who regularly drink water, beer or cider which has accidentally been contaminated by lead from the piping it has passed through or in the vessels in which it has been kept.

To take two examples, *painter's colic* is a type of lead poisoning found in men working with old fashioned lead paint, while *Devonshire colic* used to occur in cider drinkers living in parts of Devon where cider was kept in lead containers.

Among children, lead poisoning is commonest in young infants who suck at or chew lead paint on their cots; the habit of eating strange substances is called *pica*. It is particularly dangerous where children are allowed to play with old lead accumulators and similar lead-containing objects; another hazard occurs if such things are flung on a fire or bonfire, and the fumes inhaled.

The principal symptoms of lead poisoning are colicky pain in the abdomen (hence the name *painter's colic*), the appearance of a curious blue line on the gums, and certain serious effects on the nervous system. These include a peripheral neuritis (see **neuritis**), characterized by weakness of the muscles around the wrist *(wrist-drop)*, and a severe brain disorder called lead encephalopathy (see **encephalopathy**) which leads to mental deterioration and fits. Lead poisoning also tends to make the victim anaemic.

Treatment consists in lowering the level of lead in the body, which can be done by means of drugs, and in finding the source of the poison and eliminating it — for instance, replacing the lead paint on a child's cot with safe paints.

LEECHES are slug-like animals which live mainly in ponds. If a person wades in water containing leeches, he is liable to find several of these curious creatures sticking firmly to his skin. They do this by means of a powerful sucker and hook-like teeth. Once attached to the skin, they suck blood out in quantities large enough to make their bodies grossly swollen. While having this happen regularly would, of course, make a person anaemic, leeches appear otherwise to have no ill-effects on human beings.

For this reason, they were for many hundreds of years employed by physicians to bleed patients — bleeding being a therapeutic measure highly thought of in the

these, there are the 26 smaller bones of the foot and toes.

The muscles of the leg are the most powerful in the body — particularly those of the thigh and buttock. The gluteus maximus muscle, which runs between the pelvis and the back of thigh-bone, is the largest of all muscles; in cattle it forms the basis of the cut known as rump steak. The hamstrings (at the back of the thigh bone) and the quadriceps (at the front of the same bone) are also very powerful indeed. The strength of these muscles is such that holds with the legs are completely banned in sports such as judo, because of the very real danger of severe injury to an opponent.

The blood supply of the legs is mainly through the femoral artery, which leaves the abdomen at the point in the groin where a very powerful pulse can be felt beating.

The main nerves which supply the limbs are the femoral and sciatic nerves. The latter runs from the buttock down through the back of the thigh. Pain felt in it is called *sciatica.*

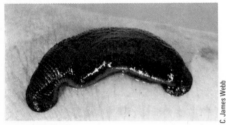

A leech attached to the skin by its powerful sucker, drawing up blood from the tissues.

Middle Ages. Indeed, leeches were occasionally employed by doctors as late as the Second World War. It was because of their use of these creatures that doctors themselves were for long referred to as 'leeches'.

LEG is the lower limb of the body, from the hip joint to the toes (though curiously enough, anatomists employ the word to mean only the lower leg, below the knee).

The leg contains three long bones — the femur, or thigh-bone, the tibia, or shinbone, and the fibula, a slim bone which runs vertically beside the tibia. Beyond

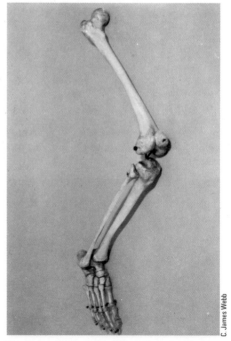

The bones of the leg and foot. From top: femur, tibia, fibula, tarsals, metatarsals, phalanges.

LEISHMANIASIS is an infection which occurs in certain tropical areas, notably the Mediterranean, the Middle East, Central and South America and many parts of the Orient. It is caused by a microscopic parasite of the group known as Leishmania which is transmitted to man through sandfly bites.

Leishmaniasis can be of various types, depending, among other things, on the species of Leishmania involved. One of the commonest forms of the disease is kala-azar (see **kala-azar**), caused by the species known as Leishmania donovani.

Other types of Leishmaniasis include the *cutaneous* variety. Known as Oriental sore, Delhi boil or Aleppo button, it produces unpleasant ulcers on the skin. It is never fatal, however. The causative organism in this case is Leishmania tropica.

American leishmaniasis, known also as espundia and forest yaws is caused by Leishmania braziliensis. It can be mild and produce only skin ulceration, or much more serious, destroying the mucous tissues of the body particularly those of the mouth and nose. All types of leishmaniasis are treated with compounds of the metal antimony.

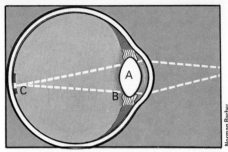

Section of the eye, showing *A* the lens, *B* the suspensory ligaments, *C* light focused on retina.

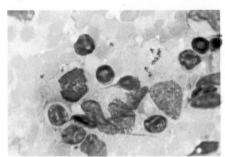

Smear of cells from the spleen of a patient with Leishmaniasis, showing small parasites.

LENS is the structure in the eye which is responsible, in part at least, for bringing rays of light to a focus on the retina, or screen, at the back of the eyeball. In fact, a good deal of the bending of light takes place in other layers of the eye, but the lens has the remarkable property of being able to alter its shape, so that the eye can 'accommodate' to near or far away objects.

LEPROSY is one of the least infectious, but perhaps the most unreasoningly feared, of all diseases caused by germs. It was once common throughout the world, but is now increasingly rarely seen. The germ which produces the illness is called Mycobacterium leprae. All efforts to discover exactly how it is transmitted from person to person have so far failed, but it is never passed on except after prolonged and close contact between two people, usually over a period of months or years. Typically a child may catch the disease from his mother. Nothing, therefore, could be further from the popular idea (inherited from mediaeval times) that leprosy is a wildly contagious disease.

There are two main types of leprosy: *tuberculoid* and *lepromatous.* Both types are characterized by a long incubation period, but the lepromatous variety runs a rather more rapid course than the tuberculoid, and tends to affect the skin in particular. It produces highly disfiguring nodules which may give the patient a hideous appearance. The tuberculoid variety, on the other hand, tends more to affect the nerves supplying the skin; the result of this is that areas become numb and devoid of feeling. Tuberculoid leprosy is so benign that it may even 'heal itself' in the end; however, very rarely, it may lead to gross ulceration or deformity of the part supplied by a particular nerve.

The results of the treatment nowadays are extremely good. The disease can always be arrested with drugs called *sulphones,* and in many cases a complete cure is effected. After a certain stage of treatment, the patient can usually leave

213

the hospital or leprosarium, since he is no longer infectious, and can live in the outside world in perfect safety.

LESBIANISM is female homosexuality. It is so called after the Greek island of Lesbos, most of whose inhabitants in classical times were apparently homosexual. The incidence of lesbian tendencies is totally unknown, but most experts in this field believe that true lesbianism occurs in less than five per cent of women, although it has been shown that (as in the case of male homosexuality) a considerably larger proportion of the female population have had trivial escapades of this sort – often, for instance, in adolescence.

True lesbians are sometimes (but by no means always) rather masculine in appearance, with close-cropped hair, and a tendency to wear suits and smoke pipes. Others may seem perfectly feminine in appearance. Sexual contact between them consists mainly of genital kisses and caresses, though sometimes a 'male' type of lesbian equips herself with a loin harness to which is attached an artificial phallus.

Treatment of lesbianism is almost impossible, except in the rare cases where the woman herself actually wants to convert to heterosexuality: here a psychiatrist may be able to help. (See also **homosexuality**.)

LESION means any kind of localized injury or disease process.

LEUCOCYTE means a white blood cell. These are much less numerous than are red blood cells *(erythrocytes)* in the bloodstream, but there are still roughly seven thousand of them per cubic millimetre of blood. They form an important part of the body's defence mechanisms. However, doctors do not yet fully understand the origin or function of all types of leucocyte.

Neutrophils normally make up about 65 per cent of all white blood cells in adults. Their numbers are greatly increased when the body is attacked by bacteria.

Eosinophils normally make up less than 3 per cent of the total. They increase in number when the body responds to an allergic challenge – for instance, in many cases of asthma.

Basophils make up less than 1 per cent of all white cells. Little is known of their function.

Lymphocytes make up about 25 per cent of the white cells. They may increase in number in certain virus infections and in tuberculosis.

Monocytes usually number less than 7 per cent. They increase in number in the disorder known as *infectious mononucleosis* (glandular fever).

Several types of white blood cell also increase greatly in number in various kinds of leukaemia (see also **blood**).

LEUCODERMA is a white discoloration of the skin, due to loss of the pigment melanin.

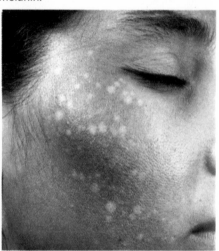

Typical appearance of the skin in leucoderma, showing discrete areas of depigmentation.

LEUCOTOMY is an operation in which certain white nerve fibres in the brain are severed. Although it is of some benefit to certain patients, particularly those suffering from schizophrenia and paranoid states, the operation is nowadays performed far less frequently than it used to be.

However, in selected patients it reduces emotional tension and anxiety, and allows the patient to take more interest in everyday practical matters than in his illness. It has no effect on his memory or his intelligence.

214

LEUKAEMIA is a form of cancer of the white blood cells, or leucocytes (see **leucocytes**). It may take various forms, but the cause of each is unknown; however, some cases have followed exposure to ionizing radiation. Leukaemia may be acute or chronic.

Acute leukaemia may involve any of the types of white blood cell present in the body, but the clinical picture is much the same in each case. It usually begins quite suddenly, with fever, great weakness, bleeding from the nose or throat or the formation of mouth ulcers. Anaemia is usually severe. Examination of the blood shows that there are anything up to ten times as many white cells as normal present. Untreated, the patient dies within a few weeks. New methods of therapy are constantly being introduced, but with rare exceptions all these can do at present is to prolong life for a relatively short period. Tragically, this disease very often affects young children.

Chronic leukaemia, on the other hand, is often a disorder of adults. Chronic lymphatic leukaemia is commonest in the age group 40–65, and occurs more frequently in men than in women. Its onset is slow and insidious, and it is characterized by enlargement of the lymph glands – most obviously seen in the groin, armpit and neck. The glands remain quite painless, however. Examination of the blood shows an increase in white cells of up to 50 times the normal value; most of these cells are of the type known as *lymphocytes*; which normally constitute only about 25 per cent of the total number of leucocytes. Chronic lymphatic leukaemia usually produces death in about four years, but modern methods of treatment may extend the life span appreciably, and make the exacerbations of the disease easier to bear.

Chronic *myeloid* leukaemia occurs in a slightly younger age group, and is equally common in men and women. Again, the disease is insidious in onset.

The main features include severe anaemia and weakness, both of which are related to invasion of the bone marrow by leukaemic cells. There may, however, be many diverse symptoms. Examination of the blood shows an increase in white cells many times over, the particular type affected being the neutrophil leucocyte (see **leucocytes**).

It is usually about 3 years before death occurs, and again treatment may considerably prolong life.

Although the outlook is at present bleak, nonetheless, since patients with chronic leukaemia can expect to survive several years, there is always hope that continuing research will produce a cure within the lifetime of anyone found to have the disease.

LICE are minute insects which very readily infest human beings. They produce extremely unpleasant itching, and, in some countries, can also carry very serious diseases.

Lice are divided into three types – those which infest the head, those which infest the body generally, and those which infest the genital regions. In all cases, the creatures shelter under hairs, and attach their eggs to them. Transmission is by contact with an infested person, and there is literally no protection against it, however high one's standard of personal hygiene. Anyone who suspects that he may have acquired an infestation with lice, should consult a doctor as rapidly as possible, before this infestation is passed on to someone else. The doctor will probably recommend treatment of the skin or hair with a DDT preparation, coupled with careful de-lousing of the clothing. Bedding is likely to form a reservoir of infection, and must also be de-loused.

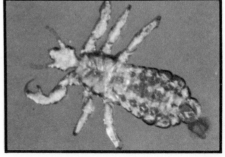

James Webb

The type of louse which affects the human head, seen magnified about twelve times normal size.

LIGAMENTS are tough fibrous bands which bind bones together, especially in the region of joints.

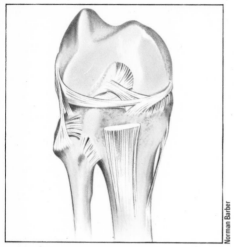

The complex of ligaments which surrounds the knee joint seen with the knee-cap removed.

Norman Barber

LIGHTNING is responsible for a considerable number of deaths every year. Some of these are avoidable – for instance, if a person insists on either standing out in the open or, worse still, sheltering under a tall tree, in a heavy thunderstorm, he greatly increases his chances of being struck. It is much safer to take shelter under bushes, low trees, or any structure that does not 'stand out' and attract lightning. Most authorities believe that holding a metal object is also dangerous – the worst possible situation, therefore, is that of a golfer with a metal trolley and bag of clubs who takes shelter under a lone tree.

Nonetheless, lightning is so unpredictable in its behaviour that some deaths are quite unavoidable – people sitting in houses are struck quite frequently; lightning conductors do, however, reduce this risk.

Essentially, a lightning strike is a severe electric shock, and tends to stop the heart just as current from the mains does. *First aid:* if there is no pulse, start compressing the chest (cardiac massage), as described under 'drowning'; get someone else to give mouth to mouth artificial
216

respiration till breathing is restored. Keep both these measures up without ceasing till medical help arrives.

LIGNOCAINE is a local anaesthetic. It is also known as xylocaine. The first widely used local anaesthetic was cocaine, which dentists found extremely effective for filling and removing teeth, and which surgeons used for minor operations such as stitching up cuts or removing small lumps from the skin. Cocaine, however, had many dangers, not least the fact that it is a highly dangerous drug of addiction.

During the last twenty years, therefore, it has been entirely replaced by chemically related compounds of which lignocaine is the most widely used. Injected into the tissues, lignocaine produces anaesthesia in the surrounding area for periods of twenty to sixty minutes. It can also be injected close to a nerve to 'block' (or deaden) it; this is the technique most widely used in dentistry, since it banishes all pain sensation from the entire area supplied by the nerve.

Lignocaine has few drawbacks; it is important, however, not to inject it directly into the bloodstream, since large doses reaching the brain may cause fits.

LINCTUS means any medicine made up as a syrup in order to make it palatable.

LINEA ALBA is the anatomical name applied to the 'white line' of tissue running down the mid-line of the abdomen and through the umbilicus. Along this line, the muscles of the two sides of the abdomen join. (See also **linea nigra**.)

LINEA NIGRA literally means 'black line'. Down the middle of the abdomen runs the 'white line', or linea alba (see **linea alba**). In pregnancy, the region of this line becomes progressively darker, owing to deposition of pigment, until, toward the end of the nine months, the linea nigra appears as a very distinct blackish line or band running from the lower end of the breast bone to the top of the pubic hair.

LINIMENTS are oily external applications also known as 'embrocations'.

LIPOMA means a fatty swelling or tumour; the word 'tumour' does not imply cancer, incidentally, and lipomas are benign growths. They are extremely commonly seen in almost any area of the body.

Diffuse lipomas tend to occur under the skin of the neck. They are said to be associated with excessive beer-drinking, and, according to one of Britain's leading surgical authorities, are less commonly seen nowadays, owing to the increased price and diminished strength of beer.

Circumscribed lipomas are very common. They are felt as small lumps, usually just under the skin; they have a clearly defined edge, and it may be possible to feel the separate lobules of fat. Circumscribed lipomas may also grow in the region of the scalp, around joints, in muscles, in glands, and, indeed, anywhere in the body where fat occurs.

A particularly common form of circumscribed lipoma is the *pedunculated* variety. These tumours grow out from the skin at the end of a slim stalk, giving them a rather bizarre appearance, which may be alarming to the patient. However, it is an extremely simple matter for the surgeon to divide the stalk and remove the tumour.

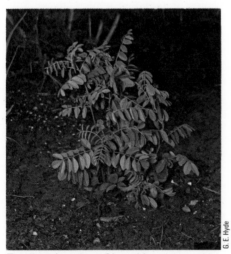

The liquorice plant *Glycyrrhiza glabra*, which grows in Mediterranean countries.

LIQUORICE is a plant root, widely grown in the Mediterranean region. Apart from its use in confectionery, liquorice has some importance in medicine. It has had a reputation for well over a hundred years as a folk remedy for stomach ailments, and also as a mild laxative. Until quite recently, however, doctors prescribed it only as a flavouring ingredient in medicines.

It was not until a group of medical researchers decided to investigate what basis there was for its reputation as a folk medicine that it was discovered that liquorice contained an ingredient of very considerable value. An extract of this substance, known as *carbenoxolone* has been shown to be the only drug which has any effect whatever on the healing of gastric ulcers. It may also be of value in promoting the healing of other types of ulcer, including duodenal ulcer, but in the latter condition it has so far proved difficult to find a satisfactory way of bringing the substance into contact with the ulcer.

LITHIUM is a metal which is chemically related to sodium and potassium. It has recently been claimed to be of value in the treatment of mental illness. In fact, it was one of the earliest drugs to be tested by psychiatrists, being first tried out in the treatment of depression in 1897.

Lithium was then largely forgotten, however, and it was not until 1949 that an Australian researcher carried out experiments with guinea-pigs which suggested that it might have a tranquillizing effect on disturbed human beings. Since then, a number of psychiatrists have published work suggesting that lithium is useful in the treatment of patients with the disorder known as mania. It is also believed in some quarters that it has a beneficial effect on patients with depression, though this view is not widely accepted.

LITHOTOMY means removal of stones or calculi (see **calculi**) from the body. Almost invariably, the term is used to refer to operations to remove urinary stones, as opposed to other types of stone.

The oldest bladder stone of which we have knowledge was found in an Egyptian mummy which was believed to be over 6,000 years old. Whether the Egyptians tried to remove such stones is not known, obtained what seems to have been at least some measure of success. They used what nowadays seems a crude and somewhat brutal operation, involving driving a knife into the mid-line of the perineum (the area between the genitals and the anus) and extracting the stone with a finger.

This operation was used more or less unchanged for 1500 years. In Elizabethan times, it was regularly carried out all over Europe by itinerant lithotomists. Many of these men were not medically qualified, and they frequently plied their trade at fairgrounds; they would have moved on to the next 'pitch' before there was time for a patient to complain of any after effects.

During the next two or three centuries, considerable improvements were made in technique. Samuel Pepys had a stone the size of a tennis ball removed in 1658 and enjoyed good health for many years thereafter. Men like Frère Jacques, the famous lithotomist who practised around 1680, made the operation considerably safer, though it was not until the advent of anaesthesia in the 1840s and of antisepsis in the second half of the 1800s that lithotomy became a safe, and usually effective, operation.

Nowadays, there are a number of techniques of removing urinary stones. Soft stones may be crushed by means of a special 'claw' attached to a cystoscope (the 'telescope' which can be pushed up the urinary passage and into the bladder). This process is known as 'lithotrity'. A similar instrument can be used to catch small stones and draw them out via the urethra. Larger stones are usually removed nowadays by making an incision in the lower abdomen and opening the bladder. More complex techniques are used to deal with stones stuck in the upper parts of the urinary passages (the ureters and kidneys).

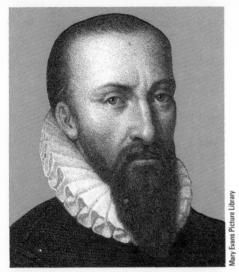

Mary Evans Picture Library

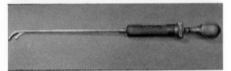

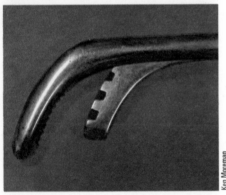

Ken Moreman

Above Ambroise Pare, French surgeon of the sixteenth century, and an adept at lithotomy.
Below The lithotrite, an instrument introduced into the bladder to grip and crush stones.

but the ancient Greeks certainly did. In fact, the celebrated oath of Hippocrates forbids doctors to 'cut for the stone', which suggests that the results of the operation of lithotomy in 400 BC were not too good.

From Roman times up until the middle ages, however, lithotomists (as surgeons who carried out lithotomy were known)

LITMUS is a chemical whose special value to medicine (and many other forms of science) is that it changes colour depending on whether it is placed in an acid solution or an alkaline one. In acids, it goes red, while in alkalis it goes blue. Litmus paper consists of little strips of reagent paper impregnated with litmus solution.

LIVER is a large organ which lies in the upper right-hand corner of the abdomen immediately under the diaphragm. It is the largest gland in the human body, weighing about $3\frac{1}{4}$ pounds in an adult male, and slightly less in a female. Even in children, the organ is very large in comparison to the size of the body. For instance, it constitutes about one twentieth of the entire weight of a new-born baby, and for much of babyhood it is so large that its lower edge may be felt well below the lower margin of the child's ribs on the right-hand side.

In adults, however, the whole of the liver normally lies under the lower ribs, which protect it from injury. If the edge of the organ is felt any lower than this, then the liver is either enlarged or pushed down by a low diaphragm.

The liver is purplish-brown in colour, and, although solid, is composed of relatively fragile tissue. In fact, it bears a very considerable resemblance in appearance and consistency to the type of animal liver which is seen in butchers' shops. Its shape has been described as that of a triangular prism, with the right angles rounded off. Anatomists refer to the organ as having two main lobes (right and left); the right lobe is very much larger than the left one. There are also two much smaller lobes situated between the right and left major lobes.

Although the tissue of the liver is soft, the whole organ is protected by a strong capsule, which renders damage to it less likely. Once this capsule is breached, however (as may occur in the type of violent strains the body undergoes in car accidents), the consequences are likely to be severe, since the internal tissue will tear very readily. A ruptured liver may easily prove fatal, because of the very considerable amount of blood loss which can take place from the torn hepatic tissues. However, the organ has such powers of regeneration that it heals rapidly.

The liver is very closely situated to several other abdominal organs – notably the stomach and duodenum, which lie just underneath it, and the gall bladder, which is attached to its under surface.

Among the most important functions of

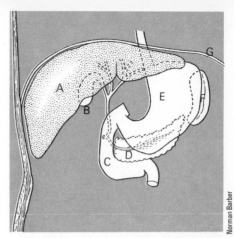

The relation of the liver to other organs. *A* the liver; *B* gall bladder; *C* duodenum; *D* pancreas; *E* stomach; *F* spleen; *G* diaphragm. Note how the ducts from the liver unite into one duct, which joins with the duct from the pancreas and opens into the duodenum.

Norman Barber

the liver is the production of bile (see **bile**). The hepatic cells produce roughly three pints of fluid each day, and it flows out of the organ via a slim tube known as the hepatic duct. This duct joins in a Y-junction with the cystic duct, which leads to the gall-bladder – a small pear-shaped organ which acts as a reservoir and as a concentrator of bile. From the Y-junction, the common bile duct leads down to the duodenum, the first part of the small intestine, in which bile is mixed with food to aid digestion.

In addition to producing bile, the liver has dozens of other functions, but only a few of them are of considerable importance to doctors.

In particular, the liver plays a vital role in the process of absorption of food into the body. Broken-down (digested) food passes through the walls of the small intestine and the tiny molecules of nutriment enter the bloodstream. They are carried by a large vein, called the portal vein, to the liver, which, in a sense, 'masterminds' their subsequent fate in the body.

Carbohydrates, in the form of glucose, reach the liver and are stored there in an altered form called 'glycogen', or 'animal

219

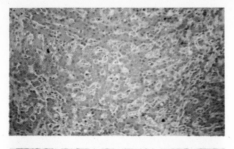

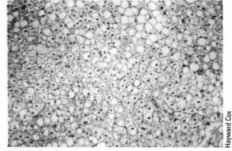

Microscopic sections of the normal liver *(top)* and the cirrhotic liver *(bottom)*, showing how the fibrous tissue replaces normal cells.

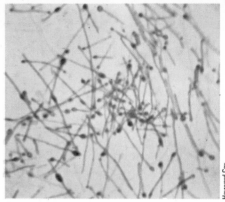

The organisms responsible for tetanus – *Clostridium tetani* – typical 'drumstick' shapes.

starch'. The liver releases glucose (which is the body's basic fuel) from this store of glycogen as it is needed.

The liver also 'organizes' the conversion of the breakdown products of proteins and fats to the forms in which they will be used by the body. It also breaks down alcohol.

The liver is also a major storage organ, containing large quantities of vitamins A, B_{12}, D and K and also of iron and copper. Finally, it breaks down or otherwise renders harmless many chemicals, including potentially dangerous drugs and certain poisonous substances. (See also **hepatitis**.)

LOBECTOMY means cutting out a lobe of an organ. It is particularly applied to the removal of lobes of the liver or the lung. The former operation is uncommon, and usually carried out for cancer. Removal of a lobe of the lung is, however, a more frequently-performed operation, either for cancer or for the presence of a chronic but often localized lung disorder known as bronchiectasis.

LOCKJAW is the common name for tetanus (see **tetanus**). This disorder is caused by infection with a germ known as *Clostridium tetani*, which normally exists in the faeces of man and, more particularly, domestic animals such as the horse. Human beings become infected when the germ enters a cut in the skin; this may readily occur, for instance, if a person sustains even a very slight break in the skin while gardening. The disease is commonest in agricultural countries, but still causes a substantial number of deaths in industrialized nations. Most doctors feel, therefore, that it is wisest for everyone to be immunized against lockjaw.

The earliest symptom of the disease is 'trismus' – a painless spasm of the cheek muscles, occurring some days after the original injury. The rigidity spreads over a matter of hours until spasms affect all the muscles of the body. In particular, the facial muscles are drawn into a hideous grin, and the muscles of the back are so violently contracted that the patient's whole body is arched backwards each time a spasm occurs.

A very high percentage of untreated cases of lockjaw prove fatal. Treatment consists in giving penicillin and anti-tetanus serum (A.T.S.), together with sedatives and muscle relaxants. Even with the most skilled and careful nursing, there is an appreciable death-rate, which is all the more reason why it is wise to take the precaution of being fully immunized.

LOCOMOTOR ATAXIA is one of the late manifestations of the venereal disease syphilis. It is also known as *tabes dorsalis*.

In this particular form of the disease, the organisms causing syphilis (tiny germs called *Treponema pallidum,* or *Spirochaeta pallida*) attack the patient's central nervous system. As a rule, this does not happen until many years after the original infection. It is, therefore, mainly a disorder of middle-aged or elderly people.

Syphilis attacks particularly those portions of the spinal cord which receive messages concerning sensation from the limbs and body. Very often, therefore, the first symptoms of locomotor ataxia are 'lightning pains' in the legs or trunk. These can be so severe that patients are occasionally admitted to hospital with suspected appendicitis because of them. Before very long, the patient usually develops a tendency to stagger when he walks; he finds that he cannot keep his balance when his eyes are shut, and may actually fall about if, for instance, he gets out of bed in the middle of the night. This is because the damage to the part of his spinal cord that deals with sensation is preventing information about the position of his body from reaching his brain.

Damage to the region of the spinal cord which supplies the bladder very often leads to urinary retention (which is characteristically painless). If the infection has spread to the brain (as occurs in 90 per cent cases) then the pupils of the eye are affected in a characteristic manner, and double vision may be present.

Eventually, the patient loses all sense of position in his legs and feet, and as a result he walks with a curious stamping gait. To the observer, he appears to be banging the feet down forcefully on the ground, but he himself feels as if he is stepping on a thick layer of cotton wool. There may well be mental changes, depending on how far the spirochaetes have penetrated the brain tissues.

The advent of penicillin 30 years ago has dramatically reduced the incidence of locomotor ataxia. Unfortunately, however, once the disease has attacked the central nervous system, penicillin can usually do no more than arrest its further progress.

LORDOSIS is an abnormal curvature of the spine forwards (as opposed to kyphosis, where the curvature is backwards).

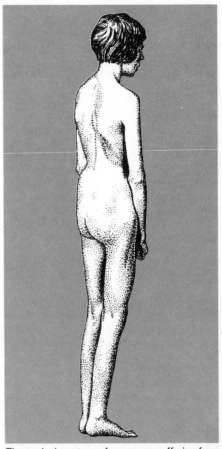

Norman Barber

The typical posture of a person suffering from the spinal curvature known as lordosis. The back becomes hollowed, the stomach protuberant.

LOVE PLAY, or fore-play, is the type of excitatory behaviour (in the form of kisses, caresses and so on) which takes place before sexual intercourse.

It is fair to say that neglect of this aspect of marital relations is the cause of a very great deal of sexual frustration in marriage. It is the universal view of experts on this subject that both husband and wife should be well versed in the simple techniques of love-play. All too often, however, what happens is that both husband and wife are quite unaware of these methods of enriching their relationship, and the result may be that sex is totally unrewarding for both parties.

To take an example, many men have, because of ignorance, simply no idea at all of how to arouse their wives. They therefore make a habit of commencing intercourse without any preliminary caresses whatever, get the whole thing over with as rapidly as possible, and then turn over and go to sleep — probably leaving a frustrated and wakeful wife. It is no wonder that until recent years a very high proportion of wives simply never reached a sexual climax (orgasm) at all. It is now widely recognized that most women are perfectly capable of (and probably need for their mental well-being) not one but several climaxes during love-making. The object of the husband should therefore be to arouse his wife slowly for a period of time (say, 5, 10 or even 20 minutes) before actually beginning intercourse. He can do this very easily by means of kisses and caresses of the whole body, including the lips, breasts and the genital region.

Conversely, many women have no idea at all of how to excite their husbands. Widespread knowledge of the simple fact that to caress the penis is an essential part of love play would, among other things, probably greatly reduce the incidence of impotence (see **impotence**). Many men are affected temporarily or permanently by this disorder. It is the view of sexologists that what has been called 'mistress-like' behaviour on the part of the wife (involving 'taking the lead' in love play) greatly helps men with this psychological difficulty. (See also **intercourse**.)

LUMBAGO means pain in the lower back. It is not, as most people imagine, a disease in itself. (See **backache**.)

LUMBAR PUNCTURE is the procedure whereby cerebrospinal fluid (see **CSF**) is tapped from the lower part of the back. The patient lies on his side, and a small quantity of local anaesthetic is injected into his skin over the spine. A needle is then pushed through the anaesthetised area and between two of the lumbar vertebra, and a little of the fluid, which sur-

rounds the spinal cord, is investigated.

LUNG is one of a pair of organs which take up most of the chest cavity. In these organs, air which has been breathed in gives up some of its content of oxygen to be absorbed into tiny blood vessels called capillaries. At the same time, 'stale' blood in the capillaries discharges carbon dioxide (the waste gas of the body's tissues) to be breathed out by the lungs.

Disorders of the lung are dealt with under their own headings, with the exception of *cancer of the lung*.

This disorder is now the commonest cancer among men in many western countries, and among both men and women the incidence is rising steeply. There is not the slightest doubt that this alarming increase (which has been going on for over a quarter of a century) is due in the main to the rising consumption of cigarettes. Any heavy smoker stands a good chance of getting lung cancer, and the disease is quite common among those who only smoke moderately. The best preventative, therefore, is not to smoke cigarettes.

The commonest symptoms of the disease are cough, chest pain, and blood-stained sputum, but anyone over the age of 35 who develops a chest infection which fails to clear up in a couple of weeks should have a chest X-ray *at once*; the only chance of curing lung cancer is if it is caught early.

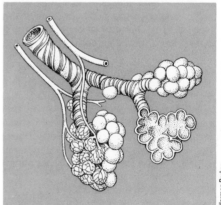

The fine structure of the lung, showing the small air sacs in which each bronchiole ends, and the network of bloodvessels surrounding them, carrying blood for reoxygenation.

LUPUS VULGARIS is a form of tuberculosis which affects the skin. Like all manifestations of this disease, it is far less frequently encountered than it used to be, but until the advent of streptomycin and other anti-tuberculous drugs, in the early 1950s, lupus vulgaris was a common sight.

It usually affects the skin in the region of the cheeks and nose, although it can occur in other sites as well. The characteristic appearance is that of a raised semitransparent nodule which bears a strong resemblance to a blob of apple jelly. This nodule may be present for many months or years without altering in form. However, the patient usually develops other manifestations of tuberculosis in due course: there may be local complications such as skin ulcers, often with considerable destruction of the face; on the other hand, there may be evidence of tuberculosis in other parts of the body, for instance, the lungs.

Lupus vulgaris is theoretically infective but, in practice, it is rare for someone else to catch tuberculosis from a person in whom the disorder is confined to the skin. Nonetheless, prompt treatment with antituberculosis drugs should be instituted, to save the patient from the unpleasant complications of the condition.

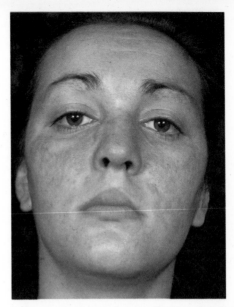
Lupus erythematosus, one of the collagen diseases, with a characteristic 'butterfly rash'.

LUPUS ERYTHEMATOSUS is one of the group of disorders known as the *collagen diseases*. It has nothing whatever to do with lupus vulgaris, and it is not caused by tuberculosis, though some lay people still invariably associated the word 'lupus' with tuberculosis.

The collagen disorders are a group of diseases which affect the connective tissue of the body. Their cause is completely unknown, but it has been suggested that they may occur because of some error in the body's normal mechanisms of immunity.

Lupus erythematosus can occur in two forms – localized *discoid* lupus erythematosus and disseminated (*systemic*) lupus erythematosus (see also **DLE**). However, differentiation is often difficult, since, like all the collagen diseases, they tend to merge one into another.

Localized *discoid* lupus affects females much more commonly than males. It occurs in the form of a red, scaly butterfly-shaped rash across the bridge of the nose. This rash is exacerbated by sunlight; very often, it occurs one summer, then disappears, only to recur again the following year. Things may continue like this for many years, and the rash may spread no

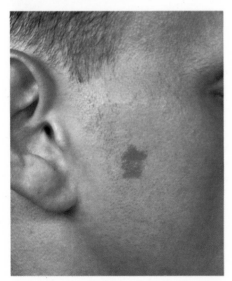
Tuberculosis of the skin, or lupus vulgaris, is now rarely seen, thanks to modern drugs.

223

further. On the other hand, it may progress to involve other areas of the skin which are exposed to sunlight – for instance, the lips. Rarely the disease may progress until it becomes disseminated lupus erythematosus.

Treatment of discoid lupus consists mainly in giving the antimalarial drug chloroquine, since it was discovered quite by accident that this has a beneficial effect on the rash. Possibly this is because one of the actions of some antimalarial drugs is to protect the skin against sunlight.

Disseminated (systemic) lupus erythematosus is, as the name implies, a generalized disease, which may involve not only the face but many tissues of the body, and the kidneys in particular. A fuller account is given under the heading **DLE**.

LYMPH is the fluid which circulates in the body's lymphatic system and lymph glands (see **lymph glands**). It is a thin, colourless fluid which contains white blood cells, fats and many chemicals. Essentially, it is the 'drainage fluid' of the body.

All tissues contain a great deal of water and waste products, and although some of this material is carried away by the bloodstream, the blood circulation is simply not capable of coping with all of it. All the tissues of the body are therefore drained by a fine network of tiny lymph channels. These are demonstrated quite clearly if a dye, such as Indian ink, is injected into the tissues. Within a few minutes, the lymph channels draining that particular region can be picked out as dark, spidery tracks across the skin. As a rule, the only time when a person is likely to see evidence of the existence of his own lymph channels is if he has a poisoned finger, or other severe inflammation of the hand. Under these circumstances, red streaks are likely to appear, running up the length of the arm. This condition is called **lymphangitis**, and there is likely to be simultaneous enlargement of the lymph glands in the armpit.

The lymphatic system can, however, be blocked. Such blockage occurs in certain infections with parasitic worms (filariasis), and also when the tissues are damaged by radiotherapy. The effects are quite dramatic, since the affected part becomes

grossly swollen. This condition is known as elephantiasis; its occurrence is an indication of damage to the important lymphatic drainage system.

LYMPH GLANDS are the small glands (see **glands**) at the connecting points of the body's lymph system (see **lymph**). When infection or inflammation occurs in the tissues which a particular group of glands drain, then those glands swell up.

The main sites at which lymph glands occur in the body are as follows: the arm pits, above the collarbones, at the sides of the neck, at the angle of the jaw, in the groins, and behind the knees.

LYMPHANGITIS is inflammation of the lymph channels. It is most commonly seen as a series of red streaks which run up the arm when a person has a poisoned finger, as the infecting organisms spread.

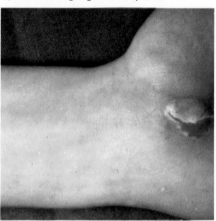

Infection travelling along the lymph channels from a wound may show up as red streaks.

LYSERGIC ACID, or **LSD**, is a potent hallucinatory drug (see **hallucinogens**). Known to its users as 'acid', it produces the most bizarre and extraordinary disorders of perception. It is not a drug of addiction, but most doctors condemn its use, save under controlled conditions, because of the danger of producing serious, possibly permanent, psychiatric illness. It may also damage the chromosomes in the sex cells, and thus pose a threat to unborn children.

MCBURNEY'S POINT is the anatomical landmark which, in the majority of people lies over the region of the appendix (see **appendix**). It is therefore in the region of McBurney's point that surgeons generally make their incision when operating for appendicitis. The point lies two thirds of the way down a line between the navel and the front prominence of the hip-bone.

MALARIA is one of the world's commonest infectious diseases. It occurs almost entirely in the tropics and sub-tropics, wherever conditions are suitable for the breeding of the anopheline mosquito. The infected mosquito carries the parasite which produces the disease in man and injects this organism whenever it bites a human being in order to suck blood.

The parasite carried by the mosquito may be of four different types, and each type produces a different variety of malaria. The four species of parasite are called *Plasmodium vivax*, *Plasmodium ovale*, *Plasmodium malariae* and *Plasmodium falciparum.*

Plasmodium vivax and Plasmodium ovale both produce what is called 'tertian' fever, in which the patient's temperature goes up every other day, Plasmodium malariae produces 'quartan' fever occurring every third or fourth day, and Plasmodium falciparum produces a more or less continuous fever.

In each type, the cycle which occurs is as follows: a female mosquito feeds on the blood of someone with malaria. The parasites are drawn into the mosquito's stomach with the blood, and there they mate. One to three weeks later, their offspring are ready to infect anyone bitten by the mosquito. A week or more later, the infected person starts to feel cold and shivery. However, his temperature is in the region of 104°F. This attack of fever comes on as the parasites (which up till now have been 'resting' in the liver) are released into the blood.

After his initial bout of shivering (known as a rigor), the victim starts to feel extremely hot and usually has to take to his bed. Headache and vomiting are prominent features at this stage, and the patient may become delirious. After some hours,

he breaks out into a very heavy sweat, sufficient to drench the bedclothes. The immediate attack is then past, the temperature drops and the patient feels well until the next peak of fever comes, two or three days later.

In the case of infection with Plasmodium falciparum, the fever tends to be continuous and prolonged, and the characteristic cold, hot and sweating stages do not occur. This type of malaria is highly dangerous. It does, however, have the advantage that, since all the parasites are present in the blood, it can be entirely wiped out with anti-malarial drugs such as chloroquine. In the other types of malaria, some of the parasites remain in the liver, where they are immune to chloroquine, and are thus liable to produce relapses. However, newer drugs such as primaquine are effective in banishing the parasite from the liver.

People going to areas where malaria is very common should always take a suppressive drug, such as proguanil, every day from about a week before they enter the area until a month after they leave.

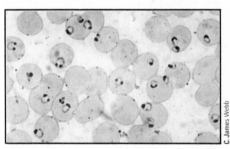

Malaria parasites in typical ring shapes, in the red blood cells, during severe infection.

MALATHION is an organo-phosphorus insecticide. Although these chemicals are extremely useful in agriculture and gardening, they must be treated with great respect, since they are highly toxic to man as well as to insects. Although malathion is not as dangerous to human beings as the related compound parathion, nonetheless it should never be allowed to get on the skin, and must at all costs be kept locked up and out of the reach of children.

The manifestations of poisoning include blurred vision, increased production of saliva, sweating, nausea, vomiting, diarrhoea and cramp. These are followed by paralysis. Contaminated clothing should be removed, and contaminated skin washed clean as rapidly as possible. A doctor should be called at once, and he will commence treatment with atropine injections and remove the patient to hospital.

MALIGNANT is a term which is principally used in medicine to refer to cancerous growths. Non-cancerous growths are referred to as 'benign'. The word 'malignant' does not, of course, imply that death is inevitable or even necessarily likely, since many malignant growths are curable.

MALIGNANT HYPERTENSION has nothing to do with cancer. It is an old and rather unfortunate term used to describe an especially severe form of raised blood pressure in which there is a particular type of change (called 'papilloedema'), noted on examining the retina, at the back of the eye. This sign is an indication that immediate energetic treatment, normally involving hospitalization, is called for. (See also **hypertension**.)

MALLET FINGER is a fairly common deformity seen after injury to a finger, for instance, after catching a cricket ball. (In fact, the condition is known as 'baseball finger' in America.)

What happens is that a sharp blow on the end of the finger bends it so violently that the tendon on the back of the finger is torn, and it can no longer straighten the joint which is nearer to the nail.

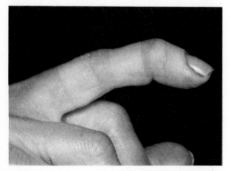

Typical appearance of the finger following rupture of the tendon which straightens it.

226

Treatment of this injury is difficult and not always successful. It involves splinting the finger so that it is flexed at the joint nearer the hand itself but straightened at the one nearer the nail. The object of this is to rest the torn tendon for a period of about six weeks.

MAMMARY GLAND is the structure, possessed by all female mammals, which produces milk. In women it is, of course, the breast (see **breast**). The mammary glands in any mammal are situated somewhere down the so-called 'milk-line', which runs from the middle of the collar-bone to the groin. Many human beings (including men) have tiny rudimentary nipples along this line, and occasionally patients are seen with an extra fully developed breast somewhere along it.

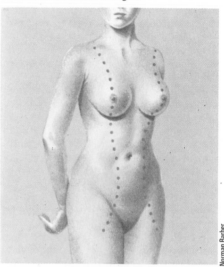

Norman Barber

The 'milk-lines' of the human body. Along these lines extra, rudimentary nipples may grow.

MAMMOGRAPHY means X-raying the breast. The object of this technique is primarily to determine the nature of breast-lumps which could be cancerous, but whose nature is not clear from simply examining the patient. In America, mammography is sometimes also used on apparently normal breasts as a matter of routine examination, in case a small growth is present but is 'missed' at physical examination. (See also **breast**.)

MANDIBLE is the anatomical name which is applied to the lower jaw (see **jaw**).

MANIA is a state of mental disorder in which the patient is excited, over-active, and usually irrationally happy. It may seem odd to say that a person who is mentally ill may be extremely happy, but in manic states of this type, the characteristic mood is one of wild elation, super-optimism, and great confidence. The patient feels he can do almost anything he wants to, regardless of his own abilities. His air is that of a triumphant superman, who can become Prime Minister or win an Olympic gold medal next week if he wants to. When mania is severe, the patient may become quite delirious.

Hypomania is a milder form of the same condition. Because of this the patient can often get along for days or even weeks before someone realizes that something is seriously wrong. He seems constantly in the best of spirits, talks a great deal and is full of over-optimistic plans. He may spend money like water, and buy things he cannot possibly afford. He may be arrested for some offence, since he is likely to believe that laws are for mortals, not for people like him.

Very occasionally, a hypomanic person may achieve some remarkable feat, particularly if he is in any way artistic. For instance, he may paint something of considerable beauty, never having done anything of equal value before. In such instances, what has happened is that the repressions of his mind have been broken through, and, for a brief moment, allowed him to express himself.

In general though, the manic or hypomanic person has to be protected from himself. This may be difficult, as such a person will almost certainly feel that he is perfectly well and healthy. In severe manic states, admission to mental hospital will be necessary, though this is not necessarily so when the patient is merely hypomanic; it may be possible to merely calm him with tranquillizers.

In any case, the outlook in most patients who suffer a single attack of hypomania or acute mania is good, particularly when there is some obvious precipitating factor, such as the death of a loved one. However ill the patient seems at the time of an acute attack, it is perfectly possible that, within a few months of psychiatric care, he can be returned to a normal state of mind.

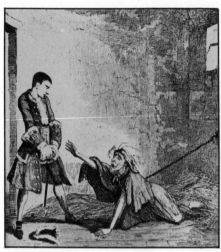

A drawing by Cruikshank of a miserable patient consigned to Bedlam. Patients with severe mental disorder, only a century ago, were liable to be chained and treated in an inhumane way.

MANIC-DEPRESSIVE PSYCHOSIS is an illness characterized by alternate bouts of mania (see **mania**) and depression. In fact, such an occurrence is rare, but there are many people who are prone to episodic illnesses, which are sometimes depressive in nature, and which sometimes have hypomanic features. It seems that a liability to such illnesses is to some extent inherited; they seem also to occur in people whose bodies are described as 'endomorphic' — plump and stocky in build. Often, their personality prior to the onset of the illness has tended to be very much 'up-and-down', with a characteristic over-response to life's failures and successes.

The outlook varies in patients with this type of illness, but with the advent of new drugs and the skilled use of electro-convulsive therapy (ECT), it has improved in recent years.

MANTOUX TEST is a type of skin test which is of considerable value in the

227

control of tuberculosis. In many countries, it is carried out as a routine on all children of about the age of fourteen, and also on anyone who is likely to be exposed to tuberculosis — for instance, nurses, medical students, hospital doctors, and sanitorium workers.

The fluid used for Mantoux testing is a protein-containing liquid obtained by sterilization of a laboratory medium on which tubercle bacilli have previously been grown. This fluid is entirely harmless, but when small quantities of it are injected into the upper skin layers of the forearm of a person who has tuberculosis, a reddish swelling develops at the injection site within two or three days.

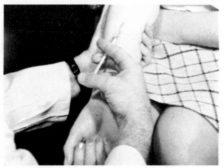

Above Receiving an injection for the Mantoux test, in the arm, and *below* a strongly positive reaction in the presence of tuberculosis.

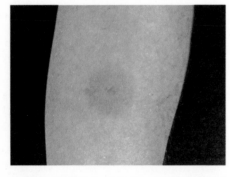

About half the adult community in most countries have had at some time in the past a mild tuberculous infection which has passed totally unnoticed, since their bodies' defences have overcome the germs. In all these people, the Mantoux test will also be positive, though the red-228

ness and swelling of the skin are likely to be very slight compared with the reaction found in someone who actually has the disease.

As a rule, school children who prove to have negative Mantoux tests (and who have therefore never had a tuberculous infection) are offered vaccination against the disease, using BCG vaccine. Those who *have* overcome such infections in the past do not need such vaccination.

The *Heaf test* is essentially a modern modification of the Mantoux test. It involves spreading a slightly different fluid on the skin, and then pressing a device called a 'multiple puncture gun' down on it. This is practically painless, which makes it much pleasanter for use with children. The interpretation is essentially the same as for the Mantoux test itself.

MAPLE SYRUP DISEASE is an uncommon disorder of babies. It is an inherited defect of metabolism which, if untreated, leads to mental deficiency. It gets its name from the fact that the child's urine has a very penetrating aroma of maple syrup.

MARGARINE is, strictly speaking, any form of imitation butter. Most margarines are just as nutritious as butter, provided that they have had appropriate amounts of vitamins added. This is likely to be so in most Western countries, where strict statutes usually insist on the addition of appropriate quantities of vitamins A and D to these products.

More important, an increasing number of medical men now suspect that, in the long run, margarine is very much better for the health than butter is. This is because butter, as an animal product, consists of the type of fats (called *saturated* fats) which are suspected as being a cause of arterial disease and coronary heart disorder. These diseases now constitute a virtual epidemic threatening Western man.

Margarine, on the other hand, is usually made from vegetable oils only (though this is not always so; some margarines contain a percentage of butter or whale oil). This type of fat is *unsaturated*, and is thought not to cause these widespread and often fatal disorders (see also **fats**).

MARIJUANA is an extract of the leaves of the plant Cannabis sativa (see **Cannabis**). It is much weaker than the other and less commonly used extract, *hashish*, or Cannabis indica, which comes from the flowering tops. It is widely used in many areas of the world, and it is noteworthy that medical investigators fail to agree about possible ill-effects it may have on the human mind or body. It is not a drug of true addiction.

It thus falls into the class of 'soft' drugs, and is probably less dangerous than either nicotine or alcohol. Its main drawback at the present time seems to be that it is used by social groups (e.g. the hippies) in whom taking of 'hard' drugs (such as heroin, cocaine and the amphetamines) is commonplace. These drugs *are* addictive, and are also potential killers. Some people fear that to use marijuana may lead on to taking 'hard' drugs. In fact, there is no evidence at the present time that such escalation is inevitable. In the light of these facts, it seems probable that the harsh penalties which exist in the United States (and, to a lesser extent, in other Western countries) for use or possession of marijuana may well be relaxed in years to come. There are certainly drugs more dangerous.

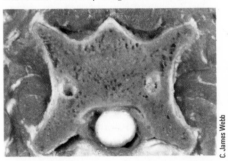

A cross-section of a spinal vertebra shows the spongy marrow in the compact outer layer.

MARROW is the soft matter found in the middle of bones. It is of two types – red marrow and yellow marrow. The red marrow is found in the interior of the smaller and flatter bones of the adult body, and also at the ends of the shafts of the long bones, such as the thigh bone, shin bone and so on. The yellow marrow occupies the remainder of the shafts of the long bones in adults; it is yellow because much of it is made up of fat.

The red marrow, on the other hand, is very rich in the cells which are responsible for the formation of blood. In children, the whole of the long bone shafts are taken up by this red marrow, but it gradually shrinks and gives place to yellow marrow as adulthood approaches. If, however, an adult has urgent need of new blood formation (for instance, when he is anaemic, or after a severe haemorrhage), then the red marrow will expand again to meet the demand.

MASOCHISM, called after L. von Sacher-Masoch, is a form of perversion (see **perversions**). Its characteristic feature is that the sufferer cannot achieve sexual satisfaction unless pain is being inflicted upon him, for instance, by flagellation. Contrary to popular belief, masochists frequently have sadistic tendencies as well, and may find it necessary to inflict, as well as to receive, painful stimuli to find sexual release. In fact, like all perversions, masochism is frequently associated with still other varieties of perverted sexuality, notably leather fetishism.

While it is perfectly normal for human beings to wish to give and receive what may be described as minor pinpricks of pain (e.g. 'love-bites') during love-making, nonetheless when a desire for this sort of thing becomes so excessive that the infliction of considerable pain becomes a necessity, then a very serious psychological illness is present. The causes of such a perversion of the sex instinct are believed to be related to abnormal experiences in infancy; psychiatric treatment may help.

MASS X-RAY is a widely employed and highly effective method of radiological examination of the chests of large numbers of people.

Mass miniature radiography (MMR) units are normally housed in large vans, which travel from place to place, often making stopping points at schools or factories for several days at a time. The apparatus is capable of X-raying about 60 to 100 people an hour. The films which are produced are miniature ones, measuring only a few inches square, but they are

229

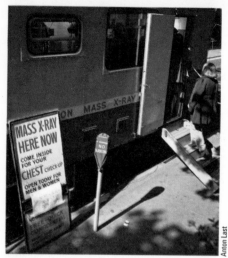

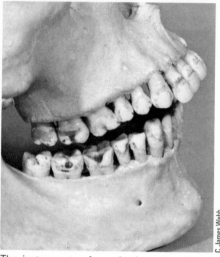

Mass X-ray vans were a common sight in most large towns. The miniature films that were produced indicated to the radiologist whether a further, more detailed examination was required.

The instruments of mastication, the grinding back teeth (molars) show clearly on this skull.

a most valuable guide to the radiologist who examines them to see whether any chest disease, especially tuberculosis, is present.

However, very often all the radiologist can do is to note that there is some slightly abnormal appearance on the miniature film. The person concerned will then be asked to have a full-size chest X-ray taken. Frequently this reveals that the 'shadow' is of no significance, but it may, of course, show that the patient is in need of treatment for a hitherto unsuspected chest condition.

Routine mass X-ray methods played so great a part in the dramatic reduction in the incidence of tuberculosis that the units are now less needed.

MASTICATION means chewing of food. It is an essential part of the process of digestion, by which the food is rendered suitable for the next stage, which takes place in the stomach. The powerful muscles of the lower jaw, aided by those of the cheeks and tongue, churn the food as it is cut up by the front (incisor) teeth, and ground up by the back (molar) teeth. At the same time, it is mixed with saliva, which contains chemicals which initiate the
230

breakdown process that renders food suitable for absorption into the body from the small intestine.

MASTITIS means inflammation of the breast. Although there are various types of breast inflammation (including, for example, breast abscesses), the term 'mastitis' normally implies a *diffuse* inflammation of the mammary tissues.

Among the types of such diffuse inflammation which may occur are the following.

Infantile mastitis occurs in babies of both sexes, and usually resolves itself. *Puberty mastitis* is also common in both sexes, and requires no treatment other than reassurance. *Local irritation mastitis* is seen in women who wear over-tight brassières, and also occasionally in men who wear braces. *Milk engorgement mastitis* occurs particularly at weaning, when the breasts are 'choked' with milk. While uncomfortable, it rarely lasts very long. *Premenstrual mastitis*, causing slight pain in over-tense breasts before the period, is very common indeed. Treatment for a few days with a drug to reduce the amount of fluid in the body (a *diuretic*) may help. *Mastitis due to infection* is dealt with under the heading **breast**. So too is *mastitis due to chemicals*, such as silicones.

MASTOID literally means 'breast-shaped'. The term is particularly applied to a projection of one of the bones of the skull, which can be felt directly behind the lobe of the ear.

The particular importance of the mastoid process is that it contains air cavities which communicate with the cavity of the middle ear. Middle ear infection (*otitis media*), producing earache and fever, is common in childhood, and it is very easy for the infection to spread into the mastoid process. When this occurs, the condition is known as mastoiditis.

Up till about 20 years ago, severe mastoiditis was extremely widespread and many children suffered long periods of ill health as a result. It was often necessary to perform an operation which involved chiselling away the infected bone. The resultant scar behind the ear was a very common sight.

Fortunately, things are different nowadays. The advent of antibiotics, and the recognition that their prompt use in middle ear infections is essential, has reduced the incidence of severe mastoiditis to virtually nil. In order to avoid this unpleasant condition, parents should ensure that any child who has an earache, especially if there is tenderness over the bone behind the ear, is seen promptly by a doctor. He will inspect the child's ear-drum with an auriscope, determine whether middle-ear infection is present, and, if so, prescribe an antibiotic, either by mouth or injection.

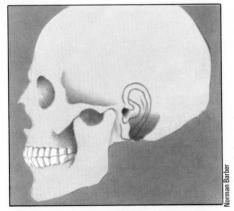

Mastoiditis is infection which has spread to the spongy bone behind the ear.

MASTURBATION means stimulation of the genitals by hand or other means to produce sexual pleasure. Strictly speaking, the term includes the caresses which are a feature of love-play, but, as a rule, it is used only to indicate *self*-stimulation of the genital areas.

There are few subjects on which ignorance and misinformation has been more widespread than this one. Regrettably, this ignorance has been responsible for considerable harm and anxiety being caused to the minds of parents and children in the past. Fortunately, in the last 20 years or so, a much more enlightened attitude has begun to prevail.

Masturbation in infancy is extremely common, and a normal feature of the young child's development. Only if it becomes excessive is some form of child guidance necessary; in such circumstances it is usually an indication of some deep-seated anxieties. Otherwise, a child should simply be left alone if he or she is noted to be masturbating. There are obvious exceptions to this rule, of course, and if on a particular occasion, the situation makes it socially undesirable that the child should continue (for instance, if visitors are present), then his or her attention should be distracted. This is very simply done by proffering a toy or any other means: fortunately infants are the most readily distractible of all human beings. *On no account should the child be slapped or subjected to dire threats.* A generation ago, it was common practice to threaten to castrate young children found masturbating; the psychological consequences of this sort of parental behaviour can be disastrous.

In years gone by, masturbation during puberty and adolescence was widely regarded with horror. Victorian fathers sometimes engaged attendants to stay with boys day and night, and make sure they did not engage in what was referred to as 'self-abuse'. Worse still, apparatus was devised for children to wear to keep them from masturbating, and sometimes operations were undertaken with the same aim.

All this was because there was an extraordinary idea in most Western countries

231

(particularly the United States and Great Britain) that masturbation caused insanity or blindness. Even in the 1940s, sex education books hinted that it had frightful consequences.

In fact, all these ideas were complete nonsense, though the harm they did was incalculable. It is now recognized that masturbation is a perfectly normal part of growing up, and indeed, apart from nocturnal emissions, the only form of sexual release available to the young at a time when the sex glands are far more active than they will ever be again. (See also **puberty**.)

MAXILLA is the upper jaw-bone, which carries the upper set of teeth (see **jaw**).

MEASLES is one of the common infectious diseases of childhood. It is caused by a virus which spreads from child to child in tiny droplets expelled from the mouth or nose during talking, laughing, coughing or sneezing. (This is the standard method of transmission of many viral diseases.)

The characteristic features of the disease are as follows. About 10 days after exposure, the child develops symptoms rather like that of a cold, with catarrh, sneezing and red eyes. At this stage, it may be possible to discern the first manifestation of the rash; this takes the form of tiny blueish-white spots (see **Koplik's spots**) inside the cheeks. After about 3 or 4 days (i.e. about 2 weeks after the original exposure), the skin rash itself develops. This usually begins behind the ears, but it rapidly spreads to cover the whole skin. The spots are blotchy and pinkish-brown in colour; they are usually thickest on the face.

At this stage the child usually feels rather unwell, and the worst of the disease is largely over. He gradually gets better over the course of a week or two, and the areas of skin affected by rash slowly become a pale brown and flake off.

Complications of measles are fortunately fairly uncommon in Western countries, though the disease can very often be a killer in underdeveloped lands where the children are suffering from malnutrition.

No treatment is necessary, or indeed possible, in the uncomplicated case; antibiotics have no effect on viruses and are therefore not given.

Immunity against measles: most people have had measles and one attack probably gives life-long immunity, but since it is so easy at times to mistake these childhood rashes for other conditions, a person who thinks he has had the disease as a child is not necessarily safe from infection. Babies of up to about six or nine months are usually immune, thanks to antibodies they receive from their mothers (assuming, of course, that the mother has had measles in the past). A vaccine against measles has become available in the last few years, and in countries where it is used the incidence of the disease has dropped dramatically. It is certainly worthwhile having a child immunized (unless the doctor advises against it), since complications of measles, while uncommon, can be severe and even fatal.

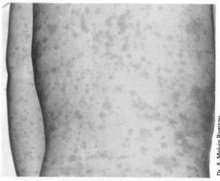

Typical appearance of the rash which appears during an attack of measles, with many spots.

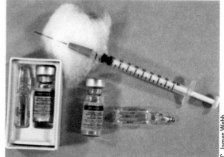

Immunization with measles vaccine gives protection against the disease for several months.

232

MEAT is the flesh of animals. It forms the richest of all sources of proteins, (see **proteins**) which are contained principally in the 'lean' meat, or muscles. There are no significant differences between the various types of animal meats (e.g. beef, lamb, pork, etc.) in this respect. Lean meat is also very rich in iron, so that the likelihood of either protein deficiency or anaemia is considerably reduced in those who get adequate quantities of it in their diet; unfortunately, of course, lean meat is expensive the world over, so that the poor in many countries get little of it.

Fatty meat is a rich source of fat (see **fat**) and little else. In view of the general feeling among doctors that animal fat intake may be related to arterial and coronary disease, fatty meat has little to recommend it at the present time, except that it is, like other fats, a good source of energy.

The third group of meats which are widely eaten are organ meats, such as heart, kidneys and sweetbreads. As a rule, the quantity of these meats taken by any one person is so small as to have no significant influence for good or ill on him. Liver, however, is rich in protein, iron and certain important vitamins including B_{12}, the vitamin which combats pernicious anaemia. In order to absorb a valuable amount of vitamin B_{12}, however, it is necessary to eat liver in far larger amounts than are ever taken by the average person.

MECKEL'S DIVERTICULUM is a pouch found in the wall of the small intestine in two per cent of the population. Its significance is that (a) it may contain tissue very similar to that of the stomach, and thus ulcers may develop in it; (b) it may be the cause of intussusception, a particular type of bowel obstruction; (c) it may become inflamed and produce symptoms which mimic those of appendicitis. In each instance, the treatment is surgical.

MECONIUM means the dark, semi-liquid motions of a newly-born baby. Since the infant has never swallowed anything solid, meconium consists of bile and cells shed from the intestinal wall. If meconium is not passed after a baby is born, the doctor or midwife will be alerted to the possibility that there is some obstruction of the bowels, especially if there is abdominal distension and vomiting.

Meconium should not be passed *before* the baby is born. If it appears during the latter part of labour, this is an indication that there is *foetal distress*, and that measures should be taken to ensure that the baby is delivered promptly.

MEGALOMANIA literally means 'great madness'. Although, like many psychiatric terms of several generations ago, it still appears a good deal in novels, it has more or less dropped out of medical usage. It does not imply any particular psychiatric illness, but rather a group of symptoms in which the most characteristic feature is an unshakeable belief in one's own greatness or power. It is claimed that some of the more remarkable business tycoons of history have had megalomaniac tendencies.

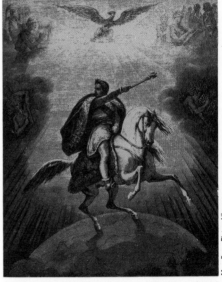

A print depicting Napoleon and his sensational rise to fame, by conquest. It has been suggested that he suffered from a form of megalomania.

MELAENA means black motions. This important symptom, which always demands medical investigation, is dealt with under the heading black motions.

233

MELANIN is the dark pigment found in everybody's skin (except albinos). It is also present in the hair and eyes, whose colour it determines. Those who have plenty of melanin in their tissues, for instance negroes or dark-skinned members of the 'white' race, are likely to have black hair and brownish eyes. This is not invariably so, however; a few negroes have green, grey or even bluish eyes (especially in the West Indies, where many people have some European ancestry).

On the other hand, people who have very fair skins, and therefore little melanin in the tissues, are likely to have fair or blonde hair, and blue eyes. The blueness of the eyes is due to a very small amount of pigment.

Under the influence of sunlight, the melanin-producing cells in the skin are stimulated to secrete more of the pigment; this is why the skin becomes tanned.

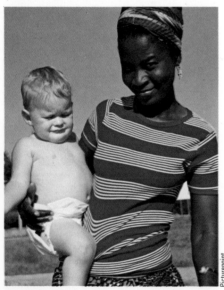

The difference in skin coloration from race to race is dependent upon the melanin content.

MELANOMA is a tumour of melanin-producing cells. As melanin is the dark pigment of the body, such tumours are usually black. They may be either benign (non-cancerous) or malignant (cancerous).

Benign melanomas are commonly seen in the form of pigmented moles or warts on the skin. Occasionally they become malignant, and if any dark wart or mole starts to enlarge in size, to bleed or to cause irritation, a doctor should be consulted without delay.

Malignant melanomas occur in the skin, the intestine, and the pigmented parts of the eye. On the skin, a melanoma is seen as a black growth which usually increases rapidly in size, or which produces dark secondary deposits nearby. In the intestine, melanomas tend, like other bowel growths, to produce a relatively sudden change in bowel habit, and perhaps bleeding. In the eye, malignant melanoma is the most commonly seen ocular tumour among adults. It occurs mainly in elderly people, and usually produces blindness in one eye.

MENARCHE is the age at which the periods, or menses, start. The age varies very considerably. On average, in Western countries, it is probably around 12 to 13, but a high proportion of girls reach the menarche at 11 or 14 and a rather lower percentage at 10 or 15. If the menarche occurs before the age of 9, this is highly unusual, but not necessarily abnormal: however, a doctor's advice should be sought. Similarly, although many girls do not have their first period until they are 16 or 17, a doctor should be consulted if the onset is delayed beyond the 17th birthday.

Often anaemia can be responsible for delayed or absent periods, and it may be that a simple blood test to check the haemoglobin level will reveal this easily corrected condition. It is possibly because anaemia is now much less frequent than it was 60 or 70 years ago (thanks to improved diet in most sections of the population) that the age of menarche seems to have become appreciably younger since the turn of the century. Evidence suggests that, at that time, the average age of onset of the periods was about 15 or 16. Anaemia is not the whole explanation, however, and there are probably other factors involved in this apparent change; at the present time, doctors are not clear as to what these factors are (see also **puberty**).

MENDEL was the founder of the science of genetics (see **genetics**). He was the abbot of Brno in what is now Czechoslovakia, and he spent much of his spare time breeding plants of various types in the monastery garden, and observing the results, which he recorded carefully in his notebooks. From years of study of these findings, he was able to formulate the basic laws of heredity.

MENIÈRE'S DISEASE is a disorder of the balancing apparatus of the inner ear (the **labyrinth**). Its cause is unknown.

The disease is characterized by sudden attacks of vertigo, in which everything seems to the patient to be spinning round him. He has to cling to the nearest article of furniture for support. At the same time, he feels nauseated and may vomit repeatedly. (Nausea and vomiting are characteristic of all conditions in which something disturbs the balancing apparatus – for instance, as in sea-sickness.)

Other features of Menière's disease are tinnitus (noises in the ears) and deafness. Since the cause of Menière's disease is unknown, it is extremely difficult to treat. Quite good results are at present achieved by giving anti-emetic drugs of the same type as those used for travel sickness. These seem to 'damp down' the activity in the inner ear in some way, and thus alleviate both the nausea and the giddiness. It has been claimed that directing ultra-sonic waves at the inner ear has a beneficial effect on the condition, and some ear, nose and throat surgeons believe that a low salt diet alters the chemical composition of the fluids inside the labyrinth and so lessens the incidence of attacks.

MENINGITIS is an inflammation of the membranes surrounding the brain and spinal cord. In the vast majority of cases, it is caused by infection, either by bacteria or, less commonly, by viruses. Children are more frequently affected than adults.

The common features of most types of meningitis are severe headache, fever, vomiting, stiffness of the neck, and dislike of bright lights. In all cases, admission to hospital is essential. There the patient can have a lumbar puncture, a procedure in which a needle is inserted into the lower back region to tap off cerebrospinal fluid (CSF). Tests on this fluid will confirm which type of germ is responsible.

Meningococcal meningitis is caused by bacteria known as meningococci. These germs are believed to be spread from person to person in tiny droplets expelled from the nose and mouth during talking, coughing, sneezing or laughing. The disease sometimes occurs in small epidemics, especially where people are living in overcrowded conditions. However, the adult or child who catches it will not necessarily be known to have been in contact with a case of meningitis; very often, the germs are passed on by symptomless 'carriers'.

The features of meningococcal meningitis are as described above; in addition, there is usually a skin rash which comes out on about the second day of the illness.

Although this is a very serious condition, the chances of recovery are fairly good once treatment with antibiotics is instituted.

Acute pyogenic meningitis is very similar in clinical features to meningococcal meningitis, except that there is usually no skin rash. A variety of different bacteria may be responsible, some being more common in certain parts of the world than others. Prompt lumbar puncture and institution of treatment with antibiotics is lifesaving in the majority of cases.

Tuberculous meningitis was once very common in western countries, but is now fortunately seen less frequently. It invariably starts as a result of a tuberculous infection somewhere else in the body (e.g. the lungs); this primary infection may at times be so minor as to have passed unnoticed.

The onset of tuberculous meningitis is usually very slow, which often makes it difficult to diagnose, especially in children who cannot give a good account of their symptoms. During the first few days, the patient feels generally unwell, and then slowly develops a headache and possibly some vomiting. There is slight fever and, after a few days, some stiffness of the neck. The diagnosis is made on the findings of the lumbar puncture, and immediate treatment with antituberculous drugs is started.

Virus meningitis is uncommon. The clinical features depend on the type of virus involved but are usually similar to those of the other varieties of meningitis.

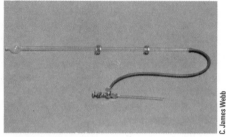

The equipment used to perform a lumbar puncture and take samples of the cerebrospinal fluid.

MENINGOCOCCI are the bacteria (see **bacteria**) which are the cause of a common type of meningitis (see **meningitis**). They affect the brain and spinal cord.

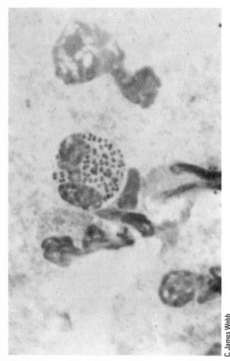

Meningococci, which are often responsible for meningitis, seen under the microscope.

236

MENOPAUSE is strictly speaking the time when the periods cease; in a broader sense, the term is often used to incorporate the whole episode of months or even years when a middle-aged woman experiences 'menopausal' symptoms, such as hot flushes. This entire time is sometimes referred to as 'the climacteric'. The age at which the menopause occurs varies very greatly. There is some evidence that if a woman has a late menarche (or onset of the periods), she is likely to have an early menopause. Some women's periods stop as early as 38 or 39, and in other women as late as 50 years of age. Occasionally the menopause occurs outside these age limits, but, if it does, it is wise to check with a doctor that all is well.

Ability to have children may sometimes go on well beyond the menopause, though this is not common, and most women can safely regard themselves as most unlikely to become pregnant when a year has passed since the periods stopped.

The question of how the periods should cease at the menopause is very important indeed. Ignorance of the facts about this point is undoubtedly responsible for the deaths of many women who simply do not recognize what may be the symptoms of cancer.

The main problem is that there is a widespread and entirely erroneous belief that the periods usually stop after a spell of irregular bleeding. This belief is not only wrong but highly dangerous. The most vital thing for any woman approaching the menopause to know is this: any type of irregular bleeding, at this or any other time, needs full investigation by a gynaecologist.

There are only three ways in which the periods should cease. These are as follows:

(a) they stop suddenly and never return;

(b) the interval between them grows steadily longer and longer until they stop; or, (c) the flow of blood at each period gradually becomes less and less, until it finally stops altogether.

It cannot be stressed too strongly that any other sequence of events should be regarded as being abnormal, and should be fully investigated as soon as possible.

MENORRHAGIA means heavy periods. It is difficult to assess how heavy a period may be without it becoming abnormal, but the following may be stated as basic general rules.

(i) Bleeding should not normally go on for longer than about 5 days, though traces of 'old' blood may still appear for a day or two afterwards.

(ii) Although there is no reason why periods should come every 26 to 28 days, and many women have 21 day or even 14 day cycles, nonetheless blood loss is likely to be excessive if there are 7 or 8 days bleeding in a calendar month.

(iii) Blood loss is also likely to be more than it should be if a woman finds she is using more than about half a dozen pads a day, though it is hard to generalize about this, since factors such as pad absorbency vary so much.

In any case, the best criterion of whether periods are too heavy or not is the presence or absence of anaemia (weakness of the blood).

The average woman's blood is appreciably weaker than that of the average man, and this fact is due almost entirely to the blood loss all women undergo at the periods. When menorrhagia is present, actual anaemia invariably follows, and, in fact, heavy periods are the commonest of all causes of anaemia.

Severe anaemia is marked by considerable pallor of the skin and of the body's mucous membranes (e.g. the normally red mucous membrane which is exposed when the lower lid of the eye is turned down). Milder degrees of anaemia may only be associated with tiredness and very slight pallor, but a blood test will rapidly detect the presence of the condition.

Various types of gynaecological treatment may be necessary in patients with menorrhagia, depending on the degree of the blood loss; all patients will, however, require iron tablets (or possibly injections) to correct their anaemia.

MENSTRUATION, a term derived from the Latin word for 'month', means the regular process of shedding the lining of the womb, accompanied by bleeding. This process most people call 'the period'. It is a regular cyclic phenomenon, which need not necessarily occur every calendar month at all. Although some women expect their periods to turn up 12 times a year, in January, February, March and so on, in actual fact, the average interval between most women's periods is only about 26 days. Some women have shorter cycles, in which the menses occur only 14 or 21 days apart, but when the interval is very short, anaemia is likely to result. In some cases too, the interval between periods is very long, and quite healthy women may menstruate at 40 or 50 day intervals. This does not matter: the important thing is that the periods should be *regular*. If their onset is not predictable (within a few days at most) then a doctor's advice should be sought.

Rather more important is the subject of *bleeding between the periods*. Any such intermenstrual bleeding, including *bleeding after intercourse*, is definitely abnormal and needs urgent full investigation by a gynaecologist. It may, of course, be due to some trivial condition, but it is also the classic symptom of cancer of the cervix, or neck of the womb, which most commonly starts in the 28–40 age group and kills many women every year. Cure is only possible if the disease is caught early, so that it is essential for *anyone* with irregular bleeding of this type to seek medical help at once.

Pain during the periods occurs at times to the vast majority of women, but gives the most trouble by far to teenagers. This in itself is an encouraging point, since it means that menstrual pain tends to ease up as a girl gets older. There are various means of treating it, and if taking a couple of aspirin does not usually relieve the symptoms, it is best to ask the family doctor's advice.

Menstrual or pre-menstrual tension is also very widespread. If mild, it should be accepted as a normal phenomenon, but, if more severe, the family doctor will again be able to advise on the best treatment.

Education about menstruation: every girl should be frankly told by her mother about the process of menstruation when she is about nine years old. If this is not done, what often happens is that the child

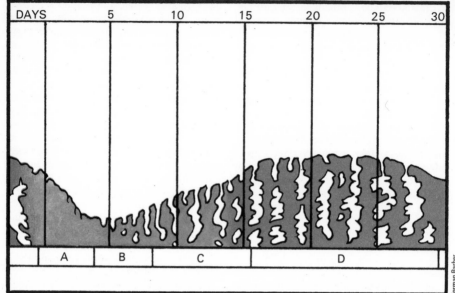

| DAYS | 5 | 10 | 15 | 20 | 25 | 30 |

| A | B | C | D |

Diagrammatic representation of the changes in the lining of the uterus during the different stages of the menstrual cycle. During the menses, A, the lining is shed. Then follows a repair phase, B, and a growth phase, C, as the lining returns to its full thickness. From the 15th to the 28th days the lining is in the secretory phase D, and the process is repeated when the lining is again shed around the 28th day. If pregnancy occurs, the cycle stops.

starts her first period when she is away from home (for instance, in the classroom); this may be an exceedingly frightening experience for her.

Until quite recently, there were so many 'taboos' about the whole question of menstruation, which was widely regarded as an 'unmentionable' subject, that mothers often shirked the duty of telling their daughters about it properly. This should no longer be so. Furthermore, when a girl's periods do start, it is very important that her parents, her family, her schoolteacher and, indeed, her boy-friend, if she has one, should treat her with sympathy and understanding. It is inevitable that the period time will always be a slightly trying one for a girl or a woman, and it is essential that her family and those close to her recognize that this is so and treat her accordingly.

MENTAL DEFICIENCY is a state of arrested or incomplete development of the mind which includes subnormality of intelligence. These words are taken from the
238

British Mental Health Act of 1959, one of the most advanced pieces of legislation in the world dealing with mental deficiency and other mental disorders. The Act divides the mentally deficient into two groups — the subnormal and the severely subnormal. Essentially, the difference between the two is that a person in a state of severe subnormality is (or will be when he is an adult) incapable of living an independent life or of guarding himself against exploitation.

There are many causes of mental subnormality, and it is possible that about five per cent of all children born fall into this category, though many of these die in the first few years of life. In the adult population, the incidence is probably less than two per cent.

Among the causes which may be listed are inheritance from parents of very low I.Q. (who tend themselves to have children of low intelligence); birth injury or asphyxia at birth (which are still fairly common and often unavoidable); maternal German measles during pregnancy; mongolism; cretinism (which is now rarely seen); and the inheritance of specific genes for particular types of mental deficiency (for instance, phenylketonuria, a congenital disorder of metabolism).

MENTAL ILLNESS, whether major or minor, affects a surprisingly high percentage of the population at one time or another during their lives. One of the greatest advances of recent years has been the realization by many people that mental disorder *is* an illness like any other. Many types of mental disorder are curable, and most can be appreciably helped by careful psychiatric treatment. Anyone who feels that a member of his or her family is in need of such treatment should not hesitate to suggest gently that the affected person talks the subject over with the family doctor.

It is impossible to provide a satisfactory classification of mental illness. One reason for this is that it is rarely practicable to attribute one particular cause to a particular illness. For example, if we were dealing with *physical* illnesses, we could usually say, 'this man's pulmonary tuberculosis was caused by infection with the tuberculosis bacillus'; even here, we should be only half right, because other factors are involved, including such matters as the previous condition of the man's lungs, his general physical fitness, his state of immunity to the tubercle bacillus, the environment he was living in, and so on.

However, with *mental* illness, we cannot even be as accurate as this — firstly, because so little is known of what goes on in the mind, and secondly because there are almost invariably many factors responsible for the development of a psychiatric illness. A Victorian novelist would say of his heroine (with complete confidence in his own diagnosis): 'she went mad because her lover left her for another'. On the other hand, the modern psychiatrist would perhaps say: 'This 20-year-old girl is of above average intelligence, but of a rather immature personality, related probably to excessive dependence on her father (who died a year ago) and to the fact that she has a somewhat hysterical mother; she herself exhibited severe hysterical symptoms (involving leaving home in a 'trance') when she was jilted by her boyfriend; a recent severe bout of pneumonia is also likely to have played a part in the precipitation of the illness.'

This may seem a somewhat cumbersome way of making a diagnosis, but it does demonstrate the enormous number of factors which play a part in the causation of mental illness, and which therefore make satisfactory classification so difficult.

However, among the more important psychiatric disorders, the following may be listed:

Anxiety states (see **neurosis**);
Obsessionalism (see **neurosis**);
Hysteria (see **hysteria**);
Depression (see **depression**);
Mania and hypomania (see **mania**);
Schizophrenia (see **schizophrenia**);
Paranoia (see **paranoia**);
Delirium (see **delirium**);
Dementia (see **dementia**);
Mental deficiency
(see **mental deficiency**);
Psychopathic states
(see **psychopathic**).

MEPACRINE is an antimalarial drug (see **malaria**). It is a yellow dye which was introduced during the Second World War as a replacement for quinine in the treatment of acute attacks of malaria. It remains an extremely effective drug, but prolonged dosage may lead to yellow staining of the skin, and to intestinal upsets.

MEPROBAMATE is a widely-used tranquillizer. Its main effect is to produce a calm state of mind in people who are anxious or disturbed.

MEPYRAMINE is one of the antihistamine group of drugs. These drugs combat the effects of histamine, a chemical which is released in the tissues in certain allergic conditions — for instance, urticaria and seasonal hay-fever. Mepyramine is of considerable use in this type of disorder. It is also, like other antihistamines, a potent anti-emetic — that is, a drug that combats nausea. It is employed for this purpose in sea-sickness and other types of travel-sickness, and in the persistent vomiting which often occurs in early pregnancy.

Mepyramine, like other antihistamines, has certain potentially serious side-effects. When taken by mouth, it can produce severe drowsiness. This may make it dangerous to those driving cars or operating machinery: furthermore, under no circumstances should it be taken with alcohol, which will exacerbate this drowsiness and increase the danger.

Skin applications containing antihistamines may produce dermatitis if used regularly.

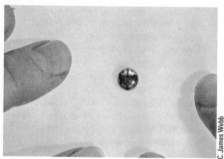

Mercury has an attractive appearance, but handling it is dangerous, causing poisoning.

MERCURY, or quicksilver, is a heavy metal which is liquid at normal temperatures. Its compounds have been used in medicine for centuries, but are now falling almost entirely out of use. Those which are still used include certain external preparations which have an antiseptic effect, and are thus used on cuts and grazes. Internally, a mercurial purgative is still occasionally prescribed. Injections of mercury-containing diuretics (substances which increase the flow of urine, and hence reduce dropsy, or oedema) still have some place in medicine, but are now being replaced by newer diuretics introduced during the 1960s.

In past times, up till the introduction of salvarsan in the early part of this century, mercury was probably the most widely used treatment for syphilis (see **syphilis**). Whether it had any effect on the disease is not entirely clear.

Poisoning by mercury has become much less common as mercurial compounds have been less and less used in medicine.
240

It still occurs at times, however, particularly where someone attempts suicide by swallowing the antiseptic perchloride of mercury. Those who work with the metal may also be affected by chronic mercurial poisoning.

The usual symptoms of acute poisoning due to mercury are severe pain, rapidly followed by vomiting and blood-stained diarrhoea. As soon as the metal is absorbed, it poisons the kidney cells, and this causes the flow of urine to shut down.

Prompt treatment by washing out the stomach is essential; the patient is then given a preparation called B.A.L. (British Anti-Lewisite), which 'binds' the metal into a harmless compound.

Chronic mercurial poisoning produces symptoms like those of acute poisoning, but milder and more insidious in nature. Teething powders containing mercury were probably the cause of 'pink disease', an unpleasant condition affecting young children. The most characteristic feature was a pink, scaly condition of the hands and feet. Since mercury-containing powders were banned, pink disease seems to have virtually disappeared.

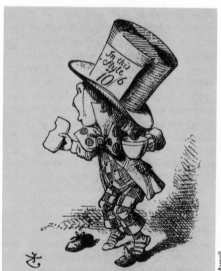

The 'Mad Hatter' in Lewis Carroll's 'Alice in Wonderland'. The fur used in hat-making was treated with mercury compounds, and hatters often developed mercury poisoning – including bizarre mental and nervous changes.

MERSALYL is a compound of mercury. It is used in the form of an injection to treat oedema (dropsy), which it relieves by increasing the volume of fluid excreted by the kidneys. In the last ten years or so, it has been used less commonly than formerly, because of the introduction of newer drugs. (See **diuretics**.)

MESCALINE is a chemical derived from a cactus which is found principally in Mexico. This cactus has been used by the Central American Indians for many hundreds of years in religious and magical ceremonies, because the mescaline content is powerfully hallucinogenic (see **hallucinogens**). Like the drug lysergic acid (see **lysergic acid**), and also like certain unidentified chemicals found in mushrooms in Central America, mescaline gives rise to states of ecstasy, in which the person taking it sees fantastic and colourful visions. While these visions are mainly pleasurable, they are also sometimes extremely frightening, and psychiatrists regard mescaline and similar hallucinogenic drugs as highly dangerous to the mind, and not to be used except under medical supervision.

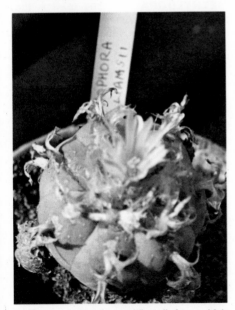

The cactus Lophophora williamsii, from which the drug mescaline may be extracted.

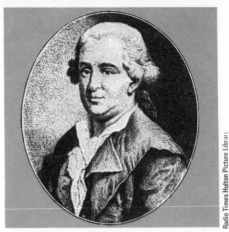

The German physician Friedrich Anton Mesmer, inventor of 'animal magnetism' or mesmerism.

Radio Times Hulton Picture Library

MESMERISM, so-called after Friedrich Mesmer, a famous German physician, is another term for hypnotism (see **hypnosis**), or 'animal magnetism'.

METABOLISM literally means 'change'. The term is applied to all the processes of chemical change which take place in the body. *Anabolism* is that part of human metabolism which is concerned with change through 'building-up' of chemical units. By this is meant such constructive processes as the building up of the various tissues of the human body (bones, muscles and so on) from the basic raw materials provided by food. *Catabolism*, on the other hand, is that part of human metabolism which is concerned with chemical breakdown — for instance, the 'burning' of fuel within the body, and the destruction of unwanted compounds to form waste products.

The *metabolic rate* is an expression of the rapidity at which the body's chemical turnover takes place. It tends to be rather low in slow moving people who tend to put on weight easily, and rather high in thin, active people who can readily burn up food without growing fat. It is extremely low in those who suffer from underactivity of the thyroid gland (hypothyroidism or myxoedema), and extremely high in those who suffer from an overactive thyroid (hyperthyroidism or thyrotoxicosis).

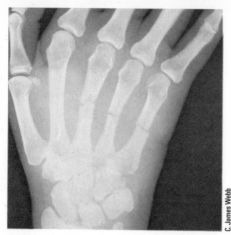

An X-ray of the hand, showing clearly fractures of three of the metacarpal bones.

METACARPAL is the term applied to the five bones which lie more or less side by side in the palm of the hand, and which connect the small bones of the wrist to each of the five fingers.

The metacarpals are particularly liable to damage in boxing, since the force of most blows with a clenched fist is transmitted through the outer ends of the metacarpals at the points where they meet the bones of the fingers to form the first row of knuckles. Particularly vulnerable in this respect is the fifth metacarpal, which lies at the base of the little finger.

'Metacarpal' literally means 'beyond the wrist' and the very similar word 'metatarsal' means 'beyond the heel', and is thus applied to the five corresponding bones in the foot.

METHADONE is a powerful analgesic (i.e. pain-relieving drug), which has properties rather similar to those of morphine (see **morphine**). Like morphine and a number of related drugs, it not only relieves pain, but also has a depressant effect on the cough reflex; it can therefore be used as a cough suppressant. Unfortunately, however, such drugs tend to be addictive, and must be used with extreme caution.

METHOHEXITONE is an injectable anaesthetic which has become very widely used in the last decade. Like thiopentone 242

(see **thiopentone**), which is also a barbiturate anaesthetic (see **barbiturates**), methohexitone is injected into a vein, reaches the brain, and produces complete and rapid unconsciousness. The patient will remain unconscious for a few minutes, which is sufficient only for procedures such as a rapid dental extraction; if any longer operation is contemplated, it is necessary either to give intermittent additional injections of methohexitone, or (much more commonly) to continue anaesthesia with a gas or mixture of gases.

Methohexitone can also be administered very slowly, or in dilute form, into a vein to produce mental relaxation. This technique, which is proving very useful in psychiatry, is also described under the heading *barbiturates*. (See also **anaesthesia**.)

METHOTREXATE is an extremely valuable drug used in the treatment of certain types of cancer. In one particular form of this disease called *chorionepithelioma*, an unusual malignant growth which affects the womb, methotrexate has effected cures in cases which would otherwise have been hopeless.

METHYLDOPA is a drug used in the treatment of hypertension, or high blood pressure (see **hypertension**). First introduced in the early 1960s, it has rapidly become one of the most widely used of all the drugs in this condition.

Methyldopa has a complex chemical action which results in a relaxation of the blood vessels, and hence a lowering of the blood pressure. Like other drugs used in this disorder, it has certain side effects, but most of these are relatively harmless, and disappear when dosage is reduced. Sometimes, however, the drug has to be withdrawn. The side-effects include drowsiness, mild depression and stuffiness of the nose.

More important, however, is an unusual type of anaemia. Although patients normally recover from this, once methyldopa is stopped, many doctors feel that in patients taking the drug it is wiser to perform a blood test every few months to check if such anaemia is likely to develop. This test is known as the *Coombs test*.

METRONIDAZOLE is a drug which is very widely used in the treatment of a common form of vaginal discharge, caused by a microscopic organism called Trichomonas vaginalis (see **Trichomonas vaginalis**). Trichomonas usually produces a profuse yellow discharge. There are often erosions on the cervix (neck of the womb) and upper vagina, and irritation of the vulva. Treatment was rather unsatisfactory until the 1960s, when metronidazole was introduced. It is usually given three times daily by mouth, and rapidly clears up the infection.

It is, however, important that the affected woman's husband should also be treated with metronidazole. This is because, although he will probably have no symptoms whatever, he is very likely to be harbouring the organism in his own genital tract. Until this fact was realized, relapses were very common, due to persistent reinfection of wives by their husbands.

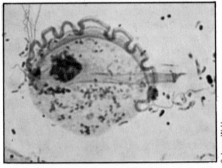

Microscopic appearance of Trichomonas vaginalis, an organism killed by metronidazole.

METROPATHIA HAEMORRHAGICA

is a relatively common condition of women. It causes abnormal bleeding from the womb, whose lining becomes thickened (hypertrophied) and full of cysts, so that its appearance is said to resemble that of Swiss cheese. At the same time, the musculature of the womb increases in size, so that on internal examination it is possible to feel that the whole organ is bulkier than usual.

These changes are due to an abnormal condition of the ovaries, whose hormones normally control the state of the uterus. For instance, in the first half of the menstrual cycle, ovarian hormones prepare the lining for the reception of an ovum (egg). In the second half of the month, other ovarian hormones break the lining down so that menstruation occurs if the egg is not fertilized.

In metropathia haemorrhagica, the ovaries produce only the hormone responsible for the changes of the first half of the cycle, so that the lining of the uterus receives persistent over-stimulation.

The result is that the patient may go for some weeks without having a period. The grossly hypertrophied womb lining then breaks down of its own accord, and heavy and irregular bleeding takes place.

It is usually necessary to scrape the womb to be certain of the diagnosis. (This very frequently performed gynaecological procedure is known as dilatation and curettage, or 'D and C'.) Hormone treatment is helpful; in very severe cases, removal of the womb (*hysterectomy*) is sometimes necessary.

MICROCEPHALY means smallness of the head. It is a fortunately uncommon condition of young babies, in which the size of the skull is so small that the brain has no room to grow. At birth it is approximately the same size as that of a normal baby four or five months *before* delivery, and it grows only very slowly thereafter.

Many such babies die during infancy; the outlook for those who survive is very bad, as they are almost invariably severely mentally deficient.

MICRO-ORGANISM means any living thing of microscopic size, including, of course, those which produce disease in man. Micro-organisms include bacteria, viruses, Rickettsiae, yeasts, fungi, and protozoa. All these are discussed under the heading **bacteriology.**

MICTURITION is the act of passing water, or urination. The bladder receives urine from the kidneys via two slim tubes called the ureters. As a rule, the urine remains in the bladder (unless the person makes a conscious effort to expel it) until the volume present begins to approach the amount which the organ can comfortably contain. At this stage, the fibres in the wall of the bladder begin to be stretched, and thereupon they transmit messages via the bladder nerves up to the spinal cord. In a young baby, or in a person paralyzed below the waist, a reflex emptying of the bladder then takes place. In most people, however, inhibitory impulses from the brain pass down the spinal cord, and prevent the bladder emptying until circumstances are suitable. When this happens, the brain cuts off the inhibitory impulses, and the muscles of the bladder wall contract forcefully. At the same time, the muscles of the sphincter, or neck, of the bladder relax, so that urine can pass out into the tube called the urethra which leads to the exterior. In women, this tube is very short indeed, which is one reason why women are liable to pass small quantities of water without meaning to when they cough, laugh or sneeze.

This is called 'stress incontinence', and is common in women who have borne several children, and whose pelvic tissues are rather lax.

If a person does not micturate when he or she feels the need to do so, the fibres of the bladder wall are capable of considerable expansion, increasing the capacity of the organ very greatly. Eventually, however, the stimuli from the bladder to the spinal cord will become so powerful that reflex micturition will take place.

MIDWIFE is a nurse who practises obstetrics (midwifery). In underdeveloped countries, midwives are often completely unqualified, but in most western countries, the midwife is a highly-trained person. In the United Kingdom, for instance, she normally spends some years in becoming a registered nurse (SRN), and must then undergo considerable further training over a period of a year before taking the State Certified Midwife's examination (SCM). Only when she has passed this is she legally entitled to call herself a midwife. It is noteworthy that such was the opposition to women practising midwifery in English-speaking countries that the United Kingdom was over 100 years behind France and several other European countries when it brought in registration of midwives in the early part of this century. In the United States the midwife has today more or less ceased to exist, all obstetric work being carried out by doctors. Midwifery will, however, continue to offer a worthwhile and rewarding career in most other countries outside the United States.

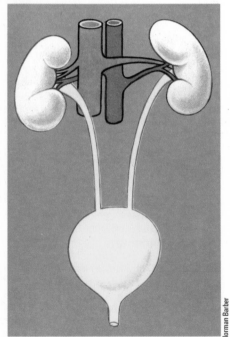

Norman Barber

Urine passes down the ureters from the kidneys and is stored in the bladder until micturition.

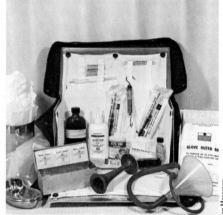

Ken Moreman

The midwife's bag, containing all the equipment necessary to assist at the birth of a child.

MIGRAINE is a disorder characterized by recurrent severe headaches, often preceded by symptoms of transient disturbance of the circulation to the brain, and associated with bouts of vomiting.

The disease is more common in women, and seems to affect especially people who are intelligent and highly conscientious. It may run in families. Attacks usually begin somewhere around the time of puberty, and may be greatly eased in severity and reduced in frequency in middle age.

Attacks frequently begin in the morning, and the first symptoms may be blurring of vision or the apparent presence of coloured dots or lines before the eyes. Sometimes, such visual disturbances affect only half the field of vision. They are due to spasm of the branches of the main artery supplying the brain.

After these initial symptoms, a violent throbbing headache comes on. Characteristically, it affects only one side of the head to start with, but it may spread to both sides. It occurs because the blood vessels which were initially in spasm are now markedly wider than normal; the throbbing sensation is due to blood pumping its way through them.

Attacks usually last a few hours and are often relieved by going to sleep, where this is possible. Occasionally, a severe attack may go on for two or three days.

Attacks, once started, are difficult to stop, so that the first basis of treatment is to try to ward them off. This can often be achieved by giving a patient regular daily medication with a drug called ergotamine, which contracts the blood vessels. Attacks are also treated with this drug, given by mouth or by suppository, or with injections of one of its derivatives. The patient should, if possible, lie in a darkened room and try to sleep even if only for an hour or two.

It is widely felt that some cases of migraine, at least, have a background of psychological upset. Where this is so, medical help in resolving mental problems may also relieve the symptoms of migraine.

MILK is the liquid produced during lactation (see **lactation**) by the mammary glands of all mammals. Mother's milk is, of course, the ideal food for young babies, and vastly superior to any form of prepared milk. Cow's milk is also an excellent food, for children past the age of weaning, though doctors no longer believe that drinking it in large quantities is necessarily good for the health of adults. This is because it is extremely rich in animal fats, which are widely suspected as being among the causes of coronary disorder and other arterial diseases. Unfortunately, a belief in the innate 'goodness' of both milk and butter (to which the same objections apply) is now so deeply rooted in most people's minds that it will probably be many years before public thinking changes on this matter. In the United States, however, where the population is very 'coronary-conscious' (and with good reason), consumption of both milk and butter among adults is now appreciably lower than it used to be.

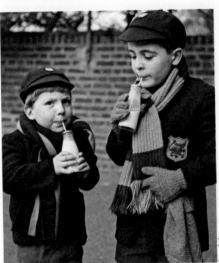

Milk provides valuable dietary protein for growing children.

For children, however, both cow's and mother's milk provide a good source of protein, calcium, vitamin A and several of the B group vitamins. Milk also contains some vitamin C, and a varying amount of vitamin D — in the case of cow's milk, the content of this vitamin varies with the type of cattle and with the season of the year, being higher in the summer months.

245

In general then, while not a complete food, milk does contain most of the constituents of a healthy diet, with the notable exception of iron.

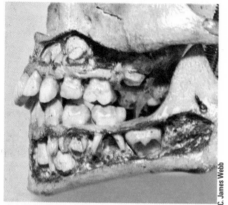

The skeleton of the jaw, showing how the milk teeth develop above the permanent dentition.

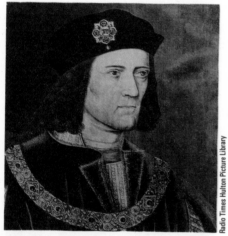

King Richard the Third is said to have been born with a complete set of milk teeth.

MILK TEETH, or deciduous teeth, are the temporary teeth of children. Although an occasional child is born with one or two teeth, they usually appear first at about six months of age. Most commonly the incisors (cutting teeth) of the lower jaw come through first. The molar (grinding) teeth appear at about the age of a year, the canine (eye) teeth at about 18 months, and the second molars at about 2 years. The milk teeth start to be replaced by the

permanent dentition from about the age of five onwards.

MISCARRIAGE means expulsion of the foetus from the womb before the 28th week of pregnancy. Nowadays, it means exactly the same thing as abortion (see **abortion**) in medical usage, though at one time the latter meant expulsion of the foetus before the fourth month of pregnancy, and *miscarriage* meant expulsion between the fourth and seventh months. Neither term implies any suggestion of interference from outside; a very high proportion of miscarriages occur quite spontaneously.

Threatened miscarriage (threatened abortion) means that while there is a slight vaginal bleeding and perhaps some pain, the pregnancy can still be saved. The doctor does not examine the expectant mother internally, for fear of making things worse, but usually orders strict bed rest under heavy sedation until at least three days after the bleeding ceases.

In *inevitable miscarriage* (inevitable abortion), there is copious bleeding and much pain; it is evident that there is no hope of saving the pregnancy, and it is often necessary to scrape the womb in hospital (curettage). The patient may need blood transfusion and other urgent treatment if blood loss is heavy.

MITRAL VALVE is one of the valves of the heart (see **heart**). It lies between the left upper chamber (the left atrium) and the left lower chamber (the left ventricle). Blood pumped from the atrium to the ventricle goes through the valve, which should prevent it from returning. If the valve is congenitally deformed or (more commonly) deformed by rheumatic fever, it may become *incompetent*, and allow blood to leak back into the left atrium.

Like mitral incompetence, narrowing of the mitral valve, or mitral stenosis, is a very frequent sequel to rheumatic fever. The narrowed valve dams back blood in the upper chamber of the heart, and creates back pressure on the lungs. Heart failure may be produced as a result. Nowadays, mitral valve disease can often be cured by operation.

MOLAR TEETH are those which carry out the grinding of food. There are three on each side of the upper and lower jaws, making twelve in all.

MOLES are raised, pigmented spots or lumps on the skin. The vast majority of all moles are completely benign, but a very small percentage are cancerous or eventually become so.

Anyone who suspects that he has this type of skin cancer should see a doctor *at once*, since prompt surgical removal of malignant skin tumours is usually curative; delay may be fatal.

The symptoms which may suggest malignancy are as follows:

(i) Sudden increase in size of a mole; (ii) Occurrence of bleeding; (iii) Persistent itching; (iv) Development of 'daughter' moles in the region of the original one; (v) Marked darkening in colour of a mole.

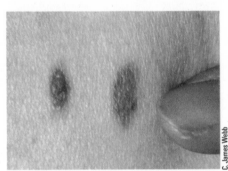

Moles are accumulations of brown melanin.

MONGOLISM is a tragic and not uncommon condition in which a child is born with a very characteristic face whose features include eyes that bear a superficial resemblance to those of people of the Mongolian races of Asia; there is invariably severe mental deficiency, and frequently gross heart malformation as well. This last feature is often responsible for the early death of mongol children.

Mongolism is due to an abnormality of the chromosomes, the tiny threads which carry genes. Some cases occur for no apparent reason, but there is a high incidence of the condition in children of older mothers, particularly those over 35. It has recently become apparent that there may

be a higher incidence also in the children of older fathers.

Although mongols are mentally defective, they are usually very affectionate and often fond of music.

MONILIA is a type of fungus which lives a parasitic existence on human beings. It is also known as Candida albicans. It affects babies, producing *thrush* in the mouth. Rarely, it causes lung infections, and under certain circumstances it can colonize the bowel. This is likely to happen if the harmless germs normally present in the bowel are wiped out by certain antibiotics, notably the tetracyclines.

Perhaps the most common illness caused by monilia is a type of vaginal discharge. This can usually be cleared up by the use of nystatin pessaries, which kill the fungus.

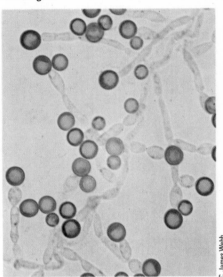

The organisms of the fungus Monilia cause 'thrush' in babies and vaginitis in women.

MONOZYGOTIC TWINS, or monovular twins, are those which develop from one single egg (ovum). They are therefore identical, and, of course, always of the same sex, since they have exactly the same genetic inheritance. It seems that such twins occur because a fertilized egg splits entirely in two in the very early stages of intra-uterine life.

MORBILLI is another name for measles (see **measles**).

MORON is a term which was at one time applied to mentally defective people whose mental age was that of a young child, so that they were capable of life outside an institution, but needed the constant care and protection of relatives. The term has now dropped out of medical use.

MORPHINE or morphia is an extract of opium, and hence a derivative of the Indian poppy; opium contains roughly 10 per cent morphine. The drug is usually administered medicinally in the form of the hydrochloride or the sulphate. The dose of these preparations is about 10 mg in an adult patient.

Morphine is of immense value in the relief of severe pain, and also in the premedication of patients for operation. It also depresses the cough reflex, and is thus sometimes used as a cough supressant. It decreases the motility of the bowel, and can therefore be employed in small doses (usually as a mixture with kaolin) to relieve diarrhoea.

The great drawback with morphine, as with other related drugs such as pethidine, is that there is an immense risk of addiction if a patient has repeated doses of it. There have been tragic instances of such 'therapeutic addiction' when young and healthy people who have sustained severe injuries in accidents have been given morphine repeatedly for relief of chronic pain. Nowadays, therefore, the drug is used as sparingly as possible.

MOUTH is the cavity which makes up the first part of the alimentary canal, and in which the food is chewed and mixed with saliva as the first part of the digestive process.

The back of the mouth communicates with the pharynx, another cavity more or less corresponding to the 'throat'. From there, the gullet, or oesophagus, passes down to the stomach, while, just in front of it, the voice-box (larynx) and windpipe (trachea) lead to the lungs.

There are many diseases of the mouth. Ulcers may be due to poorly-fitting dentures, to jagged teeth, to thrush (a fungal infection common in children) and probably to general constitutional ill health. Recurrent ulcers necessitate medical advice. Large, or rapidly-growing, or 'hard' ulcers, particularly those occurring on the tongue may be cancerous. Immediate medical help is needed.

Lumps in the mouth may also be cancerous, but there are a multitude of other causes; it is, however, safer to consult a doctor about any such swelling.

Persistent bleeding around the teeth, or the oozing of pus from the tooth sockets are invariably symptoms of gum disease. A dentist should be consulted about such symptoms at an early date; regrettably, many people simply ignore these symptoms, with resultant disastrous effects on their teeth.

Gumboils are abscesses developing in the region of the root of a decayed tooth; they produce swelling of the gum and pain when the tooth is tapped sharply. Again, it is essential to consult a dentist as soon as possible.

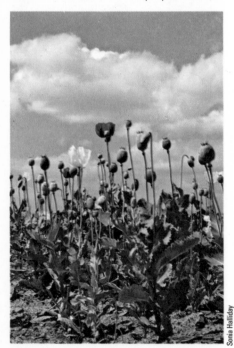

Sonia Halliday

This field of poppies yields a harvest of opium, from which the drug morphine is extracted.

MUCOUS MEMBRANE is the term applied to a large number of membranous structures throughout the body, all of which are kept moist by a flow of mucus. Such mucous membranes line the inside of the nose, the mouth, the throat, the windpipe and air passages leading to the lung, and many other organs.

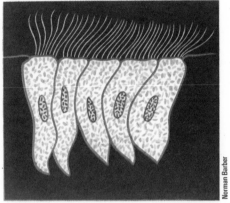

Diagram of the cells in the mucous membrane of the nose, showing the fine hair-like cilia.

MUCUS is the name given to the semi-liquid substance produced by the mucous glands of the body's many mucous membranes. Normally, it is produced only in sufficient quantities to lubricate the membranes, but where there is inflammation present, the volume of mucus may be very considerably increased. For instance, in chronic bronchitis inflammation leads to the production of copious amounts of thick tenacious mucus. Similarly, when a person has a cold, the mucous membranes of the nose pour forth large quantities of the substance.

MULTIPLE SCLEROSIS is another name for disseminated sclerosis (see **disseminated sclerosis**).

MUMPS is a common infectious disease caused by a virus. In most cases, it affects the parotid salivary glands, which lie just in front of the ear, but the virus can also cause inflammation in other tissues.

Mumps, or epidemic parotitis, occurs all over the world. It is probable that three-quarters of all city-dwelling children catch the disease at some time or other. Young adults are also prone to it, but it is rare in the middle-aged and elderly. The virus is principally spread in the tiny droplets of fluid sprayed out during talking, laughing, coughing, or sneezing.

The incubation period is usually in the region of three weeks, but varies by as much as a week in either direction. As a rule, the child starts to feel generally unwell over a period of about four days. He has a raised temperature and is off his food. It may be possible to detect tenderness in the parotid glands by pressing the cheek just in front of the ear.

Often, one parotid gland swells up before the other (and, indeed, the swelling may be on one side only throughout). The face now takes on its characteristic globular appearance. The child feels very unwell. Pain in the cheeks is troublesome, and becomes much worse on attempting to eat. This is because chewing stimulates the infected gland to produce saliva.

As a rule, both temperature and swelling subside after a few days. Complications are fairly common, however. The virus may affect the other salivary glands, which are situated in the neck region. It can also cause inflammation in the sex glands. In girls, this is fairly uncommon; it causes only an ache in the lower abdomen, and seems to have no unpleasant consequences in regard to the future ability to bear children.

In adolescent boys and young men, however, the mumps virus not infrequently causes orchitis, or inflammation of the testicles. (Before puberty, orchitis is rare.) This complication is both painful and alarming for the patient. For many years, it was believed that sterility could be caused by mumps orchitis, but it now seems very doubtful indeed whether there is any truth in this belief, and it is essential to reassure the patient on this point.

The virus also affects the central nervous system in a small proportion of cases. It may cause a benign form of meningitis (which is nonetheless very unpleasant for the sufferer over several days); in a smaller percentage of patients, an encephalitis, or inflammation of the brain is produced (see **encephalitis**).

Treatment of uncomplicated mumps consists only of measures to make the patient comfortable. A moderately warm pack or well-wrapped hot water bottle applied to the side of the face often brings some relief. Eating makes things worse, and so the child should suck milk or fruit juice through a straw until he is able to chew again. There is no point in giving antibiotics since these have no significant effect on viruses.

MUNCHAUSEN SYNDROME is a term which was invented in the early 1950s to describe a group of symptoms which had been familiar to doctors for hundreds of years.

Baron von Munchausen is a popular character in German fiction: his particular speciality was the telling of wildly improbable stories. Patients who suffer from the Munchausen syndrome do much the same thing, but the principal object of their tales is to get themselves into hospital for a long period, even if this means undergoing an operation, or perhaps a whole series of operations.

This condition, which has also been called 'hospital addiction' is, of course, a serious psychiatric illness, and the reason for its occurrence is not well understood. The typical sufferer is usually something of a wanderer, travelling from town to town in search of a hospital which will admit him. When he arrives in a Casualty Department he may complain of weird and bizarre symptoms, or, if he has acquired some medical knowledge, he may simulate the classical signs and symptoms of some well-known disease. He will go to almost any lengths, including faking high thermometer readings or surreptitiously inserting substances into his urine specimen, in order to convince the doctors that he is desperately ill and needs an operation.

The point that often gives him away is that his abdomen is likely to be already covered with a fantastic collection of operation scars. This, coupled with the fact that he has usually come from another town, may arouse suspicion of the Munchausen syndrome, and a phone call to the hospital there may well establish that he
250

was in *their* Casualty Department the previous night — with a completely different set of symptoms!

Such patients are to be pitied rather than blamed; psychiatric treatment may help them.

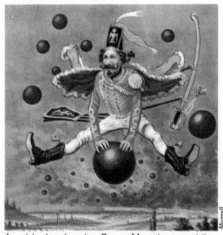

An old print showing Baron Munchausen riding on a cannon ball — one of the incredible tales he asked his readers to believe. Patients seeking hospital admission may spin yarns, too.

MURMUR is a rumbling or hissing sound produced by the heart and heard when a doctor listens with his stethoscope.

Murmurs are caused by turbulence in the blood passing through the heart. Such turbulence may be caused by deformity of the heart valves, or by the presence of abnormal communications, such as a 'hole in the heart'. It is nowadays appreciated, however, that many murmurs are of no significance whatever and are *not* an indication of heart disease.

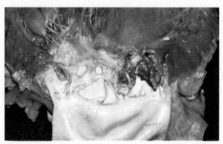

The post-mortem appearance of the heart valves; distortion causes blood turbulence.

MUSCLE is the 'lean' meat of animal bodies; as such, it is rich in protein. This is why a child requires plenty of protein in its diet in order to develop strong, healthy muscles.

Muscles are composed of fibres, whose outstanding property is the ability to contract. In the case of the group of muscles which are described as *voluntary*, this property of contractility enables them to move the various parts of the body. Voluntary muscles are also called 'striped' muscles because of the appearance of their fibres under the microscope.

Involuntary muscles, on the other hand, with the notable exception of the heart muscle, appear unstriped under the micro-

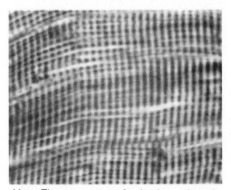

Above The appearance of striped muscle under the microscope, contrasted with that of plain muscle, *below*; heart muscle bears a resemblance to both types, with branching fibres.

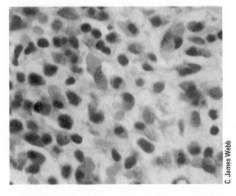

scope. Such muscles, which, as the name implies, are not under the control of the will, are found especially in the coats of such hollow organs as the stomach and intestines. Contraction of their fibres may, for instance, help such organs to empty themselves of their contents.

MUSCULAR DYSTROPHY is a term applied to any member of a group of inherited muscle diseases, or myopathies, in which there is weakness and wasting away of muscle groups. These diseases affect only the muscles, and not the nerves supplying them. The wasting is always symmetrical, i.e. present equally on both sides of the body. These points help to distinguish muscular dystrophies from other muscle disorders.

Unfortunately, several different classifications of the muscular dystrophies are in use, and doctors differ in the names they give to each condition. However, in many parts of the world it is customary to refer to *three* distinct types of muscular dystrophy. These are:

(i) The *pseudo-hypertrophic* type: this is common, and occurs only in males; the wasting begins in the first five years of life, and starts in the hip and buttock region, so that the child's walking muscles are weak, giving him a characteristic waddling gait; he also finds it difficult to stand up from a sitting position; at first, the muscles, although weak, appear very bulky;

(ii) The *limb girdle* type: this affects both boys and girls, and tends to appear in adolescence; it affects mainly the muscles of the hip and shoulder regions, and its progress is slower than that of the pseudo-hypertrophic type;

(iii) The *facio-scapulo-humeral* type: this is also hereditary, but may start at any age; it affects both males and females, and normally starts in the face muscles, later spreading to the shoulders and arms; its progress is very much slower than in the other types of muscular dystrophy.

Although no cure is at present known for muscular dystrophy, affected persons can be considerably helped by physiotherapy and the use of special appliances. Research continues on this problem and indeed may possibly produce a cure within the lifetime of present-day sufferers.

MUSHROOM POISONING—see **fungi**.

251

MYASTHENIA GRAVIS is a disease in which certain of the muscles of the body are abnormally weak. There was no treatment until the 1930s, when it was discovered that this weakness was due to insufficient amounts of the chemical which transmits instructions from the nerves to the muscles. This chemical, acetyl choline, is broken down in the body by an enzyme called choline esterase, and it was found that giving injections of neostigmine, a chemical which inhibits choline esterase, greatly alleviated the condition.

Myasthenia gravis usually appears in early adult life or middle years. Its most typical feature is that certain muscle groups become abnormally fatiguable; that is to say, they are strong when first carrying out a movement, but become abnormally weak within seconds. Very often, this fatiguability is first noted in the chewing muscles, or in those which keep the eyelids open. A simple chemical test usually confirms the diagnosis. From then on, neostigmine by mouth, or sometimes by injection, will greatly help most patients.

Occasionally, myasthenia gravis is associated with a tumour of the thymus gland, which lies in the front upper part of the chest. Removal of such a tumour may relieve the symptoms.

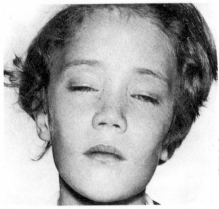

The drooping eyelids of a patient suffering from the condition called myasthenia gravis.

Institute of Ophthalmology

MYCOPLASMA is a term applied to a micro-organism which has undergone considerable investigation in the last few years. It is a cause of one type of pneumonia, and is also suspected of being the agent responsible for certain other infectious diseases.

MYELITIS means inflammation of the spinal cord. This may be due to a wide variety of causes including infection, especially with viruses such as that of poliomyelitis.

MYOPATHY literally means 'disease of muscles'; usually, the word implies wasting of muscles, and, in particular, wasting due to muscular dystrophy. There are, however, other causes of myopathy, for instance, the wasting and weakness frequently associated with lung cancer.

MYXOEDEMA is a condition of underactivity of the thyroid gland (hypothyroidism). It is characterized by slowness, both physical and mental, and by increase in body fat. The deposition of fat affects the face in particular, so that the features take on a curious bloated, coarse appearance. One of the most striking phenomena in medicine is the extraordinary return to normal of the face once treatment is underway.

Myxoedema may or may not be associated with a goitre (swelling) or with an inflammation of the thyroid gland, which lies at the front of the neck. It may occur after the gland has been removed by operation or partially destroyed by radiotherapy (usually as treatment for previous *over*-activity of the gland). The disorder is far more common in women than in men, and tends to occur in middle age. The patient may not realize she is ill, and may attribute her altered appearance to the change of life. If she is not treated, her physical condition will deteriorate: the skin becomes dry, as does the hair, which may fall out. The appetite is poor, though the patient puts on weight. She feels cold all the time, and may experience chest pain due to coronary heart disease.

Fortunately, all this can be prevented by giving extract of thyroid gland, or one of its newer chemical derivatives. Within a few weeks, improvement will begin, and the patient is frequently restored to normal in two or three months.

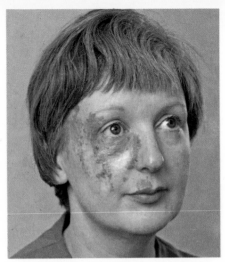

Pharmaceutical and cosmetic manufacturers have devoted much time and money to research into really effective preparations to hide unsightly scars and naevi. Here the efficacy of a modern covering cosmetic is shown.

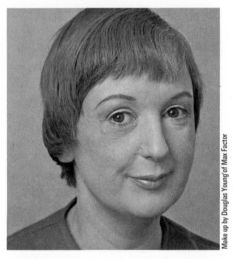

Make up by Douglas Young of Max Factor

NAEVUS is a birthmark (see **birthmarks**). In particular, the term is applied to those birthmarks which consist of dilated blood vessels — either veins (in which case the naevus is described as 'cavernous') or capillaries, the smallest blood vessels of all (in which case the naevus is simply described as being 'capillary').

Many naevi diminish in size as the years go by, while others can be readily removed

or dealt with by ray therapy. Some can be hidden with special cosmetic preparations, but others, like large 'port wine' stains, are a more serious problem. However, it is encouraging that the vast majority of people with such conditions come to terms with them, and usually regard them as of little importance.

NAILS are basically modifications of the same tissue which, in the embryo, gives rise to the hair and the skin. This tissue is called the ectoderm. The nails contain exactly the same layers as does the skin, but some of them have been modified.

This process of modification makes the nail strong and firm. Just like the claws of birds and animals, nails are of immense value for gripping objects, in a way that the soft tissues of the fingers could not possibly achieve by themselves.

The nail is subject to many disorders, most of which are the province of the dermatologist, or of the surgeon.

Perhaps the simplest and most common disorder is physical injury to the nail. This can be extremely painful, as the tissues protected by the nail are very sensitive. Gross tears of the nail may require surgical removal of any parts of it which are sticking up or flapping loose. This operation need not be painful, as it is very easy for the doctor to 'numb' the area by injecting a 'ring block' of local anaesthetic round the base of the finger. Although a considerable area of tender tissue may be laid bare by such a partial nail removal, this tissue rapidly hardens over in the next few days, until it can be touched without producing pain.

Blows on the nail are often followed by bleeding under it — seen as a brown or black discoloration. Very infrequently, there is enough bleeding to produce considerable pain, due to pressure under the nail. This pressure can be relieved by the simple operation of drilling through the nail with a needle. Sometimes, however, the bleeding is such that the whole nail sloughs off. Here again, no harm is done, as the tender area underneath hardens over, and a new nail grows. (In about six months' time.)

Ingrowing nails are very common indeed

253

in the toes, but are rare in the fingers. Badly-fitting shoes are possibly a factor in producing this condition; it is also traditional to say that clipping away the corners of the nails, instead of cutting straight across, predisposes to ingrowth, though this is difficult to prove. Many doctors feel that where a nail is only moderately ingrowing, treatment should consist simply of cutting it straight across; this is difficult, however, where the corners of the nail are buried deep in grooves lying along each side, as is often the case. Sometimes attempts are made to lift these corners by packing a small amount of lint under them, but very often ingrowth is so severe that it is necessary to remove half or even the whole nail under local anaesthetic. This gives a respite for six months or so, but if the nail returns to its former condition, then it may be necessary to perform a rather more extensive operation. In this, the whole nail bed is obliterated, so that the toe nail never regrows. Although this looks slightly odd, it does no harm whatever, since toe nails, unlike finger nails, have long since lost their function.

Whitlows are small collections of pus at the side or root of the nail. It is necessary to let the pus out, and this is done by incision, though half the nail may occasionally have to be removed.

Fungus infections of the nails are common in people whose work involves getting their hands wet. They require prolonged treatment with anti-fungal agents.

The common skin disease psoriasis also frequently affects the nails. Treatment is along the same lines as for psoriasis (see **psoriasis**), possibly with the addition of steroid injections into the nail bed.

Spoon-shaped nails (koilonychia) are a sign of iron-deficiency anaemia.

The widespread belief that white marks on the nail are a sign of lack of calcium is not borne out by the facts.

NALIDIXIC ACID is a drug, introduced in the last decade, which has proved of considerable value in the treatment of urinary infections caused by certain germs (called 'gram-negative' because of their appearance in stained microscopic preparations). Nalidixic acid is also sometimes used in certain gastro-intestinal infections. It occasionally produces nausea or vomiting, and abnormal sensitivity to sunlight. It must be used with caution in people with liver disease, but is nonetheless a most useful drug in eradicating dangerous bacteria from the urine (see **urinary infections**).

NAPPIES, or diapers, are of two main types—disposable and non-disposable.

Disposable nappies are a relatively recent development. They are extremely convenient, and of course dispense with the problem of washing. However, they are not always as absorbent as the non-disposable type, and do not fit the contours of the baby's body so well.

Non-disposable nappies are, of course, the traditional type. They are oblong shaped pieces of cloth (normally towelling or gauze), which are usually folded into a triangle and secured with one pin (as is common in the United Kingdom), or into a kite shape, and secured with two pins (as is common in the United States).

Whichever type of nappy is used, it is important that it should be changed reasonably frequently; allowing urine to lie around on the skin may produce nappy rash (see **nappy rash**).

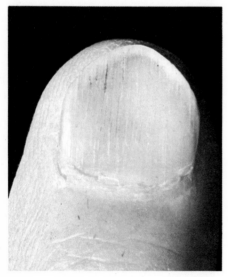

The appearance of the nail in the condition known as koilonychia — almost spoon-shaped.

NAPPY RASH is a common skin eruption which affects the napkin area in babies. The inner sides of the thighs, the genitals, and the buttocks are red, and often excoriated and tender. There is usually considerable itching, and when the child's nappy is off he scratches the skin, so making things worse.

Nappy rash is usually caused by the irritation of persistent contact with nappies which are wet with urine. It is, of course, extremely difficult to keep a baby's napkin area free of urine, however often the nappies are changed.

Treatment often starts with the use of soothing and protective applications such as calamine lotion or zinc and castor oil cream. At the same time, it is absolutely essential that urine in the nappies is given a chance to evaporate; *this can only be so if plastic covering pants are entirely discarded until such time as the rash is entirely better.* The mistake most mothers make is continuing to use such pants.

Meantime, the nappies should be changed as frequently as possible; in severe cases it may be necessary to do without them altogether. This makes considerable difficulties for the mother (though at least it dispenses with the washing of nappies), but it means that urine is no longer in contact with the skin.

Washing of the nappy area should be kept to a minimum, and the skin should be carefully dried afterwards with a soft towel. The family doctor will advise on whether any special precautions are necessary in washing towels and nappies: some chemicals such as washing soda, may be an irritant to the skin. The doctor may also prescribe creams containing steroids and antibiotics to apply to the inflamed area; these often have a very good effect indeed.

NARCISSISM means excessive admiration of oneself. It is so called after the classical legend of Narcissus, who fell in love with his own reflection in a pool of water.

Psychoanalysts describe the state of mind of a very young infant as 'primary narcissism'. In this instance, the term has a rather different meaning: it implies that the infant's ego has not yet emerged as a reasonable and rational part of the mind, and the baby is therefore an almost unthinking organism, capable only of screaming until its needs are gratified. Psychoanalytic theory holds that people with the very common form of mental illness called schizophrenia regress to this state of primary narcissism in the later stages of the disease, although many psychologists regard this as an over-simplification.

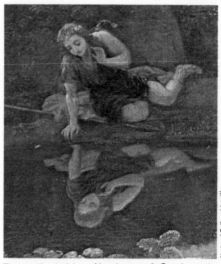

The self-admiring Narcissus of Greek mythology, who lent his name to modern psychology.

National Gallery (detail)

NARCOLEPSY is a fairly uncommon condition in which the sufferer tends to fall asleep quite suddenly during the day. The onset of these attacks is quite irresistible, but the patient does not have any sort of convulsion or fit. He merely sinks into what to all appearances is a perfectly normal sleep, and then, after an interval of some minutes, he wakes up, usually feeling refreshed and well.

Narcolepsy usually, but not always, begins in the teens, and it affects men more often than women. Attacks occur more frequently when a person is tired or drowsy. There are sometimes associated disorders of sleep at night — for instance, sleep-walking or persistent nightmares. These features are not common, however. Also rare is the complication called *catalepsy.* This is a condition in which the narcoleptic person does not fall asleep, but suddenly collapses onto the ground, usually for a period of seconds only. Frequently, attacks of this sort are provoked by laughing.

Narcolepsy is, of course, very embarassing for the patient. It also means that he or she cannot ride a bicycle or drive a car. Otherwise, however, there seem to be no ill-effects. Treatment usually consists of giving stimulant drugs to ward off the attacks.

NARCOTICS are, literally speaking, substances which produce sleep. It is in this sense that the word is used in the United Kingdom and most Commonwealth countries.

Such narcotic drugs include the barbiturates, the derivatives of opium and many newer synthetic preparations. These drugs are also known as 'hypnotics'.

In the United States, the word 'narcotics' often has an entirely different meaning. Owing to a basic misunderstanding of the term by the legislators who originally brought in laws to control drug-addiction in the USA, all addictive drugs (and, indeed, all banned drugs) were erroneously described as 'narcotics'. This has since, of course, led to very considerable confusion.

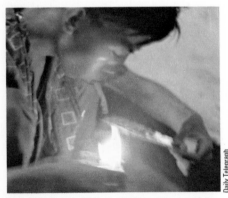

The 'lighting-up' ritual of the narcotic addict, seeking solace in the fumes of opium.

NATURAL SELECTION is a term first popularized by Charles Darwin (1809–1882), the father of the theory of evolution. Before Darwin published his book *The Origin of Species* in 1859, many other

256

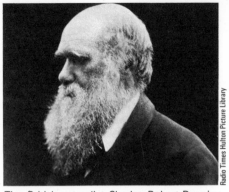

The British naturalist Charles Robert Darwin; originator of the theory of Natural Selection.

people had put forward the idea that Man was descended from a line of more primitive animals, stretching back over hundreds of thousands of years to the beginning of life itself. It was extremely difficult, however, to understand just how this process of evolution took place. Why had living things slowly increased in complexity, so that from the earliest simple life forms, existing only in the sea, there had developed land animals, and, eventually, an ape-like creature which was the common ancestor of Man and monkeys? Why had this 'missing link' eventually given rise to primitive Man? And why, indeed, had primitive Man slowly changed into a rational being, capable of speech, writing, and reasoned thought? The answer, Darwin pointed out, lay in *selection*.

Almost all living things in their natural state produce many more offspring than can ever survive long enough to reproduce themselves. This 'survival of the fittest' was true of Man until quite recently in his history (and is still true of some primitive peoples today).

But if a sudden beneficial genetic change (called a 'mutation') occurs, so that an animal's offspring has some advantage over its fellows (for instance, if the mutation results in a more efficient brain), then that offspring will have a better chance of survival. It will also have a better chance of passing the advantageous characteristic on to its own offspring. So, by this mechanism of 'natural selection', the process of evolution very gradually takes place.

NAUSEA means a feeling of sickness. It is, of course, frequently followed by vomiting or retching.

Nausea, like vomiting, may have many causes. In general, these causes may be divided into two groups. In the first, the basic origin of the trouble is located in the abdomen, and in the second, nausea is due to stimulation of centres in the brain.

Within the abdomen, stomach disturbances may very frequently produce nausea: anything which causes gastric irritation (for instance, an excess of alcohol, or infection by the type of germs which produce gastro-enteritis) leads to a feeling of sickness. If actual vomiting follows, then the irritant substance is expelled from the stomach, so that, very often, the feeling of nausea diminishes and the patient feels better.

Other much less common intra-abdominal causes of nausea include bowel obstruction and irritation of the peritoneum, the membrane which lines the abdominal cavity (as occurs, for instance, in appendicitis). In these conditions, vomiting almost invariably follows the feeling of nausea.

Within the brain, there are certain centres which, if stimulated, cause both nausea and vomiting. Such stimulation is readily caused by sea-sickness. In these disorders, the balancing mechanisms of the inner ear are disturbed by constant motion, and the constant flow of nerve impulses sent from them to the brain triggers off the sensation of nausea.

Certain drugs, for instance morphine can also stimulate these brain centres, as can raised pressure inside the skull. Such raised pressure can be produced by a cerebral tumour, but it should be emphasized that this is a very rare cause of nausea. Much more common is *psychogenic* (or nervous) vomiting and nausea. Many people experience this when they are under some form of nervous strain; very commonly, the patient feels literally 'sick with fear' on the morning of a day on which he has to face some anxiety-provoking situation — for example, an examination.

Finally, any kind of stimulation of the back of the throat, as is well known, produces nausea. If the stimulation is continued, vomiting results. This is due to the fact that nerve impulses travel from the back of the throat to the brain centres we have mentioned. This reflex is obviously of considerable value in protecting a human being against anything becoming jammed in the throat and choking him.

NAVEL is the umbilicus. This small pit in the abdomen marks the site at which the umbilical cord (which joins the baby to the placenta, or afterbirth) is attached in the unborn child (see **umbilicus**).

NECK is the part of the body connecting the head to the trunk. It contains many structures of vital importance, which is why any penetrating injury to the neck is likely to be serious.

The neck is supported by the seven cervical vertebrae which make up the topmost part of the spine, and to these bones, and to the base of the skull itself, are attached powerful muscles. These not only move the head and neck, but provide considerably protection for the vital structures which they enclose.

The foremost of the structures is the trachea, or windpipe, which lies only a

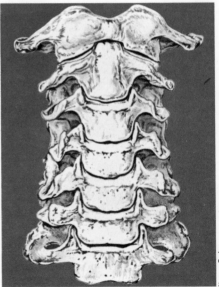

The atlas bone, which meets the skull, the axis, and the other vertebrae of the neck.

257

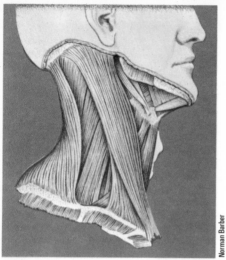

Dissection to show the neck muscles. Prominent is the sterno-mastoid, to turn the head.

short distance under the skin of the front part of the neck; the rings of cartilage in its walls can clearly be felt with the fingers.

Behind the trachea is the oesophagus, or gullet, which conveys food and drink from the mouth to the stomach.

Directly behind this are the seven cervical vertebrae themselves. Contained in the canal which lies within them is the upper part of the spinal cord, which transmits almost all the nerve impulses between the brain and the body. If the topmost part of this section of the cord is severely damaged (as is the case, for instance, in judicial hanging) then death is almost immediate.

Under cover of the pair of very prominent muscles (called the sterno-mastoids), which lie one on each side of the neck, are several extremely important blood vessels. These include the common carotid artery, which supplies blood to the head, and also the internal jugular vein, which collects 'used' blood from the brain, and certain other areas of the head and neck, and returns it to the heart.

Among the many other structures lying within the neck are the thyroid gland and a large number of extremely important nerves. The neck is therefore one of the most susceptible areas to injury in the entire body.

258

Stiffness of the neck, with painful contraction of one or more muscles, and limited movement, may result from injury to, or disease of, the cervical vertebrae or the numerous nerves in that region.

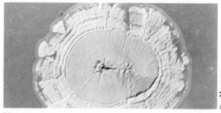

Neomycin is obtained from the fungus Streptomyces griseus, shown here growing in culture.

NEOMYCIN is an antibiotic derived from the same group of fungi from which we obtain streptomycin. It has certain properties in common with the latter antibiotic (for instance, if given by injection, it could produce deafness), but, unlike streptomycin, it is not used in the treatment of tuberculosis.

It is, however, very useful in the treatment of bowel infections, and is also often given by mouth to sterilize the bowel prior to an abdominal operation. This sterilizing effect is also employed in the treatment of coma due to cirrhosis of the liver. Neomycin creams and ointments are used in cases of skin infection.

As pointed out, injections of neomycin may produce deafness by damage to the nerves. They also cause kidney damage, and the drug is therefore practically never administered in this way.

NEONATAL MORTALITY is the death rate of infants under four weeks old. It is calculated in terms of the number of deaths per 1,000 live births, and provides a very good indication of the adequacy or otherwise of maternity services in a country. In certain developed countries, for instance the United Kingdom and Scandinavia, the neonatal mortality rate is now usually around 12–14 per thousand live births, but in underdeveloped lands the rate may be as high as 50 or even 100 per thousand. The mortality was as high as this in many developed countries at the turn of the century.

NEPHRECTOMY means removal of a kidney (or part of a kidney) by surgical operation. As a general rule this procedure is carried out by making an incision in the back, immediately under the lowest rib. This results in a fairly unobtrusive scar. Very occasionally, however, a kidney is removed through an incision in the front of the abdomen. There are various possible reasons for carrying out a nephrectomy. These include tuberculous disease of the kidney, growths and stones. In many cases, nephrectomy is likely to be *partial* rather than *total*, and only a small part of the kidney may be removed.

An increasingly common indication for total nephrectomy is the offer of a kidney to be transplanted into someone else's abdomen. The donor is frequently a twin or a close relative of the recipient of the kidney, because of the fact that the tissues are likely to 'match' better; however, tissue matching does sometimes show there is likely to be a good chance of success in transplants between unrelated persons. Provided the donor's other kidney is healthy, it will readily take over the work of the one which has been removed.

In the 1950s and early 1960s, it was very common for people to have partial or total nephrectomies for high blood pressure (hypertension), where it was suspected that localized kidney trouble was the cause of the disorder. The results were not as good as was first hoped, however, and the operation is now less frequently performed for this purpose.

NEPHRITIS means inflammation of the kidneys. It is not one disease, but many.

Strictly speaking, the word 'nephritis' covers both glomerulonephritis (which is inflammation of the substance of the kidney) and pyelonephritis, or pyelitis (which is inflammation mainly of the part of the kidney called the pelvis, from which urine is carried away by the ureter to the bladder). Almost invariably, however, doctors mean the former group of conditions when they use the word 'nephritis'.

Nephritis meaning glomerulonephritis or pyelonephritis may be *acute* or *chronic*.

Acute glomerulonephritis has been classified as either 'type I' or 'type II'.

Type I nephritis is a fairly benign condition, mainly occurring in children and young adults. It is a disease of abrupt onset. The patient's face suddenly becomes puffy, because of retained fluid (oedema). He usually feels very poorly, and may have a headache and a temperature. His urine is usually rather scanty and blood-stained.

The cause of this illness is not definitely known, but in a high percentage of cases the patient has had a bout of tonsillitis or a throat infection about two weeks previously. It is widely believed that the inflammation of the kidneys is due to a hypersensitivity reaction to the Streptococcus germ, which is the cause of many throat infections.

The great majority of people with type I nephritis recover after a week or so in hospital. A small proportion of patients develop a more chronic inflammation, however, so that careful treatment and observation are essential.

Type II nephritis has a much wider age distribution, and the outlook is not so good as in type I nephritis. The disorder is characterized by massive dropsy (oedema), which produces a persistent and progressive swelling of all the tissues (and not just the face, as in type I nephritis). The urine is rarely blood-stained but contains large quantities of protein. As a result, the blood is severely deficient in protein.

The cause of type II nephritis is completely unknown. However, this group of symptoms, which are collectively described as 'the nephrotic syndrome' (see **nephrotic syndrome**) is occasionally caused by diseases such as diabetes, or by poisoning with certain metals. Certain drugs have also been blamed.

Treatment again involves a stay in hospital, often for a considerable period. Some varieties of type II nephritis respond well to the steroid group of drugs.

Chronic nephritis is a long-standing inflammation of the kidneys. Some cases may result from a previous episode of type I or type II acute nephritis, but others occur without a history of any previous illness. The features of the condition are related to a progressive failure of the kidneys to clear poisonous substances from the body.

There may be weakness, thirst, nausea, anaemia and high blood pressure. Dietary and other treatment can nowadays be augmented by the use of the artificial kidney (see **kidney – artificial**).

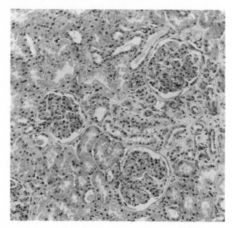

Contrast the normal microscopic appearance of the kidney, *above*, with that of the kidney in nephritis, *below*. The structure of the glomeruli, or filtration units, is completely altered.

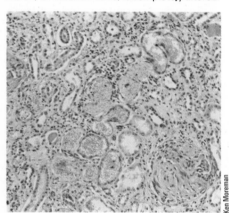

Ken Moreman

NEPHROTIC SYNDROME is a general name for a group of symptoms comprising massive dropsy (oedema), heavy loss of protein in the urine, and corresponding deficiency of protein in the blood.

Most commonly, the nephrotic syndrome is due to type II acute nephritis, which is described under the heading **nephritis**. It may also, however, occur as a complication of diabetes, of a condition called 'amyloidosis' (which results from a

260

chronic suppuration in the body), of poisoning by certain metals, or of disseminated lupus erythematosus (see **lupus**). It can also be due to blockage of the veins which carry blood away from the kidneys.

NERVES are the bundles of fibres which form the 'wiring system' of the body, carrying electrical impulses around it.

The nervous system is divided into various parts. The central nervous system comprises only the brain and the spinal cord. A very large number of pairs of cranial and spinal nerves run out from the brain and spinal cord to supply nerve impulses to the various parts of the body and others carry impulses in the reverse direction, to convey information from the distant parts of the body to the central nervous system.

Other nerves make up the autonomic nervous system, which is not under voluntary control, but essential for the proper working of many of the organs of the body, especially the glands and organs of secretion.

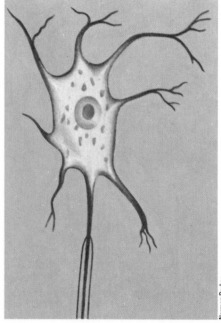

Norman Barber

Diagram to show the structure of a nerve cell. The delicate processes reaching from the body of the cell make contact with other cells. At the bottom, the beginning of the nerve fibre.

NERVOUSNESS, or anxiety, occurs at some time to all human beings. As such, it is often a beneficial phenomenon, since it prepares the individual's body to deal with the situation he is facing. For example, an athlete about to run a race may feel nervous, but that same nervousness produces changes in his body which send the blood coursing rapidly round it, bringing much needed oxygen and nutriment to the muscles. At the same time, the blood vessels of the muscles increase in size, so that not only is it easier to supply these materials for the effort to come, but it is also easier for the blood to carry away the waste products produced by muscular activity. At the same time, the mind becomes alert and concentrated on the task in hand.

Nervousness can, however, become so severe and recurrent as to constitute an actual illness. Such anxiety states are very common indeed, and may be very disabling to the patient. Fortunately, in many cases, such illnesses are self-limiting, and the symptoms disappear entirely after a short time. Where they do not do so, however, the family doctor will usually refer the patient for psychiatric help, which, in the majority of cases, effects considerable improvement and often a complete cure.

NEURALGIA literally means pain in a nerve. In fact, *all* pain is felt as a result of impulses running up nerves and reaching pain centres in the brain. It would therefore be more accurate to say that neuralgia is pain actually arising in a nerve. At one time, all sorts of aches and pains were referred to as 'neuralgia', which was thought to be due to exposure to cold and damp. It is now realized that this is not so, and that only a relatively small number of conditions can properly be described as neuralgia.

These include tic douloureux, or trigeminal neuralgia, which is an extremely painful condition of the trigeminal nerve, which supples the skin of the face. The patient suffers recurrent paroxysms of pain in one side of the face; these attacks may be brought on by touching the cheek, or by eating, and they can be almost unbearably agonizing. If treatment with pain-killing drugs is not effective, the ganglion from which the nerve springs can be numbed by means of an alcohol injection. It is sometimes necessary to cut through the nerve entirely, but this has the disadvantage that the side of the face becomes permanently 'dead' to all sensation.

In recent years, a new drug called carbamazepine has become available for the treatment of trigeminal neuralgia, and promising results are claimed for it.

Another form of neuralgia occurs during and after attacks of herpes zoster, or shingles (see **herpes zoster**). Particularly in older persons, this pain may be very trying.

NEURASTHENIA is a psychological condition in which the patient feels exhausted and irritable. He has many fleeting symptoms which are suggestive of bodily disorder but which are in fact due to his mental state.

This condition was diagnosed very frequently in years gone by, but now seems to be very rare. This is probably because the term 'neurasthenic' was loosely used at one time to describe people with chronic depression and many other types of mental disorder. However, there is some evidence that in Edwardian days, among wealthy people with nothing to do, the condition probably was rather commoner than it is today.

NEURITIS means inflammation of a nerve. Such inflammation may affect only one nerve, or many throughout the body.

Inflammation of a particular nerve is usually due to something pressing on it. Sciatica, for instance, is usually the result of pressure on the roots of the sciatic nerve (often by a so-called 'slipped' disc); this produces pain in the distribution of the nerve, i.e. down the back of the leg.

Generalized inflammation of many nerves is called polyneuritis, peripheral neuritis or peripheral neuropathy. Its features are usually numbness and tingling of the hands and feet, often followed by pains in the legs and difficulty in walking. The muscles may be tender, and may become weak, so that there is 'wrist-drop', a condition in which the hands flop limply and can only be straightened at the wrists with difficulty if indeed moved at all.

There are many causes of this type of polyneuritis. It may be due to absorption of poisonous substances, such as arsenic, lead, gold, mercury and carbon tetrachloride. It may also be due to deficiency of the B vitamin group, as occurs in beriberi and alcoholism. It can also be caused by certain infections, including diphtheria, and by diabetes. In some cases, the cause is completely unknown.

Neuritis of an extremely serious sort occurs when the fatty myelin layer of the nerves starts to degenerate.

NEUROSIS, or psychoneurosis, is a state of disturbed personality adjustment, in which the stability of the patient's mind is threatened by stresses. As a result, he produces what are called 'ego defences', and these take the form of behaviour which, while unusual, is in no sense 'insane'. To this extent, at least, neuroses are *minor* mental illnesses, though they may be extremely unpleasant for those suffering from them.

The neuroses include hysteria (see **hysteria**) and anxiety and obsessional states. Some psychiatrists include neurasthenia (see **neurasthenia**) in this group of disorders.

Anxiety states (which are also discussed under the heading nervousness) are characterized by tremendous emotional tension which may centre round some particular situation (say, being in a lift, or in an open space); alternatively, the anxiety may be 'free-floating' — by which is meant that it is always with the patient, and does not centre round any one situation.

Obsessional states are a form of neurosis in which the patient either cannot avoid thinking repetitively about certain unpleasant ideas, or alternatively feels compelled to keep carrying out certain actions in a repetitive manner. For instance, a man may feel that he has to carry out some minor ritual, such as washing his hands, several times every hour.

In all types of neurosis, it is essential that medical help be sought as soon as possible to aid the patient to restore the adjustment of his personality to normal. (See also **mental illness**).

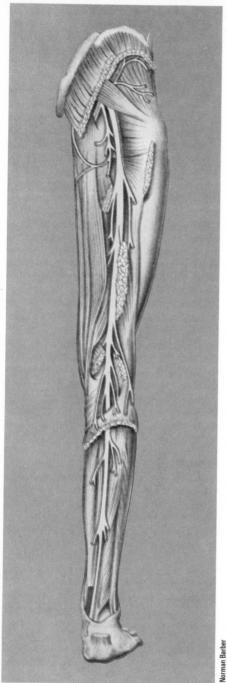

Norman Barber

Dissection of the back of the leg, to show the distribution of the sciatic nerve. Pressure on its roots in the spine may cause sciatica.

NIGHT BLINDNESS means inability to see properly in a dim light. In absolute darkness, none of us can see anything at all, of course, but where there is even a minute amount of light, a healthy person's eyes can detect it. The image he forms will be in black and white, however. This is because we perceive colour by means of tiny receptors, called cones, in the retina, the screen at the back of the eye. These cones need a considerable amount of light to stimulate them, and therefore we can only detect colour in daylight or moderately good artificial light.

There are also another set of receptors called rods. These are much more sensitive, but though they can be stimulated by very small amounts of light, they do not detect colour.

In some disorders, the function of these rods is interfered with, and so, although the patient can see perfectly well in the daytime (thanks to his cone receptors), at night or in faint light, he is blind.

Such night-blindness occurs in vitamin A deficiency (see **deficiency diseases**); this is a condition which occurs in people whose diet lacks carotenes, chemicals which are found in high concentration in carrots. For this reason, it was at one time the practice, during the Second World War, to give pilots a diet rich in carrots, with the object of improving their night vision. Unfortunately, there was no evidence that this worked.

Night blindness also occurs in a number of other diseases, notably retinitis pig-mentosa, an inherited defect in which large areas of the retina are covered with black pigment.

Night blindness may also be the temporary result of over-exposure to a very bright light — for instance, where a person has been looking at an eclipse of the sun without wearing dark glasses. In this case, the symptom is due to exhaustion of the supply of a pigment called visual purple in the rods. A return to normal vision can be accelerated by giving vitamin A, from which this pigment is formed provided permanent retinal damage has not been done.

NIGHTMARES are frightening dreams. Although all of us (even those who think that they do not dream) probably have nightmares at times, the occurrence of persistent and very terrifying dreams of this sort usually has an underlying cause. Where a person has been through a frightening experience, or is undergoing some considerable stress, nightmares may, to some extent, provide a useful 'safety valve' for the mind. However, if such dreams are very troublesome, it is wisest to consult a doctor. This is particularly so in young children, since it is very important in these formative years to try to resolve any stresses which are troubling the child.

NIPPLES are the teats of the breast (see **breast**). The word is almost invariably taken by most people to include the circular pigmented area called the areola, but this is not so. The word 'nipple' actually refers only to the projecting teat in the middle of the areola.

In the female, the nipple contains the tiny openings of about 20 'lactiferous ducts', from which the baby sucks milk. The nipple is mainly composed of erectile tissue; that is to say it is capable of stiffening as a result of stimulation. The stimuli which most commonly cause this phenomenon are, of course, breast-feeding and sexual excitement; exposure to cold has a similar effect.

The areolas and nipples are, of course, of tremendous importance to the primitive mind of the young baby. Freudian theory suggests that it is for this reason that

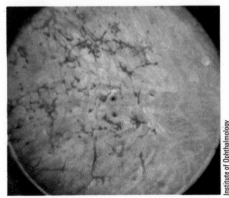

The appearance of the retina in the disease called retinitis pigmentosa.

Institute of Ophthalmology

263

these areas have always been regarded as of immense sexual significance. For example, the nipple and areola are widely regarded as the 'taboo' areas of the breast. While in most countries of the world, it is socially acceptable to show the rest of the bosom, exposure of any part of the nipple or aerola tends to be forbidden or at least frowned on.

NITROFURANTOIN is an extremely useful drug employed in the treatment of urinary infections, such as cystitis or pyelitis. Occasionally, nitrofurantoin causes rashes or symptoms rather similar to asthma. It can also produce an unusual type of anaemia in people of the negro race. In general, however, it is a safe and effective agent against the germs which so commonly enter the urinary tract. (See **urinary infections**.)

NITROUS OXIDE is the proper chemical name for 'laughing gas', (see **laughing gas**) which is very widely used in anaesthesia (see also **anaesthesia**).

NOSE. The nose is not only the organ by which we smell things, but it is also important in respiration, since a considerable proportion of the air we breathe in enters via the nose.

The nose may be divided into two parts — external and internal.

The external part contains only a small amount of bone, which forms the hard 'bridge' of the nose. Below this, the rest of the skeletal support of the nose is made up of cartilage, which has the advantage of being firm yet pliable. This is important, because most males, at any rate, suffer quite a considerable number of blows to the nose during sporting activities, for instance. The cartilages can be dislocated from each other by violence, but this is not nearly as important as breaking a bone would be.

The two nostrils open the way into the interior of the nose, which basically consists of two cavities divided by a thin layer of bone and cartilage. The two cavities, which are very narrow, run backwards until they communicate eventually with the naso-pharynx, a wider space
264

which leads directly into the back of the throat, or pharynx.

From the interior part of the nose, fibres of the two olfactory nerves carry messages regarding smell up to the appropriate centres in the brain.

The exact mechanism by which different sorts of smell are distinguished from one another is at the moment still a mystery, although it is known that the free ends of the olfactory cells in the mucous membrane each have six to eight protruding 'hairs' which have been shown to contain a high proportion of fatty substances – lipids – in which many odorous substances are known to dissolve readily. It is possible that the different substances that we smell, in the form of extremely small particles, or perhaps even molecules, dissolve in the mucous secretions covering the olfactory membrane, and react with different sensitive receptors to produce a characteristic nerve-impulse pattern which the brain interprets according to past experience.

Many researchers believe that there are in fact only a few basic odours, and that all other sensations of smell result from various combinations of these odours. Last century there were thought to be as many as nine basic odours, but a simpler classification is just into four categories: fragrant, burning, cheesy and putrid.

All odours of course disappear when the nose is blocked, and air cannot reach the nerve endings in the olfactory membrane.

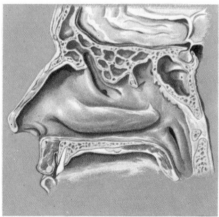

Norman Barber

A cross section of the head, to show the nasal cavity, and the cavities of the sinuses.

NOTIFIABLE DISEASES are those whose occurrence is required by the law of a country to be reported to the appropriate authority — usually the medical officer of health. This procedure of notification is one of the most important features of any public health service. The reason for this is obvious: if a case of a serious disease, capable of starting an epidemic, is notified to the public health authorities immediately it is diagnosed (or suspected) then there is a much greater chance of preventing the epidemic. In the instance of some notifiable diseases, there is no actual risk of an epidemic, but the very occurrence of one case of the disorder is usually an indication of some breakdown in hygiene.

The actual diseases which are notifiable vary a little from country to country depending on prevailing health conditions, but the following list of infectious diseases which should be notified in England and Wales may be taken as typical: Anthrax; Cerebro-spinal fever (meningitis); Cholera; Diphtheria; Dysentery; Encephalitis; Enteric fever; Food poisoning; Infectious jaundice; Leprosy; Leptospirosis; Malaria; Measles; Ophthalmia neonatorum; Plague; Poliomyelitis; Relapsing fever; Scarlet fever; Smallpox; Tetanus; Typhus; Tuberculosis; Whooping cough.

There are also a number of non-infectious *industrial* diseases which, in many countries, must be notified to the authorities, but the nature of these varies very greatly between different nations. (See **occupational diseases**.)

NURSES have been part of the health team since the earliest days of medicine. However, although there must undoubtedly have been many good individual nurses in the distant past, there was no proper training provided in nursing anywhere in the world until well into the nineteenth century. In fact, by about 1850, the profession had fallen into considerable disrepute in many countries. In England, nurses were noted only for immorality, ignorance and incompetence.

Florence Nightingale began to set this state of affairs to rights when she took her small party of nurses to the Crimean

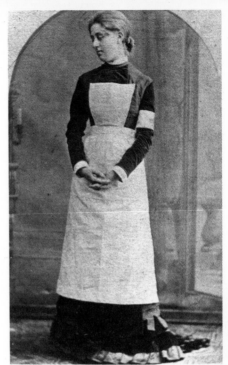
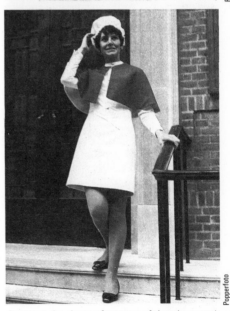

Radio Times/Hulton Picture Library

Popperfoto

Contrast the dress of a nurse of the nineteenth century, starched, stiff, stifling, with the neater and infinitely more hygienic type of uniform seen in hospitals everywhere today.

War. On her return to England, she set about organizing the training of nurses to standards which were subsequently accepted throughout the British Empire. It was not until very much later, however, that proper standards were established in the United Kingdom for the training of midwives (see **midwife**).

Nowadays, the word 'nurse' can mean a number of things in various parts of the world. In many countries, there are 'academies' which guarantee to turn a young woman into a 'practical nurse' after a course of only a few weeks, often by postal instruction. The 'diplomas' of such institutions are, of course, quite worthless.

However, most reasonably advanced countries have some system of training whereby a girl studies for approximately three years and then becomes a Registered Nurse (RN) or State Registered Nurse (SRN). A lower academic standard of entry is normally required of girls who wish to take a two year course and become an Enrolled Nurse (EN) or State Enrolled Nurse (SEN).

To obtain either of these types of certificate requires a very considerable amount of time spent in hard work in the hospital wards, together with a good deal of study. Most of all, it requires an immense amount of dedication to an extremely difficult and responsible job, which in most countries brings very little in the way of financial reward. There are a great many openings, offering first-class nursing training combined with the additional possibility of travel abroad, in the medical services attached to the armed forces.

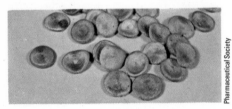

The seeds of the plant Strychnos nuxvomica, source of the alkaloid strychnine.

NUX VOMICA is a preparation which was in widespread use in 'tonics' until

266

relatively recent years to improve appetite. It contains a small amount of the poison strychnine, and has an extremely bitter taste. It is extracted from the seeds of an Eastern tree called *Strychnos nuxvomica*.

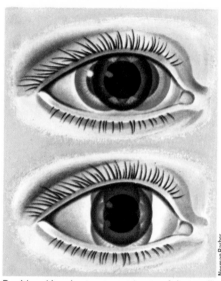

Rapid and involuntary movements of the pupil, either vertically or horizontally, may indicate disturbance of the balancing organs and faulty coordination of brain and eye.

NYSTAGMUS is a rapid jerking of the eyeballs, usually from side to side, but occasionally in an up and down or rotary direction.

Nystagmus is an important finding, because it is often an indication of disease of the balancing mechanisms, and, in particular, of that part of the brain known as the cerebellum. Disorders of the nerve which connects the cerebellum with the inner ear, or of the inner ear itself (the labyrinth) commonly produce the symptom also.

Nystagmus can also be due to overactivity of the thyroid gland (hyperthyroidism), and occasionally to a type of eye-strain seen particularly in people who work in the dark, such as miners.

NYSTATIN is a drug which kills fungi. Fungal infections of the body are common, particularly in the mouth and vaginal areas. Nystatin is probably most commonly used, in the form of pessaries, to treat a very widespread form of vaginal discharge due to the fungus known as *Candida albicans* or *Monilia* (see **monilia**).

OBESITY

OBESITY is a state of being overweight. Well over 2,000 years ago, the Greek physician Hippocrates wrote that those who are fat are much more liable to sudden death than those who are thin.

This observation remains entirely true today. In addition, it is known that obese persons are far more likely to suffer from diabetes mellitus, coronary heart disease, high blood pressure, osteoarthritis, varicose veins, gall-stones and a number of other conditions.

The life expectancy of a man who is 25 pounds overweight at the age of 45 is 25% less than that of a healthy man.

It is therefore essential that anyone who is obese should make every effort to lose weight by reducing his intake of food. This simple fact is not widely understood, and far too many obese people regard their fatness as more or less inevitable. Anyone who finds that he or she is 10% or more overweight by the tables at the end of the dictionary should start reducing immediately for his health's sake.

OBSTETRICS

OBSTETRICS, or midwifery, is the art and science of delivering babies, and also of caring for the mother and her unborn child during pregnancy.

Obstetrics is practised by midwives (see **midwife**) and by obstetricians. In many countries of the world (excepting the United States), midwives undertake much of the routine care of mothers during pregnancy, and also deliver the vast majority of all babies. Deliveries which are in any way complicated, however (for instance, breech presentations, multiple deliveries, and those requiring forceps) are almost invariably dealt with by obstetricians. These are doctors who have had special training in obstetrics after qualifying.

In the United States, however, *all* deliveries are dealt with by doctors.

OBSTRUCTION OF THE BOWEL

OBSTRUCTION OF THE BOWEL is a common surgical condition. There are many possible causes, but the most common are hernias (ruptures), adhesions (which are fibrous bands that develop within the abdomen following a surgical operation), diverticular disease (see **diverticular disease**), and cancer of the bowel.

The features of acute obstruction are distension of the abdomen, pain, constipation, and vomiting.

Where the obstruction is in the *small intestine* (which is the upper part of the bowel), abdominal pain is likely to be the first symptom. It tends to be colicky in nature, with attacks lasting perhaps only a few minutes, but returning every half hour or so. Vomiting may occur with each bout of pain, or only with the first attack. If the obstruction is not relieved, however, vomiting eventually becomes severe and recurrent. Distension is not very marked in the early stages of this type of obstruction, but it may be possible to see the wave-like movement of distended loops of bowel progressing across the abdomen. Constipation may be the last symptom of obstruction of the small intestine, and it may be preceded by a normal bowel action or by diarrhoea.

Conversely, obstruction of the large intestine or colon (the lower part of the bowel) is usually characterized by constipation, which may occur well before the advent of either pain or distension. Vomiting is unlikely to occur until the very late stages of the condition.

Both types of obstruction are of considerable seriousness, and require urgent hospital treatment. In some cases, it may be possible to relieve the condition by the procedure known as 'suction and drip'. This means putting a tube through the patient's nose or mouth and down through his stomach into the intestines, so that the fluid collecting there as a result of the obstruction can be sucked out. At the same time, the patient has a 'drip' of replacement fluid, usually into an arm vein.

Alternatively, it may be necessary to relieve the obstruction by means of a surgical operation. Even in these cases, however, it is essential for the patient to

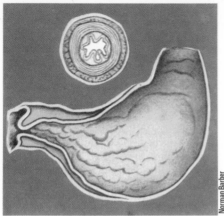

Diagram to show abnormal narrowing of the stomach, which may cause obstruction in babies and require surgical correction.

Norman Barber

the air passages, caused by the spasm of muscle fibres in their walls. Bronchospasm is a feature of asthmatic attacks, and often of chronic bronchitis.

Obstruction may also be due to inflammation of the inner walls of the air passages. Such inflammation leads to the formation of fluid, which swells the walls, so that air cannot get through. This kind of obstruction also occurs in asthma, and in chronic bronchitis as well. It may happen where a person has inhaled an irritant dust, gas or smoke into the lungs. Inflammation may also lead to outpouring of mucus into the air passages, and this frequently causes obstruction in people with chronic bronchitis.

Where there is loss of elasticity of the lungs (as occurs in the common condition called emphysema), it is even more difficult for air to be driven out past the obstruction in the airways.

Chronic obstructive airway disease may therefore be the result of chronic bronchitis (see **bronchitis**), of emphysema (see **emphysema**), and of asthma, if attacks are recurrent and prolonged (see **asthma**). It can also be caused by such conditions as pneumoconiosis, which is due to long-standing irritation of the lungs by coaldust, and which is very common in miners, causing extreme distress.

The features of such chronic obstruction are as follows. There is very considerable *wheeze*, as the air tries to force its way past the obstruction. At the same time, there is increasing *breathlessness*. The patient has *reduced exercise tolerance*, and the slightest exertion may make him distressed, and either pink or blue in the face. He often becomes *barrel-chested*, as a result of the distension of his lungs by air which cannot escape, and his chest X-ray will demonstrate this hyperinflation. He will also have the other features of the original disease — e.g. a persistent and productive cough if he has chronic bronchitis.

Chronic obstructive airway disease requires careful observation and regular treatment. The patient should take especial care to avoid respiratory infections in winter, and should, at all costs, give up smoking.

have the 'suction and drip' regime of treatment both before and after the operation. Though unpleasant, this may be lifesaving.

It should also be mentioned that obstruction of the bowels may occur in newborn children. In such cases, the common causes are stenosis (narrowing) or atresia (congenital blockage) of the intestines; in many cases of atresia, a section of the intestine consists only of a cord-like stretch of fibrous tissue, and nothing more. Rapid surgical treatment is always necessary to save the child's life.

Other causes of obstruction in children include volvulus (a condition in which the intestines become tightly twisted round each other) and intussusception (a disorder in which part of the bowel actually enters the next portion, and becomes jammed in it). Here surgery is life-saving.

OBSTRUCTIVE AIRWAY DISEASE is, in general terms, any condition in which there is interference with the flow of air entering or leaving the lungs. However, most doctors use the expression to indicate only a condition in which there is a long-standing obstruction of the lower airways — that is, the smallest air passages which lead directly out of the lung.

Such obstruction may occur because of bronchospasm, which is a constriction of

OCCIPUT is the back part of the head, just above the junction with the neck. The underlying bone, called the occipital bone, forms a joint with the atlas bone of the neck – the atlanto-occipital joint.

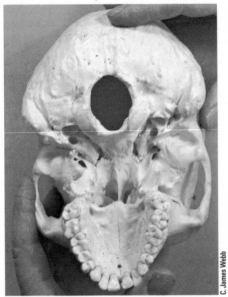

The skull seen from below, to show the bony ring formed by the occipital bone.

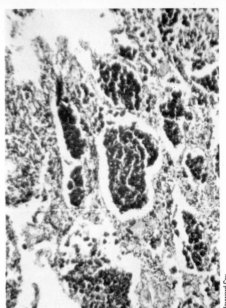

Very heavy deposits of coal dust are seen here in a section from a miner's lung.

OCCUPATIONAL DISEASES are those which occur as a direct or indirect result of a person's job. There are literally hundreds of such diseases. To name but a few: miners are prone to the chest condition known as pneumoconiosis (and, indeed, several other disorders); doctors and nurses in sanatoria are more liable than other people to tuberculosis; racing drivers are liable to all kinds of violent injury; and sewer workers are prone to leptospirosis (a serious form of jaundice passed on by rats) also known as Weil's disease.

Many people who suffer from occupational diseases are eligible for compensation as a result of contracting them; however, the arrangements for such compensation, and the list of diseases covered, vary greatly from country to country.

In Great Britain and most industrialized countries, there are comprehensive arrangements for the prevention of indus-

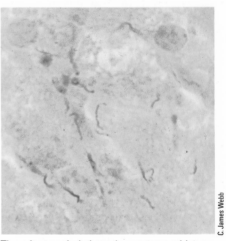

The minute spiral shaped organisms which are responsible for the dangerous Weil's disease.

trial diseases, involving cooperation between industrial medical officers, working in individual factories and plants, and a central liaison officer, called in Britain the Chief Inspector of Factories. These arrangements normally include the compulsory notification of certain industrial diseases. Naturally, these vary from

269

country to country, depending on the types of industry which are common in different parts of the world. In England and Wales, a doctor has to notify to the Chief Inspector of Factories the occurrence of any of the following industrial diseases: poisoning by lead, phosphorus, manganese, arsenic, mercury, carbon bisulphide, aniline or benzene; compressed air sickness; anthrax; toxic jaundice; toxic anaemia; chrome ulceration of the skin; epitheliomatous ulceration (cancer) of the skin. These diseases are, of course, only notifiable if there is reasonable cause to believe that they were contracted in a factory or similar premises.

OEDEMA, a word which is derived from the Greek word for 'swelling', means dropsy of the tissues – that is, swelling due to the presence of fluid which has leaked out of the small blood vessels and lymph vessels.

Oedema (which is spelt 'edema' in the United States) tends to occur mainly in those sites of the body which the overlying tissues are rather slack, so that there is room for fluid to accumulate. Oedema will also tend to collect in the lowest parts of the body. It very commonly appears at the ankles during the day, but passes off after the feet have been elevated for a few hours while the patient is asleep.

Among the commonest sites where oedema may be found are just below the eyes, below the small of the back, on the top surface of the feet, and (as previously mentioned) at the ankles. It may also occur in internal organs, such as the lung (where it will produce breathlessness), but it is, of course, only visible when it forms in tissues just under the skin. In such instances, one of its most characteristic features is that it 'pits on pressure' – that is to say, if a finger is firmly placed on the skin, and then removed, a depression remains visible at the spot for half a minute or so.

A very slight degree of ankle oedema may sometimes occur in healthy people who have been standing upright for a very long time, but otherwise oedema is usually an indication of a disorder which needs treatment.

One of the commonest causes is heart failure, in which the circulation is too sluggish to carry away the fluid in the tissues. It can also be due to many types of kidney disease, for instance most varieties of nephritis (see **nephritis**). In the latter instance, the problem is sometimes that the kidneys are failing to carry away the body's waste products, including water.

However, another mechanism which is often of importance is dependent on the fact that in certain kidney diseases, there is a very great loss of protein in the urine. This leads to a deficiency of protein in the blood; fluid then tends to seep out of the blood vessels and into the tissues.

Exactly the same thing happens in starvation and in kwashiorkor, the protein malnutrition so often seen in children from backward or war-torn lands. Because the starvation leads to a low level of protein in the blood, fluid again seeps out of the bloodstream and into the tissues.

Oedema is also a feature of hepatic (liver) failure, which occurs in cirrhosis of the liver, though in this case a number of factors are responsible, again including a low level of blood protein. In cirrhosis, and also in heart failure, certain hormones, including aldosterone (see **aldosterone**) are believed to be produced in abnormal amounts; these have a complex effect on the kidney, with the result that it excretes insufficient quantities of water.

It should also be mentioned that oedema of the ankles is one of the early signs of the common condition, toxaemia of pregnancy. The occurrence of such ankle swelling should be reported at once to the midwife or doctor, who will probably order increased rest for the expectant mother.

It is essential to determine the cause of oedema before it can be treated. Heart failure oedema can be relieved by heart 'stimulants', such as digoxin or digitalis, helped by diuretics (see **diuretics**), and other means. (See also congestive cardiac failure.)

In kidney and liver disease, the treatment of oedema depends on the precise nature of the illness, but will probably also include the use of diuretics.

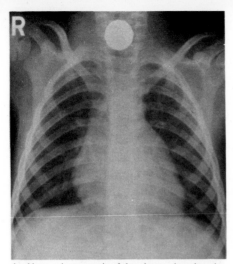

An X-ray photograph of the chest, showing the shadow of a threepenny piece in the oesophagus swallowed by accident.

OESOPHAGUS is the gullet – the tube which conveys food from the back of the throat to the stomach. It is about ten inches in length, and its upper part lies almost directly behind the windpipe (trachea); its lower part runs down through the chest and pierces the diaphragm (the tough membrane separating the abdomen from the chest) before joining the stomach.

This important structure is subject to many diseases. Most of these are dealt with under the heading 'gullet', with the exception of *cancer of the oesophagus.* This disease is relatively common, and despite modern methods of treatment is extremely difficult to cure. This is partly because the diagnosis is often difficult to make until quite late in the progress of the illness, and partly because most patients do not consult the doctor until the disease is very far advanced.

Cancer of the oesophagus is commoner in men than in women, and is more frequently encountered in oriental races (especially the Japanese) than in Western peoples. The average age of onset is about 60, but it may occur in the forties or fifties. *The first symptom is difficulty in swallowing;* the patient may feel that food sticks at some point which he can usually localize fairly accurately by pointing at his chest somewhere in the mid-line.

There may be no other symptoms apart from this, and so the patient's survival may depend on whether he realizes something is wrong and goes to a doctor right away. Unhappily, two patients out of three do not seek medical help until the symptom has been present for three months or more.

When the patient is referred to hospital, he will normally have a special X-ray in which the oesophagus is outlined with barium. If this does not make the diagnosis clear, the surgeon will pass a telescope-like device (called an oesophagoscope) down the throat so that he can examine the interior of the oesophagus. If it then seems that an operation is practicable, the growth will subsequently be removed. It may be necessary to replace the missing segment of oesophagus with a stretch of intestine or stomach, or with a piece of polythene tubing. Radiotherapy may also be employed.

OESTROGENS are a particular group of female hormones. During the first half of the menstrual cycle, these hormones are produced by the ovaries, and, under their influence, the lining of the womb is prepared to receive a fertilized egg. In fact, oestrogens are also produced in the second half of the menstrual cycle (after ovulation) as well, but the main influence during this part of the 'month' is exerted by another female hormone, also produced by the ovaries, called progesterone.

Oestrogens are first secreted in considerable quantities some time before puberty. As a result of their action, changes appear in the young girl's body at about the age of ten. The first of these changes is usually an increased prominence of the nipples, called 'budding'. Subsequently there is deposition of fat behind the nipples and eventually formation of the breasts themselves. Oestrogens also stimulate some increase in height and weight, certain changes in shape of the bones that make up the pelvis, and the growth of pubic and armpit hair. Shortly afterwards, under the influence of these hormones, the nipples (and the surrounding discs called the areolas) become more pigmented; meantime, changes occur in the internal sex organs, culminating eventually in the start of menstruation (see **menstruation**). (The order of these changes may vary considerably, however.)

When the change of life, or menopause comes about, usually in the forties, production of oestrogens falls off, and, as a result, some regressive changes take place in the genital organs. There should be no effect on sexual enjoyment, however; oestrogens do not seem to have any significant influence on this.

There are a considerable number of oestrogens, among the most important of which are oestradiol, oestrone and oestriol. Chemically-related man-made oestrogens include ethinyl-oestradiol and stilboestrol. Many such oestrogens are used in medicine — for instance, in the contraceptive pill, in a number of gynaecological complaints, and also in the treatment of cancer of the prostate gland in men.

OINTMENTS are skin applications in which an active medicament is mixed with a greasy substance such as lanolin, paraffin or vaseline.

OLD AGE is sometimes described as being a state of mind. Certainly, it is hard to say when it begins, since, while one person may have many of the characteristics of old age in his early sixties, another may be hale, hearty and young in outlook in his seventies or eighties.

The important changes which take place in old age are as follows. The body's tissues lose their natural elasticity, so that they tend to sag. Nowhere is this more apparent than in the skin of the face and neck (which are, of course, the areas where people are keenest to 'look young'). Fat lying just under the skin may be absorbed, thus increasing the wrinkling effect produced by the loss of elasticity.

Meanwhile, in most people a greater or lesser degree of degeneration appears in the weight-bearing joints of the body. If this degeneration is severe, the process is called osteoarthritis. Concurrent stiffening of the ligaments and atrophy of the muscles may lead to reduced physical activity. This in turn provokes further wasting of

muscles and other degenerative changes, so that a vicious circle may well be established.

At the same time, degeneration of the arteries may eventually lead, among other things, to impairment of the blood supply to the brain. Little can be done about this, though there is some evidence that cutting down on animal fats (such as butter) and on sugar much earlier in life may help prevent such arterial disease and so possibly help to prolong life.

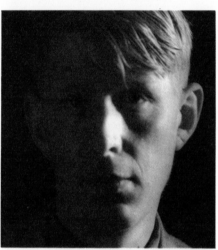

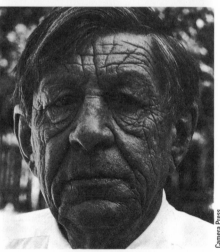

Camera Press

One of the most noticeable of the changes in ageing — wrinkling of the skin. The poet W. H. Auden at the age of 22, and some 40 years later. The elasticity of skin slowly diminishes.

OPHTHALMOSCOPE is the instrument which doctors use to examine the interior of the eye (and, in particular, the retina, or screen at the back of the eyeball). Basically, it consists of a device to produce a beam of light (which is projected through the aperture of the pupil), combined with a system of lenses, and a pinhole which enables the doctor to look along the beam at the contents of the eye.

The ophthalmoscope is, of course, of great value to eye specialists. It is, however, also an invaluable tool in the hands of the general physician, because it enables him to see in the retina not only the branches of an artery and vein (the only place in the whole body where this is so), but also the end of the optic nerve. This nerve connects the eye to the brain, and direct observation of the nerve ending gives the doctor valuable information, not only about the nerve, but sometimes about the condition of the brain itself.

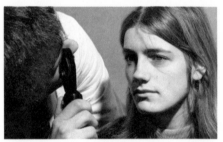

Using an ophthalmoscope, a doctor is able to look right inside the eye, and detect disorders.

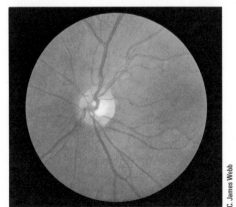

The appearance of the normal retina, as seen through the ophthalmoscope. Note the vessels.

OPISTHOTONOS is the term given to a position in which the body is so far arched backwards that only the heels and the head rest upon the bed. It is characteristic of tetanus (see **tetanus**); a similar posture is seen also at times in meningitis (see **meningitis**) and in epileptic seizures.

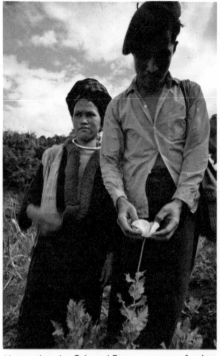

Daily Telegraph

Harvesting the Oriental Poppy, source of opium and many valuable drugs, including morphine.

OPIUM is an extract of the juice expressed from the seeds of the white Indian poppy. This plant is grown very widely in the East, from Turkey to China; in fact, very much more is grown than is needed to supply the medicinal needs of the entire world. This is because of the unfortunate fact that some governments still connive at the illegal growing of these poppies, and at the export of opium extracted from them to the criminal drug markets of Europe and America.

Apart from this, however, opium is still quite often used in some parts of the world as a medicine in its own right. In most countries, however, its employment as a potent reliever of pain has been largely

273

supplanted by the use of its derivative, morphine.

ORGANO-PHOSPHOROUS IN-SECTICIDES are a group of chemicals which are now very widely used in agriculture. They include such compounds as malathion and parathion. They are extremely effective in destroying insects, and have very largely replaced such chemicals as DDT in recent years.

However, they have been responsible for numerous cases of fatal poisoning in human beings. They are readily absorbed into the bloodstream as a result of being swallowed or inhaled in the breath. Worse still, they can penetrate intact skin; it is very common for people working in agriculture, or simply doing gardening, to spill these insecticides on themselves.

If this happens, it is absolutely essential that the area of skin is thoroughly washed with running water. Contaminated clothing must be removed *at once*, and preferably destroyed if possible. If any quantity of an organo-phosphorous insecticide has been allowed to remain on the skin for more than a second or two, a doctor should be called. This is also the case if there is a suspicion that any has been inhaled. If some of the insecticide is swallowed (as is sometimes the case if such compounds are not locked away from children), make the patient vomit immediately, and rush him to hospital.

There he will be treated with atropine injections. Large doses of this drug may be needed to block the effect of these compounds, and artificial respiration may also be necessary if the patient develops paralysis of the breathing muscles.

Other features of this type of poisoning are blurring of the vision, sweating, nausea, vomiting, increased production of saliva and nasal secretions, breathlessness, cramps in the chest and stomach, and diarrhoea.

ORTHOPAEDICS is derived from two Greek words meaning very roughly 'teaching to grow straight'. Originally, therefore, orthopaedics was a science concerned principally with the correction of deformities of children.

Nowadays, however, orthopaedics is the branch of surgery which deals with all kinds of deformities and injuries in every age group, but more particularly those which affect the limbs and backbone rather than the trunk or the head.

OSMOSIS is a process whereby when two solutions of different strengths are on opposite sides of a membrane, water is attracted through the membrane in the direction of the stronger solution. This process is of the greatest importance to all cells and many of the complex physiological mechanisms of the human body depend on it.

OSTEOARTHRITIS is a degenerative disease of the body's joints. In fact, in the United States and many other countries, it is commonly referred to as DJD, or degenerative joint disease.

Osteoarthritis is a disorder of middle and old age, and it affects a high percentage of the population. In some people, it may be a relatively minor affliction, giving only a moderate amount of pain and stiffness in one or two joints, while in other persons it can be much more severe. In certain cases, it is possible to relate the onset of osteoarthritis to some definite cause such as joint strains earlier in life, but often this is impossible.

Most of the body's joints can be affected by the disorder, but those which tend to be particularly painful are the ones which bear weight – i.e. the hips, knees, ankles, and the joints of the backbone. In addition to pain, there is usually limitation of movement, creaking of the affected joints, and often swelling as well. As a result of enforced inactivity, there is often muscle wasting, and this may throw the joint out of balance and make matters worse.

The treatment of osteoarthritis involves the use of pain-killing drugs, physiotherapy and the application of local warmth to affected joints. In overweight patients, drastic slimming is of very great importance, to reduce the load on the damaged weight-bearing joints. In some severely-affected patients (particularly those with osteoarthritis of the hip), surgery may be necessary.

OSTEOMALACIA is a condition in which the bones become abnormally soft. Though it occurs in adults, it is in many ways very similar to childhood rickets. The softening of bone, which is due to calcium and phosphorus deficiency, may be accompanied by general poor health, and the patient usually feels weak and ill.

At first, the affected person notices only a loss of appetite and some loss of weight. Soon, however, his muscles become rather weak, he develops pains in the bones, and ultimately he notices the onset of deformities of the legs, as the soft bones bend under the weight of his body.

The lack of calcium and phosphorus in osteomalacia is usually due to one or more of a number of factors. The patient may simply not get enough dietary calcium and vitamin D (a vitamin intimately concerned with the metabolism of calcium and phosphorus). In the case of women, there may have been excessive loss of calcium due to repeated pregnancies — this is because not only does an expectant mother have to contribute a good deal of calcium to her unborn baby, but she also passes on large quantities of the same mineral to him in the breast milk.

Lack of calcium and phosphorus can also be due to disorder of the small intestine, with consequent failure to absorb essential nutriments. In these cases, the patient may have recurrent diarrhoea. Similarly, excessive loss of these essential minerals in the urine, due to kidney disease, can also cause osteomalacia.

Untreated, the disorder leads to gross bone deformities, fractures and even death. However, once the diagnosis is made, the disease process can usually be reversed by dietary supplementation of calcium intake, often with the addition of large doses of vitamin D.

OSTEOMYELITIS literally means inflammation of the marrow, or central core, of a bone. In fact, the inflammation, which is caused by infection with a germ, normally involves other parts of the bone as well.

This disease is far more common in children than in adults, and boys are affected twice as often as girls. Any bone may be affected, but most commonly osteomyelitis arises near the end of a shaft of a long bone — common sites include the upper end of the shin bone and the lower end of the thigh bone.

Sometimes an attack of osteomyelitis is preceded by a blow on the bone. Occasionally, the patient has had an infected scratch or cut from which germs may enter the body. The attack begins with severe pain and swelling over the infected bone; if the pain and swelling are close to a joint, as is often the case, they may be mistaken for manifestations of arthritis or rheumatic fever. The child usually feels ill, and has a raised temperature. He may have shivering attacks (rigors).

Nowadays, as soon as the diagnosis is made, the child is treated with antibiotics, and these almost invariably clear the condition up fairly rapidly. In the past, however, the infective process frequently extended along the shaft of the bone, cutting off its blood supply and thus killing large areas of bony tissue. In those pre-antibiotic days, the disease was frequently crippling or even fatal; there is, however, little need to fear it nowadays.

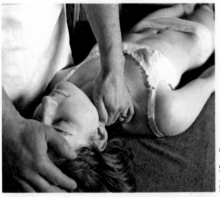

An osteopath manipulating the bones of the neck. This is dangerous without medical training and a thorough knowledge of anatomy.

OSTEOPATHS are people who practise osteopathy, a system of treating disease by musculo-skeletal manipulation. It is based on the assumption that abnormalities of the bones, muscles, ligaments or other tissues cause disease by

275

disturbing the function of adjacent nerves and blood vessels, which in turn affect other parts of the body. Osteopathy is more widely recognized as a method of healing in the U.S. than in Britain.

OSTEOPOROSIS is a condition in which the bones become gradually less dense because of loss of basic materials. It is very common in elderly people, particularly those who have been confined to bed for long periods.

Osteoporosis affects mainly the bones of the spine (the vertebrae). The symptoms occur principally in the lower back, or lumbar region, where there is quite severe aching, and sometimes incapacitating

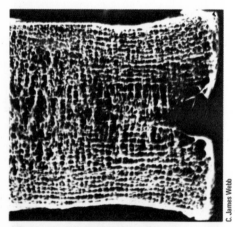

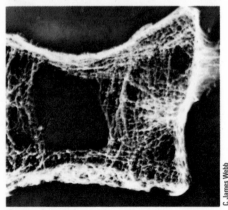

Contrast the appearance of bone from a normal vertebra, above, with that of bone from a patient suffering from osteoporosis, below. The loss of bone substance causes thinning.

276

pain, particularly after exercise. If the vertebrae become much softened, they may collapse altogether, with resultant compression of the nerves which join the spinal cord; such compression may produce pain radiating down the legs.

At the same time, deformities of the spine may develop, owing to the softness of the bones.

Mild osteoporosis sometimes occurs in rather younger people (for instance, the 40–60 age group) after long confinement in bed, but it is unlikely to produce symptoms of any seriousness in these circumstances, and will usually remit soon after the patient is up and about again. An almost identical thinning of bone is caused by the inactivity of space flights, but this too is reversed as soon as an astronaut returns to earth. It remains to be seen whether longer space flights will produce actual symptoms of osteoporosis, though this is unlikely now that the danger has been realized; spacemen now have a programme of exercises to combat the inactivity of prolonged existence in a weightless environment.

The treatment of osteoporosis consists in trying to recalcify the bones, and calcium and vitamin D are often given, and with these may be combined hormones, such as the anabolic steroids – the same agents which have gained publicity recently because of their illegal use by athletes to put on bulk. The most important part of treatment, however, is the avoidance of immobility.

Treatment by surgical operation is not usually of value in osteoporosis. If collapse of a vertebra occurs, however, the patient may be referred to an orthopaedic surgeon, who may well fit him with a plaster-of-Paris jacket or plastic support. The other common reason why a patient may need the help of a surgeon is if he fractures his 'hip', i.e. the upper end of his femur, or thigh bone. This is perhaps the most dangerous complication of osteoporosis; it is therefore essential that, while the osteoporotic patient should remain active, he should try to take no risks which might involve falling heavily and incurring this type of fracture. The healing process is considerably delayed in osteoporosis.

OTITIS MEDIA is an extremely common childhood condition. It is an infection of the cavity of the middle ear by germs; its principal symptom is earache.

In children who are old enough to speak, the diagnosis is rarely difficult to make, since they will invariably complain of severe pain in the ear. In an infant, however, all that the mother may notice is that the child is miserable and off-colour, and has a moderately raised temperature. Too often, in such circumstances, the child's illness is ascribed to 'teething', and he is left to get better on his own. If, however, the parents take the child to the doctor, he will be able to insert his auriscope (the funnel-shaped instrument used to inspect the ear-drum) into the child's ear. If the drum is inflamed, he will know that the cause of the child's illness is otitis media.

Another valuable pointer to the diagnosis of this disorder is that the child has often had an upper respiratory tract infection (e.g. a cold in the head) a few days previously; he may also hold his ear as if in pain, and sometimes there may be a little discharge from the ear. In addition, there may be slight tenderness over the mastoid bone (the hard prominence immediately behind the ear). This indicates some spread of inflammation to the mastoid air cavities: when this symptom occurs, it is important that the doctor should be consulted, and treatment started, reasonably swiftly – i.e. within a few hours.

This is because infection of the mastoid bone, or mastoiditis (which is dealt with under the heading mastoid), can be serious. Up till about 20 years ago, many children bore the ugly scars of the operation which was often necessary in order to remove the infected portion of the bone. Since the widespread advent of prompt antibiotic therapy, the complication of mastoiditis has fortunately become rare.

The standard treatment of otitis media therefore involves the use of antibiotics, such as penicillin, as early as possible. It is sometimes necessary to administer the early doses by injection, but some doctors prefer to give the child the treatment in the form of tablets or medicine. (It is not possible to treat this disorder with ear-drops, as people often imagine.) Very occasionally, so much pus may collect in the middle-ear cavity that the eardrum starts to bulge outwards under the pressure. It may then be necessary to perform a minor surgical operation (called 'myringotomy'), which involves making an incision in the ear-drum and letting the pus out. (See also **ear disorders**.)

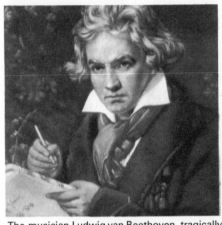

The musician Ludwig van Beethoven, tragically a victim of the disease otosclerosis.

OTOSCLEROSIS is a common form of deafness (see also **deafness**). In the past, its effects could be quite tragic, particularly as it attacks younger people very frequently. It is very probable that Beethoven suffered from this form of deafness: his hearing was already impaired when he was in his thirties, and by the time he died at the age of 50 he was unable to hear a single note.

In general, otosclerosis is seen in women more often than in men. There is often a hereditary element in the disease.

It is caused by a curious hardening process which affects the three tiny bones that transmit sound waves across the cavity of the middle ear (see **ear**). These bones (the malleus, incus and stapes) are closely linked so that they form a chain between the ear-drum (which vibrates in response to sound like the diaphragm of a telephone mouthpiece) and the hearing apparatus of the inner ear.

The hardening process reduces the mobility of the three bones, and, in par-

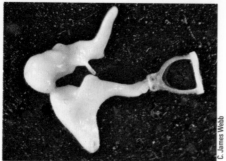

The small bones of the middle ear; from left to right, the malleus, incus and stapes.

ticular, it tends to 'fix' the base of the stapes (or stirrup-bone) at the point where it should be freely mobile to transmit vibrations into the inner ear, so that they can be heard as sound.

Nothing could be done about this condition until the 1950s, when surgeons first began to operate on these tiny bones; in the 1960s, these operations were further refined and perfected. It is now an everyday thing for an ear, nose and throat (E.N.T.) surgeon, working with the aid of a microscope, to remove the tiny stirrup-bone, and perhaps polish it to remove all the material deposited by the disease process. The surgeon may also put in a plastic bone replacement, and very often will make a new aperture through which the bones can transmit their vibrations to the inner ear. New variations of these operations are constantly being developed, and it is fair to say that the entire outlook for people with this kind of deafness has been revolutionized. In the vast majority of cases, their hearing is very greatly improved after operation.

OVARIES are the female sex glands. In the unborn child, they originate from the same tissue as do the male sex glands or testes.

Every woman has two ovaries, situated very close to the womb, one on the right side and one on the left. From each runs one of the two short tubes (called the Fallopian tubes) which carry ova (or eggs) down to the womb.

Each ovary is just over an inch long and about half an inch wide. The surface of

278

each is usually wrinkled and of a pinkish-grey colour. Each contains many thousands of eggs, only a very small proportion of which will ever be released during the woman's lifetime. One egg ripens and reaches the surface of the ovary during each menstrual cycle. From the surface, it bursts free, and finds its way to the mouth of the Fallopian tube. From there it passes down into the cavity of the womb.

The ovary is a most important source of hormones, including the group which are called oestrogens (see **oestrogens**). These are not only largely responsible for the development of such female characteristics as the breasts, but also are the main influence on the preparation of the lining of the womb during the first half of the menstrual cycle. Progesterone (see **progesterone**), another hormone produced by the ovaries, plays the most important part in the second half of the cycle. The ovary is stimulated to produce both types of hormone by the activity of the pituitary gland at the base of the brain.

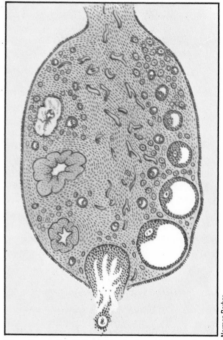

The stages (anticlockwise) of ovulation, showing how the follicles grow in size within the ovary, release ova, and turn into corpora lutea.

OVUM is the Latin word for egg. In medical use, the word means the tiny egg released during each menstrual cycle by the ovary (see **ovaries**).

All mammals produce ova (ova being the plural of ovum) which are very similar to those of a human being. Other mammals do not have a menstrual cycle in the same way as humans do, however. In many animals, the female has an episode of œstrus (or 'heat') once or twice a year, and at this time eggs are released from the ovaries. Simultaneously, there are changes in the female genital passages which allow intercourse (usually impossible at any other time) to take place; the female is also much more attractive than usual to the male during such episodes of œstrus. This system occurs in dogs, for example, but in many other mammals (for instance, in rabbits) ova are released only as a result of the stimulus of intercourse. This means that pregnancy is likely to follow a single act of mating.

Obviously, such an arrangement would be highly unsuitable for the human race. What happens in women is that each 'month' (or, to be more accurate, each 26 days, on average), the ovaries release a single ovum. This process of ovulation, as it is called, takes place, as a rule, just before the half-way point between the start of one period and the start of the next. For instance, in a woman with a 26-day cycle, the ovum is likely to be released about 12 days after the start of one period, and about 14 days before the onset of the next. The release of the ovum may be marked by very slight backache, and the precise day of ovulation can often be determined by taking temperature readings every morning; in most women, the thermometer shows a slight rise on the day the ovum is released. Calculation of this day is the basis of the 'rhythm' method of birth control, in which the object is to refrain from intercourse from about five days before ovulation until five days afterwards. Unfortunately, this method very frequently breaks down in practice.

Why is the ovum released at all? It seems that the phenomenon occurs as a result of the activity of the pituitary gland, at the base of the brain, which controls

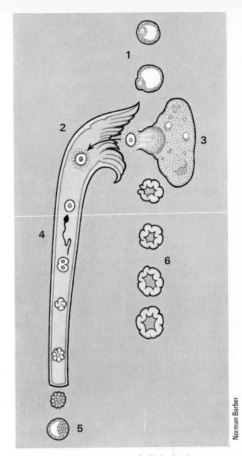

Norman Barber

Diagram to show how the follicle 1 releases an ovum 2 into the fallopian tube from the ovary, 3. While the ovum travels down the tube to be fertilized, 4, and start the new embryo, 5, the follicle turns into the corpus luteum, 6.

so much of the workings of the other endocrine glands. Under the influence of a pituitary hormone called FSH (or follicular stimulating hormone), one particular tiny egg-bearing region of the ovary, called a 'follicle' begins to ripen, and to rise toward the ovary's surface.

When it reaches the outermost layer of the ovary, it bursts and releases the ovum. From then on, the follicle is known as the corpus luteum (or 'yellow body'). Under the influence of another pituitary secretion, the luteinizing hormone (LH), the corpus luteum secretes progesterone (see **progesterone**), a hormone which is

279

of paramount importance in the second half of the menstrual cycle in maintaining the womb's lining in a state to nourish the ovum.

If the ovum has *not* been fertilized, then it will be lost in the next menstrual flow. If, however, a sperm reaches it (a meeting which is believed to occur in the Fallopian tube), then the fertilized ovum will burrow its way into the lining of the womb, and there develop in the succeeding weeks into an embryonic human being.

OXYGEN is the gas on which almost all living things depend for their very existence. With the exception of certain types of bacteria, every living form on earth lives by 'burning' fuel in its tissues in the presence of oxygen.

Various living things have different systems for bringing the oxygen into contact with the tissues. In the case of human beings, it is breathed in from the air, which contains a little over 20 per cent of oxygen (the rest being almost entirely made up by nitrogen). In the lungs, the oxygen diffuses through a thin membrane into the bloodstream, where it enters the red blood cells. Within them, it forms a compound called oxyhaemoglobin with the red cells' natural pigment (haemoglobin). Oxyhaemoglobin has a much redder colour than haemoglobin, which is why the oxygenated blood pumped round our arteries is bright red in comparison with the darker (deoxygenated) blood returning from the tissues in the veins.

Therapy with oxygen, administered from a cylinder and mask, is of use in some, but by no means all, cardiac and respiratory disorders. There are circumstances in which oxygen therapy can be very hazardous, and although it is possible to buy oxygen cylinders for self-treatment, they should not be used except under the direction of a doctor.

Hyperbaric oxygen therapy is a method of increasing the oxygen supply to the tissues by putting the patient in an environment (such as a pressure chamber) where the pressure can be increased to several times normal. Under these circumstances, large quantities of the gas will dissolve, not in the red cells (which are probably

fully saturated with oxygen in any case), but in the actual fluid component of the blood. This may be of value in certain types of infection and poisoning, and also where there is breathing difficulty in babies.

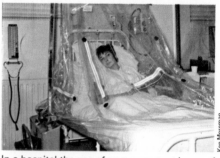

In a hospital the use of an oxygen tent is one of the most common treatments for heart disorder.

OXYURIS is the medical name for the threadworm (see **threadworms**). It is also known as *Enterobius*. Infestation with threadworms is called oxyuriasis.

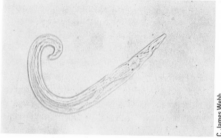

The appearance of the threadworm, Oxyuris, responsible for irritating intestinal infestation.

OZONE is a gas which is composed of atoms of oxygen arranged in an unusual fashion. It is sometimes produced by lightning passing through the air, when it may be detected by the odd tang it gives to the atmosphere. There is a slightly increased ozone content in the air at some holiday resorts, but there is no evidence whatever that this has any effect on the health, beneficial or otherwise. Even when there is sufficient ozone present in the atmosphere for its smell to be detectable (which is unusual), the actual proportion of ozone to oxygen is so minute that it cannot possibly exercise any influence on the workings of the human body.

PAS – see para-aminosalicylic acid.

PACEMAKERS are parts of the heart which control the rate and rhythm of the heartbeat by electrical impulses.

In many cardiac conditions, the heart starts to beat with an unusual rhythm, either regular or irregular. Some of these abnormal rhythms are not of great importance, but others may be life-threatening. Under certain circumstances, it is essential to use an *artificial* pacemaking device to restore normal rate and rhythm.

All these devices are designed with the object of providing a regular pulse of electricity in the region of the right atrium, at the top of the heart. If such a pulse surges through this part of the cardiac tissue 72 times per minute, then the heart responds by contracting ('beating') at this rate. The problem, of course, is how to deliver the current to this particular region of the heart.

In emergency, it is possible to simply place two large electrodes on the chest and pass a current between them. However, for short-term control of these disturbances of rhythm, an electrode on the end of a wire is usually passed through an incision in the skin of the neck, down the large vein called the jugular, and into the heart itself. Once the electrode is in the right position, it is connected to a small 'external pacemaker', which delivers a shock of about 2 volts at the appropriate rate. The pacemaker is driven by a battery, as connecting it to the mains is normally considered too dangerous.

This method is not as a rule suitable for long-term treatment, however, partly because of the risk and discomfort of having the external pacemaker under the clothing, and partly because of the danger of infection entering the bloodstream at the point where the wire pierces the skin and goes into the vein.

For long-term pacing, therefore, it is more usual for the patient to have an 'internal pacemaker'. This is a tiny device, often no larger than a latch-key, which is implanted somewhere under the skin of the body – usually in the chest wall, the abdominal wall or the arm-pit. From it, a short wire (usually insulated by a rubber

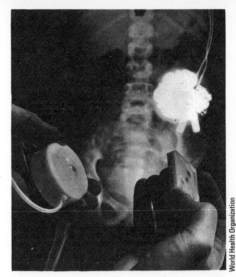

Above Two pacemakers, the one on the right the size of a book of matches; on the left a larger one, also seen in the X-ray when implanted.
Below Another view of a pacemaker's circuitry.

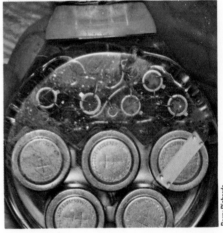

World Health Organization

Barry Richards

or plastic sheath) runs to the cathode electrode, which is attached to the heart in one of a number of ways. The pacemaker often contains its own batteries (which have to be renewed every two years or so by means of a minor operation). Some types of internal pacemaker, however, contain a receiving coil, which picks up a signal from a small external power unit, often worn on a belt round the waist; this power unit is quite bulky, and its batteries

281

have to be replaced every few weeks. It can, however, be adjusted and serviced more readily than is the case with an internal power unit.

Although artificial pacemakers are still far from trouble-free, there can be no doubt that they have saved the lives of many patients with cardiac disorders.

PAEDIATRICS is that branch of medicine which deals exclusively with the disorders of childhood. A specialist in these disorders is called a paediatrician.

PAGET'S DISEASE is a term which, owing to an unfortunate confusion, is used to describe three completely unrelated disorders, all of which were first described by Sir James Paget (1814–1899), who was a surgeon at St Bartholomew's Hospital, London. It should be stressed that none of these diseases has anything to do with the others, and the only thing they have in common is their name.

By far the rarest is Paget's disease of the penis: in this condition (which is often related to poor hygiene, or in plain words, lack of soap and water), a raw area develops into an ulcer, and eventually into a cancerous growth.

More common is Paget's disease of the breast. This condition usually occurs in women over fifty. It looks like a persistent patch of eczema over the nipple area, but it eventually develops into cancer.

Far more frequently encountered is Paget's disease of bone (osteitis deformans), which is said to affect three per cent of all people over the age of 40. In this disorder, there is thickening and deformity of one or many bones of the body. The reason why this happens is quite unknown at the moment.

The most commonly affected bones are those of the skull and pelvis, and also the shin and spine. The enlargement of the skull produces a very characteristic facial appearance, and one of the first symptoms is often that the patient finds he needs a larger size in hats. He may also notice pain and deformity, mainly of the bones of the legs and pelvis, since it is these that bear the weight of the body. Spontaneous fractures of bone sometimes occur.

At the present time, treatment consists only of measures to relieve the pain, though sometimes surgical operations are useful in cases of severe deformity. There is no known method of arresting the disease process, but very often it ceases by itself, having affected only a few bones of the body to varying degrees.

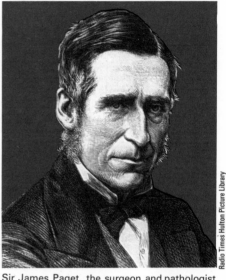

Radio Times Hulton Picture Library

Sir James Paget, the surgeon and pathologist who described three distinct new diseases.

PAIN is one of the commonest of all symptoms, and (unpleasant though it may be) it is often an essential danger-signal that warns us of trouble within the body.

Pain may be simply classified as either 'superficial' or 'deep'. Superficial pain is caused by injury to the skin or the structures immediately underlying it: it is easy for the patient to 'localize' the source of it.

In contrast, 'deep' pain, originating in the internal structures of the body, is often hard for the patient to localize accurately. This is partly because it is 'detected' by a rather different part of the nervous system. In addition, deep pain may have many characteristics – it may be 'aching', 'crushing', 'burning', 'colicky', 'knife-like', 'gnawing', and so on. Descriptions of these characteristics by the patient may be of considerable help to the doctor in making a diagnosis and deciding on the most appropriate treatment.

PAINTER'S COLIC is the name applied to an abdominal pain characteristic of lead poisoning (see **lead**). In the days when lead paints were still very widely used, poisoning was common among painters.

PALATE is the roof of the mouth. It forms a partition between the mouth and the cavity of the nose. The front part of this structure is called the hard palate: this area is hard because here the mucous membrane of the mouth overlies bone.

Further back, however, the soft palate consists only of mucous membrane overlying muscular tissue. The soft palate can move up and down, forming as it does a sort of flap which can readily close off the nose from the cavity of the throat. This movement is easy to demonstrate: if one looks into a mirror and says 'ah', the soft palate is seen to rise upwards. Doctors often ask patients to do this while examining them. The purpose of this request is twofold: the movement of the soft palate gives the doctor a better view of the back of the throat, and, in addition, it tells him whether the nerves supplying the palate are working properly.

At the middle of the back edge of the palate is the uvula, a small globular mass of tissue which seems to have no particular function. It is occasionally bifid, or 'cleft'. This in itself is of no significance, but it indicates the fact that the whole of the soft palate is formed in the unborn child from two processes of tissue, one on either side, which fuse in the mid-line. If they fail to fuse, then the result is the condition known as cleft palate. The hard palate (like the upper jaw and lip) is formed by the fusion of the same two processes and a third central one. The condition of cleft palate is dealt with under the heading **hare-lip**, since the two conditions have much the same origin, and are so commonly associated.

Contrary to popular belief, the palate has little to do with taste. This sensation is relayed through the action of special receptors on the tongue and *not* on the palate. However, quite an appreciable part of what most of us call 'taste' is, in fact, *smell*, since the aroma of food we eat can readily pass up to the smell receptors in

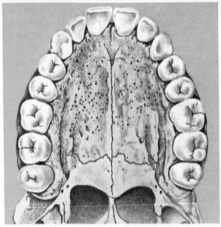

The appearance of the bony palate, seen from below. The central line of fusion shows clearly.

Norman Barber

the areas located higher, in the roof of the nose. This is why, when we have a cold, the blockage of the nasal cavity appears to diminish the sense of taste. At such times, the soft palate is usually sore and inflamed, and people tend to think that this is the reason why food is not so tasty.

PALPITATIONS are heartbeats which can be felt. Most of us experience such palpitations at one time or another (e.g. after violent physical activity, or as a consequence of excitement), and, in the great majority of instances, the symptom is of no significance whatever although causing many people unnecessary concern.

Persistent palpitations, occurring for no apparent reason, do however indicate

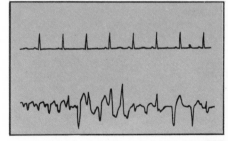

Certain forms of palpitation show up on ECG tracings as irregularities of rhythm. Contrast the normal ECG pattern, *above*, with that found in one variety of rhythm abnormality, *below*.

283

the need for a check-up by a doctor. Again, in the majority of cases, it will be found that the patient has nothing at all wrong with his or her heart. In many young men and women, the symptom is merely an indication of some mild emotional upset, very similar in nature to the condition called da Costa's syndrome (see **da Costa's syndrome**).

In a small proportion of patients, however, palpitations can be an indication of an abnormal heart rhythm, whose nature it may be possible to determine if an electrocardiogram (ECG) is taken during an attack.

PANCREAS is a gland situated in the abdomen, just below the stomach and within the loop of the duodenum. It is one of the most important glands in the human body.

The pancreas has two sorts of function — described as exocrine and endocrine.

The word 'exocrine' is used to describe glands which pour their secretions into a duct or tube, instead of into the bloodstream. The exocrine secretions of the pancreas flow down the pancreatic duct and into the duodenum (the uppermost part of the small intestine) where they mix with the food which has just been passed on from the stomach. These secretions play a most important role in the digestive process. Pancreatic juice contains three enzymes called lipase, amylase and trypsin, and these have the effect of breaking down fat, carbohydrate and protein respectively, and making them suitable for absorption into the body.

The pancreas is also an endocrine gland (see **endocrine glands**). There are probably a number of hormones which it releases into the bloodstream, but much the best-known is insulin (see **insulin**).

This chemical is absolutely essential to life, because it regulates the way in which glucose, the body's basic fuel, is 'burnt'. So important is this function that, if an animal's pancreas is removed, it dies very shortly afterwards. There is only one measure that will keep it alive, and that is the administration of insulin by injection.

Similarly, in the common condition

diabetes mellitus (see **diabetes mellitus**), in which the body's glucose metabolism gets out of control, insulin injections are often required: in a proportion of diabetics, insulin is life-saving.

When insulin was first extracted from the pancreas, in 1921, by Drs Banting and Best, the underlying cause of diabetes mellitus seemed clear - lack of the hormone, due to some defect of the islet cells, reduced the ability of the body's tissues to utilize glucose, which therefore appeared in the patient's urine. The hold-up in glucose metabolism was followed by disturbance in fat metabolism, so that substances not normally found in the bloodstream tended to accumulate, and could even be smelt on the breath. We now know that diabetes is a very much more complicated business than that. Microscope studies of the pancreas in patients with diabetes show that in at least a quarter of cases there is no readily observable change in the islet cells, although in other cases changes may be detected. Furthermore, some patients have now survived total removal of the pancreas when given only 40 Units of insulin daily — whereas many patients with diabetes from an unknown cause require well over 100 Units daily. It is clear that in the latter cases the disease cannot be due to a simple lack of the hormone circulating in the bloodstream. In early diabetes, some patients actually produce *excess* insulin.

Disorders of the pancreas. The pancreas is sometimes subject to inflammation (pancreatitis). Acute pancreatitis produces severe pain in the upper part of the abdomen, often radiating to the back. It is difficult to distinguish from the pain of a perforated ulcer, but a rapid laboratory test of the amount of amylase (one of the previously mentioned pancreatic enzymes) present in the blood may aid the diagnosis.

Cancer of the pancreas often causes severe weight-loss. There may be a boring pain in the back, and if the growth is in the region of the head of the pancreas (where it can block the common bile duct) there will be obstructive jaundice (see **jaundice**). The treatment is surgical, but it is usually only successful in cases where the growth is caught early.

PAPILLOMA is the general name for a benign stalk-like growth, most commonly occurring on the skin. These tumours are invariably quite harmless and can be readily removed from the skin by a very minor operation under local anaesthetic; sometimes, in fact, the stalk of the tumour becomes so long that it outgrows its own blood supply, and the papilloma falls off of its own accord. Very occasionally, a papilloma (like any other lump on the skin), may change its nature and become malignant; the symptoms of such an occurrence are bleeding and extension of the growth *sideways*, i.e. across the skin.

Papillomas can also occur in other sites, notably in the cervix (neck of the womb) or in the body of the womb itself. Multiple papillomata of a rather different nature occur inside the wall of the bladder, where they give rise to bleeding into the urine. This type of bladder papilloma must be kept under careful observation by the urological surgeon (urologist), since they can very readily invade and destroy the bladder wall. The surgeon usually burns away as many as he can with a special instrument which is passed up into the bladder; subsequently, he checks the condition of the bladder wall at frequent intervals with the aid of a telescope-like device called a cystoscope.

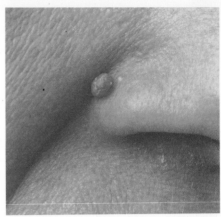

A papilloma at the angle of the nose. Sometimes unsightly, they are rarely dangerous.

PARA-AMINOSALICYLIC ACID, or PAS, is a most valuable anti-tuberculous drug. Together with two other drugs, streptomycin and INAH (isoniazid), PAS has completely changed the outlook in tuberculosis, and what was once a killer disease is now a relatively rare cause of death in most western countries.

PAS is normally taken by mouth. It has a rather unpleasant taste, and is therefore supplied in a wide variety of forms such as in cachets and granules. It is usually not difficult to find one of these preparations which is palatable to the patient.

PAS tends to cause such gastro-intestinal upsets as nausea, vomiting, diarrhoea and sometimes abdominal pain, but its value is so great that anyone taking it should make every effort not to discontinue it if possible. Unfortunately, if all three of the common anti-tuberculous drugs (PAS, streptomycin and INAH) are not taken together, the germ which causes tuberculosis may develop resistance (see also **isoniazid**, and **streptomycin**).

PARACETAMOL is one of the most commonly used of all pain-killing drugs, mainly because it is available to the public without prescription. Its effect in relieving pain is roughly equivalent to that of aspirin, and, like aspirin, it also has the effect of lowering the temperature in feverish patients. The drug's principal

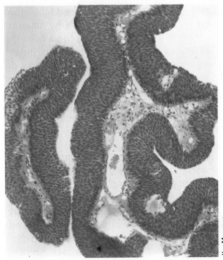

Ken Moreman

Magnified view of a papilloma removed from the bladder. Many take bizarre shapes.

285

advantage is that, unlike aspirin, it does not seem to cause irritation of the stomach, and hence it can be safely used in patients with ulcers. (Aspirin is so irritant that it can readily provoke stomach bleeding even in those who do not have ulcers).

Paracetamol seems to be a relatively safe drug, but, on the basis of past experience, most doctors feel that no pain-killing drug should be used repeatedly or in large quantities without advice from a medical practitioner.

PARAFFIN is the general name for a large group of chemicals. The type of paraffin used as fuel is extremely dangerous and a number of deaths occur each year among children who swallow it.

The medicinal form of paraffin, often referred to as 'Liquid paraffin' is a laxative. It exerts its action by lubricating the inside of the bowel.

PARANOIA is a type of mental disorder. The condition is very closely related to paraphrenia and paranoid schizophrenia (see **schizophrenia**) and some psychiatrists regard all three disorders as being basically the same condition.

Paranoia is characterized by delusions of persecution. These often start from some very minor wrong (or imagined wrong) which the patient has suffered. Before long, however, he elaborates these ideas so greatly that he starts to believe that he is the victim of a world-wide conspiracy, or that the government and all its forces are working to suppress him. All attempts to convince him that he is wrong are futile : he will merely conclude that whoever tries to reason with him is part of the conspiracy. Sometimes, his anger and suspicion are directed against a readily-identifiable ethnic group — for instance, Jews or Negroes. People with paranoid tendencies have played no small part in arousing racial or religious hatred in the past.

The paranoiac patient may be able to conceal his illness from the world for some considerable time, but eventually his delusions are so gross that his illness becomes apparent to other people. Fortunately, it is only rarely that he reveals himself by violent action, such as an assassination attempt.

The outlook in many patients with paranoia is poor, but there are so many varieties of this group of disorders that it is difficult to generalize about the likely outcome. The best chance a patient has of improvement in his symptoms lies in early psychiatric treatment. Therefore, anyone who finds that a relative is beginning to exhibit the type of systematized delusions characteristic of paranoid behaviour should not hesitate to call in medical aid.

PARAPLEGIA is paralysis of the lower part of the body. Paraplegic patients cannot move their legs, and frequently have no conscious control of the bladder and rectum. In men, sexual function is likely to be interfered with.

This tragic condition is common in young people nowadays, the majority of cases being the result of spinal cord injuries sustained in motor car accidents. Many diseases of the nervous system can, however, cause paraplegia.

What is so surprising (but also so encouraging) is that very many paraplegics learn to cope with their illness with the utmost bravery, and go on to lead rich and full lives despite this disability.

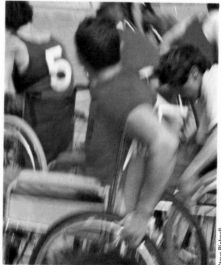

Steve Bicknell

Despite their disabilities, paraplegic patients are still able to enjoy some sporting activities.

PARASITES are organisms which live off other forms of life. These organisms may be either plants or animals. Although Man is subject to parasitic infestation by primitive organisms, such as fungi and germs, it is usual in medical practice to confine the use of the word 'parasite' to fairly complex members of the animal kingdom, such as worms, insects and arachnids (a class of creatures closely related to the insects).

The parasitic worms which infest Man are divided into two classes, the flatworms and the roundworms.

The flatworms fall into two different groups or 'orders'. The first of these (the trematodes) includes liver-flukes, lung-flukes and the schistosomes, the parasites which cause the extremely widespread tropical disease bilharzia (see **bilharzia**). The other 'order' of the flatworms is the cestodes, which include the common tape-worms (see **tape-worms**) and also the Echinococcus (see **Echinococcus**), the parasite which affects men who work with sheep and sheep-dogs.

The class of roundworms (see **roundworms**) includes such parasites as the common roundworm (*Ascaris lumbricoides*), the thread-worm, the whipworm and the hook-worm.

Insects which commonly live as parasites on Man include lice (see **lice**), fleas (see **fleas**) and bed bugs (see **bed bugs**).

The parasitic arachnids are mainly mites and chiggers. Perhaps the most frequently encountered is *Sarcoptes scabiei*, which causes 'the itch' or scabies (see **scabies**).

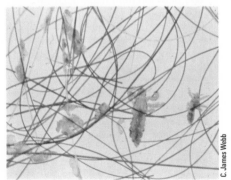

Magnified view of head lice, seen in the hair. Once a common finding in poorer communities.

PARATHION is one of the organo-phosphorus group of insecticides. It is a useful but highly dangerous compound. It must be kept out of reach of children, and should on no account be swallowed or allowed to touch the skin. Treatment of poisoning is discussed under the heading **organo-phosphorus insecticides.**

PARATHYROIDS are small glands lying close to the thyroid gland in the neck (see **thyroid**). They are usually four in number.

The parathyroids are among the most

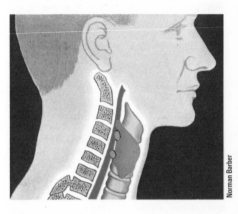

The position of the parathyroid glands (blue), in relation to the thyroid (red) in the neck.

important glands in the body, but because they are so small, very little was known about them for many years. In fact, in the early days of thyroidectomy (surgical removal of the thyroid), the parathyroids were often accidentally removed as well, with disastrous results. Nowadays, however, surgeons are extremely careful to ensure that the parathyroids are not removed when they perform this operation.

The parathyroids are endocrine glands — that is, they release their hormones directly into the bloodstream. We still do not entirely understand the nature and workings of these hormones, but they are intimately concerned with the metabolism of the mineral calcium.

A man weighing eleven stone (roughly 70kg) has about 2lb of calcium in his body. 99 per cent of this is in his skeleton, but the tiny proportion in his blood stream and tissues is essential for the maintenance of life. This is because (a) calcium's presence is necessary for blood clotting to take place, (b) it regulates the way in which nerve impulses pass around the body, and (c) it affects the way muscles contract – in particular, heart muscle.

The best known of the calcium-regulating hormones is parathormone or PTH. If the level of calcium in the blood falls (perhaps because of dietary deficiency or the demands on the mineral caused by breast-feeding a baby), then the parathyroids react by pouring out more PTH. The hormone mobilizes calcium from the bones to keep up the level in the blood. This action, while life-saving, is of course, only a temporary expedient; if fresh sources of calcium are not found eventually, the bones will become thin and soft (see also **osteomalacia**).

PTH also affects the metabolism of the mineral phosphorus, apparently increasing its excretion in the urine; less is known about this hormonal action.

We are now in a position to see what happens when there is under or over-activity of the parathyroids. Under-activity (*hypoparathyroidism*), occurs after accidental surgical removal of one or more glands, or simply as a failure of function of gland tissue. The level of calcium in the blood falls, and the level of phosphorus rises. The patient develops tetany (see **tetany**), a curious muscular spasm; if the calcium deficiency is severe enough, he may go into convulsions and even die. In emergency, the condition is

treated by giving calcium injections. On a longer term basis, the calcium can be given by mouth, and the patient can also be treated with vitamin D (which keeps up the level of the mineral in the body).

Over-activity of the parathyroids (*hyperparathyroidism*) is not uncommon. It is sometimes due to a growth (almost always benign) in one parathyroid gland. As a result of the increased output of PTH, the level of calcium in the blood is too high, while the phosphorus level is low. There are many possible symptoms of this disorder. For instance, the effect of the excess calcium on the nerves and muscles of the body may lead to sluggish motility of the intestines, with constipation, and

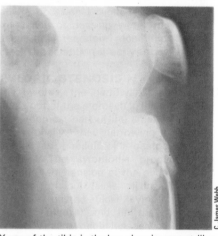

X-ray of the tibia in the leg, showing a cyst-like space due to loss of calcium from the bone.

sometimes vomiting; it may also affect the brain, causing mental disturbances.

The excess calcium may be deposited in the kidneys in the form of stones, and these may give rise to pain or to bleeding into the urine.

The transfer of calcium from bones to the blood and tissues may lead to softening of the skeleton, formation of cysts and fractures of the weakened bone.

Finally, for reasons which are not clear, people with hyperparathyroidism seem liable to develop peptic ulcers. For these reasons, American physicians call it the disease of 'stones, bones and abdominal groans'.

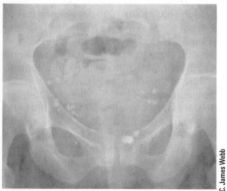

Small white shadows in an abdominal X-ray, due to stones in the urinary tract.

288

PARATYPHOID FEVER is a severe infection of the intestinal tract, caused by a germ known as *Salmonella paratyphi*.

As the name implies, paratyphoid is very similar to typhoid fever (which is caused by a germ called *Salmonella typhi*), and the two conditions are often called 'the enteric fevers' (see **enteric fevers**).

There are three different types of paratyphoid germ, and these are described as A, B, and C. Type A occurs in the far east, type B mainly in sub-tropical countries (e.g. the Mediterranean region) and type C almost exclusively in the region of Guyana in South America. Although there are minor differences between the effects of three types of germ, the symptoms are very much the same. In fact, the clinical picture is not much different from that of typhoid (see **typhoid**), except that in paratyphoid the onset of fever is more rapid, the temperature may rise higher, there is a much greater tendency for the patient to develop a rash, and, most important, the risks of serious complications and death are considerably less. Treatment and prevention of the two disorders are identical.

PAREGORIC is an opium preparation once widely employed as a cough mixture.

PARKINSON'S DISEASE, or Parkinsonism, is a disorder of the central nervous system, once called 'the shaking palsy'. It occurs mainly in elderly people – men more than women. The characteristic features are muscular rigidity and a shaky 'pill-rolling' movement in the hand and arm in particular, together with immobility of the facial muscles. This latter feature gives the patient an impassive, stony-faced look, and people may mistakenly think because of this that sufferers from Parkinsonism feel little emotion or are mentally impaired.

The rigidity and shaking usually affect only one arm at first, but, as the years go by, may spread to the other limbs, so that the severely affected patient has considerable difficulty in walking. He tends to break into a rapid, automatic and almost uncontrollable trot each time he steps forward, and has difficulty in stopping without falling over.

The cause of most cases of Parkinsonism is unknown, but the symptoms are undoubtedly due to damage to a particular internal region of the brain. In a small proportion of patients, this damage seems to have been due to a previous attack of encephalitis (brain inflammation) occuring many years before. Viruses which cause this type of inflammation were responsible for a number of epidemics of encephalitis which swept round the world between 1918 and 1930.

Some other patients develop Parkinson's disease following brain damage due to arterial degeneration, poisoning by household gas and certain metals, head injuries, or tumours. In young patients, an uncommon disorder of copper metabolism called Wilson's disease produces rather similar brain damage and symptoms.

Treatment of Parkinsonism consists in the first place of administration of drugs to control muscle rigidity and tremor. Combined with physiotherapy if necessary, these drugs work reasonably well in some patients.

A great advance in recent years has been the development of surgical techniques in which a probe is passed into the affected area of the brain to destroy certain nerve fibres. In a high percentage of patients there is immediate benefit. The operation is completely painless, and frequently performed with the patient fully conscious.

PAROTID is the name applied to the pair of salivary glands which lie, one on either side of the face, just in front of the ear. The parotid gland pours saliva down a short duct which runs within the substance of the cheek to open into the mouth opposite the molar teeth.

The saliva secreted by the parotid glands, together with that of the other salivary glands, is mixed with the food during the process of mastication, both to moisten it in preparation for swallowing and to initiate the process of digestion. It is tasteless, clear, sticky and slightly alkaline (and is therefore neutralized when it is swallowed and meets the acid contents of the stomach). The digestion of foodstuff starts in the mouth, when the enzyme ptyalin begins to break down chemicals classified as starches — those contained mainly in cereals, bread and potatoes — into simpler chemical substances of the class called sugars. Because of the relatively short time that the enzyme has to work on the starches, very little breakdown can occur before the food is swallowed.

Inflammation of the parotid is called 'parotitis'. The most common form of this inflammation is mumps (see **mumps**) which is caused by certain viruses infecting the gland. Other types of parotitis may, however, be caused by bacterial infection. The gland may also become inflamed and swollen if a stone forms within it, and blocks the flow of saliva down the duct. In all types of parotitis, the swelling at the back of the cheek becomes worse, and there is more pain, when the patient attempts to eat food, because eating stimulates the flow of saliva from the gland.

PASTEURIZATION is a process devised to kill germs in milk. It is so called after Louis Pasteur, the great French investigator who was the founder of the science of bacteriology (see **bacteriology**).

There are various methods of pasteurizing milk but a common one involves heating (to 150° F) for half an hour, and then rapid cooling (to below 55° F). This kills all the germs likely to infect milk.

It is no exaggeration to say that pasteurization of milk has been one of the most important developments of the last 100 years in the control of disease. A good deal of 'raw' unpasteurized milk still on sale today carries very definite risks, and should on no account be given to children. The fact that it is 'straight from the cow' is no guarantee against infection. Unfortunately, any cow-shed (however carefully it is cleaned) is bound to be teeming with germs, and a proportion of these cannot fail to get into the milk. Cows themselves carry infections which can be passed on to human beings in milk; in 1961, for instance, the British Ministry of Agriculture found that 25–30 per cent of all herds contained animals with the infectious disease called brucellosis.

290

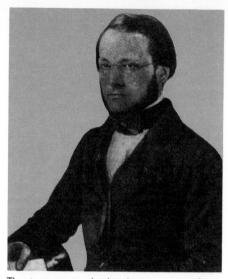

The term pasteurization became part of our language following the discoveries about the nature of organisms causing infection made by the French chemist Louis Pasteur (1822–95). His earlier work was concerned mainly with the processes of fermentation and wine-making.

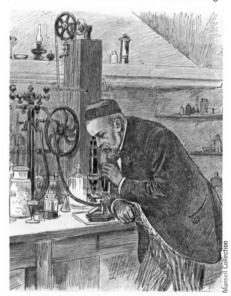

Pasteur is here seen at work in his laboratory in Paris. The development of his fundamental discoveries and their application to medicine came about through the researches of other workers — such as Koch and Roux — who with him founded the science of bacteriology.

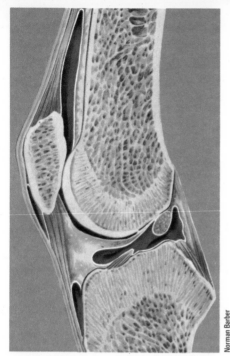

Diagram to show the relationship of the patella to the other bones meeting at the knee-joint.

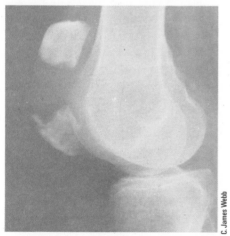

X-ray of a knee-joint, showing a fractured patella with the fragments widely separated.

PATELLA is the knee-cap. This small, shield-shaped bone lies in front of the knee joint and forms a protection for it.

The patella may be fractured either by a direct blow on the knee or, sometimes, as a result of a sudden violent contraction of the leg muscles. It is sometimes possible to operate and 'wire' the broken bone together, but if badly shattered it may have to be removed altogether.

PATHOLOGY is the study of disease. This often sounds slightly puzzling to a lay person, since, in a sense, medicine itself is the study of disease. However, pathology is concerned only with the actual processes of, and changes caused by, disease, rather than the whole patient. It is therefore essentially a laboratory subject.

Pathology is divided into several sub-specialities. *Bacteriology* (see **bacteriology**) is the study of germs and other micro-organisms. *Haematology* is the study of the blood and its disorders. *Chemical pathology* is the study of chemical changes in disease. *Morbid anatomy* (*histopathology*) is the study of the changes in body structure produced by disease, including study of these tissue changes under the microscope. A pathologist is a doctor who specializes in one (or sometimes more than one) of these sub-specialities.

PAUL-BUNNELL REACTION, or Paul-Bunnell test, is a laboratory procedure used in the diagnosis of glandular fever, or infectious mononucleosis (see **glandular fever**). Most people who have this condition produce a chemical factor in the blood which can make the red blood cells of sheep agglutinate, or 'clump'. It is, however, true that people with certain other conditions show a positive reaction to this test, and so the result has to be interpreted with caution.

The Paul-Bunnell reaction usually becomes positive a few days after a person goes down with glandular fever, and becomes negative again about three months later.

PELLAGRA is a disease caused by lack of nicotinic acid (one of the B group of vitamins) in the diet. It occurs in the warmer areas of the world, mainly between the latitudes of the American cotton belt in the northern hemisphere, and of Chile, Argentina and Uruguay

291

in the southern hemisphere.

This type of deficiency tends to occur when people's diets consist largely of maize. To provide adequate quantities of nicotinic acid, a person needs such foods as eggs, milk, meat and cereals other than maize. For complex biochemical reasons, pellagra only develops if there is a deficiency of protein (which is found in meat, cheese, fish, milk, peas and beans) as well as a lack of nicotinic acid.

In many areas of the world, it is extremely difficult for poorer people to obtain the foods necessary to prevent pellagra. However, the United States has shown in the last few decades that it is possible to banish the disease almost entirely by the simple process of adding the missing vitamin to bread.

Pellagra appears only after many months of dietary deficiency. Its three cardinal symptoms are usually described as 'dermatitis, diarrhoea and dementia'.

The dermatitis of pellagra is a generalised dark brown pigmentation of the skin, coupled with pain, itching, redness and thickening of those parts exposed to sunlight, notably the hands and forearms.

Diarrhoea is associated with other disturbances of the alimentary tract: the mouth and tongue become inflamed, there may be pain on swallowing, and the patient may suffer abdominal colic.

The 'dementia' of pellagra is not a true dementia (see **dementia**), since in most countries this term implies a permanent mental disorder. However, pellagra does cause all sorts of brain disturbances, which are usually minor at first, but which eventually lead on to confusion and delusions.

The treatment of pellagra is relatively straightforward, and consists in administering nicotinic acid. Naturally, it is also essential to ensure that the patient receives adequate amounts of vitamin B and protein for future prevention, and this may be far more difficult. (See also **deficiency diseases.**)

PELVIS, which is the Latin word for 'basin', is the name applied to the group of bones which surround and protect the organs of the lower part of the trunk, forming a somewhat basin-shaped structure.

The pelvis also forms the only link, at the hip joint, between the vertebral column (the spine), whose weight it supports, and the long bones of the leg.

The back part of the pelvis is actually formed by the bones of the lower end of the spine: the sacrum and the coccyx. The sacrum can be felt under the skin, just above the cleft of the buttocks, while the coccyx is immediately below the sacrum.

At the sides and in front, the 'basin' is completed by the right and left hip-bones. Each side of the pelvis actually consists of three smaller bones fused together. These are called the ilium (which is the bone we can feel under the palm when we stand with hands on hips), the ischium (whose prominence, or 'tuberosity') can be felt deep under the muscle of the buttocks, and, finally, the pubis. This last bone forms the front of the pelvis; it runs across to form a joint with the pubis of the opposite side, immediately under the upper pubic hair, and just above the genitals.

The organs contained within the pelvis include the bladder, the rectum, and, in women, the ovaries, Fallopian tubes and uterus (womb).

The bones of the pelvis vary slightly in shape between the two sexes; this is, of course, because a woman's pelvis has to accommodate a baby's head during labour. Deformities of the female pelvis (for instance, caused by rickets) may cause the condition known as obstructed labour: in such circumstances, a Caesarian delivery will be necessary.

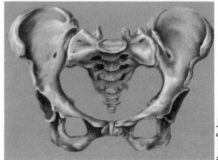

The bony structure of the pelvis. Note the sockets for the heads of the thigh bones.

292

PENICILLIN was the first, and remains the most valuable, of all antibiotics.

Men have searched for hundreds of years for agents to combat disease. It was not till the great work of Louis Pasteur (see **pasteurization**) in the nineteenth century, that this search was placed on a serious scientific basis. Pasteur showed that germs were the cause of infectious diseases, and from his time onward, men such as Robert Koch, the brilliant German bacteriologist, advanced the study of germs and the ways in which they produce disease.

Many of these investigators made attempts to find ways of inhibiting the growth of germs in laboratory experiments, and we now know that a number of men (including Lord Lister, the founder of antiseptic surgery) noticed the curious fact that many types of bacteria would not grow when in close proximity to a fungus called *Penicillium*.

Penicillium is an extremely wide-

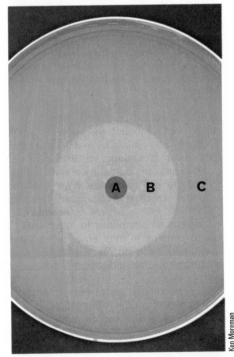

Ken Moreman

A bacterial culture, showing how penicillin stops growth. A. penicillin disc, B. zone of no bacterial growth, C. bacteria growing normally.

spread organism. It is most commonly seen on mouldy bread, but its spores can drift considerable distances in the air, which is why it so frequently turns up on the bacteriological 'plates' used in laboratories.

Unfortunately, none of the early investigators realized the significance of their findings, and it was not until 1929 that a Scottish pathologist, Sir Alexander Fleming, having found the same chance occurrence on one of his 'plates', investigated and extracted the active substance, penicillin, from cultures of the mould, although at first it was not sufficiently pure or concentrated for the purposes of study. It was not till just before the Second World War that a team of investigators, including Sir Howard Florey and Professor Ernest Chain, took up this work once more.

After much intensive research, some of which they had to carry out in the United States, because of the lack of facilities during the War in the United Kingdom, this team isolated penicillin from the fungus and developed a process for producing it in large quantities. The results of its use were dramatic: patients suffering from a wide range of severe infections caused by bacteria were rapidly cured.

The advent of penicillin was of immense value in wartime, and it probably saved many thousands of lives among injured soldiers. In addition, it provided for the first time a way of fighting many bacterial infections, which so often killed children and young people before the war.

This type of penicillin was called *benzylpenicillin*, and it had to be given by injection. In 1953, an oral penicillin (penicillin V) was developed.

However, by the late 1950s, an increasing number of bacteria were developing resistance to penicillin. Fortunately, at this time a group of research workers at the Beecham laboratories in England found that it was possible to isolate the actual chemical nucleus of penicillin, and to add various compounds to it, thus making what are called the *semi-synthetic penicillins*. This was a tremendous advance, as it meant that there was virtually no limit to the number

293

of new penicillins which could be produced. Many of these are effective against bacteria which have developed resistance to ordinary penicillin, and others are capable of killing bacteria against which the original penicillin had no effect.

. The penicillins have few direct side-effects compared with most other antibiotics (some of which can be highly dangerous). However, doctors are reluctant to use them without good reason, firstly because some people are hypersensitive to penicillin (and a few have even died as a result of reactions to it), and secondly because indiscriminate use of the drug encourages the development of resistant strains of bacteria. Unfortunately, some patients believe so strongly in the value of penicillin that they try very hard to persuade their doctors to prescribe it in all sorts of inappropriate conditions (e.g. colds, on which *no* antibiotic yet discovered has the least effect).

PENIS is the male organ. It consists mainly of three cylindrical masses of erectile tissue (see **erection**). These are the two corpora cavernosa, and the corpus spongiosum: These three masses are so placed that the penis is more or less triangular in cross-section when erect.

The corpus spongiosum carries within it the urethra (the urinary passage which runs down from the bladder). The urethra reaches the exterior at the tip of the penis, where it emerges near the centre of a smooth, cone-shaped expansion of the corpus spongiosum which is called the glans. The glans is the most sensitive area of the penis and in children who have not been circumcised (see **circumcision**) and, to a much lesser extent, in adults, it is protected by the foreskin or prepuce (see **foreskin**).

Within the trunk, the urethra is also connected not only to the bladder, but to the two vasa deferentia, tubes which carry seminal fluid up from the testicles. The prostate (see **prostate**) gland also contributes to this fluid, which is forcibly squirted from the penis during the process known as ejaculation (see **ejaculation**).

There are fortunately relatively few disorders which affect the penis. *Balanitis*

(see **balanitis**) is probably the commonest. *Cancer* of the penis is very rare among people who wash themselves carefully and is practically unknown in those who are circumcised at birth. *Impotence* (see **impotence**) is rarely due to a disorder of the penis but almost invariably to psychological causes.

An extraordinarily large number of men worry quite unnecessarily about the size of the penis (see under **virility**).

PEPTIC ULCERS are ulcers of the stomach (see **gastric ulcers**) or duodenum, the uppermost part of the small intestine, which leads out of the stomach. Occasionally they occur in other sites.

Both gastric and duodenal ulcers occur because the gastric juices, whose function is to digest food, start to digest the lining of the stomach or duodenum instead. Why this happens is not known. In duodenal ulcers, the output of acid by the stomach is usually high, and it is thought that this may be related to the emotional stress which sufferers from this type of ulcer often exhibit. Smoking may also make things worse.

The symptoms of both types of peptic ulcer are somewhat similar, and are discussed under the heading **ulcers**.

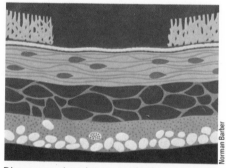

Diagram to show how a peptic ulcer erodes the intestinal wall, and then the muscle layers.

PERCUSSION is the technique of tapping with the finger tips which doctors use to determine the density of internal structures such as the lung. It works on exactly the same principle as that employed when one raps on a panel of wood to see if it is hollow.

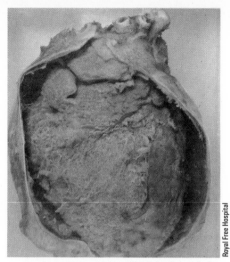

In pericarditis the outer wall of the heart is inflamed and roughened. As seen at post mortem.

PERICARDITIS

PERICARDITIS is inflammation of the pericardium (see **pericardium**). It is quite common, and may be due to a variety of causes. These are broadly classified as dry pericarditis, pericarditis with effusion, and constrictive pericarditis.

Dry pericarditis occurs in the course of such disorders as rheumatic fever and myocardial infarction (the medical term for a 'heart attack' or 'coronary thrombosis'). It may also follow injury to the chest. The principal symptom is pain, which may be felt in the chest, or in the shoulder. It may be worse on deep breathing or coughing. The patient is usually feverish. The doctor can detect a 'friction rub', or grating sound, when he listens with his stethoscope over the region of the heart, and he can confirm the diagnosis by means of an electrocardiogram, or ECG (see **ECG**).

In *pericarditis with effusion*, the inflammation of the pericardium is accompanied by an outpouring of fluid around the heart. This occurs when tuberculosis and other infections, and also cancerous growths, attack the pericardium: other causes include stab wounds of the chest, and heart failure. The outpouring of fluid makes the work of the heart very difficult, so that there is a fast pulse, distension of the veins of the neck, and breathlessness. The results of the doctor's examination are confirmed by taking X-rays, which show a very rapid apparent increase in the size of the heart, due to the accumulation of fluid.

Constrictive pericarditis is due to tuberculosis. The pericardium becomes less and less elastic over a period of months or years, until it forms a rigid sheath around the heart. The main symptoms are breathlessness and oedema.

The treatment of pericarditis depends largely on the cause of the disorder (e.g. tuberculous pericarditis will probably need to be treated with antituberculous drugs). In addition, pericarditis with effusion may necessitate tapping off the fluid through a needle, while constrictive pericarditis will require a surgical operation to cut away as much as possible of the ensheathing pericardium hindering heart action.

PERICARDIUM

PERICARDIUM is a double membrane enclosing the heart. Inflammation of it is called pericarditis (see **pericarditis**). The underlying heart muscle is termed the **myocardium**, and is lined with **endocardium**.

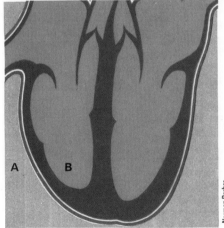

The layers of the pericardium *A* envelop the muscular heart walls of myocardium, *B*.

PERINEUM

PERINEUM is the region which lies between the genitals in front, and the opening of the bowels (the anus) behind. It is very frequently torn during the delivery of a baby, or incised surgically by the obstetrician just before the baby's head is born; this operation is called an 'episiotomy' (see **episiotomy**). In either case, the perineum is repaired by means of stitches shortly after delivery.

PERIODS are the menses – the regular episodes of bleeding from the womb which occur in most women in cycles of approximately 28 days. Bleeding between the periods, pain during the periods, tension occurring at period times, and education about menstruation are all dealt with under the heading **menstruation**. Heavy bleeding during periods is discussed under the heading **menorrhagia**.

Abnormal vaginal bleeding is frequently mistakenly thought only to be due to a period. For bleeding after the change of life, see **menopause**; for bleeding after intercourse, see **menstruation**; for bleeding in early pregnancy, see **miscarriage**, and **ectopic pregnancies.**

PERITONITIS is inflammation of the peritoneum (see **peritoneum**). Such inflammation may be caused by a wide variety of abdominal disorders. The common feature of each, however, is that some material (for instance, pus, blood, gastric juices, or faeces) leaks into the abdominal cavity and produces intense irritation of the peritoneum. The result is very severe abdominal pain, often accompanied by collapse.

Among the causes of peritonitis are perforation of a gastric or duodenal ulcer, the bursting of an inflamed appendix or of a bowel abscess due to diverticular disease (see **diverticular disease**), leakage of blood from a ruptured ectopic pregnancy (see **ectopic pregnancy**), and penetrating injuries to the abdomen.

PERNICIOUS ANAEMIA is a relatively uncommon type of anaemia.

It was first described in the mid-1800s by Thomas Addison, a physician at Guy's Hospital, London. He called it 'pernicious' because at that time, the disease was invariably fatal. This remained true till 1926, when Murphy and Minot found that including very large quantities of raw liver in the diet saved the lives of sufferers.

In 1948, vitamin B_{12} was discovered; injections of this vitamin (usually given every few weeks throughout the patient's
296

life) gave complete control of the anaemia. This treatment was obviously much preferable to eating anything up to a pound of liver every day of one's life.

Usually, the first symptoms of pernicious anaemia are related to the 'weakness' of the blood common to all types of anaemia; the patient, who is almost always middle-aged or elderly, feels tired and ill, and has little energy for exertion.

In addition, the tongue becomes sore, smooth and red, while the skin has the characteristic pallor of anaemia, and also develops a slightly lemon-yellow tinge. There may be loss of weight, and fever.

If the condition becomes far enough advanced, the patient develops neurological complications: first, nerve inflammation (see **neuritis**) characterized by tingling of the feet and hands, and then a very serious degenerative disorder of the spinal cord. In this 'sub-acute combined degeneration', as it is called, there is unsteadiness of gait, and loss of certain types of sensation in the hands and feet. If untreated, the disorder is eventually fatal. It can, incidentally, be provoked, in people who are only in the early stages of pernicious anaemia, by taking proprietary 'blood tonics' containing a chemical called folic acid. For this reason, doctors believe that folic acid should be banned from 'tonics'. (See also **anaemia**.)

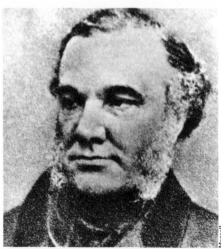

Thomas Addison, Physician of Guy's Hospital, who first described pernicious anaemia.

PEROXIDE is the name by which hydrogen peroxide is commonly known. It is a colourless liquid whose chemical properties depend largely on the fact that its molecule is similar to that of water, but with the addition of an extra atom of oxygen. This makes the molecule unstable, so that it very readily turns to water by releasing the extra oxygen, in the form of the little bubbles which appear when peroxide is used, for instance on a wound.

This property is extremely useful in medicine, since certain germs (called anaerobes) flourish in an environment where there is no oxygen. The bacteria which cause tetanus (lockjaw), for example, fall into this category, and, for this reason, peroxide is often used to disinfect dirty cuts in which the tetanus germ might have lodged.

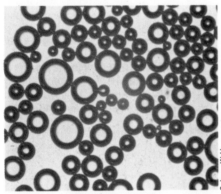
C. James Webb

A froth of small oxygen bubbles, released when blood cells contact hydrogen peroxide.

PERSPIRATION is sweat. It is a fluid secreted by a vast number of tiny glands, called sudorific glands, situated all over the skin. Its function is to evaporate, and hence to cool the body.

The sweat glands are of two main types, one of which occurs in ordinary skin, and the other in the skin of the armpits and, to a lesser extent, in that of the perineum (see **perineum**).

For human beings the practical importance of this distinction is that 'ordinary' sweat has no smell, unless it is allowed to remain on the skin for a considerable time, while the perspiration found in the armpits (axillary sweat) invariably carries an aroma.

This aroma varies considerably between races (being least marked among Chinese people) and between the two sexes. Since among animals this type of secretion exercises an attraction upon the opposite sex, it is not surprising that, in human beings, *small* quantities of this perspiration can be shown to have the same effect. However, axillary sweat readily becomes offensive: this problem can be dealt with by the use of deodorants (see **deodorants**). Offensive perspiration occurring on the feet is usually an indication for more frequent washing, but deodorants may help as well.

There are a small proportion of people who produce very large quantities of perspiration from the palms and also from the soles of the feet. This condition, called hyperhidrosis, is due to overactivity of that division of the nervous system (the sympathetic) which controls the sweat glands. Drugs may be helpful, and in some cases an operation on the nervous system, called sympathectomy, in which small nerves are cut, produces good results.

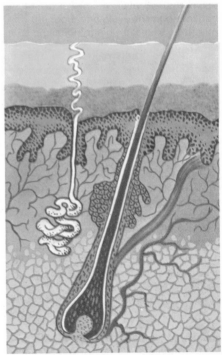
Norman Barber

The coiling duct of a sweat gland in the skin — described once as 'like a fairy's intestines'.

PERTUSSIS is the medical name for whooping cough (see **whooping cough**).

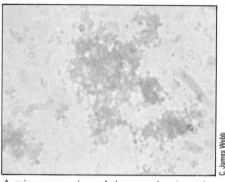

A microscope view of the organisms causing 'whooping cough' – Haemophilus pertussis.

PERVERSIONS may be broadly defined as gross abnormalities of sexual behaviour. There is, however, considerable argument among psychiatrists and psychoanalysts as to what exactly constitutes abnormality when it comes to sexual behaviour. Probably the most common aberrations from the generally accepted norm include male homosexuality (see **homosexuality**), female homosexuality (see **lesbianism**), sadism (see **sadism**) masochism (see **masochism**) and fetishism (see **fetishism**). Also frequently encountered are voyeurism (in which the individual can only get sexual satisfaction by watching other people naked or making love), exhibitionism (in which satisfaction is only achieved by the patient showing his own body to someone else, usually unexpectedly), and transvestitism, (in which dressing up in clothes of the opposite sex is the requirement for satisfaction).

It can be seen that most of these perversions are, in fact, exaggerations of the components of normal sexuality. For instance, it is perfectly normal for lovers to enjoy looking at each other (or, indeed, other people) naked, and also to enjoy showing their bodies to each other, but when a person can *only* reach a sexual climax by spying on others (voyeurism), or by displaying his nudity to some unfortunate passer-by (exhibitionism), then he is obviously suffering from a severe psychiatric illness. In many instances,

298

the illness will show the features of several perversions – for instance, sadism, masochism and fetishism (particularly leather fetishism), are very often found together. In America there exists a very large industry profiting from a traffic in books, magazines and pictures featuring leather-clad girls waving whips and wearing high-heeled boots. (In several countries, high heels are common fetish objects.)

Distortions of the sexual instinct may be due to a variety of psychological factors operating in early childhood, but it is hard to elucidate these factors.

Treatment of sexual perversion is difficult. In cases of long-established homosexuality for instance it may prove virtually impossible. However, it quite often happens that a person takes to some particular perversion such as transvestitism for only a short period, simply as an unconscious means of side-stepping a mental conflict he has been unable to resolve. Here the outlook may be good if only the basic conflict is recognised and treated.

It should be stressed that many forms of sexual behaviour other than intercourse are neither uncommon nor unnatural. Love-play such as genital kissing (fellatio or cunnilingus) is certainly perfectly normal, provided that the individual does not prefer these techniques to intercourse. Similarly, masturbation can only be regarded as abnormal if satisfaction achieved in this way is found preferable to intercourse itself.

PESSARIES are medicinal preparations designed in a form suitable for insertion into the vagina. Confusion over instructions leads with surprising frequency to such preparations being taken by mouth.

Some types of contraceptive are supplied in pessary form. Prolapse supports are still sometimes referred to as pessaries.

PETHIDINE (also called demerol) is a most useful synthetic pain-killing drug, less potent than morphine but much more so than codeine. Unlike drugs of the opium series, it does not suppress cough, nor does it cause constipation. There is a great danger of addiction developing in those to whom it is given repeatedly.

PETIT MAL is a form of epilepsy (see **epilepsy**), quite common in children. Instead of having a fit (convulsion), the child merely loses contact with the outside world for a matter of seconds. He usually stands stock still, looking vacantly ahead of him, and is quite unresponsive if spoken to. After a short time, he recovers completely, and carries on with whatever he was doing, often being quite unaware that anything untoward has happened. Such a child may also suffer from other types of epilepsy.

The diagnosis of petit mal can be confirmed by an electroencephalogram (EEG), or electrical test on the brain. Treatment with such drugs as troxidone and ethosuximide may be helpful. The child should not be allowed to go swimming unless supervised, nor to ride a bicycle because of the obvious risk of drowning or serious injury.

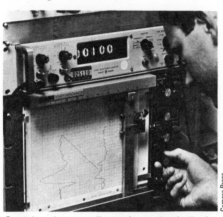

Studying the recordings of a patient's 'brainwaves' with an electroencephalograph.

PHANTOM LIMB is a phenomenon experienced by some people who have had an amputation. Impulses reach the brain from the severed nerves of the leg or arm, producing the feeling that the amputated limb is still there. Because nerves which have been cut across often generate pain impulses, the sufferer may feel intense agony in the phantom leg or arm. This type of pain is difficult to treat, but fortunately it usually passes off after a time.

PHARYNX is the medical name for the cavity behind the mouth, corresponding more or less to the word 'throat'. The pharynx joins the mouth in front, to the nasal cavity above, and the oesophagus (gullet) and the trachea (windpipe) below. *Pharyngitis* is inflammation of the pharynx.

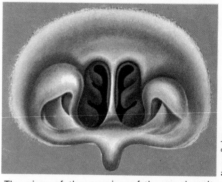

The view of the opening of the nasal cavity into the pharynx, seen in a surgeon's mirror.

PHENACETIN is a pain-killing drug, roughly of the same potency as aspirin (see **aspirin**) or paracetamol (see **paracetamol**); like them it also has the capability to lower the temperature of patients who have fever. Phenacetin is combined with aspirin (and often other drugs) in proprietary pain-killers available in many countries without a doctor's prescription. There is, however, no evidence that such combinations have any advantage over aspirin alone. In addition it should be stressed that phenacetin is potentially very dangerous. It can cause haemolytic anaemia (see **haemolytic anaemia**) and serious kidney disorder in those who make a habit of taking it over long periods.

PHENFORMIN is a drug used in the control of many cases of diabetes. As a rule, the type of patient in whom this drug is used is overweight and developed diabetes in middle age. As dietary measures alone give insufficient control, diet control is combined with the administration of phenformin or one of the other drugs which lower the blood sugar.

Phenformin's principal drawbacks are that it may cause nausea, vomiting or diarrhoea and occasionally a disorder called acidosis. (See **diabetes mellitus**).

PHENOBARBITONE is one of the barbiturate drugs (see **barbiturates**). It is an extremely useful preparation, chiefly employed for daytime sedation in various emotional disturbances, such as anxiety states, and also for the prevention of some sorts of epileptic attack.

The main drawbacks of phenobarbitone are that in large doses, it may produce coma and even death, particularly when its effects combine with those of alcohol, and that it is quite easy for a patient to become habituated to the use of the drug. Some doctors today regard phenobarbitone as a drug of addiction, since there is a noticeable tendency for some patients to show withdrawal symptoms when administration of the drug is stopped.

PHENYLBUTAZONE is a valuable drug used in the treatment of many painful inflammatory disorders, such as osteoarthritis, gout, rheumatoid arthritis, and muscle and joint strains.

Its disadvantages are that it irritates the stomach, so that is may upset people with ulcers or a tendency to 'indigestion' pain; diarrhoea is also common. The most serious side-effect is *agranulocytosis*, when the number of white cells in the blood is greatly diminished. Fortunately, this only occurs in a very small proportion of patients taking phenylbutazone.

PHENYLKETONURIA is a rare but very serious disorder of metabolism, due to an inherited genetic abnormality, which leads to the accumulation in the blood of a chemical called phenylalanine. For reasons which are not yet clear, affected children become severely mentally defective, unless the diagnosis is made very early in life and they receive a diet which is low in proteins containing phenylalanine. (Children with phenylketonuria usually have very fair hair and blue eyes.) Diagnosis is very difficult in the early months of life, and so, in many countries, a routine urine test for the disease is performed on all babies shortly after birth.

PHIMOSIS is tightness of the foreskin or prepuce (see **foreskin**). If it is severe, phimosis provides one of the indications for circumcision (see **circumcision**). *Paraphimosis* is a condition where the tight foreskin becomes constricted around the penis at the base of the glans. Medical help is needed to relieve this constriction, and it may be necessary to perform an operation called a 'dorsal slit' (which involves cutting the foreskin) or circumcision.

PHLEBITIS means inflammation of a vein. Such inflammation commonly occurs in the deep veins of the leg, particularly during pregnancy, or when a person is confined to bed for several days. The blood within the affected veins often clots, blocking the blood-flow.

Usually there is considerable pain and tenderness deep within the calf, and a raised body temperature. It may not prove serious, but does require immediate medical advice. Much more important are painless and unrecognized ('silent') vein thromboses, from which clot material may break off and cause pulmonary embolism (see **embolism**). The best way of preventing this is exercising the legs if confinement to bed for more than a day or two is unavoidable particularly in the elderly.

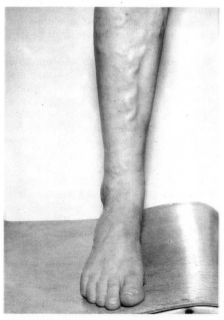

Varicose veins may become inflamed—phlebitis — but this is more serious in deep leg veins.

PHLEGM is the name many people apply to green or yellow sputum, coughed up from the lungs. Such coloured sputum is an indication of bacterial infection within the chest, and usually of the need for an antibiotic (see also **sputum**).

PHRENOLOGY is a practice which purports to analyse a person's character by means of the shape of his head. It is sometimes referred to as 'reading the bumps'. Phrenology had a considerable vogue over a century ago, but with the development of the modern sciences of neurology and psychiatry in the latter part of the nineteenth century, it rapidly lost ground. It now has no scientific support whatever.

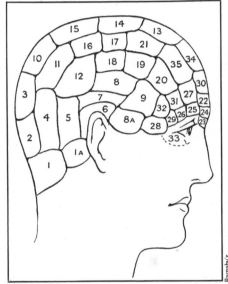

Phrenologists claimed that specific areas of the skull gave clues to one's mental make-up.

PHTHISIS literally means 'wasting'. Almost invariably, however, the term was used to imply pulmonary tuberculosis.

PHYSIOLOGY is the study of the body's workings. It is a science which is divided into many specialities. For instance, respiratory physiology is concerned with the measurement of rates of breathing, the content of various gases in expired and inspired air, the ability of blood to combine with these gases, and so on. Cardiac physiology is concerned with measuring, among other things, the rates of blood flow and the pressures within the heart, while renal physiology is concerned with the measurement of the concentrations of various chemicals at different points within the kidney, and with such matters as the rates of blood and urine flow in the organ.

PIA MATER is one of the three membranes (*meninges*) which cover and protect the brain and spinal cord.

PICA means an unusual desire to eat substances which would not normally be regarded as food. Adults sometimes exhibit this phenomenon, expressing a craving for such materials as coal dust, cinders, ice or raw flour. Although it has long been traditional to say that such cravings are common in early pregnancy, in practice this does not appear often to be so. Pica occurring in an adult is more likely to be an expression of some emotional disturbance.

In children, pica is quite common. As is well known, the young infant will chew almost anything. Until quite recently, pica most often required medical attention where children contracted lead poisoning (see **lead**), through nibbling at paint on their cots.

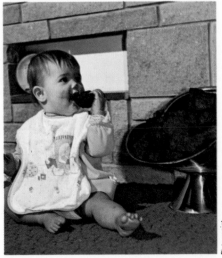

Children enjoy eating the strangest things. Coal-eating is just one form of pica.

PILES – see **haemorrhoids**.

PILL – 'the Pill' is the name by which the contraceptive pill is now almost universally known. (See also **contraception**.)

This method of contraception was introduced in the mid 1950s, and has proved extremely reliable as a means of preventing pregnancy. It is generally felt that almost all the pregnancies occurring in women who are on the Pill are due to failure to remember to take the preparation as prescribed. However, pregnancies have undoubtedly occurred in sensible, reliable women who have been absolutely convinced that they have not omitted a single dose. It is thought that some, at least, of these pregnancies may have come about because the woman has been taking a 'low-dosage' preparation designed to minimize side-effects.

It must be remembered that there are many different types of Pill. Indeed, at least 20 preparations are currently available. All contain hormones whose effect is to inhibit ovulation (the release of an ovum, or egg, from the ovary), but these hormones vary greatly from preparation to preparation. It is therefore difficult to generalize about possible side-effects.

This problem of assessing unwanted effects is further complicated by the fact that intensive research is constantly being carried out on the subject, and many of the pronouncements made only a year or two ago are now out of date.

This position at present appears to be as follows, however.

Risk of cancer. The Pill has been very widely used in various forms since 1956, and there is no evidence that it causes cancer. If it did, some cases at least should have appeared by now.

Minor side-effects. Transient nausea, headache, slight vaginal bleeding and weight gain (usually not more than five pounds) occur in some women in the early months of taking the Pill. In many cases, these symptoms pass off spontaneously.

Psychological effects. Some women complain of depression after starting on the Pill, but it is often difficult to be sure of the relationship between this symptom and the drug. It is also worth remembering that many women feel much better when on the Pill than they do normally.

Disorders of metabolism. The Pill is reported to make certain rare abnormalities of liver function worse. More important, it may sometimes alter the way in which the body deals with sugar, so that a normal woman who has a special series of blood estimations called a 'glucose tolerance test' may show a result suggestive of a pre-diabetic condition. It is, however, claimed that the test reverts to normal after stopping the Pill.

Formation of clots (thrombosis). This side-effect is giving much more concern than any other at the moment. It is possible for a clot which forms in the veins to travel to the lungs and there produce the very serious condition called pulmonary embolism (see **embolism**). Even before the Pill this disorder was said to kill about six women per million every year. *All authorities are now agreed that the Pill does increase the death rate from this cause,* although in the early 1960s, it was stoutly maintained in many quarters that the Pill had no such side-effects.

However, argument now centres around the question of just how great the risk is. Most researchers believe that it is small, and differs with different types of pill; it has recently been stated that a woman on the Pill stands a greater chance of being killed in a road accident than she does of dying from thrombo-embolic complications. It has also been said that the risk of death occurring in pregnancy is about the same as that from embolism in 8–16 years on the Pill, and the risks in medical termination of pregnancy about 20 times as high as in taking the Pill. This may be so, but, of course, an average woman spends only two or three years of her life in a pregnant condition, while she could well take the Pill for 20 or 30 years.

At present, then, it seems that each woman should make up her mind for herself about whether she wants to use the Pill, and then consult her family doctor. It seems likely that within the next few years the whole position regarding the risk of embolism will become much clearer.

PIMPLES are small, infected 'spots' on the skin. They are very common in adolescence, when they may be a feature of acne. In general, pimples without a pus-filled 'head' should be left alone as far as possible; it may be necessary to avoid shaving the affected area. Pimples which have a head should not merely be squeezed between the fingers, as this will spread infection. If they look ugly, the best thing to do is to wash the hands carefully, sterilize a pin in a match flame, and break the pimple with it. Matter from the inside can then be squeezed out into a clean tissue, which (like the pin) is discarded. Do *not* use a handkerchief, which will simply bring the germs in contact with the face next time it is used. After the procedure, wash both hands and face very carefully indeed. If pimples keep recurring, it is best to consult the family doctor.

PINK DISEASE is a condition occurring in children, in which the infant loses his appetite, exhibits a marked dislike of the light, sweats profusely, and eventually develops a curious bright pink discoloration of the hands and feet. The skin in these areas may later become blue and peel.

The disorder was common until the 1950s, when it was first suspected that it might be due to mercury in 'teething powders'. Though this may not have been the whole answer, the abandonment of the use of mercury for this purpose has been followed by the virtual disappearance of the condition.

PITUITARY GLAND is the 'master gland' situated at the base of the brain. It is often called the 'leader of the endocrine orchestra', because of the control which its hormones exercise over the other endocrine glands. (See **endocrine glands**).

Hormones are secreted not only by the pituitary gland itself, but also by its connections in the lower part of the brain. For practical purposes, the hormones produced by these connections and by the back part of the pituitary itself are referred to as 'posterior pituitary hormones'.

This group of hormones includes the antidiuretic hormone (ADH), lack of which

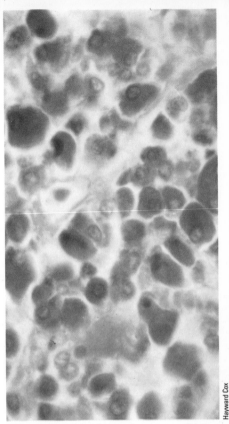

Hayward Cox

The pituitary gland contains many different sorts of cell, seen here under the microscope.

produces the disorder called diabetes insipidus (see **diabetes insipidus**), and oxytocin (which stimulates contractions of the womb, and promotes secretion of milk from the lactating breast).

The anterior (front) part of the pituitary gland produces numerous hormones. Growth hormone, as the name implies, stimulates the growth of children and adolescents. ACTH (adrenocorticotrophic hormone, or corticotrophin) plays a vital rôle in stimulating the adrenal glands (see **adrenal**) to produce steroids. Thyroid stimulating hormone (TSH) encourages the formation and release of the thyroid gland's own hormone, thyroxine (see **thyroid gland**). Follicular stimulating hormone (FSH) and luteinizing hormone (LH) stimulate the ovary during different stages of the menstrual cycle: they probably also

303

have some effect on the male sex glands.

There are probably other anterior pituitary hormones as well, but their precise nature has not yet been elucidated.

It can be seen that most of the pituitary gland hormones have the effect of stimulating some other gland elsewhere in the body. As a general rule, the stimulated glands then produce their own hormones, and when the concentration of these reaches a certain level, the stimulus from the pituitary is then cut off; this is called a 'feedback' mechanism.

PLACEBO means a 'dummy' medicine, tablet or injection — i.e. one which has no therapeutic effect. When a new drug is being investigated, its action is often compared with that of a placebo. In such circumstances, neither the doctor nor the volunteer patients will usually know whether the drug or placebo is being given in any one particular case. Only at the end of the experiment is the 'code' broken. This enables the drug to be assessed objectively; otherwise there is a very real danger that the subjective impressions of the doctor or the patients will affect the interpretation of the results.

Placebos are also occasionally given to patients who absolutely insist on treatment when none is indicated.

PLACENTA is the afterbirth, or, as some mothers prefer to call it, 'baby's luggage'. It is a thick reddish disc of tissue, weighing, on average, about a pound at the time of delivery, though it may occasionally be very much heavier.

Formed towards the end of the third month of pregnancy, the placenta is a remarkable structure. It lies flat against the inner wall of the mother's womb and, at the junction between the two, the baby's blood and the mother's blood are brought into close relation with each other (though they do not actually mix). However, it is possible for oxygen and food to cross from the mother's to the baby's blood, and for the baby's waste products to be filtered off in the opposite direction.

The baby's blood of course reaches the placenta via the umbilical cord, which is attached at the child's navel, and it

304

returns to the baby by the same route.

Normally, the placenta is expelled from the mother's womb not long after the delivery of the baby (see **labour**).

PLACENTA PRAEVIA is a condition of pregnancy, in which the placenta (see **placenta**) lies much lower in the womb than it should do, so that it partially or completely obstructs the baby's way out.

The first symptom of placenta praevia is painless bleeding occurring in the last weeks of pregnancy. During these weeks, stretching of the lower part of the womb makes such bleeding from a low-lying placenta inevitable. It may, however, be slight, particularly if the placenta does not lie too near the opening of the womb; under these circumstances, it may be possible to carry out a normal delivery.

When the placenta lies *across* the opening of the womb, however, normal delivery is impossible. In bygone times, what would happen was that the placenta would separate entirely from the wall of the uterus during labour, so that the baby would almost certainly die. The womb would be unable to contract (and so control the bleeding) and the mother might die of massive haemorrhage. Nowadays, however, the lives of both mother and baby are saved by Caesarean operation.

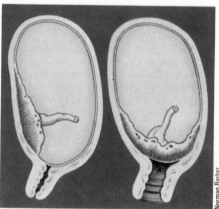

Norman Barber

Diagrammatic sections of the uterus, to show two degrees of placenta praevia. On the left the placenta, although low on the wall of the womb, does not obstruct the baby's exit through the cervix. On the right the placenta covers and blocks the cervical canal completely.

PLAGUE, is a very serious infectious disease caused by the germ known as *Pasteurella pestis.*

Plague has been responsible for many of the great epidemics of history (see **epidemic**). The worst of all was the Black Death which swept across the Western world in the middle of the fourteenth century. It probably killed about one quarter of the population of Europe. In subsequent years the disease returned again and again to Europe (though never quite on the same scale), causing, among other outbreaks, the Great Plague of London in 1665. In the centuries that followed epidemics became much less common in Europe.

In the United Kingdom, for instance, the only death from plague which has occurred in many years was that of a scientist at a Ministry of Defence biological research establishment. In the Indian sub-continent, however, plague remains endemic (that is, always present) in certain areas, and it is not widely realized that the disease is firmly entrenched in the United States, where 500 cases have been reported since 1900. It is said that in that year, plague entered America through the port of San Francisco.

In fact, when plague strikes a country, it often first appears at a port, because plague is fundamentally a disease of rats and other rodents, and throughout history ships have been infested by rats.

How does the *Pasteurella* bacterium cross from rat to Man? Usually, it is carried by the oriental rat flea, *Xenopsylla cheopsis*, a creature which is able to transfer itself from rats to human beings when the rat population starts to diminish.

What commonly happens in an epidemic of plague, therefore, is that a group of rats develop the disease; as they start to die off, their fleas have to find a new source of food, and they transfer their attentions to human beings. The germs they carry enter the human body through bite wounds made as the fleas suck blood.

Plague can at times be passed on in other ways: the bites or scratches of infected rats may give man the disease. In addition, about 350 species of animals other than the rat can carry the germ. Fortunately most of these are wild

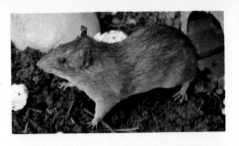

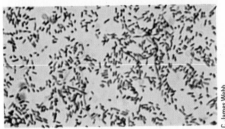

Above The rat acts as host to a variety of parasites, including fleas. When the rats die in a plague outbreak, the fleas transfer to humans. *Below* Plague organisms.

creatures with whom man has little contact in normal circumstances.

The disorder makes its first appearance in Man in the form of *bubonic plague*: that is to say, the illness is characterized by painful tender swelling (buboes) of the lymph glands. There is also fever, headache, vomiting, delirium and a tendency to bleed into the cavities of the body. Untreated, many patients die in the first weeks of the disease.

Plague in its bubonic form is not passed on from man to man, however. In an epidemic, what happens is that about five per cent of those with bubonic plague develop pneumonia. The complication is invariably fatal without treatment, but, before the patient dies, he is liable to pass on *pneumonic plague* to any number of other people. The germs are carried into their lungs in tiny droplets which the original sufferer sprays out as he coughs or even breathes out. From then on, the epidemic spreads in explosive fashion.

Fortunately, if the diagnosis is made early enough, plague can nowadays be cured by the antibiotic streptomycin. In order to contain an outbreak, patients must of course be isolated, and every

C. James Webb

effort must be made to find the source of the disease — whether it be a group of rats in a newly-arrived ship or a disused building, or sometimes a colony of wild animals infected by plague. Every means available is used to destroy such creatures, as well as the fleas they carry. If the control measures are not thorough, disaster may threaten the community.

PLASMA is the fluid portion of blood, i.e. blood without the red cells. If it is dehydrated, it can be kept in powder form and easily reconstituted with sterile water. Such dried plasma 'keeps' far longer than actual whole blood, and can be given to any patient without the need for checking his blood group. Although it does not by any means have all the life-saving properties of whole blood, plasma has proved of immense value in emergency surgery, particularly in battlefield conditions.

PLASTIC SURGERY is the branch of surgery which deals with the reconstitution of damaged or deformed parts of the body. This speciality came first into prominence during the 1930s, and received a tremendous impetus through the new techniques which had to be developed in the Second World War to deal with such terrible injuries as the burns suffered by airmen who had been engulfed in flames when their planes crashed. Nowadays, plastic surgery techniques are also used widely for cosmetic reasons such as the alteration of unpleasing facial features.

PLATELETS, or thrombocytes, are small cells which occur in the blood. They are vital to the process of coagulation (clotting), and deficiency of them leads to one

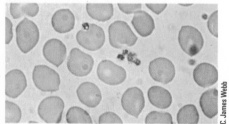

The small, dark-staining platelets of the blood, seen surrounded by the larger red blood cells.

C. James Webb

form of haemorrhagic disorder (see **haemorrhagic disorders**).

PLEURA is the membrane which lines the thoracic (chest) cavity and covers the outside surface of each lung.

PLEURISY is inflammation of the pleura (see **pleura**). Such inflammation very frequently occurs as a result of infection. Normally, this infection will start in the lung, for instance in the form of pneumonia or tuberculosis, and then spread outwards to the pleura. Sometimes, however, infection comes from outside the chest cavity, for instance, through a stab wound, or from an abscess in the upper abdomen. Pleurisy can also be due to non-infectious causes, such as the spread of a cancerous growth into the pleura, or, quite commonly, as the result of a pulmonary embolism (see **embolism**).

The result of the pleural inflammation may be the formation of an *empyema* (an abscess between the layer of the pleura covering the lung and the layer lining the chest cavity), or it may be a *pleural effusion* (a collection of fluid between the two layers) — both these conditions will necessitate some form of drainage, and probably antibiotic treatment. More commonly, however, pleural inflammation results in *dry pleurisy*. This condition causes the patient 'pleuritic pain', which is stabbing and made worse by deep breathing. Often the doctor can hear a grating 'rub' when he places his stethoscope over the area of pleurisy. Treatment naturally depends on the underlying condition: when there is infection, it will usually consist principally of antibiotics of the appropriate kind.

PLEURODYNIA — see **Bornholm disease.**

PNEUMOCOCCI are the bacteria (see **bacteria**) which are responsible for lobar pneumonia (see **pneumonia**). They may also sometimes cause infection of the middle ear (see **otitis media**), endocarditis (see **endocarditis**), pericarditis (see **pericarditis**), peritonitis (see **peritonitis**) and certain other disorders. Treatment with antibiotics is usually called for.

PNEUMOCONIOSIS means lung inflammation due to dust. In the broadest sense, most people who live in towns have at the very least a trace of pneumoconiosis. However, as a rule it is customary to restrict the use of the term to those instances in which people have sustained quite appreciable structural damage to the lung — usually to the stage where production of abnormal fibrous tissue (fibrosis) has occurred.

Owing to a further confusion of terminology, the word 'pneumoconiosis' is used by some people to refer only to the lung disease produced by coal dust. This common form of the disorder is perhaps better referred to as *coal-workers' pneumoconiosis*. It is extremely common among miners, especially those working on the coal face. In its early stages, it does not affect lung function very much, but it does render the patient more liable to infection by tuberculosis. In the later stages, progressive fibrosis leads to breathlessness, wheezing, cough and sputum. The patient may well have chronic bronchitis as well, which will make the symptoms worse.

Silicosis is another form of pneumoconiosis. It is caused by exposure to silica dust, and is found in miners who drill rocks, men who handle slate, silica bricks or sandstone, pottery workers who use ground silica, and foundrymen who are employed in the process of sand-blasting. Its manifestations are very much the same as those of pneumoconiosis.

Asbestosis is a rather similar condition occurring in those who work with asbestos (which is itself a compound of silica). It too produces lung fibrosis, but this may be followed by cancer of the lung, and also by another type of cancer, rare outside the asbestos industry, mesothelioma.

Byssinosis is a lung disease caused by the dust generated when raw cotton is cleaned. It produces symptoms akin to those of bronchitis and asthma.

Usually it takes 5–10 years for a man to develop any kind of pneumoconiosis. At this stage the lung damage can never be reversed, and all that can be done is to treat complications, such as tuberculosis or bronchitis as they occur. It is, of course essential that dust prevention measures are employed in mines and factories; the fact that there are still several thousand new cases of pneumoconiosis in England and Wales each year suggests that these measures are not as rigorously applied as they ought to be.

PNEUMONIA means inflammation of the lung. The alternative term 'pneumonitis' is widely used by doctors, especially in the United States.

Lobar pneumonia, also called pneumococcal pneumonia, is common in children. The pneumococcus germ which causes it enters the body via the mouth or nose, and finds its way to the lungs, where it produces an inflammation confined to one lobe. (The right lung consists of three lobes, and the left of two lobes and a small additional piece of tissue.) The result is fever, combined with cough (often associated with a little rust-coloured sputum) and chest pain, due to pleurisy (see **pleurisy**). In children, vomiting is very frequent, and the rate of breathing is markedly increased. Some patients develop a patch of herpes (see **herpes simplex**) on the upper lip.

This type of pneumonia was once a frequent killer of children and young people; fortunately, nowadays it can usually be cured by penicillin.

Bronchopneumonia is also common in children, and in elderly people. It is a more generalized inflammation of the lungs, associated with an inflammation (acute bronchitis) of the bronchi (the tubes which lead into the lungs from the windpipe). The patient starts with a cough, and probably a sore feeling in the upper front part of the chest (these being the features of acute bronchitis). After a day or two, as inflammation spreads, he becomes much more ill, and the temperature and rate of breathing increase considerably. Cough is severe, and associated with green or yellow sputum. Antibiotic treatment produces a cure in the majority of cases, but the death rate is high in old people. In children, bronchopneumonia may lead to the chronic chest disease called bronchiectasis (see **bronchiectasis**), particularly where (as quite often happens) bronchopneumonia has followed on an attack of whooping cough or measles.

Recurrent attacks of any type of pneumonia demand careful investigation to ensure that lung cancer is not present.

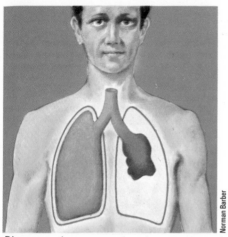

Diagrammatic representation of pneumothorax. Air outside the lung allows it to contract.

Norman Barber

PNEUMOTHORAX means air in the chest cavity, between the lung and the chest wall. When pulmonary tuberculosis was common, a pneumothorax was often artificially produced as part of the treatment: the object was to collapse the affected lung.

Pneumothorax may also be due to a stab wound in the chest, or to a 'burst lung', a not uncommon accident in people who go aqualung diving without proper training.

By far the commonest cause, however, is spontaneous pneumothorax, a condition which very frequently occurs in apparently healthy young men; it is believed to be due to an inherent weakness at one point in the wall of the lung. The patient may often be taking some form of exercise, such as a game of football, when he feels a sudden tightness, or even pain, in the chest, associated with breathlessness.

If the hole in the lung is small, it will close up as the lung collapses, and the air in the chest cavity will be absorbed over a period of weeks. This condition is called a 'closed' pneumothorax.

If the hole is larger, however, there may be an 'open' pneumothorax, in which

308

the air entering the lungs flows freely to and fro through the hole and thus in and out of the chest cavity. Infection will probably lead to the formation of an empyema (see **empyema**), an abscess.

Thirdly, the hole in the lung may be covered by a flap of tissue, so that a valve is formed. The result is that more and more air enters the chest cavity, the lung becomes increasingly compressed, and the patient's breathlessness becomes rapidly worse. This 'pressure pneumothorax' is a most serious emergency, and a needle has to be inserted into the patient's chest and connected to an apparatus which will enable the rapidly increasing quantity of air in the chest to be tapped off.

POISON IVY is a plant whose leaves cause very intense irritation of the skin. Some people also develop an allergic rash after contact with the plant. Skin irritation of this type is extremely common in the United States and some other countries; it is unknown in the British Isles, where poison ivy does not grow.

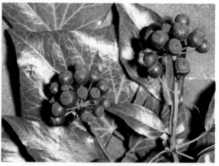

G. E. Hyde

The fruit and leaves of Poison Ivy, capable of causing intense irritation when touched.

POISONS – the treatment for almost any poison, *except corrosive agents (strong acids and alkalis)*, is to make the patient vomit at once, and then to rush him to hospital. In the case of corrosives, *do not induce vomiting.* If bicarbonate of soda is to hand, it may be administered in acid poisoning; similarly, vinegar may be given in cases of alkaline poisoning – however, do not delay in searching for these. *It is much more important to get the patient to hospital than to search for antidotes.*

POLIOMYELITIS, polio, or infantile paralysis, is an acute infection of the central nervous system by a virus. This organism destroys certain nerve cells in the brain stem and the spinal cord, with resultant paralysis of the muscles supplied by those nerve cells.

Polio is a disease which became more and more common during the first half of this century. By the 1950s, the situation was so bad that, in the United States, Scandinavia and Great Britain, the 'polio season' had come to be dreaded by every parent. Every year, literally thousands of children (and adults too) were paralysed or even killed by the disease.

The clinical picture was fairly constant. In the *pre-paralytic* stage, the patient simply felt ill and had a slight fever. Two or three days later, he developed a headache, together with pain and tenderness in the legs and back. Some patients then got better, but others went on to the *paralytic stage*. When this happened, all movement was lost in a particular group of muscles — often most of those of one limb. Sometimes however, the paralysis would affect more than one limb, or perhaps the muscles of respiration. This was one of the most serious complications of polio, since once it happened the patient could only breathe with external aid. Also of grave significance was paralysis of the muscles of the throat and voicebox (larynx).

In patients who survived, the tenderness of the muscles would pass off in about a month. Some recovery of function in the paralysed muscles could be expected for a year or so, but in the majority of cases, the patient was left with a wasted, and often largely useless, leg or arm.

In the 1950s the situation was revolutionized, through the development by Dr Jonas Salk of a highly effective polio vaccine. This was given by injection, but subsequently, Dr Sabin introduced oral vaccine, and this is now in general use.

Owing largely to a disaster following a mistake in the manufacture of one of the early batches of Salk vaccine, people were rather slow to take advantage of it.

In Britain, it was not till a popular football player died of polio that vast queues developed outside immunization clinics.

Since then, there has been routine polio vaccination in infancy, and the incidence of the disease has dropped to practically nil in those countries where it was once most prevalent. It should be very strongly stressed, however, that polio is still extremely common in many parts of the world, and could easily return to the countries where it is a rarity if adults, as well as children, do not keep their protection up to date. Anyone going to the Mediterranean or any of the warmer regions of the world should make certain he is fully immunized against the disease.

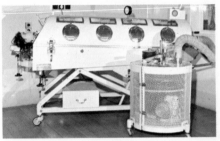

The 'iron lung', a respirator which has saved the lives of many paralysed polio patients.

POLYARTERITIS NODOSA is one of the collagen diseases (see **collagen diseases**). Its main feature is a generalized inflammation of many of the small arteries of the body. It can produce a multitude of signs and symptoms, including fever, a raised pulse, anaemia, kidney disorder, raised blood pressure, skin rashes and asthma. The disease is treated with steroid drugs (see **steroids** and **ACTH**).

POLYCYTHAEMIA is a condition in which the number of red cells (see **erythrocytes**) in the blood is increased. This can be a natural phenomenon (for instance, it occurs when a healthy person goes to live at a high altitude), but the condition called polycythaemia vera is an actual disease, characterized by headache, marked redness in the face, episodes of bleeding and a tendency to thrombosis (clotting) in the blood vessels of the brain. It is treated by simple blood-letting, and by the administration of radio-active phosphorus or other drugs which keep down the number of red cells.

POST MORTEM, p.m., autopsy or necropsy is the thorough examination of a dead body. Such an examination may provide valuable information about the illness from which the patient suffered.

POTASSIUM is a metal which is chemically related to sodium. The balance between these two elements is absolutely vital to our existence. In general, potassium is contained *within* the cells of the body, while sodium exists in the fluid surrounding the cells.

POTT'S DISEASE, called after the English surgeon Percival Pott, is a severe angular deformity of the spine, producing a hunchbacked appearance. It is caused by tuberculosis.

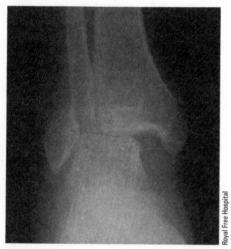

Royal Free Hospital

Pott's fracture, showing the broken end of the fibula *left*, and the displaced tibia, *right*.

POTT'S FRACTURE is a break across the lower end of the tibia (shinbone) and fibula, the two long bones which run between the knee and the ankle. At the same time, the adjacent ankle joint is dislocated. This very common injury is usually treated by manipulation under general anaesthesia, followed by immobilization in a plaster cast for some weeks. Sometimes, the broken bones are operated on to try to pin them together. Like Pott's disease, Pott's fracture is called after the English surgeon Percival Pott, of St Bartholomew's
310

Hospital, who wrote the first complete 'text-book' description of the condition while himself recovering from it.

POULTICES are hot, moist applications used on the skin. At one time, they were used very extensively in medicine, for the relief of pain, and with the object of hastening the resolution of certain inflammatory conditions.

PREDNISOLONE, like prednisone, is a synthetic corticosteroid drug. (See **prednisone**, and **steroids**.)

PREDNISONE, like its close chemical relative prednisolone, is a synthetic corticosteroid. This means that it produces actions very similar to those of steroid hormones secreted by the adrenal glands (see **steroids**). It is a most useful drug in the control of such disorders as rheumatoid arthritis and some cases of asthma.

PREGNANCY, or cyesis, is the time during which a woman carries her child. The average duration of pregnancy in a human being is 40 weeks or 280 days (roughly nine months and one week), as calculated from the first day of the last menstrual period. (Which means, of course, that the real age of the child – the time elapsed since fertilization – is about two weeks less than this.)

Few women are delivered on exactly the appointed day, and most obstetricians regard it as quite normal for a mother to over-run her expected date of delivery by as much as two weeks. It is hard to say what the absolute upper limit of pregnancy really is, but in legitimacy and divorce cases, the courts have accepted figures of up to about eleven months.

For diagnosis of pregnancy, see **pregnancy testing**; for bleeding in early pregnancy, see **miscarriage**, and **ectopic pregnancies**; for vomiting in early pregnancy, see **vomiting**; for ankle swelling in pregnancy, see **toxaemia of pregnancy**; for urinary troubles in pregnancy, see **urinary infections**; for development of unborn child, see **foetus**; for breast changes in pregnancy, see **lactation**; for delivery, see **labour**.

PREGNANCY TESTING can be carried out by either biological or chemical means, though the former (rabbit tests, toad tests, etc.) have very largely fallen into disuse since the development of accurate and convenient chemical tests during the 1960s, and now in worldwide use.

The first inkling a woman has that she may be pregnant comes when she misses a period; within the next week or two, she may experience a sense of fullness or tingling in the breasts, and subsequent to this some nausea or vomiting in the mornings. It is still difficult, however, for a doctor to tell if she is going to have a baby simply by examining her, as the womb is not much enlarged until she is about eight weeks pregnant.

The answer can almost always be found by sending a small specimen of urine for a

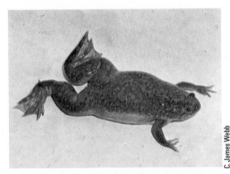

The toad Xenopsis laevis, once used as a test animal to diagnose pregnancy in humans.

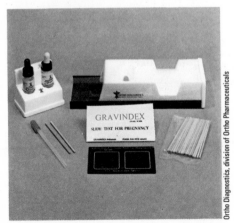

A more modern form of pregnancy diagnosis relies on serum agglutination reactions.

chemical test (or, to be more precise, an immunological test). The result should be back in a day or two, and it is almost always accurate. It should, however, be noted that misleading results do occur in a small percentage of cases — mostly where the patient has some disorder of the reproductive organs, or where she is approaching the change of life, or when she sends the specimen in too early (before the period is at least 12 days overdue).

PREMATURE CLIMAX occurs when a man reaches his orgasm or climax (see **climax**) much too early in the act of love; indeed, sometimes it may occur before intercourse has even started.

Except in the case of young and inexperienced couples (in whom such mishaps are common), premature climax is very often a source of considerable emotional strain — on the husband, because it makes him feel inadequate, and on the wife, because she is likely to achieve no satisfaction. It must be realized that the persistent occurrence of this type of premature ejaculation is basically a psychological problem. It is not (as many men think) an indication of 'over-eagerness', but may be the reverse. Deep down, the man may be reluctant to have intercourse (perhaps because of long-forgotten childhood ideas that sex is 'dirty'). Not surprisingly, this condition is very commonly associated with partial impotence (see **impotence**).

In mild cases, the condition can clear up and never return. A frank discussion between husband and wife of the difficulties he is experiencing, coupled with a loving and understanding attitude on her part, can together work wonders. Mild bedtime sedation (even, for instance, in the form of alcohol) can often reduce the man's nervousness and so help him prolong intercourse. Until such time as he is better, it is wise for him to ensure, by simple techniques of love play, that his wife is sexually satisfied despite his disability. In severe cases, the husband should under no circumstances 'just put up with it': if the condition persists for more than a few months, he needs psychiatric help; this is discussed further under the heading **impotence.**

311

PRE-MED is an accepted abbreviation for pre-medication — the drug (or, more usually, combination of drugs) given to a patient shortly before operation. The object is usually twofold: (a) to sedate the patient and produce a relaxed state of mind, and (b) to dry up the secretions of his air passages, which makes anaesthesia easier and safer. This is why most pre-medications produce not only a pleasant, drowsy sensation, but also a dry mouth.

PREPUCE – see **foreskin.**

PRESCRIPTION is a doctor's written order for drugs. Contrary to widespread belief, prescriptions in English-speaking countries have not been written in Latin for many years, though occasional words, such as *mitte*, meaning 'send' still survive.

PRICKLY HEAT is a term applied to skin irritation occurring in some Europeans living in the tropics.

PRIMIDONE is a useful drug employed in the treatment of epilepsy (see **epilepsy**). It is mainly administered to protect the patient against attacks of grand mal epilepsy (generalized convulsions), but it is also used in the treatment of certain other varieties of the disorder.

Primidone is closely related chemically to the barbiturates (see **barbiturates**) and may be converted to phenobarbitone once inside the body. For this reason, it must be prescribed and used just as carefully as the barbiturates; it is important not to exceed the prescribed dose.

PROBENECID is a drug which has two very useful functions. Firstly, it reduces the rate at which penicillin is excreted from the body, and it can therefore be given to increase the concentration of the antibiotic in the tissues when a patient is suffering from a very severe infection.

Secondly, probenecid is employed in the treatment of gout (see **gout**). Gout is associated with a high level of uric acid in the bloodstream, and probenecid has the effect of keeping this level down.

PROCAINE is a synthetic substance which is closely related chemically to the local anaesthetic cocaine, but without the dangers which caused the latter drug to be abandoned. It can be used by itself as a local anaesthetic, but has found other uses as well. Combined with penicillin, it makes injections of the antibiotic very much less painful than they would otherwise be; furthermore, this 'procaine penicillin' has a much longer duration of action than ordinary penicillin.

Compounds of procaine are also used in the control of certain dangerous disturbances of heart rhythm. The best known of these is procainamide, which since its introduction has saved very many lives.

PROGERIA is premature senility. It is a condition of very great rarity; characteristically the sufferer is a young child who goes very rapidly through the ageing process one would expect to see in a man of 70 or 80. The cause is unknown and death is inevitable. It may be that progeria is due to something going wrong with the 'biological clock' we all carry inside us.

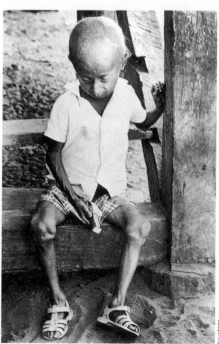

A child doomed to death from old age. All of the ageing processes in progeria are speeded.

PROGESTERONE is a female hormone. It is produced by the adrenal glands, by the placenta (afterbirth), and by the ovaries (see **ovaries**).

In the ovaries, it is the corpus luteum (or 'yellow body') that provides the source of progesterone. After an egg (see **ovum**) is released from the ovary half way through the menstrual cycle (an event which is described as *ovulation*), this 'yellow body' remains at the site which the egg previously occupied. During the second half of the 'month' (i.e. during the 12 or 14 days that remain before the next period), it is stimulated by the pituitary gland to produce progesterone.

Progesterone output rises during the latter part of the 'month' and, under the influence of the hormone, the lining of the womb undergoes a change (called *decidual reaction*) which makes it much more suitable for receiving and nourishing the egg. If a fertilized ovum embeds in the lining this decidual reaction persists; if it does not, then the lining breaks down, and a period occurs. It is believed that the occurrence of menstruation is associated with a drop in the levels of both progesterone and oestrogen (see **oestrogens**), the other female hormone produced by the ovary.

If pregnancy continues, the level of progesterone remains high until after delivery, much of it coming from the placenta (afterbirth).

In recent years, many synthetic compounds with progesterone-like activity have been isolated; these are often called *progestogens*. They are sometimes used in the treatment of premenstrual tension, painful periods and certain other conditions.

They are also employed, almost always in combination with an oestrogen, in the contraceptive pill (see **Pill**).

PROGNOSIS means the outlook in any particular disease: for instance, a condition in which there is every likelihood of recovery is said to 'carry a good prognosis'.

PROLAPSE means descent or protrusion of one of the organs of the body. Although the word is sometimes used to describe an abnormal descent of the rectum, it usually implies the condition called *prolapsus uteri*, or prolapse of the womb.

This common condition is due to weakening of the tissues which support the uterus. Since almost all cases of prolapse occur in women who have borne children, it is thought that this weakening is due to strain during labour. The more children a woman has, the more likely she is to develop a prolapse in middle life.

Depending on where the greatest weakness lies, either the cervix (neck of the womb), or the front or back wall of the vagina may descend towards, and even protrude through, the vulva. Where the walls of the vagina descend, they will tend to form a 'pouch' containing part of either the bladder or the rectum. In the former instance, quite severe urinary symptoms may be produced. In any case, the condition is extremely uncomfortable for the patient.

When an operation is impracticable (for instance, in the very old and infirm), it is possible to hold a prolapse in place reasonably satisfactorily with a solid intravaginal device called a pessary. In the vast majority of patients, operation is greatly preferable. As a rule the type of operation used is a straightforward repair of the weakened tissues, which gives very good results. Sometimes, however, a hysterectomy (removal of the womb) may be needed to resolve the problem.

PROSTATE is a gland, found only in men,

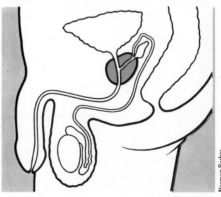

The position of the prostate gland (in blue). Its enlargement may cause retention of urine.

313

which lies close by the neck, or exit, of the bladder. It is about the size of a chestnut and is pierced by the urethra, the passage which carries urine from the neck of the bladder to the exterior. The prostate gland pours its secretions into the urethra, where they mix with the secretions of the testicles to be ejaculated as seminal fluid.

The prostate enlarges in middle or later life, and about 20 per cent of men over the age of 60 develop urinary obstruction (see **urine-stoppage of**) as a result. This may well necessitate the operation of prostatectomy, or removal of the prostate, through an incision in the abdomen. Sometimes it is possible merely to 'nibble' parts of the obstructing gland away by means of a special cutting device inserted into the urinary passage.

Cancer of the prostate gland (which produces the same symptoms) is common, and may be cured by prostatectomy if it is caught early enough. It can also be kept in check, often for many years, by the use of drugs. This cancer is so widespread that many doctors, particularly in the United States, feel that all men over the age of 50 should have a yearly rectal examination, and perhaps other tests as well. (When a doctor performs a rectal examination, he can feel the prostate gland with his finger, through the front wall of the rectum and can assess its size, shape and consistency.)

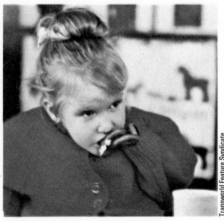

An artificial arm is one example of a prosthesis. Here a thalidomide child shows its uses.

314

PROSTHESIS means an artificial replacement for any part of the body, e.g. a glass eye or artificial leg.

PROTEINS are a group of chemicals which are of vital importance to the body. Together with carbohydrates (see **carbohydrates**) and fats (see **fats**), proteins form one of three basic types of food in our diet.

Good sources of protein include lean meat, fish, cheese, and milk. Lesser amounts are found in eggs, peas and beans.

Protein is needed to build and maintain healthy muscles and strong bones. Proteins are themselves built up from chemicals called amino acids, a number of which are essential to life itself, since they play a part in certain bodily chemical reactions of tremendous importance. Protein foods, such as meat, which contain all the essential amino-acids are sometimes called 'first class proteins'.

For protein in the urine, see **proteinuria** below.

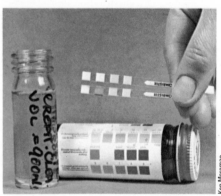

Simple and rapid tests for the presence of protein in the urine use dyes which change colour.

PROTEINURIA (sometimes called 'Albuminuria') is the presence of protein in the urine. Although it may be of no significance (particularly in women, whose urine specimens often contain a little protein material from the vagina), it always needs careful investigation, since it may indicate disease of the urinary tract, or (in pregnant women) toxaemia of pregnancy (see **toxaemia of pregnancy**).

PROTOZOA are one-celled primitive organisms. They are very widespread in Nature, and a small number of them produce disease in Man. Among these are those which cause amœbic dysentery (see **dysentery**), malaria (see **malaria**) and sleeping sickness (see **sleeping sickness**).

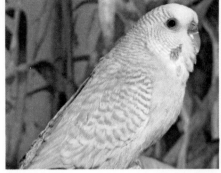

The budgerigar, a common pet, may harbour the organisms responsible for psittacosis.

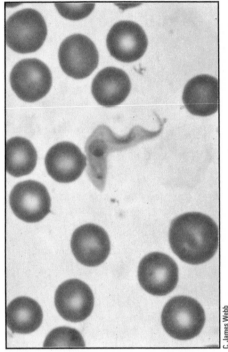

The organism responsible for producing sleeping-sickness, a protozoan, in blood.

PRUSSIC ACID is the poisonous acid from which cyanide (see **cyanide**) is derived.

PSEUDOCYESIS means 'false pregnancy'. Although the condition is relatively uncommon nowadays, in days gone by it seems to have been not infrequent for women not only to imagine themselves pregnant but apparently to develop all the symptoms of pregnancy. Among those reputed to have had this condition was Queen Mary I of England.

PSITTACOSIS is a virus disease, passed to human beings by birds. At one time, parrots were the most important reservoir of infection, but nowadays the disease is frequently caught from budgerigars.

PSORIASIS is a common skin disease, which is characterized by the occurrence of widespread rough, reddish areas, on which there are minute whitish scales. In addition, the disorder may affect the fingernails, producing quite an ugly deformity. Occasionally, psoriasis is associated with a form of arthritis rather similar in nature to rheumatoid arthritis.

The treatment of psoriasis may sometimes be very difficult. Extracts of coal-tar and preparations like dithranol are usually effective in clearing the skin of heavy encrustations. The steroid applications which have been introduced since the

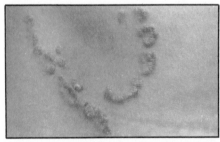

Typical appearance of the patches of thickened, reddened and scaling skin seen in psoriasis.

1950s are often effective, while, very rarely, it may be necessary to use methotrexate (normally an anti-cancer drug).

PSYCHIATRY is the branch of medicine which deals with illnesses of the mind; a

315

psychiatrist is a doctor who practises it. Psychiatry has, in a sense, been practised since the earliest days of medicine, but it was not until the advent of Sigmund Freud that study of it was placed on any kind of rational basis. Freud developed the theory of psycho-analysis (see **psycho-analysis**). Subsequently, as his teachings, and those of his successors Jung and Adler, became more widely known, the practice of modern psychiatry and of psycho-analysis spread throughout the world. Since Freud's time, various methods of treatment have been developed including electro-convulsive therapy, the use of hypnosis, the administration of tranquillizers and anti-depressant drugs, and various others. At the same time there has been a gradual realization among doctors and the lay public that a mental disorder is an illness like any other, and that a high proportion of such disorders are curable.

Nonetheless, it is true to say that psychiatry is still something of an infant science, and its state of development at the present time can perhaps be compared to that which 'ordinary' medicine had reached during the last century. However, it is also true that the advances in treatment which have occurred in the last 25 years have been the most remarkable in the whole history of psychiatry.

PSYCHO-ANALYSIS is a system of psychiatric treatment which was originally developed by Sigmund Freud. It is based on the theory that all mental disorders have their origin in disturbances of development of the mind during infancy. While this theory is far from being universally accepted among psychiatrists, many of its principles are widely regarded as valid.

Psycho-analysis proper is a form of treatment which takes several hours a week over a period of years. In each session, the patient, who lies on a couch, 'opens his mind' to the psycho-analyst and talks about anything and everything which occurs to him; this process is called 'free association'. The object of this is that, over a long period of time, the patient will have laid bare all the neurotic conflicts in his mind, and so come to terms with them through

greater self-awareness.

It is obvious that from the point of view of time alone, relatively few patients can have full psycho-analysis. For instance, there are only about 2,500 properly qualified psycho-analysts in the United States, and since none of them could possibly cope with more than ten patients under analysis, it is obvious that the very maximum number of people currently being psycho-analyzed in the very country where this system of treatment is most popular is only 25,000.

However, psycho-analytic methods have been very widely accepted throughout the world, and are used in such techniques as group therapy and analytical psychotherapy.

PSYCHOLOGY is the study of human behaviour. Some psychologists (e.g. those working in child guidance clinics) deal with disorders of human behaviour, but others (for instance, industrial psychologists) are more concerned with the application of psychology to life as a whole and the way in which Man's environment can be best adapted to suit him.

PSYCHOPATHIC is a word used to describe a small percentage of the population who have a serious disorder of personality which (in the words of the British Mental Health Act of 1959) 'results in abnormally aggressive or seriously irresponsible conduct'. In everyday terms, such people have no conscience whatever. That part of the mind which regulates most people's conduct (the superego) has simply failed to develop. The psychopath therefore lies and cheats his way through life from his early childhood; he sees no reason to do anything except what is of immediate advantage to himself. The result is that, by the time he is grown up, he is likely to have fallen foul of the law many times, to have been continuously in trouble at school and work, and to have shown signs of violence and ruthlessness towards others. It is thought that this personality defect may come about because in infancy the psychopath is not taught the difference between right and wrong as most of us are.

PSYCHOSOMATIC is a word applied to disorders in which the mind is said to play a part in producing a disease of the body. Some doctors hold that emotional strain is a factor lying behind many apparently 'physical' diseases, while others think that there are certain bodily diseases which are in themselves so likely to produce emotional upset that it is difficult to tell which came first. Among the very few conditions which are regarded by most people as, in part at least, of psychosomatic origin is duodenal ulcer. It does seem quite likely that the anxiety and stress shown by so many people with this condition tend to increase the outflow of acid from the stomach and hence to make ulcer formation more likely.

PTOMAINE POISONING is a term which still turns up regularly in books, but which has dropped out of medical use. Essentially, it corresponds to the term 'food-poisoning', which years ago was thought to be due to chemicals called ptomaines. It is now known, of course, that food poisoning (while occasionally due to other types of chemical contamination) is usually caused by germs, or their toxins, which enter food through lapses in hygiene (see **food poisoning**).

PUBERTY is the time of life at which an individual becomes sexually mature. It is a time at which tremendous changes take place in both the body and the mind; as a result, the boy or girl may need considerable help and understanding to get through what may be a very awkward and trying time. It is, of course, also an exciting time, when childhood is at last being left behind and adulthood begins.

In girls, puberty occurs on average at about the age of 12, though very considerable variation is quite normal. For reasons which are not entirely understood, the age of puberty seems to be getting steadily earlier in recent times. The changes which occur in the body are due to the influence of female hormones called oestrogens and are discussed under that heading. Basically, these changes lead to an alteration in the configuration of a girl's body, making it that of a young woman, rather than of a child. During this process, the menarche (see **menarche**) or start of the monthly periods occurs. (See also **menstruation**.)

At the same time, the girl's mind undergoes alterations. She becomes, for the first time, interested in the opposite sex, though, depending on the environment she is brought up in, this interest may or may not be obvious. Simultaneously, she is likely to develop a new awareness of the world around her, and cultivate, often for the first time, interests in art, music, literature (often romantic in nature), religion, and even sport. Many psychologists believe that these interests develop because of what is called 'sublimation' of the sex instinct — that is, its redirection into other channels.

In boys, puberty tends to occur a little later; there is not the same 'spread' in incidence over a period of years as there is in girls, and in the vast majority of boys, puberty comes between the ages of 12 and 15. As with girls, puberty is usually accompanied by an increase in height and weight. At the same time, the genitals become larger, and there is marked growth of pubic and armpit hair, together with the first development of a beard. The larynx (voice-box) changes in shape, so that the 'Adam's apple' becomes more prominent: a further result of this is that the boy's voice (often after a period of 'breaking') becomes deeper and more masculine. The occurrence of erections becomes very much more frequent, masturbation is virtually universal, and the boy experiences night-time emissions (see **emissions**). These last features are liable to worry him unless it is explained to him that such occurrences are perfectly normal and harmless.

At the same time, he too experiences marked changes in personality. While some boys find puberty a period of relative tranquillity, to many others the world seems to have undergone a complete revolution as a result of which everything in life takes on new values. Very often, it is the case that, until the 'glandular storm' of puberty is over, a boy can think of practically nothing, night and day, but Woman — a mysterious and desirable creature who is all too obviously out of his reach. Once this initial period is over, things become easier, but very often the adolescent boy is moody and difficult for his parents to deal with for a year or two. Sometimes, just as in the case with girls, he 'sublimates' much of his energy into other fields, such as sports. This, of course, is what many schools try to encourage, but it is more important that he receives understanding from his family.

It is also essential that both boys and girls have a proper knowledge of the changes which are about to take place in them when they come to puberty (see also **sex education**).

PUERPERIUM is the time during which a mother is recovering from labour (see **labour**). She should, of course, remain under the doctor's or midwife's care during this time, as there are a number of disorders which may affect her, for instance phlebitis (see **phlebitis**), urinary infections (see **urinary infection**), inflammation of the breast (see **mastitis**), and breast abscesses (see **breast**). In general, any feverishness, or any bleeding from the vagina, occurring at this time, should be reported at once to the doctor.

PULMONARY EMBOLISM is a serious condition in which a plug of matter (usually a clot, or thrombus, from the veins of the legs or pelvic region) blocks the blood vessels supplying the lungs. It is described under the heading **embolism**.

PULSE is the thrust which can be felt as the surge of blood caused by a heart-beat

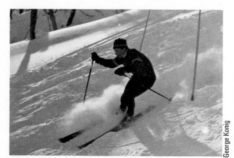

The pulse rate in skiers has been known to reach as high as 190–200 during slaloms.

passes through the body's arteries. It is usual to feel it over the radial artery, which runs just under the skin of the wrist. The pulse should be taken with the examiner's middle finger, and not his thumb (in which

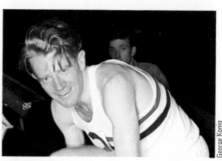

Trained athletes often have very slow resting pulses. In the runner Chris Chataway it was 40.

he is liable to feel his own pulse beating).

The normal pulse rate is about 70 beats a minute in adults, though it may be much slower in trained athletes. Slow pulse rates are also found in certain uncommon heart conditions, and in underactivity of the thyroid gland. Fast pulse rates are commonly found during violent exertion, when a person is anxious or excited, and also in patients with *over*activity of the thyroid, and a number of heart disorders.

An *irregular* pulse requires checking by a doctor, but it may well be of no significance at all.

Apart from assessing the *rapidity* of the pulse during his examination, the doctor will also be estimating its *quality*, for with experience it is possible to tell the state of the arterial wall by the slight differences in sensation which are imparted to the fingertips. The state of the artery wall changes gradually during life, and can be drastically changed by several diseases. In a young person the wall is thin, so that it is possible, with only moderate pressure from the fingers, to prevent the passage of blood through the artery. In older persons the artery wall becomes much thicker, and loses its elasticity, so that the artery feels like a hard cord which can be rolled under the fingertips. In certain degenerative diseases, also, the wall becomes hardened, and the passage of blood may be impeded by deposits.

PUPIL is the dark circular hole in the centre of the iris (see **iris**), the coloured part of the eye. It is through the pupil that light is admitted from the exterior.

The size of the pupil is regulated by contraction or relaxation of the iris. Dilated (large) pupils are caused by excitement and emotion, by drugs such as atropine, an extract of belladonna (see **belladonna**), and also by certain disorders of the nervous system. Very small pupils may be normal, but may also be due to disease affecting the nervous system. If a pupil is irregular, rather than round, a doctor's advice should be sought, as this too may be a sign of neurological disease.

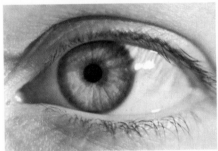

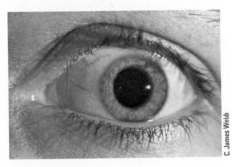

Pupil changes in response to light of strong intensity (above) and subdued light (below).

PURGATIVES – see **laxatives.**

PURPURA means the occurrence of reddish or purple spots on the skin, due to bleeding into it.

Purpura is very common and may have various causes. It may occur because of defects in the walls of the small blood vessels, or capillaries. This is the mechanism of senile purpura – the red spots which quite often appear on the legs and feet of debilitated old people. In the same way, scurvy (lack of vitamin C) and certain poisons and infections can affect the walls of the capillaries.

Lack of blood platelets (see **platelets**) can also cause purpura; this 'thrombocyto-paenic purpura' can occur as a disease in itself, or be due to such conditions as leukaemia. It may also be due to the administration of drugs to which the patient reacts in an abnormal way.

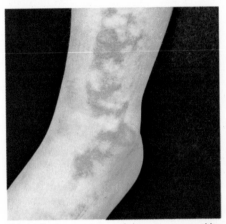

The typical appearance of the spots caused by bleeding into the skin in the disorder purpura.

PUS is a fluid found in abscesses and on infected surfaces. It is most commonly yellow, but may be white, green, or even red, depending to a large extent on the nature of the organism producing the infection. It consists of very large numbers of white blood cells, or leucocytes (see **leucocytes**), together with cells shed from the surrounding tissues, and dead bacteria.

The white cells have accumulated in the area in order to fight the threat of infection. As a general rule, where there is pus under tension (as in an abscess), the infection has been met and coped with, so that it is time to relieve the pressure by allowing the pus to escape. For this reason, there is an old surgical dictum which still holds good: 'where there is pus, let it out'.

PYELITIS means inflammation of the part of the kidney from which urine flows

319

C. James Webb

out to commence its journey down the ureter to the bladder. Such a condition is almost always accompanied by inflammation of the substance of the kidney itself. In the past, doctors have made a distinction on the basis of whether the involvement of the kidney substance was slight or gross, referring to the former as *pyelitis* and the latter, which was regarded as more serious, as *pyelonephritis*. Since one may shade imperceptibly into the other, we shall make no distinction here.

Acute pyelitis (or acute pyelonephritis) is very common, particularly in women, and more especially in pregnant women. In men, it is uncommon unless there is some structural abnormality of the urinary passages. One reason why the condition is common in women is that the female urethra (the tube leading from the bladder to the exterior) is very short indeed, and germs (particularly bowel germs, from the region of the anus) can very readily find their way to the bladder, and thence up to the kidney.

The symptoms are fever (in the region of 103°F or more), shivering (often amounting to the uncontrollable shaking called rigors), and pain and tenderness low down in the back, just below the ribs and to one side of the backbone — in fact, over the kidney. There may be some vomiting, and there is often a history of urinary symptoms (such as frequency of micturition and pain on passing water) during the previous days.

In a small proportion of cases (the pyelonephritis rather than the pyelitis group), the patient becomes very ill indeed, as the function of one or both kidneys is impaired. In most cases, however, the prompt administration of sulphonamide drugs, or sometimes one of the newer antibiotics, will kill the organisms responsible. Before he starts this treatment, however, the doctor will send a specimen of carefully collected urine to the laboratory in order to determine the nature of the germ. The result will be back within 48 hours, and he can then change his treatment or continue with it, depending on the information the laboratory gives him. After the symptoms disappear and the patient feels better, he will send another urine specimen to the laboratory to ensure that the infection has gone — it is, unfortunately, not sufficient to rely on the cessation of symptoms as a guide.

Full and careful treatment of the acute condition is essential, because otherwise it may lead on to *chronic pyelitis (chronic pyelonephritis)*, which is a serious disease with far-reaching effects on the patient's lifelong health and well-being. It has been shown that 10 per cent of all persons whose kidneys are examined after death have the changes of this condition. Sometimes the disease occurs because of the presence of a stone or other obstruction to the urinary tract. The symptoms tend to be mild — backache, a feeling of being run-down, occasional slight fever, and some frequency of passing water may all be seen. It is therefore most important to catch the condition as early as possible.

PYLORIC STENOSIS is a narrowing of the pylorus, the narrow passage which leads out of the stomach to the duodenum (the topmost part of the small intestine). Occasionally, this narrowing occurs in adults, as a result of a gastric ulcer or cancer. The symptoms produced are vomiting, distension of the abdomen and belching of foul gases, all in addition to ordinary gastric ulcer symptoms (see **gastric ulcers**) and (in the case of a cancer) severe weight loss as well.

Pyloric stenosis is commonest in young babies, however. The narrowing is the result of hypertrophy (overgrowth) of the ring of muscle at the pylorus, and the symptoms are projectile vomiting (in which the food is literally squirted some feet away from the baby), together with some constipation and failure to gain weight. A knotty lump can be felt in the upper abdomen, and waves of contraction passing across the stomach may be seen next to it.

Pyloric stenosis is commonest in boys of about 3–5 weeks of age; it is rare after the age of 10 weeks. Some children can be treated by medical means, but a high proportion will need an operation to relieve the obstruction: this procedure gives very good results.

Q FEVER is a disease caused by a germ called Rickettsia burneti (see **rickettsiae**). It occurs throughout the world, but is commoner in rural areas, because it is transmitted to Man from sheep and cattle. Often it occurs in small epidemics within such communities as nurses' homes. The features include fever and pneumonia, and the condition responds to tetracycline or other antibiotics.

QUADRIPLEGIA means paralysis of both arms and both legs. Such a condition is fortunately rare, but it may be due to severe injury to the spinal cord – as often occurs, for instance, with a broken neck.

QUARANTINE is the isolation of a person or animal with an infectious disease (or coming from an area where the disease is prevalent) until he can no longer pass it on to others. The word comes from the Latin for 'forty', since at one time, it was usual to detain travellers from epidemic-stricken areas for a period of 40 days. In the case of most infectious diseases, this was certainly a more than adequate period. Nowadays, when far more is known of the nature of infectious diseases, quarantine periods, when used at all, are usually very much shorter, although in the case of such diseases as rabies (see **rabies**) it is vital to err on the safe side.

QUICKENING is the first sensation which a mother-to-be feels of the baby moving within her womb. Where a woman is unsure of the date of her last period (which happens frequently), the time of quickening sometimes provides a useful guide as to what stage the pregnancy has reached. In cases where there is some doubt about whether the baby is alive or not, the occurrence of quickening is also helpful as an indication of life.

In mothers who are pregnant for the first time, quickening does not usually occur till the 22nd to 24th week after the last menstrual period. In other mothers, however, quickening usually comes much earlier – about the 17th or 18th week.

QUINIDINE is a drug which is closely related to quinine. It is used to control certain abnormal heart rhythms, though it is employed less frequently nowadays than it used to be, partly because of the availability of other drugs, and partly because quinidine carries certain risks. It may affect the heart adversely, and it is therefore nowadays often given only in hospital where a careful watch can be kept on the heart by means of an electrocardiogram (ECG). Other side-effects are similar to those of quinine (see **quinine**).

QUININE is a drug obtained from the bark of the Cinchona tree. South American indians used to use this 'Peruvian bark' to treat malaria, and they passed this knowledge on to the Jesuit priests who came over with the Spanish occupation of Latin America. Quinine was the most widely used antimalarial drug up until the Second World War, but it has since largely been replaced by newer drugs (see **malaria**).

The quinine content of tonic water was one reason for the long-standing popularity of this drink in the tropics: there was probably a grain of truth in the belief that tonic water helped prevent malaria.

The side-effects of quinine include nausea, vomiting and ringing in the ears.

QUINSY is the popular name for a peritonsillar abscess – that is, a collection of pus occurring in the throat immediately next to the tonsil, usually in the tissues of the soft palate.

Quinsy is fortunately rare in childhood; it is commoner in men than in women. Although it is not life-threatening, it is an extremely unpleasant and distressing condition. The patient feels a great deal of pain from the intensely sore throat. At the same time, he finds that the abscess rapidly grows so large that he cannot swallow. This is as distressing as the pain, because saliva continually gathers in his mouth and tends to produce a choking sensation while he sleeps. The inflammation is such that he cannot open his mouth properly – a condition which is known as 'trismus'.

In the early stages, a quinsy may be treated with antibiotics alone, but once pus starts to accumulate, it is usually necessary to incise the abscess surgically.

RABIES is a virus disease caused by a bite or lick from an infected dog or one of a great many other animals. (Certain bats harbour the virus and may pass it on by spraying urine as they fly.) It is perfectly possible for an infected dog to appear completely healthy. If the person who has caught the virus realizes what has happened in time, it is possible to protect him by immunization. Once the symptoms appear it is too late, and the disease is then invariably fatal in human beings. (It has, however, been reported from South America that one woman has survived after the onset of symptoms, but details of this case are not so far clear.)

The symptoms of rabies (which may take many weeks to come on) are fever, headache, vomiting, sore throat, cough, tingling sensations, pain near the site of the bite, and then agitation and restlessness. The patient becomes wildly apprehensive and irrational, and develops muscle contractions and convulsions. Violent spasms of the throat occur if he tries to drink; eventually these come on at the very sight (or even the thought) of water. This phenomenon is called hydrophobia from the Greek 'water-fear'.

Rabies is still very common throughout the world: in Europe, the incidence in wild animals such as foxes has been rising alarmingly in recent years. However, in certain countries, such as Great Britain, Australia, the various nations of the West Indies, and the Scandinavian countries, strict quarantine regulations have ensured that infection of human beings (apart from fully immunized quarantine kennel workers) does not occur. In Great Britain no fully developed case of human rabies has been seen for nearly 50 years; however, the quarantine period for incoming dogs was increased from 6 to 12 months in 1969. This was because it became evident that dogs could harbour the disease for more than 6 months without showing symptoms. Unfortunately, vaccination of dogs is not very effective.

RADIOTHERAPY is treatment by various forms of radiation, and includes X-ray, cobalt and radium therapy. This type of treatment is widely used to combat various forms of tumour, both benign and malignant. It can also be used in other diseases, for example, ankylosing spondylitis, a common form of arthritis affecting the spine. Radiotherapy is often alarming to the patient, because the devices used to direct the rays are frequently large, complex and rather awe-inspiring. However, radiotherapy is a completely painless procedure.

RADIUM is a radio-active element which has long been used in the practice of radiotherapy (see **radiotherapy**). In recent years, it has tended to be superseded by the introduction of new methods, such as the use of radio-active cobalt and caesium. It is still, however, widely and very effectively employed in the treatment of cancer of the cervix (neck of the womb).

RAYNAUD'S DISEASE is a relatively common condition in which the patient, often a young woman, suffers recurrent attacks of extreme whiteness of the fingers. This is followed by a blue discoloration (cyanosis) and finally, by a bright red flush.

Raynaud's disease appears to be due to spasm of the arteries which supply the fingers with blood. The cause of this spasm is unknown, but in men it is said to be often associated with exposure to severe and prolonged vibration of the limbs (e.g. use of a pneumatic drill).

Raynaud's phenomenon is a precisely similar change in colour of the fingers, occurring in the course of certain uncommon disorders, in some of which the spasm is due to pressure on the nerves which supply the arteries of the fingers. In these cases, treatment is directed to the

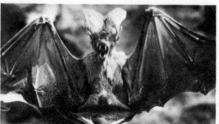

Bats in many areas of the world act as carriers of rabies – a fact only recently realized.

Australian News & Information Bureau

basic disorder, but in Raynaud's disease itself, treatment may be very difficult: it usually consists in wearing warm gloves and taking drugs intended to dilate (widen) the arteries of the fingers. In some cases, an operation on the nerves supplying these arteries may help.

RECTUM is the last part of the large intestine, which runs down through the pelvis to the anus. It is about eight to ten inches in length.

Cancer of the rectum is a common form of cancer. The great majority of cases occur in the over-40s. The symptoms are bleeding from the back passage (all too often mistaken by the patient for piles), pain in the lower left abdomen, and a change in bowel habit (i.e. diarrhoea or constipation). The patient does not necessarily have all these symptoms together, and it is essential that anyone who has any suspicion that he may be suffering from cancer of the rectum sees his doctor at once, as *early* cases of this disease can very frequently be cured.

The doctor can examine the first four or five inches of the rectum with a gloved finger, but, to exclude cancer further up, examination with a device called a sigmoidoscope and a special X-ray (a barium enema) will be necessary. These procedures will normally be carried out at hospital rather than in a surgery.

REFLEX is a muscular response to a stimulus, occurring without conscious thought. This is because the muscular movement depends on a short reflex 'arc' — or nervous circuit — rather than the receiving of a message by the brain followed by the conscious sending out of a signal to perform a particular movement. The reflex action is thus much quicker than a conscious, planned response.

We see a clear illustration of this in what happens when a person accidentally puts his finger on a very hot surface. The rapidity of action of the reflex arc is such that he has actually pulled his hand away before his brain consciously registers that he has been burnt.

There are many reflexes throughout the body, and checking certain important ones (e.g. the knee jerks) is part of the basic examination of the nervous system.

REGIONAL ILEITIS – see **ileitis**.

REITER'S DISEASE is a condition in which a particular type of eye inflammation is associated with arthritis and inflammation of the urethra.

RENAL COLIC is a type of colic (see **colic**) caused by a stone jamming in the ureter (one of the pair of tubes which run from the kidneys to the bladder). Renal colic is characterized by excruciating pain, often described as running 'from the loin to the groin', i.e. from the kidney region in the small of the back, round the flank, and down to the groin. Such pain usually requires the use of powerful drugs to relieve it. Sometimes the patient passes the jammed stone out in his urine, but often an operation is necessary. This will be preceded by a special X-ray to locate the stone's exact position.

RESPIRATION means the mechanism whereby the body absorbs and uses oxygen and gives off carbon dioxide. This is achieved firstly by the process of breathing (see **breath**), and secondly by what is called *tissue respiration*. In tissue respiration the oxygen brought from the lungs by the bloodstream and transferred to the tissues combines chemically with glucose (the sugar which is the body's basic fuel), releasing the energy we need to power our every movement and every bodily process. The combination of oxygen and glucose gives rise to water and to waste carbon dioxide. The carbon dioxide is carried back to the lungs by the bloodstream, and is there breathed out.

RETENTION OF URINE – see under **urine – stoppage of**.

RETINA is the screen at the back of the eye on which images are focused just as they are on the film of a camera. This mechanism is discussed further under the heading **eyes**.

The retina is composed of tiny light receptors called rods and cones. The former are basically responsible for black-and-white vision, while the later are responsible for colour vision (see also **colour blindness**).

Detachment of the retina may follow a blow to the eye. The result is partial or complete blindness on the affected side. Various new techniques to replace the detached retina, including the use of photocoagulators and the laser beam (see **laser**) have greatly improved the outlook in this condition.

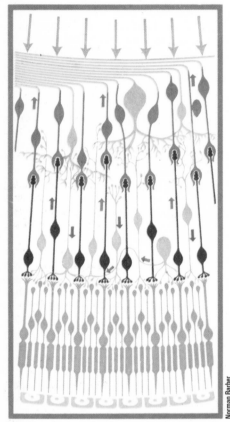

Diagram to show the layers of the retina. Light which has entered the eye passes through the nerve fibres which take impulses from the receptors (blue) *below*, to the brain. The receptors are of two sorts, rods and cones, and have separate connections with the brain.

RHESUS FACTOR is one of the blood group factors. In most western countries, about 85 per cent of the population are

Rhesus positive. If a Rhesus negative mother has a child by a Rhesus positive man, it is possible that Rhesus positive red blood cells from the baby may escape through the placenta (after-birth) into the mother's circulation, and there set up antibodies. In the last few years, a simple test has been developed to determine, shortly after delivery, if this has, in fact, occurred.

When such a 'sensitized' mother has another Rhesus positive baby, blood tests during pregnancy may show that the level of antibodies in her blood is rising rapidly. If so, the baby is likely to be affected, and early delivery may be necessary. Even so, the baby may become jaundiced and anaemic (see **haemolytic disease of the newborn**) and require an 'exchange transfusion', or change of all its blood, to cure the anaemia, and prevent the serious complication of kernicterus (see **kernicterus**).

Mothers may also be 'sensitized' by being given Rhesus positive blood in error during transfusion, but this is, of course, rare nowadays.

Since 1966, it has been possible to give 'at risk' mothers an injection shortly after delivery to prevent antibody formation. The injection, prepared from the blood of mothers with very high antibody levels, 'soaks up' the challenge offered by the red cells which have leaked through from the baby, before antibody production can be provoked. This discovery is of tremendous significance.

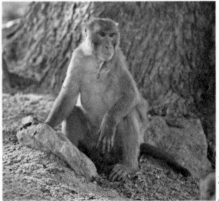

The Rhesus factor is named after Rhesus monkeys, in which it was first discovered.

RHEUMATIC FEVER is a serious and not uncommon condition which occurs most frequently in children between the ages of 6 and 15, though it is also seen in young adults.

Its great importance is that it is liable to cause disease of the heart valves (see **heart disorders**), and at one time was probably the commonest cause of cardiac troubles in those under 60. Nowadays, however, rheumatic fever seems to be encountered less frequently in Western countries than it used to be.

The features of rheumatic fever are as follows: the child usually has a sore throat or bout of tonsillitis, and then recovers from it. About 12 days later, he starts to feel generally unwell. He runs a slight fever (usually around 100°F), and develops joint pain. The characteristic feature of this pain is that it is 'flitting' — that is to say, it starts in one joint, such as the knee, ankle, elbow or wrist, and then, a day or two later, it shifts to another one. The 'flitting' process may go on for a week or more.

There are other less common features of rheumatic fever, including the appearance of nodules under the skin, and also rashes of various kinds.

In a high proportion of cases, the child develops disease of the heart valves during the weeks that he is ill.

It should, however, be stressed that many children are found to have heart disease which must almost certainly have been caused by rheumatic fever, but neither they nor their parents can remember any such episodes. The only other cause of rheumatic heart disease is chorea (see **chorea**).

The cause of rheumatic fever appears likely to be some form of hypersensitivity to a constituent of the germ (the streptococcus) responsible for the original throat infection.

Patients are treated by complete rest in bed, together with aspirin or sometimes steroid drugs, and penicillin to ensure that the infection does not recur. It may be weeks or months before the child is completely better. Following an attack, he will usually have to take penicillin tablets for some years.

RHEUMATISM is a rather vague term which has now almost entirely dropped out of medical use, though rheumatic fever (see **rheumatic fever**) is sometimes referred to as 'acute rheumatism'. Rheumatic fever has, however, no connection with what the average person means by 'rheumatism'. Like the word 'fibrositis', this term is widely used to cover almost any kind of muscle, tendon or ligament strain, or indeed the minor degrees of arthritis which are so common in the elderly.

RHYTHM METHOD is a form of birth control (see **contraception**) based on guessing the 'safe period' of a woman's menstrual cycle. The word 'guessing' is used advisedly, since the method is rather unreliable. It is widely employed, however, partly because it is convenient for people who, for some reason, do not have other means of contraception available, and partly because it is currently the only method to have the full approval of the Roman Catholic Church.

There are various ways of determining the 'safe period'. Although expensive calculators can be bought for this purpose, for most women they are not really necessary.

If a woman has a 26-day menstrual cycle (which is about average), it is likely that her ovulation (the release of the egg from the ovary) will take place just before the half-way point — i.e. about twelve to thirteen days after the start of a 'period'. The day of ovulation may be marked by slight backache. The best indication is given by keeping a regular chart of the morning temperature over several months; the day of ovulation will usually be found to be indicated by a slight increase in the thermometer reading.

The 'danger time', when conception is most liable to occur, is usually reckoned to be the five days before ovulation and the four or five days after it. For a woman with a 26-day cycle, whose ovulation occurs about the 12th or 13th day after the start of a period, this means that the 'danger time' is from the seventh to the 17th day. The 'safe period', which is rather the time when intercourse is

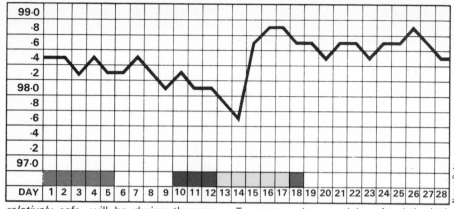

| DAY | 1 | 2 | 3 | 4 | 5 | 6 | 7 | 8 | 9 | 10 | 11 | 12 | 13 | 14 | 15 | 16 | 17 | 18 | 19 | 20 | 21 | 22 | 23 | 24 | 25 | 26 | 27 | 28 |

Norman Barber

relatively safe, will be during the menstrual flow (and, in fact, up to the seventh day after it starts), and during the last nine days before the next menses.

Temperature change and time of ovulation (*yellow*). *Red* indicates period, *green* possible lifetime of sperm (intercourse on day 10), *blue* life of ovum. Days 10–18 are thus the most fertile.

RIBS are the 24 bones (12 on each side) which form a cage enclosing and protecting the cavity of the chest. All of them run from the spine (backbone) forwards and downwards round the side of the chest wall. The topmost seven on each side join with the breastbone or sternum at the front of the chest; the next three on each side are joined to the ribs above by cartilage, but the lowest two are usually 'floating' – that is, their front ends are free and unattached.

Fractures of the ribs are painful but rarely serious (except where violent injuries cause the condition of 'stove-in chest'). Most rib fractures require only strapping, and heal within five weeks or so.

RICKETS is a disorder in which a child's bones become abnormally soft, due to a deficiency of vitamin D.

Rickets usually but not invariably occurs between the ages of six months and two years. The first symptoms are sometimes failure to sit up or stand at the expected age; the baby may be excessively fretful, and it may be noted that his limbs are abnormally flexible at the joints.

If the child is not yet crawling at the time of onset of the disease, the softening of bone is most likely to be obvious through the development of skull and rib deformities. At the crawling stage,

rickets produces bending of the bones of the baby's arms. Once he is standing, however, the weight of his body will produce very obvious bending of the long bones of the legs. Unless prompt treatment is given, the deformity may become permanent.

The ordinary type of rickets is due to lack of vitamin D in the diet. This vitamin is essential for the body to make proper use of calcium and phosphorus – two of the most important constituents of bone. Vitamin D is normally obtained either in the diet or from a chemical reaction which takes place under the skin when the sun shines on it.

Nowadays, in many developed countries, vitamin D is added to all types of dried milk; breast-milk and ordinary cow's milk also contain a variable quantity, which is usually lower in the winter. However, in cloudy climates (and particularly in industrial countries) very little sunshine may get through a child's skin; this is a particular problem in coloured children, whose pigment tends to keep the sun out.

Many doctors recommend, therefore, that all infants should have vitamin D supplements from about the age of three months to two years: this may be given in the form of cod liver oil or halibut liver oil, but it is best to take the doctor's advice about this.

326

RICKETTSIAE are a group of micro-organisms. They have nothing to do with the disease called rickets, but are called after a Dr Ricketts, who (like a number of other researchers into these organisms) died as a result of infection by them. Until quite recently, the rickettsial disorders were among the great scourges of mankind. Thanks to the research of Ricketts and others like him, and the introduction of broad-spectrum antibiotics and powerful insecticides, this is no longer so. The common rickettsial diseases include the four major types of typhus, African tick fever, trench fever, Q fever, and Rocky Mountain spotted fever. Apart from Q fever (see **Q fever**), the germs of all these illnesses are passed on to Man by ticks, lice, mites and fleas.

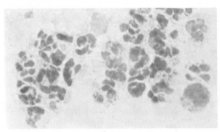

Exudate from the lung in a case of Typhus, stained to show Rickettsia organisms (purple).

C. James Webb

RINGWORM is a general name given to certain fungal disorders of the skin. Usually, ringworm is classified according to the area of the body it affects.

Ringworm of the scalp (*Tinea capitis*) used to be a common childhood condition, but seems to be less frequently encountered in developed countries nowadays. The characteristic appearance of scalp ringworm is a small area of baldness, on which the hairs have actually broken off. The scalp itself is reddened and scaly. The diagnosis can be confirmed by examining the child's head under ultra-violet light, when the affected area is seen to glow. This form needs medical care.

Ringworm of the feet (*Tinea pedis*), is dealt with under the heading **athlete's foot**. Like ringworm of the crutch area (*Tinea cruris*) and ringworm of the beard area (*Tinea barbae*) it can usually be readily dealt with by one of the modern

anti-ringworm preparations available at the chemist's. If such preparations do not cure it, a doctor should be consulted.

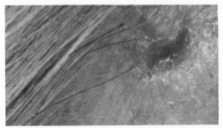

A small rodent ulcer of the skin of the forehead. Surgical removal is usually advised.

RODENT ULCER is the term applied to a very common type of skin growth, medically known as a basal cell carcinoma, which tends to occur on the cheek or nose. Although, left unchecked, many of these growths would prove immensely destructive, and even fatal, they can almost invariably be successfully removed, producing a complete cure of the condition.

RORSCHACH TEST is a simple method of psychiatric investigation. The patient is shown an ink-blot of the type readily made by folding a piece of paper with a blob of ink on it. He is asked to discuss the shapes he sees there, and from the ideas which he expresses certain conclusions about his personality can be drawn.

ROUNDWORMS are a class of parasitic worms (see **parasites**). They include the threadworm (see **threadworms**), the hookworm (see **hookworms**), the whipworm, and the common roundworm, *Ascaris lumbricoides*.

Ascaris lumbricoides tends to occur in rural areas of the world, where sanitary arrangements are poor. Infected people who have no proper toilet arrangements may deposit roundworm eggs in the soil near dwellings when opening their bowels. These eggs hatch into the form called 'larvae' if the earth is warm and moist. Particularly where the soil is cultivated, it is easy for other people to transfer the larvae to their mouths or their hands. Once inside the body, the larvae find their way to the lungs and may produce pneumonia. In the intestines, the adult worms can cause abdominal pain and other symptoms. Drug therapy is usually effective.

RUBELLA – see **German measles**.

RUPTURE is the popular term for hernias of the groin region. These may be divided into two groups – femoral and inguinal – according to their exact anatomical site.

Femoral hernias are less common than inguinal ones. They are more likely to occur in women than in men. The characteristic swelling is just on the surface of the topmost part of the thigh rather than on the trunk. It occurs because a small part of the abdominal wall bulges down a minute tunnel which runs alongside two major blood vessels passing from the abdominal cavity to the thigh.

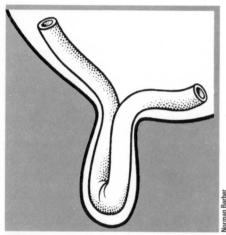

Diagram to show how a loop of intestine may be pushed outwards to fill a hernial sac.

A femoral hernia cannot, under any circumstances, be controlled with a truss; furthermore, this type of rupture is particularly likely to undergo strangulation. This complication, in which the blood supply to the hernia is cut off, with imminent risk of gangrene, is so dangerous that, wherever possible, all femoral hernias should be repaired by operation.

In inguinal hernias, on the other hand, the swelling originates slightly higher up, on the lowest part of the abdominal wall itself. This type of rupture is commoner

in men than in women. It occurs in two forms with different causes.

The first is an indirect, or oblique, hernia, in which the bulging hernial sac passes down the inguinal canal (the passage through which the spermatic cord runs upward from the testicle to enter the body). The hernia may even enter the scrotum. Most doctors think that such ruptures are due to the presence of a pre-formed sac, and not to any kind of strain.

The second form of inguinal hernia is called direct, and is less common than the indirect form. It is also smaller, as a rule, than the average indirect hernia, and tends to bulge outward, never running inward and downward into the scrotum. This type of rupture *can* be associated with strain.

All inguinal hernias are best treated by operation, but there are certain circumstances where a truss is advisable. These are (a) in very young infants, and (b) when an adult's health makes it seem doubtful that he would withstand an operation. However, it is *never* wise to send for a mail-order truss without medical advice, as many people do: it is absolutely essential that a doctor examines the rupture and advises on the best course.

Complications of ruptures: *strangulation*, which may occur with any type of hernia, has been mentioned above; *irreducible hernias* are those which will not 'go back' – although not in itself serious, this predisposes to strangulation; *obstruction of the bowel* is common when a loop of bowel is present in the hernial sac and the contents dammed back.

Contrary to widespread popular belief, ruptures have no connection at all with sexual function. This misunderstanding probably arose originally because in elderly men suffering from inguinal hernias, the abdominal musculature is sometimes so weak that it is very difficult to close the gap in the abdominal wall effectively.

Accordingly, it becomes necessary to remove the spermatic cord, which runs through this gap, and this means taking away the testicle on that side as well. This is not done without asking the patient's permission first, and, in any case, the removal of only one testicle has no effect on sexual activity.

SACCHARIN is a coal-tar derivative with a sweet taste. Although this taste is very far from being that of sugar, saccharin is nonetheless an acceptable sugar substitute for many people. It is not known to have any dangerous side-effects, and may safely be used by diabetics.

SADISM is a perversion (see **perversions**) in which the affected person cannot achieve sexual satisfaction except by inflicting cruelty on others. It derives its name from the Marquis de Sade, a deranged French aristocrat whose novels depicted scenes of revolting cruelty. Sadism is, contrary to popular belief, very often associated with masochism (see **masochism**), and flagellation — that is to say, the sufferer enjoys not only giving, but receiving pain. Sadists are very rarely dangerous, but they do need psychiatric help, if they can be persuaded to accept it.

'SAFE PERIOD' — see **rhythm method**.

ST ANTHONY'S FIRE is an old term which, owing to confusion, has been widely applied to both erysipelas (see **erysipelas**) and ergotism (see **ergotism**).

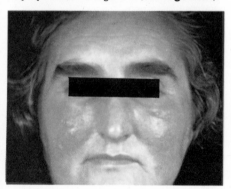

St Anthony's fire was one of the old terms given to intense inflammation of the skin in erysipelas.

ST VITUS' DANCE is the older name for rheumatic chorea, the curious attack of writhing of the limbs that is most commonly seen in children in the 10–14 age group. In fact, the term was first applied to the outbreaks of 'dancing mania' which were common in the Middle Ages; however, these outbreaks were almost certainly due to ergotism, or St Anthony's fire (see **ergotism**).

Chorea is unpleasant for the child, who usually has to stay in hospital for some weeks. It may be followed by valvular heart disease of the same kind which occurs after rheumatic fever.

SALICYLATES are a group of compounds which are closely related to aspirin (acetylsalicylic acid). First employed in the form of extract of willow-bark (which had a great reputation for the treatment of various kinds of arthritis and 'rheumatism'), salicylates are still extremely useful in medicine, thanks to their effects of relieving pain and diminishing fever.

SALIVA is spittle, the secretion of the salivary glands (see **salivary glands**). It is produced constantly by these glands, so that we have to swallow small quantities every minute or two. In response to the stimulus of chewing, however, the flow of saliva is greatly increased. It mixes with the food, and plays an important part in its digestion, mainly because it contains

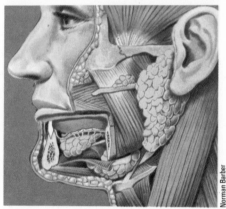

Norman Barber

The side of the face dissected to show the position of the salivary glands and their ducts.

an enzyme, called ptyalin, which breaks down starch into sugars.

SALIVARY GLANDS are the glands which secrete saliva (see **saliva**) into the mouth. There are six of these glands, three on each side. The two sub-lingual glands and the two sub-mandibular glands lie under the floor of the mouth, while the parotid glands (see **parotid**) lie just in front of each ear; these last are the glands which most commonly swell up during an attack of mumps (see **mumps**).

SALMONELLAE are bacteria (see **bacteria**) which have a characteristic fish-like appearance under the microscope (the word 'salmonellae' means 'little salmon'). Various species of these germs cause such diseases as typhoid fever, paratyphoid fever, food poisoning and gastro-enteritis. Most of them are susceptible to antibiotics, but some of

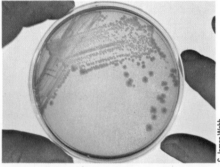

A culture of the bacteria known as Salmonella, on a specially prepared plate of gelatin medium.

them have in recent years shown a disturbing tendency to develop resistance and even to pass it on to other species of bacteria.

SALPINGITIS is inflammation of the Fallopian tubes (see **Fallopian tubes**), each of which runs from the region of the ovary to the womb. Almost invariably, such inflammation is due to infection, and infection may occur following childbirth or abortion (miscarriage), or as a result of tuberculosis or gonorrhoea. Occasionally, germs may infect the tube from some other organ in the body, such as an inflamed appendix.

Acute salpingitis is characterized by quite severe lower abdominal pain (either on one side or both, depending on whether both tubes are inflamed or not). There is fever of over 101°F, and there may be a little vaginal discharge. Often, the periods

330

have been irregular, or in some other way abnormal. Treatment will involve the administration of antibiotics in hospital; sometimes an operation may be needed.

Chronic salpingitis is likely to be associated with recurrent pelvic pain, backache and period pain. There may be persistent low-grade fever, disturbances of the periods, infertility (due to blockage of the tubes) and general ill-health. Careful gynaecological investigation is needed to determine the cause of the condition.

SALT, or, to be more exact, common salt, is sodium chloride, one of the most common of all chemical compounds, and one which is vital to life. It has been speculated that this may be because, long ago, primitive living things may have had body fluids composed largely of sea-water. Even today, the blood and many other fluids of the body (e.g. tears) are salty. The two constituents of common salt, sodium and chloride 'ions', are essential to the chemical balance of the body. Without them we cannot survive, and, in situations where the body loses a lot of either constituent (e.g. in excessive sweating, during heat stroke) life may very rapidly become threatened.

SAL VOLATILE is a mixture containing ammonia. It was once widely used in medicine, particularly as a 'remedy' for faints, since its pungent fumes rapidly woke up anyone who was semi-conscious. It is now hardly ever employed for this or any other purpose.

SARCOIDOSIS, or sarcoid, is a not uncommon disease which affects various systems of the body, but particularly the lungs. The cause of sarcoidosis is unknown. It runs a chronic but benign course, and although it may produce some fibrosis of the lungs over a period of many years, with some consequent deterioration in lung function, it is never life-threatening. Apart from its effects on the lung, it may produce an inflammation of the eyes and salivary glands.

Treatment with steroid drugs (see **steroids**) may be helpful although not producing a true cure.

SCABIES, or 'the itch', is a highly contagious skin disease caused by a small parasite called *Sarcoptes scabiei*. This tiny mite occurs very commonly among poor and over-crowded populations; it can be passed on by the merest bodily contact – even by standing next to an infected person on a train.

The chief symptom is an almost intolerable itching which is made worse by warmth. This most commonly occurs first of all on the inner surface of the wrist, or between the fingers. Within a day or two, small red inflamed areas can be detected on the skin. On close inspection, these can be seen to be the short burrows into which the female mite has crawled to lay her eggs. Scratching, which is more or less unavoidable (except to those with unusual self-control), makes the inflammation worse, so that the burrows become raised and lumpy; they may also become infected with germs.

Rapid treatment is essential, before the patient passes the disease on to others. Usually, he is prescribed treatment with benzyl benzoate, which must be applied to the whole body from the neck downwards. The doctor will give advice about laundering of clothes and bed linen. Although the parasites may all be killed in the first 24 to 48 hours, the itch itself may persist for up to a fortnight.

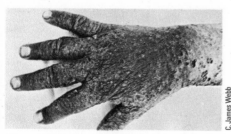

The appearance of the wrist in severe infection with scabies – itching, sore and scaling.

SCALDS are essentially burns caused by moist heat, such as hot water or steam. Steam tends to produce particularly severe scalding, because it has far more intrinsic (latent) heat than water at a temperature only a few degrees lower.

As is the case with a burn, there is no point in putting any home remedy on a scald; this cannot make things better, and even makes them worse. If the scalded area is small, it should either be left alone or protected with an adhesive dressing. If it is large, or if extensive blistering develops, then the area should be covered with a dressing (e.g. a freshly-laundered handkerchief), and the patient should consult a doctor. Blisters should never be opened except by a doctor, as infection may result. (This also applies to 'friction' blisters – e.g. on the feet, from walking long distances.)

SCALP is the covering of the top part of the skull. It consists of skin, fat, and fibrous tissue continuous with the scalp muscles.

SCALPEL is a type of surgical knife.

SCAPULA is the shoulder blade, the flat, triangular bone which, with the upper bone of the arm (the humerus), forms the shoulder joint.

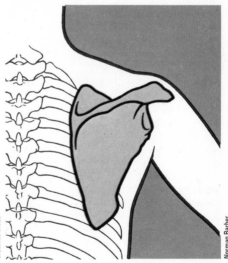

The position of the shoulder blade, or scapula, in the back. It is deeply imbedded in muscle.

SCAR is the visible remnant of an injury to the skin or a surgical incision. It contains tough, fibrous tissue. Fortunately, the vast majority of all scars heal well and cause little if any disfigurement. There may, however, be problems if the original wound was extensive, dirty or infected, or if it was caused by a large burn or scald. In

331

addition, some people develop an unusual type of raised, ugly-looking scar tissue called 'keloid'. This is particularly common in coloured people. As a rule most disfiguring scars can nowadays be removed by plastic surgery.

SCARLET FEVER, or scarlatina, is a childhood disease caused by a *Streptococcus* germ (see **Streptococci**). A century ago, it was regarded as one of the major killers of children, but nowadays it seems, in some way, to have changed its nature, so that, in most western countries, it consists of no more than a sore throat and a trivial rash in the vast majority of cases of people affected.

Scarlet fever is commonest between the ages of 3 and 12, and is rare in adult life. The incubation period is less than a week. The first symptoms are those of sore throat (or tonsillitis, if the child still has his tonsils); younger children rarely actually complain that their throats are sore, but merely vomit and develop a fever of about 102°F to 104°F. The glands at the side of the neck are likely to be enlarged, as is the case with any childhood throat infection.

On the second day of the illness, a toxin released by the germs produces a characteristic red rash on the face and body. The area around the mouth is not affected, and looks pale in comparison. After some days, the rash begins to flake off, and the child starts to get better.

Complications are uncommon except in certain areas of the world (notably eastern Europe). The most important one is a form of nephritis (see **nephritis**), and the child's urine should therefore be carefully checked in the laboratory a week or two after recovery, for signs of this condition. As is the case with streptococcal throat infections, rheumatic fever (see **rheumatic fever**) can sometimes follow about 12 days after the onset of infection.

Treatment of scarlet fever consists in giving penicillin (though it should be mentioned that not all doctors agree that this is necessary in very mild cases). Severe cases, which are rare, will need hospitalization and treatment with an antitoxin preparation.

332

SCHISTOSOMIASIS – see **Bilharzia**.

SCHIZOPHRENIA is a common form of mental illness in which there is disintegration of the personality. Owing to a complete misunderstanding of the term, schizophrenia is frequently interpreted as meaning 'split personality' or 'dual personality', meaning that the sufferer leads a 'Dr Jekyll and Mr Hyde' existence. This is completely and utterly wrong.

Schizophrenia is said to affect anything between 3 and 9 per 1000 of the population of Western countries. Its cause remains unknown, though there may be a hereditary factor. Three-quarters of all cases develop between the ages of 15 and 25.

In *simple schizophrenia*, the adolescent sufferer is usually a quiet, solitary sort of person who indulges a great deal in daydreaming, takes little or no interest in the world, and shows very little evidence of any emotion whatever. Over a period of a few years, he gradually becomes more and more withdrawn into himself until he becomes almost completely inactive.

In *hebephrenia*, the patient is also fairly young. He is less of a day-dreamer than the simple schizophrenic, but may tend instead to wrap himself up in the study of strange ideas or odd cults. Eventually, he develops hallucinations or ideas of persecution. As is the case with all types of schizophrenia, the blunting of his emotions is very marked.

Catatonic schizophrenia is characterized by episodes in which the patient becomes speechless and immobile, often remaining fixed in odd postures for hours at a time. In between these attacks, he may be wildly excited and incoherent.

Paranoid schizophrenia has many of the features of paranoia (see **paranoia**), but with the characteristic lack of emotion and withdrawal seen in all types of schizophrenia.

True schizophrenia cannot be *cured* at present. However, the advent of new tranquillizing drugs and new techniques of psychotherapy has improved the outlook, and many patients can now lead reasonably adequate lives outside a mental hospital for long periods.

SCIATICA is pain running from the buttock down the back of the leg, in the distribution of the sciatic nerve. In the young or middle-aged, such pain is likely to be due to pressure on the roots of the sciatic nerve by a prolapsed ('slipped') disc. In older people, pressure is often caused by the type of arthritis associated with degenerative changes in the spine. A much less common cause is pressure due to a tumour, either benign or malignant.

In cases of sciatica the doctor may arrange an X-ray of the lower part of the spine, and treat the condition according to its cause.

SCLERODERMA is one of the collagen diseases (see **collagen diseases**). It exists in more than one form, but its characteristic feature is curious thickening of the skin. In severe cases, the patient may suffer from Raynaud's phenomenon (see under **Raynaud's disease**), and changes in the intestinal tract which parallel those occurring in the skin.

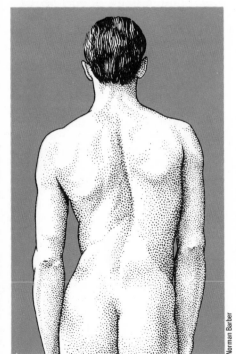

Typical appearance of a patient with the spinal abnormality known as scoliosis.

SCOLIOSIS is a sideways twist of the spine. Minor degrees of this condition are common and harmless, and most people with slight scoliosis are quite unaware of it.

SCROFULA is an old and rather vague term which is usually understood to have meant tuberculosis of the lymph glands, or 'king's evil'.

SCROTUM is the pouch which contains the testicles (see **testicles**). These glands do not produce sperms when at the temperature of the interior of the body, and so, during life in the womb, they descend into the scrotum, where the temperature is slightly lower, but where they are still afforded some protection by the walls of the scrotal sac.

The scrotum is developed from the same tissue that goes to form the labia majora (see **labia**) in the female.

SCURVY is a deficiency disease caused by lack of vitamin C, an essential constituent of human diet found in fresh fruit and green vegetables. In days gone by, scurvy was very common in sailors on long voyages, until the proof by a British naval surgeon named James Lynd that lemon juice or limes could prevent it.

Nowadays, scurvy among adults is confined to occasional cases among old people who, through poverty or ill-health, live only on bread and margarine and cups of tea. The average adult gets plenty of vitamin C in his diet, and has no need of vitamin supplements.

Among young children, however, the position is different. Cow's milk usually contains very little vitamin C, nor is there a great deal in breast milk. This is why, in Great Britain and certain other countries, free orange juice is provided for all infants. It is important not to boil the juice, as this will destroy the vitamin.

Scurvy usually makes its appearance between the ages of 6 and 18 months. The first symptom is usually severe pain in the bones of the legs, due to bleeding under the membrane (the periosteum) which covers the bone. This may be followed by bleeding and swelling in the region of the gums. The occurrence of

333

small lumps on the ribs, anaemia, bleeding in the urine, and softening of the bones are later developments.

Fortunately, the response to treatment with vitamin C is swift. Only if the disease has been neglected for a long time will the child fail to recover completely. (See also **deficiency diseases**.)

SEA SICKNESS is a very common phenomenon which is rather similar to other types of motion sickness. Although there is some psychological element (worry and apprehension about being sick making things considerably worse), the basic cause is the effect which a persistent up-and-down motion has on the body's balancing mechanisms – particularly the fluid-filled canals of the inner ear (see **ear**). Antihistamines and other drugs can be used to damp down the disturbance in these mechanisms; at the same time, they sedate the patient slightly, and thus reduce his apprehension. Continued exposure to the type of motion experienced on a ship gradually results in resistance to sea sickness, so that experienced sailors rarely suffer it except in very bad weather.

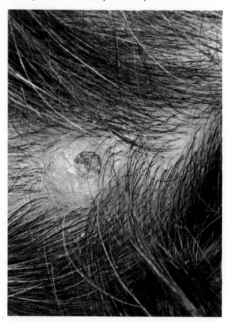

A sebaceous cyst of the scalp, due to an accumulation of sebaceous material in the skin.

SEBACEOUS means 'oily'. Sebaceous glands are found throughout the skin, on to which they secrete an oily material. Over-production of this substance is associated with acne. Sebaceous cysts are swellings, usually seen on the skin of the head; they are full of greasy material. While unsightly in appearance, they are harmless unless they become infected. However, it is usually considered better to remove them, which can readily be done by a very minor operation under local anaesthesia, leaving usually only a small scar usually much preferable to the original swelling.

SECRETION means the substance produced by a gland or group of glands.

SEDATIVES are drugs given to calm a patient. In the early part of this century, bromides were the most widely used sedative drugs, but these are now rarely employed. They were succeeded by members of the barbiturate group, such as phenobarbitone, but it is now being widely realized that these drugs carry the risk of habituation, so that there is now a tendency to use mild tranquillizers (see **tranquillizers**) instead.

SEMEN is seminal fluid, the liquid which is ejaculated from the penis when a man reaches a sexual climax (see **climax**). Most of it is produced by the testicles (see **testicles**), but some comes from the prostate gland (see **prostate**). Each cubic centimetre of semen contains a hundred million sperms or more.

SEMILUNAR CARTILAGES are the two cartilages which lie within the knee joint, and which are so readily damaged by strains, especially during sporting activities. These common injuries are discussed under the heading **knee**.

SENNA is a laxative (see **laxatives**). It is frequently used as a home remedy.

Senna may produce colicky abdominal pain and discolour the urine. It is not recommended for nursing mothers. As is the case with any other laxative, it is better not to take it regularly, or to give it in cases of abdominal pain.

SEPTICAEMIA, sometimes referred to as 'blood poisoning', is a fortunately uncommon condition in which bacteria (see **bacteria**) not only enter the blood stream, but multiply within it. Since the rate at which bacteria can reproduce is quite phenomenal, this is a very serious situation, and if prompt action is not taken, infection may rapidly spread to many parts of the body. Fortunately, with the advent of the antibiotics, the outlook has improved out of all recognition. By taking a specimen of blood and 'culturing' it, the doctor can find out in a fairly short time which germ is responsible and which antibiotic is most suitable to combat it.

SERUM is a pale yellow fluid which makes up most of the fluid content of blood.

Blood consists of red cells (erythrocytes) and plasma (see **plasma**). If fibrin, a substance necessary for clotting to take place, is removed from plasma, the remaining fluid is the serum.

Serum contains various chemicals and, in particular, antibodies (see **antibodies**), which are capable of giving protection against specific diseases to which the individual's serum has been 'sensitized'. For this reason, it is possible to give a person *short-term* protection against some infections by injecting him with serum from a horse which has been made immune to the disease in question. This type of protection is called passive artificial immunity (see under **immunity**). The method is used, for instance, in the prevention of tetanus (lockjaw), where a person has not already obtained the much preferable active artificial immunity (see under **immunity**). Serum used in this way has certain dangers. Serum sickness is a condition which develops one to two weeks after administration; its features are fever, joint pains, an urticaria-like rash, and sometimes kidney damage. Much more rarely, a patient collapses in anaphylactic shock (see **anaphylactic shock**) very shortly after an injection of serum. For these reasons, everyone should keep their immunity against such diseases as tetanus up to date, so that serum injections will not be necessary.

SEX EDUCATION is one of the most essential aspects of any child's proper development. Even though attitudes have changed radically in the last 20 or 30 years, it still remains an aspect that is all too often neglected. There are many parents who are too embarrassed to tell their children 'the facts of life'; for this, they cannot be blamed, because their embarrassment stems merely from the attitude of their own parents. However, it is perfectly easy to give a child a suitable book to read, or to ask the school biology teacher's help.

Unfortunately, there are still many people who are unwilling to take such action. Often, parents rationalize their embarrassment in the most illogical ways, claiming that it is 'bad' for a child to know about reproduction, that the fantasies of gooseberry bushes and the stork are much more 'beautiful' than the truth, or (incredibly enough) that it is healthiest for a child to learn about sex from 'dirty' stories told by his playmates. A recent survey in the United States showed that many parents thought that sex education in schools was part of a subtle communist plot to undermine Western morals.

The best way to avoid embarrassment with a child is to answer *all* his questions fully and frankly right from the start, long before he himself has had a chance to get hold of the idea that sex organs are any-

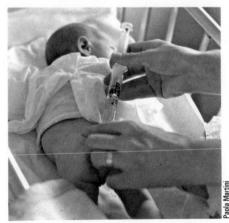

Paola Martini

A child receiving an injection of serum to confer short-term immunity with antibodies.

thing to be embarrassed about. If his mother or a friend of the parents becomes pregnant, it is helpful to explain that she 'has a baby in her tummy'. Children of three or even two years of age will accept this quite naturally. By the time he goes to school, there is no reason why a child should not have a basic understanding of how a baby is made, and where he came from. The sex education provided by an increasing number of schools nowadays can add to this knowledge.

Both boys and girls will need a good deal more information when they are aged 10 to 12 in order to prepare them for puberty (see **puberty**). A mother may find that telling her daughter about menstruation is quite straightforward, but it may be more difficult to provide either a boy or a girl with more detailed information about the sort of problems likely to be encountered in adolescence, particularly as some parents know very little of such matters themselves. Here again, the child's school may be helpful; if not, then once again an informative book will be of value.

It is unfortunately true that a considerable proportion of the population suffer from what are often called sexual 'hang-ups', while far more are less than adequate in this aspect of their married lives. There is little doubt that the cause of many of these problems is sheer ignorance, often combined with distorted ideas about sex picked up in childhood. Our own relatively enlightened generation is probably less troubled in this respect than previous ones were, but we owe it to our children's generation to ensure that they are not burdened by the difficulties that result from a lack of proper education about sex.

SEXUAL SELECTION is, like natural selection, a mechanism which enables evolution (or gradual improvement of living things) to take place. The term was coined by Charles Darwin, the father of the theory of evolution. When he published his great work, *The Origin of Species*, in 1859, he pointed out that it was principally through natural selection (or the survival of the fittest) that Man, and other species, gradually evolved over very long periods of time.

He realized that this was not the whole story, however, and in due course, he published his theory of sexual selection. Basically, this states that human beings (and, of course, other animals) who are sexually attractive are more likely to produce offspring, and pass on their own characteristics to them. In part, of course, this means that, in very general terms, people who appear fit and healthy are more likely to marry and have children than are people who do not – with obvious benefit to the human race. In addition, people with well-developed secondary sexual characteristics (e.g. girls with large bosoms and wide hips – both of which are not only attractive, but useful assets for motherhood) are more likely to reproduce, and pass these characteristics on.

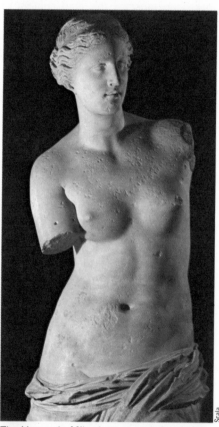

The Venus de Milo, long regarded as being a model of perfect female proportions. Well-developed secondary sexual characteristics are a distinct practical asset to motherhood.

336

SHINGLES – see **herpes zoster.**

SHOCK is a rather ambiguous term which has a variety of different meanings in medicine, depending on the context in which it is used.

The word is, for instance, widely employed to describe the state of emotional upset seen in many people who have been involved in a serious accident but who have not themselves been injured. Such people usually regain their normal equilibrium within an hour or two.

Doctors, however, tend as a rule to confine the use of the word 'shock' to circumstances in which there is a drastic physical response (usually involving extensive upset of the circulatory system) to some severe stimulus, such as a large haemorrhage, a crushing injury, a violent blow to the body, a massive allergic reaction, the influx of large numbers of bacteria into the blood-stream, overdoses of certain drugs, gross injury to the brain or spinal cord, or extensive heart muscle damage due to 'coronary thrombosis'.

In practice, most of these conditions produce a rather similar picture: the patient is likely to be very pale, with a cold, moist skin, a fast and 'thready' pulse, and a low blood pressure.

The treatment which a doctor will apply depends on the cause of this condition (for instance, if it is due to severe haemorrhage, he will replace the lost fluid as rapidly as is practicable by means of an intra-venous 'drip'). As far as the non-medical person is concerned, however, there are only a few points to remember when faced with a 'shocked' person.

First, disregard all advice given in old first aid manuals, etc., regarding giving the patient hot, sweet tea or applying hot water bottles. Give *nothing* whatsoever by mouth. Make sure the patient lies flat, preferably with his feet a little raised. If he complains of cold, do no more than cover him with a blanket or coat. Control any severe bleeding by the methods described under the heading bleeding. If the patient becomes unconscious, turn him on his side and make sure he can breathe (see also **first aid**).

SHORT-SIGHTEDNESS, or myopia, is a common condition in which the patient finds it difficult to see objects which are at a distance from him, though his near vision is normal, or even sometimes better than average. The cause is unknown and there is no cure. Attempts at improving the vision by exercises (a method popularized by Aldous Huxley) do not seem to be effective. For the time being, short-sighted people have to rely on glasses or contact lenses. However, it would be surprising if, in the future, medical science did not find a way of altering the shape of the eyeball or the power of accommodation of the lens in order to produce a cure for this condition.

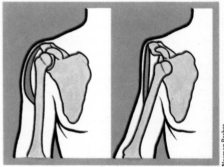

Norman Barber

The normal shoulder contour *left*, and the 'squareness' produced by dislocation *right*.

SHOULDER is the joint formed by the shoulder-blade, or scapula (see **scapula**), and the upper bone of the arm, or humerus. It is a 'ball-and-socket' joint, and is rather liable to dislocation. When this happens, it is important that the patient's shoulder be left alone until he is seen by a doctor. All too often, enthusiastic but unskilled attempts are made to 'reduce' the dislocation. As a rule, the result is increased pain for the patient, with consequent muscle spasm, hence making it more difficult subsequently for the doctor to replace the bone in its socket. Furthermore, there may be damage to the delicate structures which surround the shoulder joint.

The only exception to this general rule of non-interference occurs when a shoulder joint is so 'loose' that the patient himself has become quite used to 'popping it in' with no trouble at all.

337

In cases of recurrent dislocation, it is usually advisable to operate on the shoulder joint.

SIAMESE TWINS are identical twins whose bodies are joined together at some point. The name derives from the celebrated Chang and Ong (or Eng) Bunker, who were born in Siam in 1811. They were joined together at the lower end of the chest. Despite this, they were both healthy, and were able to make a career with P. T. Barnum's circus. Eventually, they married a pair of English sisters, the Misses Sarah and Adelaide Yates, and fathered 22 children between them. They died within a few hours of each other at the age of 64.

The occurrence of Siamese twins is very uncommon. Where there is only a narrow 'bridge' of connecting tissue, containing no vital structures, surgical separation is very easy. Unfortunately, however, it often happens that the twins may share some essential structures, such as the liver, or the blood vessels supplying their brains. Where this is the case, it is unlikely that both twins will survive.

SICKLE CELL ANAEMIA is a type of haemolytic anaemia (see **haemolytic anaemias**) which occurs mainly in people of West Indian or African extraction. It is characterized by the occurrence of sickle-shaped red cells in the blood.

In most people, the blood pigment haemoglobin (see **haemoglobin**) is inherited as a result of two genes (see **genes**), one from the father and one from the mother; these are usually represented by the letters 'AA'.

However, in the West Indies and the United States, for example, about 10 per cent of the coloured population have a type of haemoglobin which may be represented by the letters 'AS'. In fact, this appears to do them no harm at all, except that a small proportion of people with this 'sickling trait' tend at times to have episodes of bleeding in the urine.

However, where two 'AS' people marry, some of their children may have haemoglobin of a type called 'SS'. Such children have sickle cell anaemia, the incidence of

which is about 2 or 3 per thousand among West Indians. The features of the disorder are (a) anaemia (see **anaemia**), (b) growth stunting, (c) jaundice, and (d) attacks of pain, especially in the joints, which may wrongly suggest a diagnosis of rheumatic fever or other conditions.

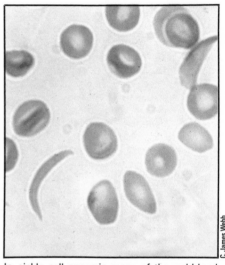

In sickle cell anaemia many of the red blood cells collapse into typical crescent shapes.

SIDE EFFECTS are unwanted effects of drugs. Despite claims to the contrary, it is probably true that *no* effective drug is entirely free from such effects, though in the case of new preparations, it may be some years before they become apparent. Wherever possible, side-effects are listed in this dictionary under the names of specific drugs.

SIGHT – see **eye**.

SILICOSIS is a form of chronic lung disorder caused by inhalation of silica dust. It is common among people who work in the brick-making industry, among potters and foundry-men, and also among miners who drill rock.

There are a number of conditions caused by the long-term inhalation of various kinds of dust, including silicosis, asbestosis, byssinosis, and coal-worker's pneumoconiosis; they are all dealt with under the heading **pneumoconiosis**.

338

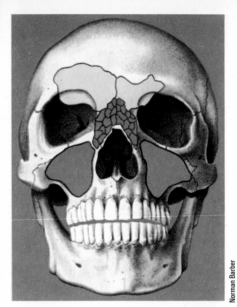

The position of the sinuses, or air-cavities, within the skull. Frontal, yellow; maxillary, green; ethmoidal, blue; the sphenoidal sinuses are deeper, behind and above the nasal cavity.

Norman Barber

SINUS means a narrow cavity or channel.

Artificially-produced sinuses (i.e. those caused by disease) are uncommon; sinuses of this type opening on to the skin may be due to an abscess within the body.

The naturally-occurring sinuses include the air sinuses, or air cavities, of the head, which so often cause trouble by becoming inflamed, in the condition known as sinusitis. Apart from the mastoid air cells (see **mastoid**), all the air cavities of the head are in close relation to the passages of the nose and drain into it. They consist of the following: (a) the frontal sinuses (one of which lies just above each eyebrow, within the bone that makes up the forehead); (b) the maxillary sinuses (one of which lies just below each eye, within the bone of the upper jaw); (c) the ethmoidal sinuses (a number of small cavities lying between the inner end of the eye and the bridge of the nose); and (d) the sphenoidal sinuses (which lie, one on each side, above and behind the cavity of the nose).

Sinusitis is due to germs infecting these cavities; as a result the lining membranes of the sinuses become inflamed and swollen, so that the narrow exit to the nose is blocked. The cavity may then fill with pus under pressure. The symptoms of sinusitis are therefore pain, tenderness over one of the sites, and fever, often following a head cold. Treatment normally consists of antibiotics, together with nasal drops to try to open up the blocked sinuses. Sometimes a 'wash-out' of the cavities via the nose may be necessary; in certain cases of recurrent sinus infection, an operation is required.

SKELETON means the hard supporting and protective tissue of the body, made up of bone (see **bones**) and cartilage (see **cartilage**).

SKIN is the tissue which covers almost all of the outer surface of the body. It consists basically of two parts – the outer *epidermis*, and the inner *dermis*.

The epidermis is thin, and is made up of several layers of cells, the outermost of which bear the brunt of the wear and tear of everyday life, and are thus continually being shed or rubbed off, and replaced. The innermost layer of the epidermis contains the pigment melanin (see **melanin**), which gives skin its colour.

The dermis is much thicker than the epidermis, being as much as an eighth of an inch deep in places. It contains nerves, blood vessels, sweat and sebaceous glands and hair-roots.

SKIN DISEASES – see **acne, athlete's foot, barber's itch, bed sores, birthmarks, boil, carbuncle, chafing, DLE, dermatitis, dhobie's itch, eczema, erysipelas, erythema ab igne, erythema nodosum, herpes simplex, herpes zoster, lupus vulgaris, lupus erythematosus, melanoma, pellagra, pimples, pink disease, psoriasis, ringworm, rodent ulcer, scabies, scleroderma, urticaria, urticaria pigmentosa, vitiligo** and **warts**.

SKULL is the name given to the 22 bones which together form a protective case for the brain, and also the skeletal support of the face.

Fractures of the skull are quite common.

339

Though such an injury may not always be a serious matter, it invariably necessitates careful observation of the patient in hospital, in case damage has been done to underlying structures, such as the brain or its blood vessels. This type of fracture can be caused quite easily, and anyone who sustains a heavy blow to the head (especially one producing even momentary unconsciousness) should always go to hospital for a check-up and an X-ray. (See also **head injuries**.)

SLEEP seems to be an absolute essential for all human beings, though it is claimed that there are one or two people in the world who can manage entirely without it. If this is so (and there is no medical evidence to prove that it is), then probably such people enter a trance-like state which is very near to sleep when they are resting. For most of us, however, symptoms of tiredness begin to come on after 16 to 20 hours without sleep. The body can readjust itself, and after 24 to 30 hours without sleeping, many people still feel quite wide awake. After 36 hours, however, efficiency begins to fall off badly. Beyond 48 hours (which means foregoing sleep for 2 nights in a row), it becomes increasingly difficult to think clearly and rationally. By 60 hours, collapse is usually imminent, and those who have managed to stay awake longer usually find that they are developing hallucinations.

These hallucinations probably take the place of dreams, which are almost certainly a necessity for the well-being of the human mind. This subject is discussed further under the heading **dreams,** as are certain other aspects of sleep.

Inability to sleep, or insomnia, is common. It is usually related to worry or depression (see **depression**), and, in fact, persistent waking in the small hours with subsequent insomnia is often an important feature of the latter condition.

Very mild cases of insomnia are not usually treated with sleeping pills. A satisfying meal an hour or two before going to bed, together with a hot drink at bedtime, or (particularly in the elderly) a 'nightcap' of spirits or sherry, will usually do the trick — psychological if not physical.

340

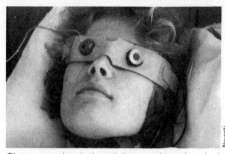

Sleep can be induced by passing electrical impulses through the eyeballs to the brain.

In more severe cases, it may be necessary to treat the underlying mental upset, as well as to give sleeping pills. As regards the latter, barbiturates (see **barbiturates**) were the most popular choice for many years. However, they are not usually suitable for elderly patients, and are quite habit-forming; in combination with alcohol, they may be dangerous. Fortunately, a number of newer preparations are now available.

SLEEPING SICKNESS is the African form of trypanosomiasis, or infection by minute parasites called trypanosomes.

Trypanosomes cause three disorders in man — Chagas' disease (see **Chagas' disease**), which is found in South America; Gambian sleeping sickness, found in West and Central Africa; and Rhodesian sleeping sickness, which occurs in the South, central and Eastern part of the continent.

The trypanosomes which cause both types of African sleeping sickness are passed on to Man by the bite of the tsetse fly. In the case of Gambian sleeping sickness, it is believed that the fly can only acquire the trypanosome by biting an infected man, but Rhodesian sleeping sickness can be passed to Man by flies that have bitten infected antelopes (and possibly other wild animals as well).

Both types of sleeping sickness can produce fever, headache, skin rashes, enlargement of the lymph glands and gross weight loss. Gambian sleeping sickness is much the more likely to produce the eventual drowsiness and coma which indicate infection of the brain, and which give the disease its name.

SLING is a supportive bandage for the arm. There are various methods of making a sling, but a simple one which is suitable for almost all circumstances is to take a triangular piece of cloth (or an oblong one folded diagonally), and tie two of the corners behind the patient's neck. His forearm rests in the loop which is thus formed, and the third corner of the triangle (which lies at his elbow) can be pinned to the front of the sling.

SMALLPOX, or variola, is a very serious and infectious virus disease. In days gone by, it wrought havoc in the Western world, and there are still areas of the globe where it is endemic (constantly present). In these days of fast air travel, smallpox can be carried almost anywhere with alarming speed. Once an epidemic breaks out, it is often very difficult indeed to contain. For this reason, most countries insist on an up-to-date vaccination certificate from all travellers from smallpox areas. Even this has, unfortunately, not proved sufficient protection in the past, and in most of the world it is probably still the wisest course for adults as well as children to keep up their protection by means of vaccination (see **vaccination**).

The features of smallpox are as follows. Roughly 12 days after infection, the patient develops headache, a fever of 103°F–104°F, and often abdominal pain and vomiting. After about 4 days, he feels better. However, at about this stage the rash appears. It consists at first of tiny red spots inside the mouth and on the upper part of the face, spreading rapidly to the extremities, and largely sparing the trunk (this distribution is in contrast to that of chickenpox, see **chickenpox**). Within a few days, these lumps or papules, have filled with clear fluid, which eventually turns to pus. The patient feels very ill when the rash is at its height, and he only starts to recover when the pustules begin to dry into scabs.

It should be stressed that smallpox can sometimes take quite a different course, depending on the strain of virus and the state of the patient's immunity. Complications are many, and the death rate is usually around ten per cent. There is no specific treatment once the disease has developed, but skilled nursing and treatment of secondary infection give the patient the best chance of survival. Isolation in a fever hospital is, of course, absolutely essential.

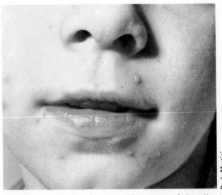

Smallpox papules in an early stage of the disease. The clear fluid later turns to pus.

SMEAR TEST is a simple and painless method of detecting cancer of the cervix (neck of the womb) *before it produces any symptoms*. It is also called the 'Pap. test', after its originator, called Doctor Papanicolaou. At a very early stage, this type of cancer can almost always be cured by a very minor operation. Since this is a disease which kills many women in their 30s and 40s (and even in their 20s), it is widely believed that *all* women over the age of about 27 should have a routine smear test each year, *regardless of the fact that they have no symptoms.*

The test itself is very simple. The patient lies on her side with her knees drawn up, and the doctor uses a device called a speculum to inspect the vagina. A small flat piece of wood called a spatula is then scraped across the upper part of the vagina and the cervix itself. The mucus and cells which are painlessly scraped off are then smeared on a glass slide and examined under a microscope. The skilled eye of the laboratory technician is usually able to detect quite readily if any further investigation is needed. (See also **cervix**.)

SMEGMA is the thick secretion which readily forms under the foreskin. Its

341

presence may be associated with chronic irritation, and boys of about the age of four upwards should be taught to retract the foreskin and wash the penis each day and thus prevent this happening.

SNAKE-BITE — see **bites**.

SNEEZE is a reaction to some irritant in the upper air passages. It is entirely a reflex action and not a conscious one, but it may, for reasons which are not entirely understood, be suppressed by exerting firm pressure along the upper lip, which has the same nerve supply as the area of the nasal passages in which irritation normally takes place.

When a sneeze occurs, the chest cavity contracts violently; at the same time, the larynx (voice-box) is kept closed, so that there is a tremendous build-up of pressure until the larynx opens. The resultant blast of air sweeps out a great deal of mucus and other material from the nose, including many germs. It is therefore quite true that 'coughs and sneezes spread diseases', and children should be taught always to sneeze into a handkerchief.

SNORING is the noise produced by vibration of the soft palate (see **palate**) as air flows past it. Except where the adenoids (see **adenoid**) are enlarged, there is very little in the way of medical treatment that can help this condition. However, snoring does no harm to the snorer, and is merely irritating to the listener. It is a relatively simple matter to induce the snorer (who is usually lying face upwards) to turn on his or her side, which will often stop the noise.

SODIUM is a metal which is closely related chemically to potassium (see **potassium**). Both are vital to life. In general, sodium is found in the fluid which surrounds the cells of the body, while potassium is actually contained in the cells. Too much sodium, however, may predispose to high blood pressure; it also causes retention of water in certain illnesses where there is a tendency to dropsy or oedema (see **oedema**). For this reason, diuretics (see **diuretics**), drugs which rid the body of excess water, often work by increasing the urinary excretion of sodium.

Our main source of sodium is common salt, or sodium chloride (see **salt**). In states of oedema it is therefore common to prescribe reduction of salt in the diet.

SOFT SORE is the ulcer which is characteristic of the venereal disease chancroid (see **chancroid**).

SOLDIER'S HEART — see **da Costa's syndrome**.

SORE THROAT, or pharyngitis, is one of the commonest of all disorders. Apart from an occasional case due to overuse of the voice (which is usually more of a laryngitis — see **laryngitis** — than a pharyngitis), almost all sore throats are due to infection. It is difficult to tell whether in any given case such infection is due to viruses (see **virus**) or to bacteria (see **bacteria**). Since viruses are completely unaffected by antibiotics, and since these drugs have certain unwanted effects, treatment with anything other than gargles and aspirin is not usually warranted in most cases.

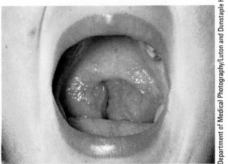

Department of Medical Photography/Luton and Dunstable Hospital

The typical appearance of the throat during a streptococcal infection: red and swollen.

SPANISH FLY, or cantharides, is an irritant preparation which has a quite unjustified reputation as an aphrodisiac. This reputation appears to be based on the fact that taken internally the drug produces intense irritation of the lower urinary passages. It cannot be stressed too strongly that Spanish fly is a deadly poison which every few years takes the life of someone to whom it has been given for its supposed aphrodisiac effect.

SPASTIC is a word used to describe any condition in which there is muscular spasm. The term is particularly employed in connection with children suffering from cerebral palsy (bodily disorder due to brain damage, which is itself usually related to birth injury). Although not all such 'spastic' children have, strictly speaking, spasm disorders, the word 'spastic' has now become widely accepted in this sense.

There are probably about half a million spastic children in the world, and the majority of these are unable to attend ordinary schools, though many of them are of perfectly normal mentality. Immense help and kindness are required to enable the spastic child to enjoy a useful and happy life; in recent years, it has been shown that careful training will work wonders in children with even the severest forms of bodily disability.

The various types of cerebral palsy are too numerous to go into here, but, in general terms, parents should take a child to the doctor if (a) at the age of ten months he is unable to hold his head up properly when his back is supported; or (b) if walking is delayed beyond the age of eighteen months; or (c) if curious writhing movements of the limbs are seen when the child first tries to walk.

In practice, most spastic children will have their condition diagnosed fairly early in countries where infants are seen routinely by the doctor, or in a clinic.

SPEECH THERAPY is available at larger hospitals in most developed countries. Among the people with speech disorders whom it may help are children with a stammer, adults who have had the larynx (voice-box) removed because of cancer, and deaf or 'dumb' children. In fact, 'dumb' children usually have the power of speech, but are very deaf, and so do not know how to use it. Speech therapy can help them to produce an adequate voice, though it will be a long and difficult process.

SPERMS, or spermatozoa, are the tiny tadpole-like structures contained in the seminal fluid (see **semen**); the union of a sperm and an ovum (egg) constitutes the act of conception (see **conception**).

SPHYGMOMANOMETER is the instrument which doctors use to measure blood pressure (see **blood pressure**).

SPINAL COLUMN, spine or vertebral column, is the 'backbone', which consists of a large number of fairly small bones, called vertebrae, piled one on top of the other. The spinal column is discussed further under the heading **back**.

SPINAL CORD is that part of the central nervous system which runs from the base of the brain down through the spinal column (see **spinal column**), and is shielded and protected by it. In adults, the spinal cord ends in the upper part of the lumbar region (the small of the back). On the way down, it gives off numerous pairs of nerves, which carry impulses from the spinal cord and brain to the rest of the body, and also transmit information in the reverse direction.

Damage to the spinal cord is normally a very serious matter. It is usually caused by severe injury involving fracture or dislocation of the spine. In general, the higher the injury, the worse is the outlook. This is why a broken neck, as occurs for instance in judicial hanging (see **hanging**), is the most dangerous spinal injury of all. Spinal cord injuries are discussed further under **back**.

SPIROCHAETES are a type of germ which have a characteristic corkscrew appearance under the microscope. Different types of spirochaetes cause the tropical disease yaws (see **yaws**), various kinds of leptospirosis including the relatively commonly-seen disorder Weil's disease (see **Weil's disease**), and the venereal disease syphilis (see **syphilis**).

SPIRONOLACTONE is a diuretic drug (see **diuretics**), i.e. one which aids the body to get rid of excess fluid. It acts by reducing the effects of the hormone called aldosterone (see **aldosterone**).

SPLEEN is an organ weighing about half

a pound which lies in the upper left hand part of the abdominal cavity, under the protection of the lower ribs. Doctors still know relatively little about its function, but it appears to play some part in blood formation, and also has some influence on the development of immunity. It is not essential to life, however, and can be surgically removed without ill-effects.

In fact, surgical removal (*splenectomy*) has to be carried out quite frequently in patients with a *ruptured spleen.*

This condition occurs after injuries to the upper abdomen or lower ribs on the left side. Blows in this area may produce only short-lived pain, but if they rupture the spleen, it will continue to leak blood, often over a period of many hours. Under these circumstances, the patient can feel perfectly well, but may literally be bleeding to death internally. For this reason, doctors now regard blows in the region of the spleen with considerable suspicion, and, if there is any doubt, admit the patient to hospital where frequent observation of pulse and blood pressure will reveal if bleeding is taking place.

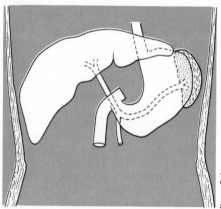

The position of the spleen in the left side of the abdomen: behind the stomach, over the kidney.

SPLINTS are supports for an injured part of the body — most commonly fractured bones. Nowadays, splints are usually made of materials like plaster of Paris, but, in emergency, anyone can make a perfectly adequate splint by using a length of wood, lashed firmly but not over-tightly

344

around the patient's limb with bandages or handkerchiefs. As a rule, the object should be to immobilize the fractured bone and, if possible, the neighbouring joints until the patient reaches hospital.

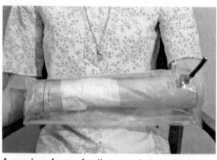

A modern form of splint, consisting of a plastic bag inflated in position around a damaged limb.

SPONDYLITIS means arthritis (i.e. joint inflammation) in the spine. Ankylosing spondylitis is a common condition which is popularly known by the descriptive term 'poker back'. Often seen in quite young men, ankylosing spondylitis usually first manifests itself as pain in the two sacroiliac joints (where the spine joins the pelvis on either side). Later the lower part of the spine becomes increasingly stiff and rigid. At this stage, the patient's X-ray shows a characteristic bamboo-like appearance. Treatment with drugs and with physiotherapy can be helpful. Patients with ankylosing spondylitis are unusually liable to certain other conditions, notably ulcerative colitis (see **ulcerative colitis**).

SPRUE is a bowel disorder of unknown origin. It is quite common in the tropics. The features include the frequent passage of bulky, pale motions, weight loss, and a red, sore tongue. There may be an associated anaemia, of a rather unusual type, and other indications of a failure to absorb essential nutriments from the intestinal tract.

Some doctors describe similar symptoms occurring in temperate regions as 'non-tropical sprue'. This condition is normally due to unusual sensitivity to food constituents such as gluten (which is found in wheat and rye). A special diet omitting gluten may prove helpful.

SPUTUM means any material which is coughed up or spat out. As a rule, however, sputum comes from the lungs.

Blood-stained or pink sputum (haemoptysis) always requires prompt investigation, including a chest X-ray, as it may be a symptom of serious disease.

Green or yellow sputum is an indication of bacterial infection, and hence, in most cases, of the need for an antibiotic.

Persistent expectoration of any kind of sputum (i.e. for more than a fortnight after an ordinary episode of cold or cough) always needs full investigation.

Sputum very often carries germs. Fortunately, the habit of spitting in public places is much less common than it used to be. It is important that any material which is coughed up should be expectorated into a handkerchief — preferably a paper one, which can be readily destroyed.

SQUINT, or strabismus, is a condition in which the eyes do not look in the same direction. This occurrence is due to some defect in the muscles which control the movements of the eyes, or in the nerves supplying these muscles.

Squint appearing for the first time in adulthood is uncommon, but needs immediate investigation, as it may well be due to some serious disorder interfering with the action of one of the nerves supplying the eye muscles.

In childhood, squint is quite common. It can only safely be ignored when it is slight and transient, *and does not persist beyond the age of six months.* After this age, it is absolutely essential that any child with a squint (even one that 'comes and goes') should be seen by an eye specialist. The earlier treatment is started, the better are the prospects of cure. Such treatment may consist of the use of glasses, of occlusion (covering) of one eye, of special exercises, or of operation. The choice of method will depend on the age of the child and the exact nature of the squint.

STAB WOUNDS are unfortunately commoner than they used to be in most countries. By the nature of the instruments which cause them, stab wounds invariably cause only a small hole at the point of entry. However, very serious internal damage may have been done, and it is essential that anyone who suffers such a wound to any part of the body should go to hospital — however slight the injury may seem, and however well he feels.

STAMMERING is a speech disorder in which there is lack of co-ordination of the normal mechanism of speech so that the sufferer has difficulty in producing certain sounds, particularly the 'plosive' consonants, such as 'B' and 'P'. Stammering responds well to speech therapy, which should be started as early as possible, both to avoid the firm establishment of this habit of speech, and to save the child the intense embarrassment so often caused by having a stammer.

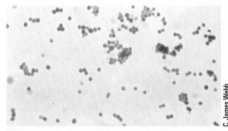

Microscopically, staphylococci *above* tend to form clusters, distinguishing them from streptococci *below* which make chain-like formations.

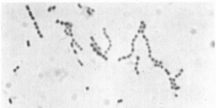

STAPHYLOCOCCI are very common types of bacteria (see **bacteria**). They cause such infections as boils, carbuncles and pimples, and may also be the source of outbreaks of food poisoning. Many people, including a high percentage of doctors and nurses, are permanent 'carriers' of staphylococci in their noses. This is why touching or picking the nose is so likely to lead to spread of infection. In the 1950s, many staphylococci became

345

resistant to penicillin, a state of affairs which created immense problems, particularly in surgical wards, where these germs were a persistent cause of post-operative wound infections. In recent years, new techniques, and the advent of a number of antibiotics to which staphylococci have, as yet, no resistance, have considerably improved the situation.

STARCH means a complex member of the chemical group called the carbohydrates (see **carbohydrates**). Starch is found in such foods as bread or potatoes. It is digested by enzymes (see **enzymes**) in the alimentary canal (see **alimentary canal**), which break it down to simpler carbohydrate compounds called sugars, which can be absorbed into the body.

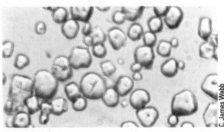

Magnified view of starch granules. Starch is a complex carbohydrate built from simple sugars.

STARVATION is going without food over such a prolonged period that bodily disease results. Provided a man has water to drink, he can usually fast for a considerable time (particularly if he is overweight) without suffering serious consequences. In fact, starvation as a treatment for obesity became widely employed during the 1960s, with varying degrees of success. However, absolute fasting (i.e. without supplements of vitamins and essential minerals such as salt) cannot be continued for many weeks; absolute fasts by political prisoners (which tend for various reasons to be the only completely genuine ones) usually result in death by starvation after 50–90 days.

The resistance of children to starvation (particularly lack of protein) is very much less than that of adults, which is why, in time of war, the death rate from this cause may be so appallingly high among infants.

346

STENOSIS means narrowing of any passage or structure in the body. For instance, mitral stenosis is narrowing of the mitral valve of the heart (see **mitral valve**).

STERILIZATION means 'making sterile'. It is used in two different senses in medicine: (a) Sterilization of instruments, dressings, fluids, etc. means ensuring that they are entirely free from live germs. This can be done fairly effectively by such means as immersion in boiling water for five minutes, or by using steam under pressure or a very hot oven. Liquids such as milk can be sterilized by pasteurization (see **pasteurization**).

(b) Sterilization of human beings is, of course, a form of contraception. (See **contraception**). Both men and women can be rendered infertile by a sterilization operation. In practice, it is far easier to sterilize a man than a woman, but (except in India, where the technique is widely used as part of the birth control programme), men tend to reject the idea because they are afraid (wrongly, as it happens) that the operation will interfere with their virility (see **virility**). In fact, male sterilization involves only the simple procedure of making a small incision on either side of the scrotum (see **scrotum**), and either tying off, or, more usually, completely dividing the two vasa deferentia, which carry sperms up from the testicles. This can be done under local anaesthetic; there is no pain, and healing is complete in a few days. Sexual performance is entirely unaffected, though any fluid ejaculated at a sexual climax will henceforth contain no sperms. The only drawback is that, should the patient ever want to have more children, re-joining the two severed ends of each vas deferens is, although possible, often difficult.

Female sterilization is a more complicated matter, as it involves opening the abdomen. It is usually carried out under general anaesthesia. An incision made in the lower abdominal wall enables the surgeon to find the two Fallopian tubes (see **Fallopian tubes**), which carry eggs from the ovaries to the womb. The tubes are tied off, or, better still, cut through, as there is less risk of pregnancy occurring.

STEROIDS are a large group of chemical compounds which have a basically similar chemical structure. The group contains many naturally-occurring hormones and other substances (such as the oestrogens produced by the ovaries, the male sex hormones produced by the testes, and certain widely-prescribed drugs, such as digitalis). However, very frequently when doctors speak of steroids, they mean the corticosteroids (the members of the group which are produced by the cortex of the adrenal gland – see **adrenal**), or synthetic compounds which are closely related to them and have similar actions.

The adrenal cortex produces a number of corticosteroid hormones. They are divided into three basic types. The first are called glucocorticoids, the second, mineralocorticoids, and the third type the adrenal androgens.

The glucocorticoids, the most important of which is cortisol (hydrocortisone), have many effects, but the most significant of these is an 'anti-inflammatory' action.

The mineralocorticoids, the most important of which is aldosterone (see **aldosterone**) play a vital part in maintaining the body's chemical balance.

The adrenal androgens are sex hormones which affect the secondary sexual characteristics and also play a part in skeletal and muscle growth.

Natural and synthetic corticosteroid preparations of the glucocorticoid type are widely used in medicine. Those available include cortisone, cortisol (hydrocortisone), prednisone and prednisolone. They are employed for their anti-inflammatory effect in such diseases as asthma, rheumatoid arthritis and the collagen diseases (see **collagen diseases**). Although they are very effective, they are not curative; furthermore, they have to be used with great care, since they have certain very important side-effects. They may produce high blood pressure, ulcers, diabetes or osteoporosis (see **osteoporosis**), or worsen these conditions where they already exist. In children, they may stunt growth very badly. Furthermore, if treatment with them is stopped suddenly (e.g. if the patient forgets to take his tablets), collapse may follow.

STETHOSCOPE is the device a doctor uses for listening to the internal sounds of the body, particularly those produced by the beating of the heart and the movement of air in the lungs.

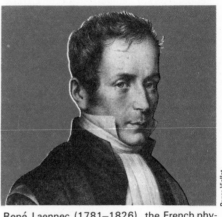

René Laennec (1781–1826), the French physician credited with inventing the stethoscope.

STILBOESTROL is a synthetic compound which has effects broadly similar to those of natural hormones called oestrogens (see **oestrogens**). It is widely used in gynaecological disorders and, in men, for the treatment of growths of the prostate gland at the base of the bladder.

STILL'S DISEASE is a form of arthritis (see **arthritis**) seen in children. Basically, it is very similar to the adult disorder rheumatoid arthritis. Both conditions cause painful inflammation and some deformity of the smaller joints of the body. In Still's disease, fever and enlargement of the spleen and lymph glands may also occur. Treatment may be difficult; there is often a good response to steroid drugs (see **steroids**), but these may cause severe growth stunting. ACTH (corticotrophin) is helpful in certain cases.

STINGS – see **bee-stings, hornet-stings, wasp-stings.**

STITCH is the popular name for a pain in the side, coming on after unaccustomed exercise. It is common in children. No treatment is necessary, as the pain passes off in a minute or two.

347

STOKES-ADAMS ATTACKS are episodes of unconsciousness which occur in the course of the disorder known as heart block. The patient usually collapses to the ground and becomes very white. After 30 seconds or so, his skin can be seen to flush bright red, and he rapidly recovers consciousness. Such attacks can sometimes be prevented by drugs; it may, however, be necessary for the patient to have an artificial pacemaker (see **pacemaker**).

STOMACH is the dilated part of the alimentary canal (see **alimentary canal**) which forms a 'bag' at the lower end of the oesophagus, or gullet. When food is swallowed, it enters the stomach, and is retained there for a variable time. While in the stomach, it is exposed to the digestive action of hydrochloric acid and enzymes (see **digestion**). At the same time, it is churned by the muscular movements of the stomach wall. When it has attained a relatively fluid consistency, the food passes out of the stomach, and into the duodenum (see **duodenum**).

Disorders of the stomach include gastritis (see **gastritis**), ulcers (see **gastric ulcer**), pyloric stenosis (see **pyloric stenosis**), hiatus hernia (see **hiatus hernia**), and cancer.

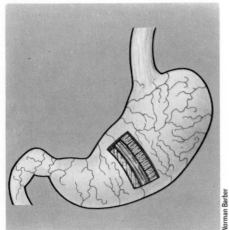

Diagram of the stomach, with the wall cut to show the different layers of muscle responsible for the complex churning movements which hasten digestion. Waves of contraction expel part-digested food into the duodenum, *left*.
348

Cancer of the stomach is common in men over 40, but is also seen in women. It is characterized by recurrent pain in the upper central part of the abdomen, often associated with vomiting (frequently of black material). The patient may also have black motions, and may have lost weight. It should be stressed that these symptoms can very readily be confused with those of an ulcer. It is therefore essential that, where there is any possibility of cancer, the patient should have a full investigation, including a barium meal X-ray (see **barium meal**). This disease can only be cured if caught very early.

STONES, or calculi, are hard concretions composed of various minerals. They are found in two main sites — the urinary tract and the biliary tract.

In the urinary tract, stones may form within the kidney itself, or, more commonly, in the ureter (the slim tube that carries urine from the kidney to the bladder). In the ureter, stones may jam, producing renal colic (see **renal colic**). Stones are also commonly found in the bladder, where they may attain considerable size, and cause intermittent blocking of the flow of urine. A stone anywhere in the urinary tract may cause bleeding in the urine, and will predispose to infection.

In the biliary tract, stones may be found in the gall bladder, the cystic duct (which leads out of it), or in the common bile duct (which carries bile down to the intestine). This subject is fully dealt with under the heading **gall stones.**

STOOLS are motions passed from the bowel. They consist of food residues, cells shed from the bowel wall and dead bacteria, mixed with bile. For the symptoms of black motions and bleeding in the motions, see under the heading **bowels.**

STOPPAGE OF URINE — see **urine**, stoppage of.

STREPTOCOCCI are a group of bacteria (see **bacteria**) which cause a wide range of disorders, including many cases of sore throat and tonsillitis, and tissue infections such as erysipelas (see **erysipelas**).

STREPTOMYCIN is an antibiotic which was first isolated in the USA in the 1940s. While streptomycin was of considerable use in the treatment of a wide variety of infections, its greatest value was that, in combination with two other drugs, PAS and isoniazid (INAH), it proved to be a highly effective cure for practically all cases of pulmonary tuberculosis, which was gradually overcome by these three drugs in the early 1950s.

Streptomycin has certain disadvantages. In particular, it is highly toxic to the inner ear, and may cause deafness, ringing in the ears, and disturbances of the balance mechanisms. For this reason, it is only rarely given to elderly people.

STRICTURE means a narrowing of any passage of the body. Most commonly, the term is applied to strictures of the male urethra, the tube which carries urine from the bladder to the exterior. Such strictures very readily cause stoppage of the urine (see **urine-stoppage of**). They are often caused by gonorrhoea (see **gonorrhoea**).

STROKES, or cerebro-vascular accidents (CVAs), are episodes in which the blood supply to the brain is interfered with in some way, producing symptoms (such as paralysis) in the area of the body supplied by the affected part of the brain.

There are three basic types of stroke — cerebral thrombosis, cerebral embolism and cerebral haemorrhage.

Cerebral thrombosis means the formation of a clot within the vessels which supply blood to the brain; cerebral embolism means blockage of these vessels by some piece of material carried in the bloodstream; and cerebral haemorrhage means bleeding from a burst blood vessel in the brain. Strokes may also occur because of spasm of the brain's blood vessels. The manifestations of strokes vary greatly, depending on the part of the brain which is involved. However, much the commonest occurrence following a major stroke is the development of a hemiplegia (see **hemiplegia**).

STRYCHNINE is a poisonous substance derived from *nux vomica* (see **nux**

vomica). It was once widely employed as a tonic but has now dropped out of use.

STYE, or *hordeolum*, is an abscess in the eyelid. Treatment with hot compresses is usually sufficient; antibiotic ointments may help to stop the infection spreading.

SUB-ARACHNOID HAEMORRHAGE is an episode of bleeding occurring between the layers of membrane which surround and protect the brain. Under one of these membranes (the arachnoid membrane) is a space, called the sub-arachnoid space, in which blood vessels run.

Most commonly, the patient has a congenital aneurysm (i.e. a swelling, present from birth) on one of the arteries supplying the brain. The swelling forms a weak point which may give way at any time. For this reason, a sub-arachnoid haemorrhage quite commonly occurs in relatively young men.

The first symptom is usually a very sudden and severe headache, which is often described as being like a blow on the back of the head. Unconsciousness may follow at once, but may be delayed. If the patient remains conscious, he complains of intense pain running from the skull down

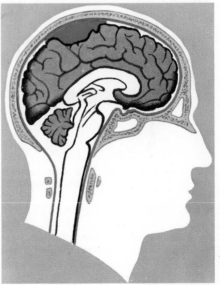

A sub-arachnoid haemorrhage, perhaps following a blow, presses on the brain tissue.

Norman Barber

the back of the neck. A lumbar puncture (see **lumbar puncture**) will reveal that the fluid which surrounds the brain and spinal cord is heavily blood-stained. The initial treatment consists of absolute rest and skilled nursing care in hospital, but after X-rays of the blood vessels of the brain have been taken, surgery may be helpful.

SUGARS are simple chemical compounds of the carbohydrate group (see **carbohydrates**). They include glucose (dextrose), fructose, galactose, sucrose, lactose, and maltose. Ordinary table sugar (cane sugar) is sucrose, while the sugar contained in milk is lactose. Both these have slightly more complex chemical structures than glucose (which is the body's basic fuel), and, like all carbohydrates, they have to be broken down to glucose before the body can make use of them.

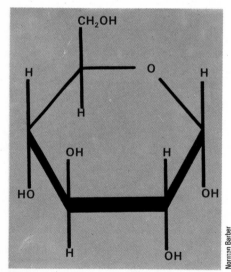

The structural formula of a glucose molecule; each angle is formed by one carbon atom.

SUICIDE is a fairly common cause of death in most countries of the world, and more particularly the industrialized ones. Contrary to widespread belief, the highest incidence of suicide in the world does *not* occur in Sweden. At the present time, Hungary has more male suicides *per capita* than any other nation, and is about 350

equal with Japan in female suicides. In every country, men are much more likely to kill themselves than are women. The highest incidence of suicides in most countries is among the elderly, and, in general, people with responsible jobs are much more likely to kill themselves than are those with few responsibilities.

The most widely used method of suicide varies from country to country and tends to change over the years. In the USA, for example, men are (not surprisingly) most likely to kill themselves with a gun. In the UK, however, there has been a change in the last 30 or 40 years, in that methods such as cutting the throat and drinking corrosive fluids have become much less frequently used, while taking barbiturates or aspirin, or inhaling coal gas are now common. The only encouraging trend of recent years has been a suggestion of a fall in the suicide rate in areas where advice services (such as the Samaritans) are available.

The widespread belief that it is pointless to save someone from suicide because 'he'll only do it again' is quite wrong. For every successful suicide, there are dozens of unsuccessful ones — and the majority of these people, once they reach psychiatric help, will not make a further attempt. Psychiatric aid is therefore important, and it is obviously best if the patient receives it *before* he tries to kill himself.

Studies have shown that the majority of people who kill themselves have talked about the possibility with someone else beforehand, but often have not been taken seriously. Anyone who has a friend or relative who talks in this way, or who seems badly depressed, should advise him to seek psychiatric advice at once.

SULCUS means any furrow in an anatomical structure, particularly the brain.

SULPHA DRUGS, or sulphonamides, were discovered in the 1930s. They were the first drugs shown to be active against a wide range of germs, and though they were partially eclipsed by the development of penicillin, they are still very frequently employed in medicine, particularly for the treatment of urinary infections.

SUNBURN is extremely common, particularly among very fair-skinned and sandy-haired people. It is advisable, even in temperate climates, to be very wary of prolonged exposure to the sun.

Mild sunburn needs no treatment, but severe burns may be very painful. It is traditional to put calamine lotion on the skin, though this has the disadvantage that in some people it forms a crust which prevents the skin from cooling. This may make the pain worse, and increase the intense itching which is often a feature of the later stages of sunburn. Antihistamine-containing creams are also widely used, but it is doubtful if they have any specific effect, apart from the cooling action of the cream itself. Probably the most effective treatment for the relief of pain is a cream containing a mild local anaesthetic. It should only be used on medical advice, however. (See also **sunlight**.)

SUNLIGHT is composed of radiation from a wide range of wavelengths of the electromagnetic spectrum. It includes the invisible infra-red rays which produce heat, the visible rays producing all the colours of the spectrum, and ultra-violet rays, which are again invisible. Excessive exposure to sunlight may cause (a) sunburn (see **sunburn**); (b) sunstroke (see **sunstroke**); (c) headache and raised temperature in children who are unaccustomed to the sun; and (d) skin growths in fair-skinned people who spend many years in a tropical climate.

SUNSTROKE is rarely seen in temperate climes, but it is not uncommon in parts of the tropics and sub-tropics. Its effects are similar to those of heat stroke (see **heat stroke**) and severe sunburn (see **sunburn**) combined. Treatment consists in putting the patient to bed in a darkened room, and gradually making good his deficiencies of salt and water, either through small sips by mouth or an intravenous 'drip'.

SUPPOSITORIES are preparations for insertion into the rectum.

SUPRARENAL GLANDS—see **adrenal.**

SUTURES are surgical stitches.

SWABS are pieces of cloth which are used to mop up blood during a surgical operation. A very large number may be needed during a major operation, and it is therefore not surprising that every year a number of cases occur in which a swab is left inside a patient's abdomen. This is likely to lead to pain, fever or abscess formation some time after the operation. In order to try and prevent this accident, it is customary for the surgeon to make a routine search of the operation area before stitching up. However, it is very easy for swabs to remain hidden behind some structure, and therefore it is essential for the theatre nursing staff to keep an accurate count of all the swabs used during the operation, and ensure the record tallies at the end. In addition, many swabs nowadays contain a thread which can, if necessary, be detected by X-ray.

SWEAT—see **perspiration.**

SWEETBREADS are animal glands used as food. The most commonly eaten gland is the pancreas (see **pancreas**).

SYMPTOMS, sometimes called 'the language of disease', are the features of an illness which the patient actually complains of. Signs, on the other hand, are the features which the doctor finds for himself on clinical examination.

SYNAPSES are the junction points between nerve cells, where the 'message'

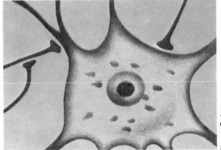

Norman Barber

The tiny spaces between nerve fibre endings and other nerve cells are known as synapses: there are tens of millions in the brain.

or nerve impulse, is passed on, not electrically, as in the nerve fibres, but chemically. The chemicals are known as *transmitters*.

SYNCOPE means **fainting.**

SYNDACTYLY is an abnormality in which two or more fingers or toes remain unseparated during development before birth. The condition is usually curable by plastic surgery.

SYNDROME is a particular collection of signs and symptoms (see **symptoms**) which, found together, constitute either a disease or a particular manifestation of one of more diseases.

SYNOVIAL MEMBRANE is the layer of tissue which lines certain joints. It produces the synovial fluid, which lubricates the joints during movement. Changes in the synovial membrane accompany some types of arthritis.

SYPHILIS is the most serious venereal disease. It has been common in all parts of the world for hundreds of years, but its incidence dropped rapidly after the Second World War, due largely to the introduction of penicillin. There is now some evidence that it may be increasing again. The main 'reservoir' of syphilis is provided by prostitutes, a high proportion of whom have and transmit the disease, but it is no respecter of persons, and the most respectable people may acquire the condition. Anyone who has the symptoms should not hesitate to go at once to a hospital 'special clinic' for treatment under conditions of anonymity. It cannot be stressed too strongly that syphilis can invariably be cured if caught early; if allowed to pursue its course, it may have the most terrible effects on body and mind.

Syphilis is caused by a germ called the *Treponema pallidum*, which is one of the group called the spirochaetes. It may be congenital or acquired. Congenital syphilis (i.e. syphilis present at birth), is now a very rare condition, thanks to routine blood testing of pregnant women.

Acquired syphilis is usually passed on by sexual intercourse with an infected person, and the first signs therefore usually appear on the genitals. This is not always so, however, and the primary stage (or 'primary chancre') is not uncommonly seen on the lips, nipples or fingers. In a widely-reported case during the 1960s, a young man with an infectious area on his lip passed the disease on to five different girls whom he kissed during a dance. However, although it is wise to regard with suspicion any hard, reddish lump which breaks down to form a skin or lip ulcer, we shall confine ourselves here to describing the much more common genital infection.

In men, the 'primary chancre' occurs on the penis, and in women on the labia (see **labia**), or sometimes within the vagina. The chancre usually occurs 10—90 days after intercourse. It is a painless, hard lump, which slowly erodes to form an ulcer. At the same time, there may be swelling of the glands in both groins.

The deceptive thing about the primary chancre is that, after a period of some weeks, it goes away. All too often, the patient assumes that he or she is cured. Unfortunately, nothing could be further from the truth.

Secondary manifestations of syphilis are seen in 80% of patients a month or two after the appearance of the primary chancre. Usually, there is a rash, often accompanied by lymph gland enlargement. Any moist, oozing area of rash will be highly infectious.

The secondary stage also passes off, and the late stage may not occur for many years. It is in this stage that there is truly terrible destruction of almost any of the tissues of the body, but in particular of the bones, liver, heart, spinal cord and brain.

The important thing to realize is that syphilis need not have these appalling consequences if the diagnosis is made early, and if treatment with penicillin is given. The way in which this therapy is administered is a specialized business, and no-one should ever try to treat themselves. It is a perfectly simple matter to attend a hospital clinic (for which no prior appointment is necessary), and anyone who has the least suspicion of the presence of VD should do so. (See also **venereal disease**.)

352

SYRINGOMYELIA is a disease of the central nervous system in which the patient loses the ability to detect pain, heat or cold in various parts of the body — usually the hands, arms and chest. As a result, the patient repeatedly cuts and burns his fingers. In the later stages, there may be wasting, and also involvement of the nerve centres supplying the palate, throat and voice-box.

TABES DORSALIS is one of the late manifestations of syphilis (see **syphilis**). It is also known as locomotor ataxia (see **locomotor ataxia**).

TABLETS are solid disc-shaped preparations made by compressing drugs with inert materials.

TACHYCARDIA means a rapid heart rate. It may be caused by exercise, emotion, anxiety, over-activity of the thyroid gland (hyperthyroidism), certain disorders of heart rhythm, and any kind of fever.

TALIPES means the deformity known as club foot (see **club foot**).

TAPE WORMS are a group of parasitic worms. The most important ones are as follows:

The beef tapeworm, *Taenia saginata*, infects cattle which graze on grass contaminated by human faeces. When the animals are killed, Man may be infected by eating the meat, particularly if it is undercooked. However, the tapeworm produces few symptoms except mild pain of the 'indigestion' type, and the patient's only complaint is often of noticing that he has passed a tapeworm (or one of its segments) in his motions.

The pork tapeworm, *Taenia solium*, is normally acquired by eating underdone pork. However, Man can also ingest eggs of this parasite if his hands pick them up through touching contaminated grass or earth. Under these circumstances, the eggs may give rise to cysts in many organs including the brain.

The dog or sheep tapeworm, *Taenia echinococcus* or *Echinococcus granu-losus,* is dealt with under the heading **Echinococcus**. Other tapeworms which are important in particular areas of the world include the fish tapeworm (acquired by eating undercooked fish) and the dwarf tapeworm, which is common in several poorer areas of the United States where standards of personal hygiene are low.

Treatment is rapidly effective in infection due to the beef tapeworm, but where a worm produces cysts in the tissues (as is the case with the dog or sheep tapeworm, and sometimes the pork tapeworm), then eradication may be very difficult indeed. In general, prevention is better than cure: all meat and fish should be thoroughly cooked before eating; carcasses in slaughterhouses should be regularly examined by Public Health inspectors for signs of cyst formation; those who work with animals or live in rural areas should take particular care about such elementary precautions as washing the hands before eating and after visting the toilet; and finally, human sewage should not be allowed to contaminate the countryside.

TASTE is a sensation felt through impulses which reach the brain from receptors called taste-buds on the tongue. The palate (see **palate**) does not play any significant part in taste, but the aromas which reach the nasal passages from food in the mouth make the nose a very important organ in the overall sensation of taste.

TEA owes its popularity to its taste (which is due largely to certain volatile oils in the leaves of the tea plant) and to the fact that, like coffee, it contains the stimulant drug caffeine (see **caffeine**, and **coffee**).

TEARS are the salty fluid produced by the lacrimal glands, which lie just above the eye. Normally the flow of this fluid keeps the surface of the eyeball clean. Part of it evaporates, and the rest is drained off into the nose through the tiny hole which can be seen on the lower eyelid, near its inner end. The drainage apparatus cannot cope with the flow of tears under two circumstances: (a) when the volume of fluid is greatly increased by irritation to the eye, or by emotion (crying); (b) when the drainage canals are blocked from birth. In the latter condition, tears constantly roll down the child's cheeks; fortunately, surgical correction is usually possible.

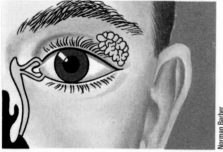

Norman Barber

The fluid secreted by the lacrimal glands passes down the tear duct behind the nose.

TEETH are the hard structures which bite and grind our food, and which also are an aid to speech. Each is composed of layers of enamel (see **enamel**) and dentine, or ivory (see **dentine**), overlying a central pulp cavity. A layer of 'cement' (a hard, bony substance) replaces the enamel over the roots of the tooth.

Milk teeth are dealt with under the heading **milk teeth**. 'Adult' teeth start to replace them in early childhood; the full adult complement consists of 32 teeth, with four incisors (cutting teeth), two canines (eye teeth), four pre-molars (small grinding teeth) and six molars (large grinding teeth) on each jaw. The rearmost molar on each side is called the 'wisdom tooth' (see **wisdom tooth**).

Decay of the teeth is one of the commonest of all diseases. The cause is still not clear, but in part, at least, it is related to excessive intake of sugar and sweet things, to failure to clean the teeth properly, and to lack of prompt attention to existing decay.

TEMPERATURES are normally measured with a clinical thermometer. No home should be without one, particularly if there are children in the house. The average temperature of a human being is taken to be 98·4°F in Great Britain, but American doctors prefer to take it as 98·6°F. Readings between 97°F and 99°F are completely normal. Tempera-

354

tures much below 97°F are usually only found either in underactivity of the thyroid (see **myxoedema**) or after exposure to cold (especially in babies). Temperatures between 99°F and 100°F may not be of much importance, especially in children (in whom such stimuli as crying may send the temperature up a little), but readings of over 100°F are almost invariably indicative of some infection (or, sometimes, some other form of inflammation). If there is not an obvious and straightforward cause, such as a cold, it is wise to check with the family doctor. Similarly, while the temperature can go as high as 103°F or 104°F in cases of cold or 'flu, such readings are beginning to get into the 'danger area', and medical advice should be sought.

Temperatures of over 107°F–108°F, if prolonged, are incompatible with life.

TENDONS are sinews – the cord-like structures which attach muscles to bones.

TENNIS ELBOW – see under **elbow**.

TENOSYNOVITIS is inflammation of a tendon (see **tendon**) and its sheath. It is common in such sites as the wrist. The principal symptom is pain on use of a particular muscle. Treatment, which may involve physiotherapy, operation or injections of steroids (see **steroids**), may take some time to produce an effect.

TESTICLES, or testes, are the two male sex glands, which lie in the scrotum (see **scrotum**). Each is developed, in early life within the womb, from the same tissue which in females gives rise to the ovaries; well before the child is born, the testes should both descend into the scrotum. If they do not descend properly, surgical advice is needed.

In adult life, the testicles produce sperms, which are conveyed to the exterior in the seminal fluid via a coiled tube called the epididymis, which connects the testicles with the vas deferens (see **vas deferens**). The testicles also produce hormones which play an important part in the sex drive, and in maintaining the secondary sexual characteristics.

TESTOSTERONE is a male sex hormone produced by the testicles. It can also be prepared synthetically, and is used in the treatment of the rare condition of under-activity of the testes (hypogonadism). Although it is administered in some parts of the world to patients with impotence, it probably has little effect on this condition, which is almost invariably of psychological origin (see **impotence**). Nor is it likely to be of help in increasing diminished sexual desire, unless this is associated with the condition of hypogonadism mentioned above.

Testosterone is not effective by mouth, and must be given by injection. Related compounds are available which may be taken orally.

TETANUS is the medical term for lockjaw. The features of the disease are discussed under that heading, and we shall confine ourselves here to methods of prevention of the disease by anti-tetanus injections.

Many people know vaguely that they have had 'tetanus injections' in the past and assume that they are fully protected against it. In most cases, this supposition is entirely wrong.

There are two ways of producing artificial immunity against an infectious disease. One is to give serum (see **serum**) containing antibodies; this is known as *passive* artificial immunity (a subject which is discussed further under the heading **immunity**). Passive immunity against tetanus is very commonly given to a patient who has cut himself by administering an injection of anti-tetanus serum (ATS). This has the advantage of producing immediate immunity, but the protection afforded only lasts a very short time. (In addition, there are dangers in the use of serum; these are discussed under the heading **serum**.)

Much preferable is to produce *active* artificial immunity (which is also dealt with under the heading **immunity**). This can be done by giving the patient a course of injections (usually three) of tetanus toxoid, a harmless vaccine. Its main disadvantage is that some time elapses before full immunity is built up. For this reason, many doctors give patients who have cut themselves both ATS and toxoid, and advise them to return for further toxoid injections to complete this course.

All too often, this advice is disregarded. The result is that, in most Western countries, the only people whose protection against tetanus is up to date are (a) those few persons who have been wise enough to avail themselves of a full course of toxoid; (b) members of the armed forces; and (c) young children (since the 'triple' vaccine given to infants in many countries contains tetanus toxoid).

It cannot be too strongly stressed that this is an unsatisfactory state of affairs. Lockjaw is a killing disease, and every child and adult should be fully immunized against it. Particularly at risk are those who may cut themselves while gardening, while performing agricultural work, or while on a sports field, since it is in the soil that the spores of tetanus are principally found.

TETANY has nothing to do with tetanus. It is a curious muscle spasm, which is most marked in the face (which twitches when the facial nerve, in front of the ear, which supplies muscles of the cheek, is tapped firmly), and in the hand, which takes up an odd cramped position, with the tips of the straightened fingers and thumb together, and in the foot.

Tetany is most commonly due to over-breathing. If a person is slightly anxious or upset about something, he tends to breathe faster than normal, without actually realizing it. Overbreathing in this fashion for some time gradually 'washes out' the carbon dioxide (see **carbon dioxide**) in the body. When it reaches a certain level, tetany results.

Tetany can also (much less commonly) be due to a low level of the mineral calcium in the blood. This can be caused by rickets (see **rickets**), osteomalacia (see **osteomalacia**), coeliac disease (see **coeliac children**), and under-activity of the parathyroid glands, or hypoparathyroidism (see **parathyroids**).

Tetany caused by overbreathing can be dealt with in a matter of a minute or so, by getting the patient to breathe and rebreathe air in a paper bag; this allows the body's level of carbon dioxide to build up again. Tetany due to lack of calcium can be terminated by giving calcium injections into a vein; subsequently, treatment of the underlying disease will be necessary.

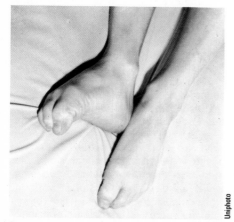

Spasm of the muscles in tetany causes the feet to assume a characteristic cramped posture; in the hand this is termed 'main d'accoucheur'.

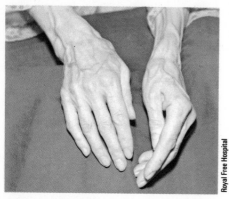

TETRACYCLINES are a group of antibiotics which have proved of great value in the treatment of many bacterial diseases during the last two decades. There are various members of the group, but they differ very little from each other in activity and effectiveness. Because of the wide range of germs against which they could be used (as opposed to the relatively narrow range of penicillin), the tetracyclines are still often referred to as 'broad spectrum antibiotics'.

356

Like all drugs, they have their disadvantages. Tetracyclines may sometimes cause upsets of the intestinal tract when given for more than a routine course of five days or so. This is because they may suppress the normal organisms present in the bowel, and thus allow others (not susceptible to tetracyclines) to take their place. In addition, tetracyclines given to a young child (or even to the mother when the child is still in the womb) may cause permanent staining of the teeth. One particular type of tetracycline is also liable to produce a rash when a patient taking the drug exposes himself to sunlight.

In general, however, the tetracyclines are among the safest and most effective of all the antibiotics so far discovered.

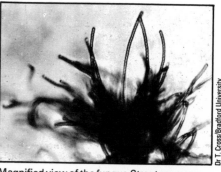

Magnified view of the fungus *Streptomyces aureofaciens*, source of one of the tetracyclines.

TETRALOGY OF FALLOT is a form of heart disease seen in children. Basically, it consists of a large hole between the two lower chambers of the heart (the ventricles), together with a narrowing of the opening of the artery which leads from the heart to the lungs; the main artery which carries 'fresh' blood to the rest of the body (the aorta) is also out of position.

The net effect is that 'stale' blood (i.e. blood which has not been through the lungs to be recharged with oxygen) is pumped round the body. As a result, the child tends to be blue in colour. He is breathless, and his growth and development may suffer.

The outlook in this condition was very bad until about 20 years ago, but it has now been greatly improved by new surgical techniques.

THALASSAEMIA is one of the haemolytic anaemias (see **anaemia**), in which the weakness of the blood is due to excessive destruction of the red cells, or erythrocytes (see **erythrocytes**).

Thalassaemia is very common in people of Mediterranean stock. It is due to the inheritance of an abnormal gene (see **gene**), and its occurrence can readily be traced in families. If a person inherits the gene from only one parent, he is said to have *thalassaemia minor*; only careful testing will show this up, however, as he is unlikely to have any symptoms.

On the other hand, if he inherits the gene from both parents, he is said to have *thalassaemia major*, and the features of the disease will be evident in his case. These features are usually first seen in infancy. They are essentially those of ordinary iron deficiency anaemia – tiredness, breathlessness and pallor – except that there is no response to treatment with iron, of which the body already has a completely adequate store. Furthermore, the child's abdomen may be distended by a greatly enlarged liver and spleen. The outlook is very poor indeed.

THERAPY means the treatment of disease. From it is derived the adjective *therapeutic* – relating to treatment.

THIAMINE is vitamin B$_1$, or aneurine. Lack of it causes beri-beri (see **deficiency diseases,** and **beri-beri**).

THIAZIDES are a very widely used group of diuretics (see **diuretics**), i.e. agents that help the body get rid of excess water. They have proved of great value since their introduction in the 1950s. They do, however, have certain drawbacks, which are as follows: (a) most of them tend to deplete the body's stores of the vital element potassium, and therefore should normally be given with a potassium supplement; (b) many precipitate a tendency towards gout; and (c) they may make the control of diabetes mellitus (see **diabetes mellitus**) more difficult.

THIGH is the part of the leg between the hip and the knee. It contains the most powerful muscles in the human body, and also the femur, or thigh-bone, which is the largest of all bones. Among the other structures in the thigh are the large femoral artery, which provides the blood supply of the leg, the femoral vein, which drains 'stale' blood back again in the direction of the heart, and the sciatic nerve, which runs down through the back of the thigh. Because of the presence of these delicate structures, penetrating wounds of the thigh may be very serious indeed.

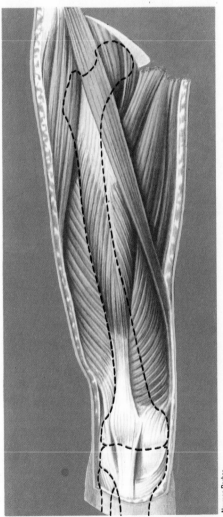

Norman Barber

The muscles of the front of the thigh. The strong *quadratus femoris* muscle, inserted into the patella, or knee-cap, straightens the leg.

357

THIOPENTONE is a widely used injectable anaesthetic of the barbiturate group (see **barbiturates**). It is sometimes erroneously referred to as the 'truth drug'.

THIRST is craving for fluid to drink. The sensation is largely located in the mouth and the back of the throat, where a 'parched' feeling develops after deprivation of water for some hours. Why thirst occurs, we do not really understand; nor do we know why it is so immediately relieved by drinking water — long before the water could be absorbed and reach the circulation. Even more puzzling, we do not know why men who need salt and other minerals as well as water (as occurs for example after exposure to extreme heat) actually thirst, not for pure water, but often for drinks containing the necessary minerals.

THORAX is the chest (see **chest**).

THREAD WORMS, or pin worms, are members of the species *Enterobius vermicularis (Oxyuris vermicularis)*. These parasites infest the human bowel (especially in children), and the commonest symptom they produce is severe itching in the region of the anus. Unfortunately, where hygiene is not too good (i.e. in families where people are not careful about washing their hands), it is very easy for the infection to be carried to the mouth of another (for instance, in food), and infect him as well. However, infection can sometimes occur even in families where the standard of cleanliness is very high.

It is usually possible to demonstrate the presence of the parasites by examining a piece of sticky tape which has been scraped across the anal region. It is often wisest to treat the entire family with a drug such as piperazine, which is said to be effective in 97 per cent of cases.

THROAT is a rather vague term which is used by most people in two senses: firstly, to indicate the region of the front of the neck, and secondly to indicate the area at the back of the mouth. Used in the latter sense, the word 'throat' more or less corresponds with the anatomical term 'pharynx' (see **pharynx**). For pharyngitis

(sore throat), see **sore throat**. Occasionally, people mean the region of the voice-box, or larynx, when they speak of the throat (see **larynx**, and **laryngitis**).

THROMBO-ANGIITIS OBLITERANS, or Buerger's disease, is an inflammatory disorder of the arteries and veins, especially those of the legs. It is commonest in men aged about 20–40 years. Smoking is believed to play a part in the development of the condition, which is characterized by thrombosis (see **thrombosis**) and eventual blockage of the arteries and veins. The symptoms include pain on walking, and this may be followed after a period of years by the development of gangrene. Treatment is a complex matter. It involves special exercises, scrupulous hygienic care of the feet, and the use of drugs to widen the blood vessels and prevent clotting; sometimes an operation may be helpful.

THROMBOSIS means clotting. Clotting of blood is, of course, a perfectly normal phenomenon (see **clotting**), and one that prevents us from bleeding to death when we cut ourselves.

Unfortunately, unwanted thrombosis in sites such as the veins of the legs is quite common, particularly among elderly people, or those who are confined to bed, especially after an operation. It also occurs more frequently than normal in pregnant women and those on the Pill (see **Pill**). Thrombosis in the leg veins is dealt with under the heading phlebitis.

Cerebral thrombosis is a clot forming in the arteries supplying the brain (see **strokes**).

'Coronary thrombosis' is a blockage of the coronary arteries which supply the heart muscle; in fact, it is rarely caused by an actual clot (see **heart attacks**, and **infarction**).

Abnormal clots may also form within the heart itself under certain circumstances, and pass either to the lungs or to the brain (see **embolism**).

THRUSH is a fungal infection caused by an organism called *Candida* or *Monilia albicans* (see **Monilia**).

THYMUS GLAND is a mass of tissue lying in the upper front part of the cavity of the chest. Although it was first described by the Roman physician Galen some 1800 years ago, remarkably little is known about its function. In young children, it is a large structure, filling much of the front part of the chest, but, about the time of puberty, it shrinks to a very much smaller size although remaining active.

It is probable that the thymus is associated with the mechanisms whereby the body produces antibodies and develops immunity (see **immunity**). Tumours or enlargement of the thymus are quite often associated with the auto-immune group of diseases (see **auto-immunization**), and removal of this gland sometimes produces a cure, or at least marked improvement, in these conditions.

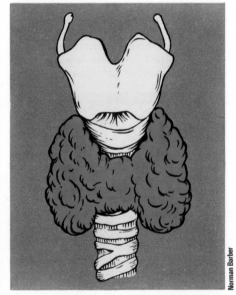

The thyroid gland in the neck — two lobes, one each side, connected by a narrow 'isthmus'.

THYROID GLAND is a structure situated in the front of the neck. It is of very great importance to the effective function of the body, since it produces a hormone called thyroxine, whose regulatory influence is essential to many chemical processes upon which life depends.

A swelling of the thyroid gland is called a goitre (see **goitre**); it may or may not be associated with over-activity of the gland, which is known as hyper-thyroidism or thyrotoxicosis (see **hyper-thyroidism**).

Underactivity of the thyroid gland, or hypothyroidism, leads to the condition called myxoedema (see **myxoedema**) in adults; in new-born babies, it causes cretinism (see **cretinism**).

THYROTOXICOSIS is over-activity of the thyroid gland. (See **thyroid gland**.) It is characterized by anxiety and irritability, a rapid heart rate, excessive sweating, a large appetite despite loss of weight, and protrusion of the eyeballs. There may also be a goitre, or painless but unsightly swelling of the thyroid. The disease and its treatment are further discussed under the heading **hyperthyroidism.**

TIBIA is the shinbone, which runs between the knee and the ankle. Fractures of the tibia are common, not only in road accidents, but in sporting injuries — for instance, skiing or football. Among the commonest of such fractures is the one known as Pott's fracture, also involving the fibula (see **Pott's fracture**).

TIC means a habitual spasm or twitch. Some cases are due to disorder of the nervous system, but many have an underlying psychological origin (but see also **tic douloureux** below).

TIC DOULOUREUX is not a tic, or habit spasm, as described under the heading tic, but a very severe form of neuralgia affecting the trigeminal nerve, which supplies the skin of the face. The condition and its treatment are fully described under the heading **neuralgia.**

TICKS are small creatures which are members of the class of arachnids (a group of living things closely related to the insects). Some of them are parasites on Man, and they may carry serious, sometimes life-threatening diseases of the rickettsial group (see **rickettsiae**).

TINEA is the medical name for the ringworm fungus (see **ringworm**).

TINNITUS means a ringing, or other unusual noise, in the ears. This common symptom has numerous possible causes.

A *throbbing* noise which is in time with the pulse, and which is heard when the ear is pressed on the pillow at night, is quite normal. If it is very troublesome, however, a doctor should be consulted, and he may consider that it is worth checking the blood pressure.

Whistling, ringing or *hissing* noises may be due to catarrh associated with a head cold. If they are more prolonged, such noises may be an indication of disorder of the ear – for instance, Menière's disease (see **Menière's disease**).

Tinnitus can also be a side-effect of certain drugs – notably aspirin (in high doses), quinine and quinidine.

TOBACCO is the prepared leaf of the plant *Nicotiana*. Its popularity is due mainly to its content of the drug nicotine, which both stimulates and depresses certain parts of the central nervous system in a combined effect that most people find quite pleasing. There are, of course, other reasons for smoking. Many types of tobacco (particularly those used in pipes and cigars) contain pleasantly aromatic ingredients which are very agreeable to the taste. Furthermore, the social pressures to use tobacco are very strong in most Western countries (especially among the young, who are usually very anxious to conform with the behaviour of their friends). In addition, many psychologists believe that the characteristic pleasure which an infant takes in putting something in his mouth and keeping it there (whether it is his mother's breast, a bottle, a dummy, or a favourite toy) is re-created by smoking.

Perhaps most important, the nicotine which we inhale from tobacco is, without any doubt, a habit-forming drug, which is why (as any smoker knows) it is so extremely difficult to abandon. The withdrawal symptoms experienced by a heavy smoker who tries to give up cigarettes can be quite unpleasant for him.

All this would not matter much, since nicotine (except in large doses) is a relatively harmless drug, and does not even 'stunt the growth' (the bogey used by past

360

generations to discourage schoolboys from taking up smoking cigarettes.)

However, the smoke which is produced by burning tobacco leaves is just as much an irritant to the lungs as is, for example, the smoke of a bonfire. Not surprisingly, this irritation has unfortunate consequences. All cigarette smokers (except those who just 'have an occasional puff' and who do not inhale) develop some inflammation of the lungs as a result. In many cases, this goes on to chronic bronchitis (see under **bronchitis**), which seems a heavy price to pay for the pleasure. If the irritation is more severe, precancerous changes can be demonstrated in the lungs and air passages. Finally, cancer itself develops in about one in eight of all heavy smokers, and in a smaller proportion of those who get through 10–20 cigarettes a day. Cancer of the lung is only rarely curable.

There are other disorders on which tobacco has a markedly adverse effect; the most important of these are duodenal ulcers and coronary heart disease.

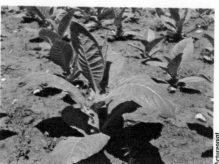

Tobacco plants growing. When ripe, the leaves are gathered and hung in bunches to dry slowly.

TOES are the digits of the feet. Unlike the fingers, the toes are relatively weak structures with practically no capacity for delicate movement. It is probable that our long-distant ape-like ancestors had such a capacity, but in modern Man the individual toes are becoming more and more useless appendages. The larger ones still play a very important part in balance, however, and in running. People who cannot use their hands can be taught to write and do other useful things with the toes.

TOLBUTAMIDE is a drug which is widely used in the control of many cases of diabetes mellitus (see **diabetes mellitus**).

As is the case with other anti-diabetic preparations which can be taken by mouth, the type of patient for which this drug is suitable is, as a rule, the person who is middle-aged and overweight, but whose diabetes cannot be controlled by strict diet alone. In these circumstances, a combination of diet and tolbutamide is often successful. If not, then other members of the same group, such as chlorpropamide or acetohexamide, may be effective. Another group of oral drugs, of which phenformin (see **phenformin**) is the best known, is also available, and if this latter group do not work, then sometimes a combination of two drugs, one from either group, may achieve effective control. If this is not the case, then the patient will have to receive injections of insulin.

Like all drugs, tolbutamide is not without side-effects, the most important of which is that it may lower the blood sugar too much and produce confusion, coma, or (rarely) death. For this reason, it is particularly important that diabetics on this drug have regular medical advice and keep a written record of daily urine sugar tests; in actual fact, *all* sensible diabetics take these precautions.

TONE is the natural state of tension in the muscles of the body. This is maintained through a reflex action which keeps the muscles slightly tense. Complete loss of tone (flaccidity) is a sign of disorder of the part of the nervous system responsible for this reflex, while a pathological increase in tone (spasticity) normally indicates injury to a higher level of the nervous system. Such spasticity may be seen, for example, after strokes, or in many spastic children who have sustained a particular kind of brain damage.

TONGUE is the muscular structure lying on the floor of the mouth. It is one of the most sensitive parts of the human body, being not only equipped to detect pain, heat, cold and ordinary touch sensation very readily, but also to taste materials which come into contact with it. This func-

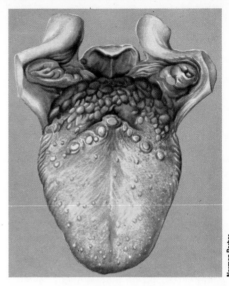

The appearance of the normal tongue. At the back are the large circumvallate papillae, while scattered over the surface in front of them are the fungiform and filiform papillae.

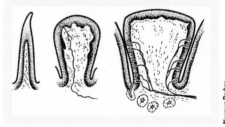

The three sorts of taste-buds. Left, filiform; centre, fungiform; right, circumvallate, showing nerves travelling from the tiny receptor cells.

tion is exercised through special receptors called taste-buds. These are hidden among the papillae, the tiny projections which cover the upper surface of the tongue.

There are three types of these papillae. The commonest are the rather pointed *filiform* papillae, which are responsible for the rough feel of the tongue.

Dotted in among these there can be seen on close inspection the small red *fungiform* papilli. Finally, at the back of the tongue (and out of sight in most people) are the much larger *circumvallate* papillae. These look like little red blobs, about the

361

size of the capital 'O' in the word 'tongue' at the head of this entry. Sometimes people see them for the first time when sticking the tongue out in front of a mirror, and go to the doctor because they think they have some strange disease.

The only common serious disorder of the tongue is cancer. This condition is rare in people under 40. It usually starts as a lump or sore patch, often at the side of the tongue, which normally develops into a wide ulcer. (This condition should not be confused with the tiny, pin-prick sized ulcers which are so common in all age groups.) Cancer is more likely to occur in people with badly-fitting dentures which constantly irritate the tongue.

Complete cure is likely, if the disease is caught early. As with any cancer, the golden rule is that anyone with the slightest suspicion that he might have the disorder should see his doctor right away.

'TONICS' as such do not really exist, though the word will probably be widely used by the public for generations to come.

In the old days when medicine had very little scientific basis, it was customary for doctors to prescribe large quantities of 'tonics' in all sorts of conditions on which the ingredients of the prescription could have had no conceivable effect. If these preparations were brightly coloured and had an unpleasant taste, then they were even more highly thought of by both patient and doctor. Many of them contained very small (and harmless) doses of poisons, which seems to have added to their impressive nature.

With the discovery of the vitamins in the early part of this century, more and more people began to ask for vitamin treatment, regardless of the fact that they were not suffering from any vitamin deficiency, nor, indeed, ever likely to be so. It nonetheless became widespread practice to incorporate a multitude of vitamins into 'tonics'.

Nowadays, doctors know that diseases must be treated with specific remedies, or at least with drugs which will have some effect on the symptoms of a disorder. If an apparently healthy person remains firm in his demand for a 'tonic' or a 'pick-me-up', then many doctors will comply by giving a prescription for something that is at least harmless. It is never wise, however, for a person to go and buy himself a bottle of 'tonic' at the chemist's — firstly, because his symptoms may indicate some disease, and secondly because some proprietary tonics actually contain chemicals which could, under certain circumstances, be dangerous.

One exception to what we have said above may be stated: young children who have been ill *may* possibly get less vitamins and iron in their diet than they need, until such times as they recover their appetites. Under these circumstances, many doctors feel that it is justified to give a carefully selected medicine containing these essential nutriments until the child is fully recovered.

TONSILLITIS, or inflammation of the tonsils, is one of the commonest ailments of childhood. Many children have numerous bouts of it (frequently without their parents ever realizing the fact), so that recurrent tonsillitis is *not* by itself any indication for taking the tonsils out, as many mothers imagine. This subject is discussed further under the heading **tonsil**.

Acute tonsillitis may follow a head cold. Children rarely complain of soreness in the throat, and the characteristic features are fever, loss of appetite, and vomiting. In fact, a feverish child who vomits once or twice and who has enlarged glands at the side of the neck is almost invariably found to have tonsillitis. Unfortunately, the vomiting may be misinterpreted, and the child may quite wrongly be thought to have some sort of abdominal trouble, such as a 'stomach upset' (gastritis).

Tonsillitis may be due to bacteria or to viruses (frequently the latter). Antibiotics have no effect on viruses, and some doctors believe it is best simply to give the child aspirin and see how he gets on. Others prefer to cover both possibilities by giving penicillin. In any event, most cases of tonsillitis get better rapidly. As with any sore throat, rheumatic fever or nephritis may very occasionally be a consequence. This is due to the spread of bacteria in the bloodstream, and the body's reaction to them.

TONSIL is one of two masses of tissue which lie on either side of the fauces (where the mouth joins the throat). In young children, the tonsils are often quite large structures; even though they are perfectly healthy, they may be so big as to touch each other and thus considerably narrow the passage at the back of the mouth. In adults they are usually smaller.

The structure of the tonsils is much like that of the lymph glands (see **lymph glands**), and, like these glands, they are believed to play an important part in combating infection. It is not yet clear whether removing the tonsils lowers a person's resistance to disease or not.

Acute inflammation of the tonsils (see **tonsillitis**) is very common. Recurrent episodes of this type are perfectly normal in childhood (just as most adults tend to suffer from sore throats two or three times a year). Therefore, a history of recurrent attacks of tonsillitis does not in itself constitute an indication for removal of the tonsils, or tonsillectomy. Many doctors think that *chronic* inflammation of the tonsils does provide a good reason for tonsillectomy, but in practice, it is extremely difficult to determine whether such chronic inflammation is present until after the tonsils have been surgically removed and can be examined under the microscope.

In fact, many doctors now believe that a high proportion of the hundreds of thousands of tonsillectomies performed each year are quite pointless. This is all the more worrying because not only do a very small number of children who have the operation die as a result, but many more are quite ill, and often emotionally upset, for some days afterwards. It seems very likely that, in a few years' time, this operation will be performed much less frequently than it used to be.

Tonsillectomy is often performed at the same time as removal of the adenoids (see **adenoid**), though the two operations can, of course, be carried out separately. Adenoidectomy seems to carry less risk than tonsillectomy. In countries where infantile paralysis is still common, neither procedure should be undertaken during the 'polio season'.

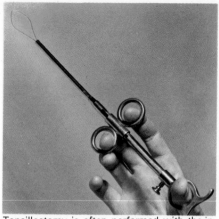

Ken Moreman

Tonsillectomy is often performed with the instrument shown here, called a 'tonsillar snare'.

TOOTHACHE is a very common symptom. It is usually an indication of decay (caries) extending into the central pulp of a tooth (see **teeth**), or of an abscess at the root (see **gumboil**). In any case, treatment of toothache is a specialized matter which should never be attempted at home; the only sensible course is to contact a dentist at the earliest possible opportunity.

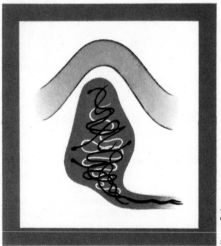

Norman Barber

An enlarged section through one of the minute touch receptors distributed throughout the skin.

TOUCH is the sensation whereby we detect objects through the pressure they exert on the skin. It is 'picked up' by tiny receptors at nerve endings distributed all

363

over the surface of the body, which relay their messages via the spinal cord to the brain. Touch is not the same thing as appreciation of temperature, pain, vibration or position, which are detected by different receptors, and relayed through different nerve fibres to separate parts of the brain. Certain diseases of the nervous system, notably syringomyelia (see **syringomyelia**) may impair some of these sensations but not others.

TOURNIQUET is a band or ligature put round a limb to arrest bleeding. However, the danger of producing gangrene with tourniquets is so great that they have been abandoned in the practice of first aid (see under **bleeding**). Tourniquets are, however, still used under carefully controlled conditions in operating theatres.

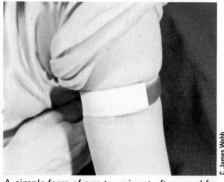

A simple form of arm tourniquet often used for such procedures as taking samples of blood.

TOXAEMIA OF PREGNANCY is a common condition, and one which must be treated with great care, firstly because it tends to lead to premature delivery of the baby, and secondly because, in a small proportion of cases, the mother develops eclampsia (see **eclampsia**), a serious and occasionally fatal disorder characterized by fits. Fortunately, the symptoms of both toxaemia (or pre-eclamptic toxaemia, as it is often called) and of eclampsia itself disappear entirely not long after delivery.

The features of toxaemia are swelling of the ankles, feet and hands (due to retained fluid), tiredness, increase in blood pressure, and the presence of protein (albumin) in the urine. Proper ante-natal
364

care requires regular examination of an expectant mother by her midwife or doctor to check for these features. If there is the slightest suspicion of toxaemia, and especially if the blood pressure is at all raised, it is absolutely essential that the mother rest more. When the blood pressure reaches a certain level, it is standard practice in most countries to admit the mother to hospital for complete bed rest under sedation.

These simple measures have had a quite remarkable effect in reducing the incidence of severe toxaemia and of eclampsia. Expectant mothers should realize the very great importance of seeing the doctor or midwife regularly for check-ups and of taking their advice regarding rest. Disregard of such advice may hazard the life and health of both mother and baby.

TOXICOLOGY is the study of poisons.

TOXINS are poisons produced by germs. Unlike the germs themselves, they may not be destroyed by heat — a case in point is the toxin of the Staphylococcus bacterium (see **Staphylococci**) which is responsible for a common type of food poisoning (see **food poisoning**) against which cooking provides no protection.

Some bacterial toxins are among the most poisonous chemicals in existence — it has been calculated by germ warfare experts that an ounce of botulinus toxin could kill the entire population of the world several thousand times over. Fortunately, the widespread use of such toxins in war poses many problems, but it is widely known that the major powers are prepared for chemical and biological warfare (CBW), and have stocks of such material, including, perhaps, toxin-smeared bullets.

TOXOIDS are toxins (see **toxins**) which have been rendered totally harmless by some process such as chemical action, or neutralization by an 'antitoxin', and which can therefore be used with complete safety to produce active artificial immunity (see under **immunity**) to a particular disease. A typical example is tetanus toxoid (see **tetanus**), also known, rather loosely, as anti-tetanus vaccine.

TOXOPLASMOSIS is a disorder which was not first described until 1939, but which has been recognized as being of increasing importance in recent years.

It is caused by a single-celled organism

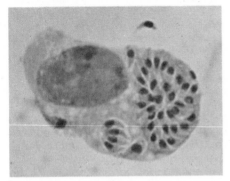

The organism responsible for the disease toxoplasmosis, *Toxoplasma gondii*, seen under high magnification in lymphatic fluid.

(or protozoan — see **protozoans**) called *Toxoplasma gondii*. This parasite is widely distributed among both animals and birds, and it is not clear how it enters the human body. However, as many as one third of the population of some American cities have been shown to have antibodies (see **antibodies**) to it, indicating past infection by the parasite. High antibody levels are also found in household pets, such as cats, dogs and guinea-pigs.

Toxoplasmosis may occur in two forms — congenital (i.e. present before birth) or acquired.

Where congenital infection occurs, the infant may be born dead; if he survives, the manifestations of infection may include jaundice, fever, rashes, inflammation of the back of the eye, and convulsions. Some infants have quite severe brain damage, and many can be shown to have a curious deposition of the mineral calcium within the skull; this can be shown up by means of an X-ray.

Acquired toxoplasmosis in older children and adults seems to produce a more benign illness, characterized principally by skin rashes and enlargement of the lymph glands. It may be confused with glandular fever, or with German measles. Sometimes, however, encephalitis (brain inflammation — see **encephalitis**) may occur. Sulphonamides, sometimes combined with other preparations, have a beneficial effect on the disease.

TRACHEA – see **windpipe**.

TRACHEOTOMY, or tracheostomy, means making a hole in the trachea, or windpipe (see **windpipe**). This operation is performed by making an incision in the front of the neck, some distance below the Adam's apple (where the rings of gristle found in the wall of the windpipe can clearly be felt under the skin). Once the windpipe is opened, the hole is prevented from closing by the insertion of a special device through which the patient can breathe; in emergency, any small tube can be used for this purpose, but it must be held in place lest it slips inside.

Tracheotomy may be a life-saving procedure in conditions where the larynx (voice-box) is blocked so that the patient cannot breathe. This may happen when a foreign body is inhaled or 'goes down the wrong way', and becomes jammed. Similarly, in diphtheria (see **diphtheria**), the membrane which forms in the throat may

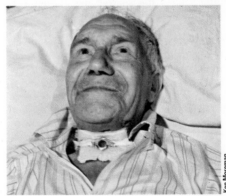

Ken Moreman

A patient with a tracheotomy tube, inserted into the windpipe from the outside of the neck. Use of such a tube is often life-saving.

block the air passages and choke the patient to death unless a tracheotomy is carried out as an emergency operation.

Tracheotomy is also used in certain cases of severe head injury, when there is a great deal of blood pouring into the throat, and in a number of conditions where it is essential to assist the patient's respiration over prolonged periods by artificial ventilation through a machine. In these instances, the device pushed into the aperture of the tracheotomy is connected directly to the breathing machine.

TRACHOMA is an eye disease, occurring mainly in those warmer areas of the world where hygienic conditions are poor. It is caused by a large virus, rather similar in nature to the organism which produces psittacosis (see **psittacosis**).

The virus first of all causes a conjunctivitis (see **conjunctivitis**) and general inflammation of the outer tissues of the eye. There is a profuse discharge of pus, and the eye-lids become badly swollen. After some weeks, the acute inflammation subsides, but is usually replaced by progressive scarring of the cornea (the 'window' of the eye). In time, this may well affect the vision and, in fact, trachoma is one of the commonest causes of blindness in the world.

In the early stages, the trachoma germ is one of the very few viruses which will respond to treatment by antibiotics. In the later stages the scarred eye tissues can sometimes be replaced by grafting.

TRANQUILLIZERS are drugs which have become used on a massive scale throughout western civilization over the last fifteen years or so.

Up until the mid-1950s, the only drugs available to cope with mental stresses and strains were the sedatives (see **sedatives**). These had certain disadvantages, the most important of which was that, in addition to reducing anxiety, the sedatives tend to make patients drowsy, and impair their concentration.

The tranquillizers which were introduced in the latter part of the 1950s and in the 1960s were intended to produce as little drowsiness as possible, though none have been entirely successful in this respect.

The first tranquillizers which were widely used were reserpine (a drug which had previously been employed for the treatment of high blood pressure), and chlorpromazine. Reserpine is now only rarely prescribed as a tranquillizer, because of its very uncertain effects, but chlorpromazine and a large number of closely related drugs called the phenothiazines are used in great quantities.

Other types of tranquillizing drug which have come into use include meprobamate, chlordiazepoxide and haloperidol.

All the tranquillizers are fairly powerful drugs, and must be used with extreme caution. The stated dose should never be exceeded, and alcohol should never be taken at the same time.

TRANSFUSIONS are infusions of one person's blood into the veins of another. Donated blood (see **blood donation**) is collected in a sterile bottle or plastic bag. With it is mixed an anticoagulant substance, to prevent it from clotting. Next, it is carefully grouped, to determine whether it is of groups A, B, AB, or O, and whether it is Rhesus positive or negative (see **blood groups**).

Before being transfused into a person who needs it, however, the blood will be carefully 'cross-matched' against a specimen of the recipient's blood; this is in case there is any incompatibility not revealed by ABO or Rhesus testing.

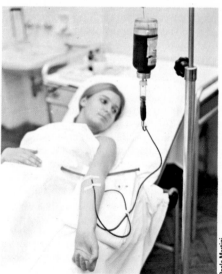

Patient receiving a transfusion of whole blood into an arm vein. Leg veins are sometimes used. The transfusion rate is carefully regulated.

TRANSPLANTS, or transplantations, are surgical procedures in which the tissues or organs of one person are grafted into the body of another.

The first operations of this type were simply ordinary blood transfusions (see **transfusions**). Those who first tried to transfuse blood found that sometimes the procedure worked without any hitch at all, but that more often than not, the person being transfused had a violent reaction to the donor blood. Fortunately for mankind, it was fairly rapidly discovered that blood could very readily be 'grouped' in a simple way (see **blood groups**), so that it was very easy to overcome this rejection problem.

However, considerable difficulties arose with tissues other than blood. Attempts were made to transplant or graft skin in cases of severe burns and similar injuries. Skin from other human beings and even animals was used for this purpose: unfortunately, it was found that most recipients rejected such 'foreign' skin after a varying period of time (which might, however, be long enough to offer some temporary protection for the damaged tissues). The best chance of a graft from another person 'taking' was if both parties were identical twins. Obviously, this was rarely a practicable possibility. Fortunately, in the vast majority of burns and severe injuries, it proved possible to borrow skin from another part of the patient's body to cover the affected area. As is the case with skin from an identical twin, the patient does not reject his own tissues either.

It was therefore clear that a human being has some means of recognizing 'foreign' tissue, and rejecting it: this mechanism we call the 'immune response'. While immunity is immensely valuable in protecting a person against many infectious diseases (see **immunity**), here it apparently acts to the individual's detriment.

So, doctors began to look around for ways of combating the immune response. Some hope was provided by the fact that it had proved possible to transplant the cornea (the tiny window at the front of the eye) as early as 1906, though, in fact, good results were not obtained on a large scale until about the time of the Second World War. However, the vast majority of corneal grafts 'took' without any evidence of rejection. It now seems likely that this is because the cornea is a bloodless area, vary largely cut off from the body's immune mechanisms. So, the body never gets a chance to recognize the foreign cornea as being 'self' or 'non-self'.

Were there any other ways of avoiding the immune mechanism? To find out, scientists looked into the way this mechanism is established. They found that it was actually developed during life in the womb, and that in mice it was possible to inject the unborn foetus (in whom the immune mechanism had not yet developed) with certain blood-forming tissues from completely unrelated types of mice. When the baby mice who had been so treated grew up, they could accept transplants from the other mice without any rejection developing: in other words, these tissues were registered as 'self', rather than 'non-self'.

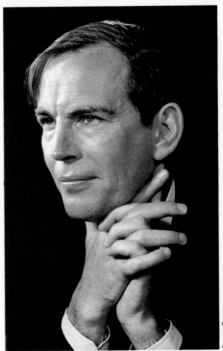

Dr Christiaan Barnard, the first surgeon to undertake transplantation of the human heart.

While this opened interesting possibilities for the future, it did not immediately help the position of people with irreversibly damaged kidneys, livers, lungs or hearts who might have benefited by transplantation. However, by various extensions of the work, it was found that the immune reaction depends to a large extent on the group of white blood cells which are known as the lymphocytes, and on the tissues which produce them. Furthermore, it was possible to suppress the activity of these tissues in various ways. It can be done by irradiation of the patient with X-rays or radio-active material; by giving him large doses of steroid drugs (see **steroids**); by treatment with anti-cancer drugs (which inhibit the workings of active tissues such as those which produce the lymphocytes); and by giving anti-lymphocyte serum (ALS), a preparation which (as its name implies) interferes with the action of lymphocytes.

Armed with these weapons, doctors began the first large scale transplantations of internal organs in the late 1950s and early 1960s.

The obvious first target was transplantation of kidneys. Many people (including those who are still young) die every year simply because their kidneys are too diseased to function properly (see **kidneys**). It is a straightforward surgical procedure to take one kidney from a healthy person and transplant it into someone with this type of chronic disease. Rejection, of course, is the problem. While almost all transplanted kidneys donated by identical twins 'took' satisfactorily, a smaller proportion of those given by close relatives (such as parents, brothers or sisters) escaped rejection. When 'random' donors (e.g. road accident victims) are used, the chances of success are rather slim, even with the aid of all the anti-immunity weapons mentioned above. In fact, the 1968 Human Kidney Transplant Registry Report found that only 45 per cent of those patients who had received kidneys from dead bodies were alive a year later. However, 75 per cent of those who had had kidneys from blood relatives were alive, and most of these would probably have died without the operation or the use of an artificial kidney (see **kidney – artificial**).

The answer seemed to lie in the process of tissue-typing, which is like a very sophisticated form of blood grouping. This became available in the mid-1960s.

It was not surprising that after a number of successful heart transplants had been carried out on animals in various countries, the first human heart transplant was performed by Dr Christiaan Barnard in 1967. This was not an outstandingly difficult technical feat for a competent heart surgeon (as witness the fact that over 100 similar operations were carried out over the next year in 19 different countries); the real achievement of Dr Barnard and his team was to keep several of their transplant patients alive for very long periods by skilful use of the anti-immunity weapons mentioned above.

Widespread use of tissue-typing has led to the transplantation of organs such as the lung and liver, but with little success at the present time. Whether heart, lung and liver transplants will be as effective as kidney transplants now are in saving lives should be known within a few years.

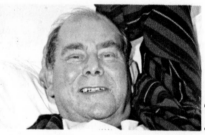

Philip Blaiberg, one of the first to receive another person's heart by transplantation.

TRANSVESTITISM, or transvestism, is a sexual perversion (see **perversions**) in which the affected person can only achieve satisfaction through dressing-up in the clothes of the opposite sex. It is much commoner in men than in women. Although any form of sexual deviation is very commonly associated with others, there does not seem (as many people imagine) to be any special connection between this disorder and homosexuality (see **homosexuality**).

368

TRAUMA, a word derived from the Greek for 'a wound', literally means an injury to some part of the body. The word is also used in a wider sense in medicine to indicate any kind of severe mental stress as well. The word 'traumatic' means pertaining to injury, or emotionally stressful.

TRAVEL SICKNESS is nausea or vomiting which develops during any kind of travel, whether by coach, car, aeroplane, train, or boat.

Though all these types of illness are rather similar, sea-sickness is a little different from the rest in that the principal factor is usually the persistent up and down motion of the boat. This has a marked effect on the body's balancing mechanism, and in particular on the fluid-filled semi-circular canals of the inner ear (see **ear**). When the fluid is subjected to continuous rhythmic disturbances of sufficient strength for long enough, nausea and vomiting are likely to follow in almost anyone.

However, in other types of travel sickness there is not this persistent up and down movement to upset the balance mechanisms, and doctors feel that in the majority of these cases, psychological factors play the most important part in bringing on nausea. No serious evidence has ever been brought forward to challenge this view, though many lay people think that car sickness, for instance, is caused by an accumulation of static electricity on the car body. While this is an ingenious theory, there is no reason at all to suppose that any significant degree of static electricity is present on the average car body. Even if there were, there is no conceivable way in which it could make a person feel sick. However, the common practice of attaching a chain to the car to drain off static electricity into the earth is quite harmless, and makes many people feel better, even if (as often happens) the chain is not touching the ground!

Doctors usually rely on slightly more orthodox methods — for instance, the use of drugs such as hyoscine, or antihistamine compounds such as cyclizine, meclozine or dimenhydrinate. Patients vary in their response to these preparations, and it is important not to be discouraged by initial failure, since it is always worth trying another drug. In addition to damping down feelings of nausea, the antihistamines and hyoscine both have a useful sedative effect, which helps to allay the sufferer's nervousness about travelling. However, this effect may also lead to drowsiness, so it is important that car drivers, for instance, should not take these preparations. (Fortunately, it is usually passengers, rather than drivers, who suffer from travel sickness, probably because the driver has so much to concentrate on.) None of these drugs should be taken with alcohol, which may greatly increase the sedative effect. Hyoscine may produce a dryness of the mouth, and blurring of the vision.

TRENCH FEVER is an infectious disease caused by the organism known as Rickettsia quintana. Like most other rickettsial diseases (see **rickettsiae**), trench fever is transmitted to Man by means of a parasite, in this case the body louse.

Lice carrying the rickettsiae infest the body when conditions of hygiene are poor, e.g. in trenches during wartime. Because of the persistent itching caused by the lice, the sufferer scratches, and thus breaks his own skin. The germs emerge from the faeces or the crushed bodies of the lice, and enter the scratches.

Trench fever was an extremely common cause of illness and debility in the First World War, in which hygienic conditions for the combatants were probably the most appalling encountered by any troops in this century. However, with the advent of powerful insecticides, and greater understanding of the need for hygiene, this disease, like many other rickettsial infections, has become a rarity in the western world.

Trench foot has been confused with trench fever by some people in the past. In fact, the two disorders have nothing at all to do with each other, except that they tend to occur under the conditions of trench warfare. Trench foot is due to immersion of the feet in water or mud for very long periods. Characteristically, the feet are cold and pulseless: very great care must be taken not to expose them to too much warmth. A precisely identical condition, occurring in shipwrecked people who have been in the sea for a long time, is called immersion foot.

TREPHINING, or trepanning, means making a hole in the skull by removing a piece of bone.

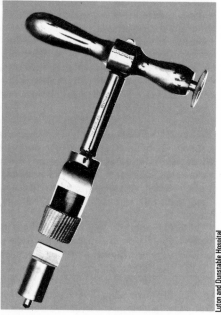

A trephine, or drill to open the skull by removing a small circular piece of the bone.

This operation seems to have been practised by Man since pre-historic times. In many parts of the world old skulls are found with neat sections chipped out. At first glance, it might appear that these were the skulls of victims of murder or ritual execution but, in fact, examination of the condition of the bone around the hole usually shows that the 'patient' was alive for a period of years after his operation. Not surprisingly, the writings of Hippocrates, which date from the fifth century BC, contain full accounts of trephining. Even today, there remain a few primitive tribes in the south western Pacific who regularly practice the operation, appar-

370

ently without any serious complications ensuing. In all these primitive societies, the general idea seems to have been to let evil spirits out of a person's skull, usually in order to relieve him of chronic headache.

Nowadays, however, trephining (or making 'burr-holes', as doctors usually call it) is mainly used in cases of severe head injury, where the surgeon wants to search for a torn blood vessel, or remove a clot. More extensive removal of bone may be needed for such procedures as draining a brain abscess, or removing a growth.

Surprisingly, having a small hole in the skull has no subsequent ill-effects, since the protective covering of the scalp over the aperture is quite sufficient.

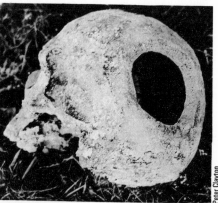

Skulls like this, from Egypt, show that trephining was practised thousands of years ago.

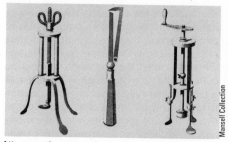

Nineteenth-century instruments used for trephining and removing portions of skull bone.

TREPONEMES are germs of the group which cause the venereal disease syphilis (see **syphilis**) and the tropical infection called yaws (see **yaws**).

TRIAMTERENE is a diuretic drug (see **diuretics**) — that is, one which helps the body to get rid of excess water by increasing the production of urine.

Triamterene was introduced to medical practice in the early 1960s. It is of considerable use in treating all kinds of dropsy (oedema), and, in particular, the type of fluid retention associated with cirrhosis of the liver. The special advantage of the drug is that, unlike most commonly-used diuretics, it does not cause dangerous depletion of the body's stores of the vital mineral potassium (see **potassium**). In fact, it may even keep the potassium level up, which can occasionally be a disadvantage. It sometimes causes mild side effects, such as nausea or diarrhoea, but, in general, it forms one of the most useful weapons in the doctor's armoury.

TRICHINIASIS, or trichinosis, is a disorder caused by eating undercooked diseased pork.

Such pork contains the larvae of a parasite called *Trichinella spiralis*. These larvae lie inside tiny cysts in the muscle fibres. Unfortunately, the cysts are so small that they cannot be detected by the routine visual examination of carcasses which is carried out by public health officials in most advanced countries; in fact they can only be seen with a microscope.

Pork which is properly cooked, pickled or smoked, or which has been frozen to at least minus 18°C for 24 hours, is safe, but it is evident that these precautions are not always taken, because the incidence of trichiniasis is very high in the United States, where there is said to be more than three times as much trichiniasis as on the rest of the globe put together. The disease is also frequently encountered in the remainder of North America and in Europe, but very rarely in the rest of the world. Apart from the popularity of pork in North America and Europe, and its low consumption elsewhere (for economic or religious reasons), there seems to be no obvious cause for the curious difference in incidence.

When a human being eats infested pork and becomes infected, he may have no symptoms at all, though many patients complain of diarrhoea in the early stages. In the succeeding weeks, larvae find their way to the patient's muscles and there form new cysts. There may be widespread muscle pain as a result, and this is usually associated with fever. The larvae may also reach the lungs and brain, but rarely cause trouble in these sites. There may also be inflammation of the heart (myocarditis).

The diagnosis of the disease is rather difficult to make, but a blood test, coupled with the removal of a small piece of muscle for microscopic examination, will usually prove helpful.

Except in the early stages, there is no specific treatment for trichiniasis. Fortunately, the death rate is very low.

Control of the disease consists largely in ensuring that all pork is properly cooked. This applies not only to pork eaten by humans, but to pork scraps which are fed to pigs; it is believed that using uncooked meat for this latter purpose is largely responsible for the continuance of the infection among these animals.

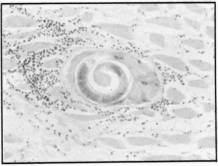

The organism responsible for trichiniasis, seen microscopically in human muscle tissue.

TRICHLOROETHYLENE is one of the most useful of all general anaesthetics (see **anaesthesia**). Since the Second World War, trichloroethylene has largely replaced ether (see **ether**) as the most important anaesthetic gas, partly because it is free from the very irritant properties of ether, and is thus less likely to lead to post-operative chest infections. Only in the 1960s did trichloroethylene come to be partly replaced by newer anaesthetic gases such as halothane.

TRICHOMONAS VAGINALIS is a very common parasite which causes vaginal discharge. It is a single-celled organism, or protozoan, with a whip-like tail.

TV, as it is frequently (though rather confusingly) referred to, is one of the most widespread parasites of the human race. It produces a profuse yellow vaginal discharge, often full of minute bubbles. There may also be severe irritation of the vulva (see **vulva**), and, when the doctor examines the upper part of the vagina, he finds that it is reddened and eroded. The cervix, or neck of the womb, may also be inflamed.

Why trichomonas produces discharge is not entirely clear. Many doctors believe that it is a natural inhabitant of the vagina in many cases, but that it will only multiply or produce symptoms under certain circumstances — possibly when the normal acidity of the vagina is lowered for some reason.

Trichomonas can be effectively treated by the insertion of special pessaries each night and morning over a period of about five weeks. It is customary to suggest refraining from intercourse during this time. Recurrences of infection are common.

However, a newer method of treatment came into widespread use during the 1960s, and seems to lead to fewer recurrences. A drug called metronidazole is given three times daily by mouth for about a fortnight; it should normally be given to the husband as well as to the wife, since he may very well have symptomless infection of his own genital tract, and may keep re-infecting his wife unless these measures are taken.

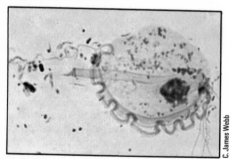

Seen under the microscope, the organism called Trichomonas vaginalis, a widespread parasite.

C. James Webb

372

TRICHONOSIS is the term for a diseased condition of the hair.

TRICHOPHYTON VIOLACEUM is the vegetable parasite that causes barber's itch (see **barber's itch**). It is a member of the genus *trichophyton*, a group of fungi that live on or in the skin or hair. The species causes various skin problems, including the ringworm infections (see **ringworm**.)

TRICHORRHOEA is the term used to describe a general falling out of the hair. It is usually caused by a disease such as typhoid, but where there is no obvious cause an investigation of scalp health may lead to a diagnosis. A certain amount of falling hair is natural.

TRICUSPID VALVE is one of the valves of the heart (see **heart**). It lies between the right auricle (atrium) and the right ventricle, and prevents blood flowing backwards from the latter to the former.

Disorders of the tricuspid valve are rather less common than those of the other heart valves. However, stenosis (narrowing) of the tricuspid is present in a small percentage of all cases of the common condition called mitral stenosis, or narrowing of the mitral valve (see **mitral valve**). Both are normally due to rheumatic fever (see **rheumatic fever**); tricuspid stenosis produces abdominal dropsy (ascites), and sometimes jaundice.

Incompetence (leaking) of the tricuspid valve is quite common. It may be due to a deformity present at birth, or, more frequently, to the back-pressure caused by disease elsewhere in the heart.

Doctors can often detect these faults by observing the blood flow in the veins of the neck and by listening for heart murmurs near the centre of the chest. Operation may be necessary in cases of severe disorder. Tricuspid stenosis can be treated by a valve to restore the full flow of blood. Serious cases of incompetence have led surgeons to replace the defective valve with an artificial one in recent years, but the long term success or failure of this complicated operation has yet to be ascertained.

TRIGEMINAL NERVE is one of the cranial nerves – that is the twelve pairs of nerves which emerge from the brain itself to supply various parts of the head, neck and trunk.

The trigeminal nerve transmits sensation to the brain from the skin of the face, and parts of the throat and mouth, including the upper and lower teeth. At the same time, it transmits 'instructions', in the form of nerve impulses, from the brain to the various muscles which are responsible for mastication (chewing).

The trigeminal nerve is particularly susceptible to neuralgia. Trigeminal neuralgia (or **tic douloureux**) is fully described under the heading **neuralgia**.

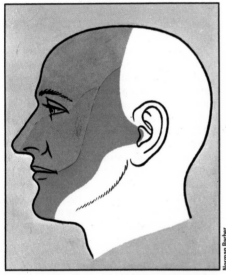

The three branches of the trigeminal nerve: blue, ophthalmic; green, maxillary; red, mandibular.

TRIGGER FINGER is a common deformity of the fingers or thumb. In adults, it normally only affects one digit, but sometimes in babies the deformity may be present in several fingers.

When a person suffering this condition 'makes a fist', and then tries to unclench it, one finger remains bent, and can only be straightened with difficulty. As the condition progresses, it becomes more severe, and eventually the finger can be straightened only by using the other hand. A click can usually be felt as the resistance is overcome and the finger straightens.

Most commonly, trigger finger is due to a narrowing of the fibrous tunnel through which the tendons of the finger pass, while on their way through the palm of the hand to the muscles of the forearm. (These muscles are actually responsible for most finger movements – see **fingers**.)

After a while, this narrowing of the tunnel makes a groove on the tendon; and this groove (which 'snaps' as it passes through) can very readily 'catch', and thus prevent the finger from straightening.

Sometimes another cause is responsible for the deformity. A ganglion, or swelling may form on the tendon, and this too may jam at one end of the tunnel.

In either case, a simple operation involving slitting the fibrous tunnel open, will cure the condition.

TRIGONE is the triangle-shaped lower part of the bladder between the openings of the ureters and the urethra.

TRIGONITIS is an inflammation of the mucous membrane of the trigone.

TRIIODOTHYRONINE is one of the two main hormones produced by the thyroid gland (the other is thyroxine). It is dependent on adequate iodine intake in the diet and on stimulation by the pituitary gland. It can be synthesized and administered intravenously in cases of thyroid deficiency (see also **thyroid gland**).

TRINITRIN, glyceryl trinitrate, or nitroglycerine, is the drug which is probably more frequently used than any other in the relief of angina – pain coming from the heart muscle and caused by degenerative disease of the coronary arteries, which supply the heart with blood.

This kind of pain usually comes on as a result of exertion, and is relieved as soon as the patient rests. Trinitrin tablets, taken under the tongue, are absorbed very rapidly, and appear to ease the pain. Why they should do this is not entirely clear. For many years, it was believed that trinitrin and similar but 'long-acting' drugs dilated (widened) the coronary arteries, and thus improved the blood flow to the

373

muscle of the heart.

However, in recent years, there has been a good deal of rethinking of this entire question. The so-called 'long-acting' chemical relatives of trinitrin are no longer widely believed to have any effect whatsoever on the coronary arteries, and it has even been suggested that trinitrin itself only produces its effect because it lowers the blood pressure slightly, and thus makes it easier for the heart to drive blood round the body. The whole situation is made more difficult to assess by the fact that patients who suffer an attack of

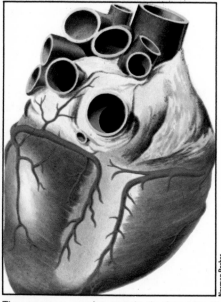

The coronary arteries supply the heart itself with blood, spreading over the muscle surface.

angina on exertion almost invariably stop whatever they are doing immediately, so that the pain passes off anyway in two or three minutes, which is about the time which a trinitrin tablet takes to reach the bloodstream after being allowed to dissolve in the mouth.

However, most doctors believe that trinitrin, unlike the 'long-acting' preparations, is definitely a very useful drug if employed properly. There is usually no point in taking it once an attack of angina starts: instead, a tablet should be chewed, and allowed to dissolve under the tongue,

about two to three minutes before an exertion (such as walking up a steep hill) is attempted. Once taken, the effect of a tablet lasts for a quarter to half an hour. It is possible to take twenty to thirty tablets a day without causing any harm, but in an individual case, a person should obviously ask his doctors advice about this.

Occasionally, trinitrin makes angina pains worse instead of better. If this happens, the tablets should be stopped at once, and the doctor consulted. Minor side effects include headache, flushing of the face, and (quite commonly) fainting, all of which occurrences are due to the widening of blood vessels which the drug produces in various parts of the body.

TRISMUS, which literally means 'grinding of the teeth', is inability to open the mouth fully.

Trismus is common in various inflammatory conditions in the region of the back of the mouth and the throat, and, most particularly, in cases of quinsy or peritonsillar abscess (see **quinsy**).

Trismus is also a prominent feature of tetanus (lockjaw). In this condition the patient's mouth may be so tightly closed over a long period that feeding him presents considerable problems, and may have to be carried out by tube-feeding, through the nose, or by intravenous 'drip'. It is, of course, because of the symptom of trismus that lockjaw got its name.

TROPICAL DISEASES are those which are commonest in the warm regions of the world. They are, however, by no means always confined to these areas, particularly in these days of rapid air travel. Some were, at one point, world-wide but have been beaten back by medical advances in temperate countries.

For specific tropical diseases see: **beriberi; blackwater fever; brucellosis; Chagas' disease; cholera; dengue; dysentery; dhobie's itch; elephantiasis; filiariasis; kwashiorkor; leprosy; malaria; parasites; paratyphoid fever; plague; rabies; sickle-cell anaemia; sleeping sickness; sprue; thalassaemia; trachoma; typhoid; yaws; yellow fever.**

374

TRUSS is a device used to support a hernia (rupture) in circumstances where an operation is, for some reason, impracticable.

Most trusses consist of a belt or spring, to which is attached a thick pad; the object is to keep this pad over the opening through which the hernia protrudes, and so keep it in place.

The great majority of trusses are inguinal ones — i.e. for hernias occurring in the region of the groin. This type of hernia is dealt with under the heading **rupture**, and it will be noted that there are certain kinds of hernia occurring in this region which simply cannot be properly dealt with by using a truss — in particular, femoral hernias.

It is, therefore, extremely unwise for a patient to buy a truss from mail order firms without seeking a medical opinion. If a truss is to be worn, it should only be after a careful examination to determine the exact nature of the hernia, an assessment of whether an operation should be carried out or not, and, finally, a proper fitting by an experienced technician. It is essential to bear in mind that the risks of leaving a rupture unoperated on are considerable, and that the complications of doing so (described under the heading **rupture**) occur quite frequently, and may be very serious. For this reason, surgeons will usually recommend cure by operation wherever possible, in preference to the use of a truss.

TRYPANOSOMES are the tiny protozoan parasites (see **protozoans**) which cause the various types of trypanosomiasis (see **trypanosomiasis**).

TRYPANOSOMIASIS means infection by parasites called trypanosomes, carried by insects.

Man is infected by three principal types of trypanosome. *Trypanosoma gambiense* and *Trypanosoma rhodesiense* are the causes of African sleeping sickness, which is dealt with under the heading **sleeping sickness**. Both are transmitted by different types of tsetse fly. *Trypanosoma cruzi*, which occurs in South America, is the cause of Chagas' disease (see **Cha-**gas' disease**), which is transmitted to Man by the bites of Reduviid 'assassin bugs'. Infection by another, but harmless, species of trypanosome also occurs in South American children.

Trypanosomes are also very important because of their effects on animals. Indeed, the depredation caused by these parasites constitutes an enormous economic problem in Africa and some other parts of the world. It is said that four million square miles of Africa cannot be developed at present because of the impossibility of raising cattle and horses there. These animals are subject to the fatal disease *nagana*, which is caused by *Trypanosoma brucei*, and transmitted once again by the bite of the tsetse fly. Fortunately, this particular species does not affect Man; nor do other species of trypanosome which produce various fatal diseases of cattle, horses, donkeys, mules and dogs in many parts of the world. Undoubtedly, one of the great problems facing Man in the last third of the twentieth century is the control and eventual eradication of the trypanosome and the tsetse fly.

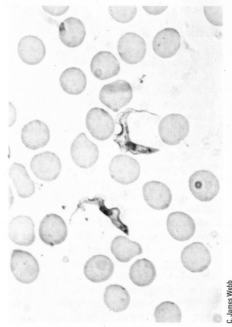

C. James Webb

Trypanosome parasites, which cause sleeping sickness, are carried by tsetse flies.

TSETSE FLY — see **trypanosomiasis**, and **sleeping sickness**.

TUBERCULIN TESTING is a means of testing children and adults for susceptibility to tuberculosis (see **tuberculosis**). In many countries, such testing is carried out routinely on schoolchildren aged 13 to 14, who can then be given a BCG vaccine (see **BCG**) if they are shown to be susceptible to the disease. Tuberculin testing is also usually performed on anyone who is suspected of having tuberculosis, or who has been exposed to the disease, or is likely to be so.

There are basically two important ways of testing — the Mantoux test and the Heaf test. Both are discussed fully under the heading **Mantoux test**.

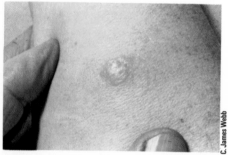

This positive reaction to a tuberculin test shows that a patient already has immunity.

TUBERCULOSIS is the disease produced by infection with the germ called *Mycobacterium tuberculosis*.

There are a number of different varieties of this bacillus, but for practical purposes, the only two important ones are the human and the bovine (i.e. cattle) varieties. The human variety is passed on from man to man, usually by inhalation into the lungs in the breath, but the bovine type enters the body in unpasteurized milk from infected cows. It remains quite a common cause of tuberculosis of the intestines, particularly in children.

Either variety of tuberculosis bacillus may spread to almost any part of the body from the original site of infection in the lungs, or intestines. The bones, joints, skin, brain and spinal cord, kidneys, and the male and female genitals are the most

frequently involved structures, and a wide variety of symptoms may be produced.

In the intestines, the primary tuberculous infection may produce persistent diarrhoea, and bowel obstruction or ulceration.

In the lungs, the primary focus of infection is a very small patch of pneumonia, which soon becomes enclosed in a capsule. At the same time, enlargement of the lymph glands inside the chest occurs.

The infection may spread no further, and, in the great majority of people, the condition heals at this stage without their knowing anything about it. However, if the infection progresses, there may be more widespread disease of the lung, or, indeed, dissemination to any of the other organs mentioned above. However, disease of the lungs (pulmonary tuberculosis) remains the most common form of tuberculosis.

Its features include persistent cough and expectoration of sputum (which may be brightly stained with blood), recurrent but slight fever, weight loss, breathlessness, tiredness, enlargement of lymph glands, and a general feeling of ill-health.

Fortunately, almost all cases of TB (except very advanced ones) respond nowadays to such drugs as streptomycin, PAS and isoniazid. Prevention and early detection depends on routine tuberculin testing (see **tuberculin testing**), BCG vaccination (see **BCG**), the use of mass X-rays (see **mass X-ray**), universal pasteurization of milk and the breeding of tubercle-free cattle.

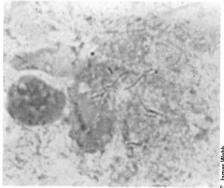

Mycobacterium tuberculosis, the germ of pulmonary tuberculosis, in human sputum.

TULARAEMIA is an infectious fever caused by a germ called *Pasteurella tularensis*, which is closely related to the organism that causes plague.

The germ is passed to Man from infected animals. A vast range of animal species may carry the disease, including rabbits, squirrels, mice, foxes, chickens, pheasants, snakes, mosquitoes and flies. Human beings may be infected by touching the carcasses of such animals (even after refrigeration), or by being bitten by infected mosquitoes and deer-flies. Those who are most frequently affected include hunters, gamekeepers, butchers, laboratory workers, cooks and housewives.

The first symptoms of the disease occur four to seven days after infection. In most cases, a reddish lump develops on the skin. This breaks down to form an ulcer, while the lymph glands in the same area of the body become grossly enlarged and painful. Sometimes, however, there is no primary lump or ulceration on the skin.

Headache, nausea and pains in all parts of the body are common. As the infection progresses, pneumonia may develop. The patient usually feels weak and ill, and he may have a fever of about 105°F over a period of weeks if his illness is not diagnosed and treated. However, the death rate is low.

Tularaemia is treated with injections of the antibiotic streptomycin, which is almost always curative. Other antibiotics such as the tetracyclines, may also be effective.

Prevention of the disease is a difficult problem. Some years ago, a vaccine was developed in Russia which gives satisfactory protection to people living in those areas of Europe and North America where the disease is very common. At present, immunization is usually only offered to hunters, gamewardens, butchers and laboratory workers. In severely affected areas, the sale of wild rabbits is usually banned. In places such as Great Britain and Ireland where the disease has not so far been a problem, it is important that stringent controls are maintained on all species of animals entering the country.

TUMOURS are swellings. In medical practice, the word means no more than this, but most lay people use it to imply cancer.

This, of course, creates considerable confusion, particularly as a patient very often overhears doctors talking about his tumour, and (quite reasonably) assumes that he has cancer.

It is, of course, true that a considerable proportion of tumours found in various parts of the body are, in fact, cancerous. It is therefore a good basic rule that any person who finds a lump or swelling of any sort on his body should go to the doctor. If it is obviously harmless, the doctor will tell him so; if there is any doubt, the matter will be investigated further, and the lump will probably be removed surgically.

The important thing is not to delay in consulting the doctor about a tumour. To take an example of what happens all too frequently, a woman may find a lump in her breast and simply do nothing about it for months on end. By the time she decides to go to the doctor, it may be too late.

The subject of malignant tumours is discussed further under the heading **cancer**. The commoner forms of cancer are dealt with under the headings of the organs in which they occur.

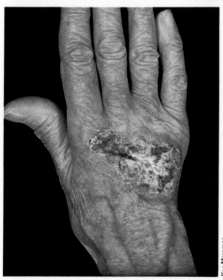

Ken Moreman

Many tumours are benign and non-cancerous. This tumour is malignant, but even so, early treatment often proves successful.

TURNER'S SYNDROME is a disorder of the genes (see **genes**). It is characterized by stunting of growth, various congenital abnormalities and maldevelopment of the sex organs.

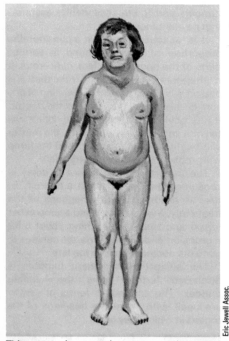

This woman's stunted appearance is caused by Turner's syndrome, a disorder of the genes affecting the body's development.

Eric Jewell Assoc.

Human beings inherit their natural characteristics through the genes contributed by their parents. These genes are arranged in lines along tiny threads of material called chromosomes. The normal human has 23 pairs of these chromosomes – i.e. 46 in all, and one of these pairs is mainly concerned with differentiation between the sexes. If the pair consists of an X and a Y chromosome, the person will be a male; if instead, there are two X chromosomes, then the individual will be female.

Unfortunately, it is not uncommon for something to go wrong with this arrangement, and the commonest abnormality is probably Turner's syndrome, in which one of this important pair of chromosomes is missing. Although the patient is female in appearance and outlook, her genetic inheritance is not 'XX', but simply 'XO' (O indicating nil), so that there are 45 chromosomes instead of 46.

Such patients are very short in stature, and tend to be obese. There is usually a deformity of the neck and the elbows, the breasts fail to develop at puberty, and there is no menstruation, as the ovaries have failed to develop properly. Fortunately, hormone therapy helps these patients considerably, and will enable them to reach sexual maturity. However, sterility is inevitable.

TWILIGHT SLEEP is a phrase which was once widely used to indicate a condition of great drowsiness induced with the object of making childbirth as painless as possible, but without making the mother unconscious. The phrase is now dropping out of use, though it is still common to induce a similar state of drowsiness towards the end of labour.

Originally, twilight sleep was produced by giving the mother large doses of morphine by injection throughout labour. This method was abandoned since it proved dangerous, not only for the mother but, more especially, for the unborn baby, since morphia crosses the placenta (afterbirth) into the baby's bloodstream, and causes profound depression of respiration at the time when (more than ever in its life) the child needs to breathe.

Nowadays, mothers may be given carefully controlled amounts of pain-killing and sedative drugs during labour. They may also, under guidance from the midwife, inhale a mixture of 50 per cent nitrous oxide (see under **laughing gas**) and 50 per cent air. Alternatively, the mother may inhale very low concentrations (less than $\frac{1}{2}$ per cent) of trichloroethylene (see **trichloroethylene**). Usually, these methods do not produce more than short periods of drowsiness (lasting, say, 30 seconds) to cover each pain of the final minutes of labour. Particularly in the United States, however, an anaesthetist (or anaesthesiologist) may give larger concentrations of anaesthetic gases and produce deeper and more prolonged drowsiness.

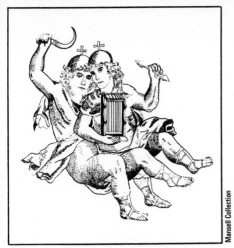

Twins were once regarded as a sign from the gods: in Greek legend, Castor and Pollux became the constellation Gemini.

TWINS occur roughly once in every 80 or 90 deliveries. The incidence of actual twin pregnancies is a little lower than this, since the chances of miscarriage are rather greater in multiple pregnancies. Occasionally, twins are found to run in families. It is recorded that a Sicilian woman gave birth to a grand total of eleven pairs, the last of whom were born in 1947. Except in unusual circumstances (e.g. a past history or a family history of multiple births), insurance companies are willing, for a small premium, to provide financial cover against the risk of having twins.

There are two sorts of twins — firstly, dizygotic, binovular, non-identical, or fraternal twins; and secondly, mono-zygotic, monovular or identical twins.

Dizygotic twins are formed from two separate eggs (ova) and two separate sperms, whereas monozygotic twins are formed from a single egg and sperm. The two types are discussed further under the headings **dizygotic twins** and **monozygotic twins.**

How does a mother know she is going to have twins? Usually, the first indication is that the womb is noticed by the doctor or midwife to be 'too big for the dates' at around the fifth month of pregnancy. There are a number of possible causes for this, however, and if the diagnosis is not clear, an X-ray will be taken in due course to settle the matter. (However, it is still true that, because the detection of this condition may be difficult, a considerable number of undiagnosed twins are born every year, to the surprise of both mother and doctor.)

Twins present a number of problems during both pregnancy and during labour itself.

In pregnancy, toxaemia (see **toxaemia**) is more common than normal, as is the less frequently encountered condition of acute hydramnios (see **hydramnios**). The relatively minor disorders of pregnancy, such as nausea, backache, and heartburn may be more troublesome. In addition, the nutritional demands of the two babies inside her may readily make the mother anaemic, so she may well have to take extra supplies of iron. She should also drink at least two pints of milk a day, to keep up her calcium intake.

Rest is of great importance during a twin pregnancy, particularly as there is a greatly increased risk of premature birth,

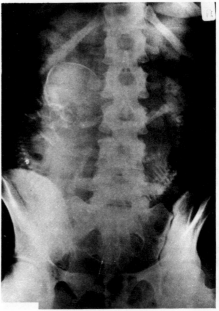

Doctors are rarely surprised by the birth of twins: if they suspect twins, an X-ray will confirm the diagnosis.

with consequent danger to the babies. For this reason, in Britain and many other countries, it is customary to admit the expectant mother to hospital at about the thirtieth to the thirty-sixth week of pregnancy. The delivery itself should, of course, always be conducted in hospital.

In labour, the problems which may arise include delay in the birth of the second twin; the mother's contractions (pains) should restart within half an hour of the birth of the first baby, and if this does not happen, the obstetrician will take measures to hasten the delivery. Occasionally, twins are actually born several days apart, but this should not normally happen. (In 1937, the British Medical Journal reported an authenticated case in which there was a delay of 92 days between the first and the second birth.)

The second twin may also become awkwardly positioned in the womb, as opposed to the normal head-first presentation.

Other complications may occur, but they are fortunately not very common. In the vast majority of cases, provided the mother attends for antenatal examinations each week from the time that twins are diagnosed, and provided she follows medical advice (particularly in regard to rest), she can expect to come through pregnancy and labour with no major difficulties whatever.

TYPHOID is one of the enteric group of fevers (see **enteric fevers**). Like the other members of this group (paratyphoid fevers A, B and C), typhoid is passed on when germs from the bowel motions (or less commonly, from the urine) of an infected person are allowed to contaminate someone else's food or drink. This can very readily happen where personal hygiene is poor, or where public hygiene (e.g. the care of water supplies and sewage, and the inspection of food factories and restaurants) is defective.

It is important to stress that the disease may be passed on by symptomless 'carriers', who, because they do not feel ill, do not bother with such simple precautions as washing the hands before preparing food or after visiting the toilet.

The germ which causes typhoid is called *Salmonella typhi*. After it enters the body, there is an incubation period of 6 to 21 days before symptoms appear. The onset is usually gradual, with headache, loss of appetite, weakness, nosebleeds and slight fever being among the commonest symptoms. It is usually a week before the fever reaches a level of 102°–103°F. By this stage the patient often has a rash, and there are usually bowel disturbances (diarrhoea being more common than constipation). As time goes on, the stools frequently become bloodstained, and perforation of the bowel or massive intestinal bleeding may be a threat to life.

If untreated, the patient either deteriorates rapidly or starts to make a slow recovery in the third week of the illness. If, however, the diagnosis has been made in good time, the great majority of patients will respond well to an antibiotic, usually chloramphenicol or ampicillin. Isolation in a suitable hospital, and careful disposal of the patient's excreta are essential. Relapses and the development of a symptomless 'carrier' state are very common, and so it is most important for the patient to have regular laboratory tests for some considerable time after he leaves hospital.

Very few patients with typhoid would die if treatment were started early, that is if the diagnosis could be made in the first week or so. Unfortunately, this is often difficult, as laboratory tests on the stools may well be negative at this time. However, the germ can often be cultured from the patient's blood in the early stages, and this constitutes the most important single test.

Prevention of typhoid depends partly on public health measures, and partly on precautions taken by the individual. Such precautions include the hygienic measures mentioned above, and also the use of antityphoid vaccination. Anyone contemplating going on holiday to regions of the world where typhoid is rife (such as North Africa) should seek immunization from his doctor *months beforehand*. Ideally, protection should be achieved by three injections over a period of six months.

TYPHUS is a name applied to a group of basically similar illnesses, all of which are caused by infection with germs of the rickettsial group (see **Rickettsiae**). It was not until the early part of this century that these diseases were clearly separated from one another, and prior to that time typhus was often confused with other fevers, such as typhoid (see **typhoid**). However, there is little doubt that typhus has been in existence for hundreds, if not thousands, of years. What was probably an outbreak of typhus was clearly described by an Italian writer in 1083, and since then typhus, in its epidemic form, has caused terrible depredations whenever war or famine have struck mankind. In Russia and Poland, for instance, typhus killed three million people between 1915 and 1922.

Only in the last 40 or 50 years has typhus become of less dreadful import to Man, partly because of the introduction of antibiotics, and partly because knowledge of the way the disease is passed on by lice, fleas, and mites has enabled countermeasures (e.g. the development of insecticides) to be taken.

Basically, there are four types of this disease. The first is *epidemic typhus*. This terrible scourge is caused by the germ *Rickettsia prowazeki* (so called after Ricketts and Von Prowazek, who both died of the infection as a result of their investigations into it). It is transmitted from man to man by the body louse, whose infected faeces get into broken skin — for instance, scratches caused by intense itching. The features consist of severe headache, chills and fever, followed, after about five days, by a pink rash over the trunk. In certain outbreaks, the death rate has been as high as 60 per cent, but a more usual figure is 10 per cent. Broad spectrum antibiotics, such as the tetracyclines, almost always produce a cure.

The second form of typhus is *Brill's disease*, or recurrent epidemic typhus. As the name implies, this condition is due to the same organism, which has been harboured in the patient's body for a period of perhaps years after an original attack of epidemic typhus. It is therefore quite often seen in relatively typhus-free countries among

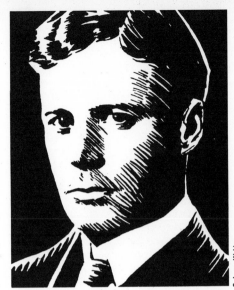

The discoverer — and a victim — of the germs that cause typhus, H. T. Ricketts.

C. James Webb

people who have returned home from other parts of the world some time before. The features are similar to those of epidemic typhus, but the disorder usually runs a milder course.

Endemic (murine) typhus is the commonest form of typhus encountered in the United States. It is caused by the germ *Rickettsia mooseri*, and is transmitted to Man by fleas, which may acquire the infection from rats. It is a more benign condition than epidemic typhus but characterized initially by much the same symptoms.

Finally, *scrub typhus*, which is seen in Asia, the Pacific and Northern Australia, is caused by *Rickettsia tsutsugamushi*, and is transmitted to Man by several species of mites, which may acquire the infection from small rodents. The features include swelling and inflammation around the site of the original bite, together with fever, headache, and enlargement of the lymph glands. The death rate, once as high as 60 per cent in certain areas, is now virtually nil where broad-spectrum antibiotics are used.

USP means United States Pharmacopeia, a volume which lists medical preparations employed in the United States.

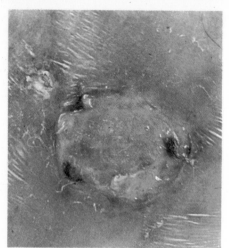

Disorders of the blood vessels may lead to the development of a varicose ulcer.

ULCERS are breaches in the skin or any of the membranes of the body. Usually, the term implies that such breaches have a tendency to become chronic and do not heal very easily.

The most commonly-occurring types of ulcer are probably *varicose ulcers* and *peptic ulcers.*

Varicose ulcers occur on the lower part of the shin, and are associated with varicose veins (see **varicose veins**). Such ulcers are very common in middle aged and elderly people; they may attain a considerable size and persist for many years. Treatment consists usually in elevation of the leg, the use of supportive bandages, and, in some cases, operation on the associated varicose veins.

Peptic ulcers are ulcers of the stomach or of the duodenum. (Occasionally, they may occur in certain other sites in the alimentary tract.) Both gastric and duodenal ulcers produce pain in the upper part of the abdomen, at or near the midline. This pain is worse an hour or two after meals, and may be relieved by eating food, or by taking alkalis. Other symptoms include vomiting of blood (see **black vomiting**) and passing black motions (see **black motions**). Sometimes, penetration of an ulcer into the abdominal cavity (perforation) may cause sudden intense pain and peritonitis (see **peritonitis**).
382

Treatment of peptic ulcers usually involves antacid therapy, rest, giving up smoking, and the eating of frequent, small meals, so that the stomach is not allowed to become empty. The object of all this is to reduce or soak up the flow of gastric juices, whose action on the mucous membrane of the alimentary tract seems to be responsible for the formation of both gastric and duodenal ulcers. However, the only drug which has been shown to have any healing effect on gastric ulcers is a preparation derived from liquorice called carbenoxolone. Attempts are now being made to use it on duodenal ulceration as well, but whether it will be effective or not is still in doubt.

Where purely medical treatment fails, peptic ulcers are treated by surgical means. Partial gastrectomy involves removing roughly the lower two thirds of the stomach, which very greatly reduces the flow of gastric juices. This operation is of use in both gastric and duodenal ulceration. It is, however, a fairly major procedure, and patients sometimes have quite troublesome abdominal symptoms afterwards.

C. James Webb

Breaks in the lining of the intestine reveal tissues below and produce peptic ulcers.

An alternative procedure is vagotomy (see **vagotomy**); this involves cutting through the two vagus nerves, which supply the stomach, so as to reduce its output of acid. It has not proved of much use in ordinary gastric ulcers, except where such an ulcer develops after a gastrectomy, but it may be very effective in duodenal ulceration. It too may produce unwanted symptoms such as diarrhoea post-operatively.

ULCERATIVE COLITIS is a disease which is characterized by severe inflammation of the large intestine (see **alimentary canal**). It occurs more frequently in women than in men. The cause is unknown, but many doctors believe it to be an auto-immune disease, that is, one in which the body for some reason produces antibodies against its own tissues. Acute attacks of this chronic disease may be precipitated by emotional stress, and, in a few patients, drinking milk is thought to cause flare-ups.

The usual history of a patient with ulcerative colitis is that the disease makes its appearance between the ages of 20 and 35. At the onset, the patient develops persistent attacks of diarrhoea. After a while, the stools are noted to contain quite a lot of blood, mucus, and pus. The patient is well intermittently, but at other times may have the bowels open as often as 30 times a day; during such attacks, he may feel very ill indeed. Without treatment, he could become badly dehydrated, or sometimes suffer a life-threatening haemorrhage or perforation of the bowel.

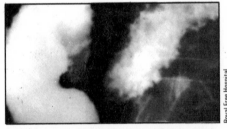

Royal Free Hospital

Barium here outlines the shape of the colon in a patient suffering from ulcerative colitis.

Fortunately, however, not all cases are as severe as this, and some patients with very limited inflammation only rarely get anything resembling the type of acute attack described above. In addition, treatment is nowadays usually very effective in controlling the symptoms of the disease.

In an acute attack, such treatment will consist of fluids and salts to combat dehydration, together with blood transfusion if bleeding has been heavy, and the administration of steroids (see **steroids**) either by mouth or (more commonly) by enema.

In between attacks, drugs such as salazopyrin, and possibly steroids as well, are believed to play a part in keeping symptoms to a minimum. Iron tablets will probably be necessary to counteract anaemia. A small percentage of patients are likely to improve on a diet which contains no milk.

In very severe cases, the operation of ileostomy (see **ileostomy**) may sometimes be of inestimable benefit to the patient's whole way of life. Sometimes it is possible to remove the affected part of the bowel, and connect the upper part of the intestine to the rectum, thus enabling the patient to have the bowels open in the normal way, instad of through an aperture in the abdomen.

There are a number of serious complications which may develop after ulcerative colitis has been present for some years. It is therefore absolutely essential that the patient sees the specialist dealing with his case at regular intervals, so that appropriate investigation of his condition can be carried out.

ULNA is one of the two bones which run parallel to each other in the forearm, the other being known as the radius. Fractures of the two bones together are quite frequently seen. The lowest part of the ulna may be snapped off in the common injury which is usually referred to as a Colles' fracture (see **Colle's fracture**). Most people call this a 'broken wrist', though, strictly speaking, it is the bones of the arm which are broken, and not those of the wrist (see **wrist**).

ULTRASONIC THERAPY is treatment by very high-pitched sound waves, well above the range of the human ear.

The note, frequency or pitch of a particular sound is measured in cycles per second. Middle C, for instance, is 256 cycles per second, and the high notes of an ordinary piano are in the range of about 2,500 cycles per second. We can hear notes which are much higher than this, however: up to about 15,000 cycles per second in an adult and even higher in a child. Some animals (for instance, dogs) can hear notes pitched considerably beyond this, and this principle is used in ultrasonic dog whistles.

However, such very highly pitched sound can also be used to penetrate tissues. In physiotherapy and physical medicine, ultrasonic waves have been widely used in recent years in the treatment of injuries to internal structures such as muscles, tendons and ligaments. The effect of this type of treatment is due to heat producing increased blood flow in the tissues.

Ultrasonic waves are sometimes directed at the labyrinth of the inner ear (see **ear**) in the treatment of Menière's disease (see **Menière's disease**). In addition, reflections of such waves can be used to produce a picture of the internal tissues of the body, and be of considerable value in the diagnosis of certain obstetric conditions.

ULTRA-VIOLET RADIATION is, like radiant heat and visible light (and many other forms of ray), a form of 'electromagnetic radiation'. The ordinary (white) light which we can see actually contains a range of colours (red, orange, yellow, green, blue, indigo, and violet) all of which are of different wave-lengths. We only see these colours separately when white light is split up in some way (e.g. by rain drops, to form a rainbow).

Radiation of slightly longer wave-lengths than that of the red part of the spectrum is called 'infra-red', and these, in fact are just ordinary heat rays.

On the other hand, rays of slightly shorter wavelength than that of the violet end of the spectrum are called ultra-violet rays. When used on the skin, ultra-violet rays have a considerable bactericidal (i.e. germ-killing) effect, and they have therefore been extensively utilised in the treatment of all kinds of septic conditions, and in tuberculosis of the skin. Ultra-violet light is also of some use in providing a screen or barrier to prevent infection entering germ-free wards. Furthermore, it produces vitamin D by its action on the skin, and, for this reason, exposure to natural ultra-violet light (i.e. in sunshine) is very important in preventing rickets (see **rickets**).

384

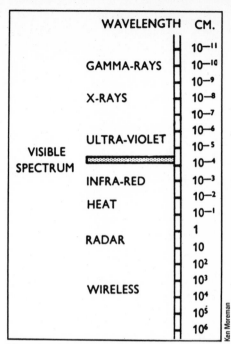

The electromagnetic spectrum of radiation. Ultra-violet rays form only a small section.

UMBILICUS is the navel, the small pit in the abdomen which marks the site at which the umbilical cord is attached in the unborn child. Within the womb, the baby receives its oxygen and all its nourishment through this cord, which connects the baby to the afterbirth, or placenta (see **placenta**).

A few moments after delivery of the baby, it is standard practice to cut through the umbilical cord (having first tied it on either side of the point where it is cut, to prevent bleeding); the baby is left with a four or five inch long 'stump' of cord which after a week or so, withers and drops off. Hygienic care of the umbilicus during the first fortnight of life is important: any infection in the area should be reported to the doctor.

Small hernias in the region of the umbilicus are common in babyhood, especially among children of African races. No treatment whatever is usually needed, as the condition normally clears up by itself. In adults, a hernia in this region frequently requires a simple operation to put it right.

UNCONSCIOUSNESS is a condition which is extremely commonly met with. When dealing with an unconscious patient, the vital thing to remember is that he must be able to breathe. Many people die needlessly while unconscious (e.g. after traffic accidents) simply because their 'airway' is blocked.

On finding someone unconscious, therefore, turn him immediately on his side. Using a finger, clear the mouth of any obstruction (e.g. blood or vomit), and remove any dentures. Then draw his lower jaw firmly forward and hold it there; this keeps the tongue from falling back and blocking the throat. If the breathing is very noisy, this indicates some obstruction; if pulling the jaw a little further forward does not help, the mouth and throat should be checked again for any material blocking the airway. If breathing stops, mouth to mouth artificial respiration should be carried out.

The commonest cause of unconsciousness in the world is said to be malaria (see **malaria**). Outside the malarial regions of the globe, however, the most frequently encountered causes are: strokes, overdoses of drugs (such as barbiturates), head injuries, insulin reactions (low blood sugar, or hypoglycaemia) in diabetics, excessive intake of alcohol, and sub-arachnoid haemorrhages (see **sub-arachnoid haemorrhage**). Quite common causes of prolonged unconsciousness (or apparent unconsciousness) are hysteria, meningitis, brain tumours, epilepsy and diabetic coma (see **diabetic coma**) — which is actually far less frequently seen in diabetics than the above mentioned condition of insulin reaction.

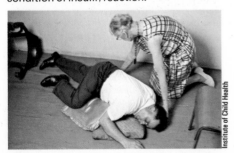

An unconscious person should be placed in a comfortable position, with breathing unrestricted.

UNDULANT FEVER is the human form of infection by *Brucella abortus*, one of the three species of germs which produce the group of illnesses known collectively as brucellosis. It is usually passed to Man in the milk of infected cattle, but a small number of cases are probably due to direct contact with animals. Thus, in the very few areas of the world where universal pasteurization of milk is the rule, the few cases which are seen occur mainly in veterinary surgeons, farmers, and meat-packing factory workers.

A fuller account of the disorder is given under the heading **brucellosis**.

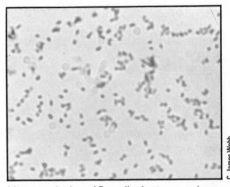

Microscopic view of *Brucella abortus* organisms, responsible for the disease undulant fever.

UNGUENTUM is the Latin word for ointment. The abbreviation 'ung.' is still used on prescriptions.

URAEMIA means a state in which there is a high concentration of the chemical urea (see **urea**) in the blood. The significance of this finding is that it indicates that the kidneys (see **kidneys**) are not functioning properly, and hence are not 'clearing' urea from the bloodstream. Urea itself is not a very dangerous chemical, but, in general, the higher the blood concentration of the substance goes, the worse is the state of the kidneys. If these organs are unable to maintain the chemical balance of the body, and, in particular, to regulate the concentrations of sodium (see **sodium**) and potassium (see **potassium**) in the blood and other fluids, then the outlook without treatment is very serious because life is threatened.

It is customary to divide uraemia into three types: pre-renal, renal, and post-renal.

Pre-renal uraemia is uncommon. It is not due to kidney disease, but occurs in severe blood loss and certain other states which fall broadly under the heading of shock (see **shock**). It can also occur in gross dehydration (e.g. in heat stroke).

Post-renal uraemia is also fairly uncommon. It is due to obstruction of the lower urinary passages (see **urine – stoppage of**), causing back pressure on the kidneys.

Much more common is renal uraemia (i.e. uraemia due to disease of the kidneys themselves). Conditions which tend to produce this state include various types of nephritis (see **nephritis**), chronic pyelitis (see **pyelitis**) and one or two rarer kidney disorders.

Treatment in each case will depend on the nature of the underlying disease.

UREA is a waste product of the body. It is chiefly formed from breakdown of proteins (see **proteins**), and it is excreted by the kidneys in the urine. Where the concentration of urea in the blood rises considerably above the normal level, this usually indicates impairment of function of the kidneys (see **uraemia**).

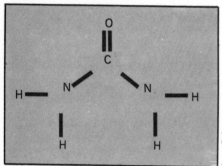

The chemical formula for urea, the chief breakdown product of proteins found in the urine.

URETER is one of the pair of tubes carrying urine from the kidneys to the bladder (see **bladder**), where it can accumulate before being discharged to the exterior when convenient.

Each ureter is about a quarter of an inch wide and is usually between 11 and 16

inches in length. It starts above the pelvis of the kidney and runs through the pelvic girdle to the base of the bladder where urine passes into the bladder through a narrow slit. This ensures that, except in cases of abnormality, fluid cannot run back up the ureter when the bladder contracts during urination.

Congenital abnormalities of the ureter (i.e. those present from birth) are seen quite frequently. They are of particular importance because they predispose to urinary infection affecting the kidneys. Treatment is by surgical operation.

Ureteric reflux is a condition which was increasingly recognized in the 1960s as being a common source of kidney trouble among children. Normally, the two ureters enter the bladder at an angle, so that they are readily closed off by the valve-like action of the muscles of the bladder when that organ contracts in order to expel urine. However, it can be shown that, in some children, this mechanism fails, so that when they urinate, the powerful contraction of the bladder forces small quantities of urine back up the ureter. This can have a harmful effect on the kidneys, particularly if the urine is infected (see **urinary infections**). If such ureteric reflux is demonstrated by a special X-ray called a micturating cystogram, then an operation on the lower end of the ureter may be necessary.

The ureters can be blocked by the development of *stones*. Although these may have no apparent cause, they are usually associated with a high level of soluble chemicals in the urine. Some of these may crystallize in the kidney and form stones. They can cause intense pain if the pressure of urine forces them along the ureter. Minor ones can be induced to 'wash away' chemically, but operation may be necessary. An ultrasonic probe can shatter small stones situated near to the kidney.

URETERITIS is the collective name of inflammations of the ureters.

URETEROGRAPHY is X-ray photography of the ureter. When obstruction of the ureter is suspected, a substance that will show up on an X-ray can be injected, and the condition inspected.

URETHRA is the tube which leads from the bladder to the exterior, and through which urine is passed.

In the male, it is about 8 inches long. It runs from the neck of the bladder (see **bladder**), through the prostate gland (see **prostate**), which opens into it, and into the penis, which it traverses to reach the exterior at the tip of this organ (see **penis**). In addition to carrying urine from the bladder to the exterior, the male urethra also carries seminal fluid or semen (see **semen**) which is composed of the fluid secretion from the prostate gland together with the sperm-containing liquid which comes up from the testicles to enter the upper part of the urethra.

In women, the urethra is a very much shorter tube — only about an inch and a half in length. This fact is of considerable significance, because it means that it is very easy for any germs (particularly from the neck passage) which enter the female urethra to ascend the very short distance to the bladder. Urinary infections (see **urinary infections**) are not surprisingly, very much commoner in girls and women than in boys and men. Since it is now realized that these infections (once thought to be trivial matters) are potentially serious, it is very important, when changing the nappies of girl babies, to wipe 'from before, backwards,' so that faecal material will be carried away from the urethra and not towards it. Similarly, little girls should be taught during toilet training to avoid contamination of the

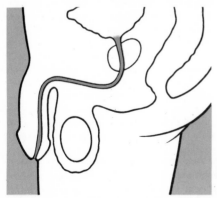

Diagram to show the extent of the urethra in the male — from the bladder to the exterior.

vulva (see **vulva**) with faeces, by wiping backwards rather than forwards.

Disorders of the urethra are quite common. In men, the most frequent is probably urethritis, or inflammation of the urethra, dealt with separately (see **urethritis**).

Among congenital disorders (i.e. those present at birth) which may affect the male urethra are pin-hole meatus (a condition where the orifice of the urethra at the tip of the penis is too narrow, and has to be widened surgically); hypospadias (a condition present in one in 350 males, in which the urethra opens on to the under surface of the penis instead of its tip); and congenital urethral valves (a not uncommon disorder in which the baby is unable to empty his bladder because of tiny folds of tissue in the upper part of the urethra). Meatal ulcer is a painful sore at the opening of the urethra, seen only in circumcised children because of the fact that they have been deprived of the protection of the foreskin against minor abrasions.

Also common is urethral stricture (narrowing of the urethra). This can be due to gonorrhoea or tuberculosis, but has other causes as well.

In women, the common disorders of the urethra again include urethritis (inflammation), which is dealt with under the heading **urethritis**. Caruncle of the urethra is a frequently-encountered disorder seen in middle-aged and elderly women; it consists of a small, tender, reddish swelling at the opening of the urethra. Like prolapse of the urethra (in which part of the lining of the tube comes down, and is felt at the opening), it can be dealt with surgically.

URETHRITIS means inflammation of the urethra (see **urethra**).

In women, one type of such inflammation is very common indeed. The symptoms are painful and frequent urination, and tenderness in the region of the front part of the vulva. Because the condition is seen so frequently just after the first sexual experiences, it is thought to be due to repeated friction (and often slight injury) around the opening of the urethra. Doctors call it 'traumatic urethritis', but the widespread lay term is 'honeymoon cystitis' (see **cystitis**). The symptoms are

387

so similar to those of a urinary infection (see **urinary infection**) that it is important to have a laboratory test on the urine.

Urethritis in women may also be due to gonorrhoea (see **gonorrhoea**), and if pain passing urine is associated with a pus-like discharge, pelvic discomfort and slight fever, this condition may be suspected.

In men, urthritis is very commonly due to this type of venereal disease, and the symptoms are discussed under the heading **gonorrhoea**. Identical symptoms are caused by another infectious condition called non-specific urethritis. It may be associated with the features of Reiter's disease (see **Reiter's disease**).

URIC ACID is a chemical which is normally present in the blood. Excessive amounts of it are, however, often associated with gout (see **gout**), though an elevated level is not invariably indicative of this condition.

In gouty people, the chemical compounds which uric acid forms in the body (urates) are deposited around the joints and in various other tissues. Fortunately, drugs are available which will keep the level of uric acid down.

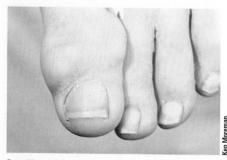

Swelling of the toe in gout, due to deposition of urates in the tissues around the joint.

URINARY INFECTIONS are extremely common. Until quite recently, these disorders were widely regarded as being of no more importance than a cold, but it is now realized that they can be of far graver significance. All too often, they can lead on to serious disease of the kidneys (pyelitis, or pyelonephritis), and, in fact, it has been found that about one in ten of all people who die have kidneys which are diseased

388

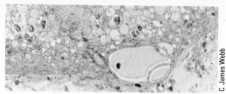

Microscope view of the tissues of the kidney in a patient who suffered from pyelonephritis.

in this way (see **pyelitis**). Therefore, when a person has a urinary infection, the most stringent precautions should be taken to ensure that it is completely eradicated. This cannot be done without full laboratory tests on the urine.

A major problem is that urinary infection may produce no definite symptoms, and surveys have shown that about five per cent of all the women in a community at any one time are likely to be suffering from such an infection without knowing anything about it. Possibly in the future women will be able to have occasional but regular routine laboratory urine tests.

The reason that urinary infections are so common in women is discussed under the heading **urethra**. Such infections are particularly likely to happen in pregnancy and the lying-in period.

The most common symptoms are pain on passing water, and frequency of urination. There may also be pain over the bladder, occasionally blood in the urine, and (if acute kidney infection develops), fever and pain in the loin (see **pyelitis**).

In all these circumstances, it is essential that a cleanly-collected specimen of urine in a sterilized container (e.g. a boiled-out screwtop jar) be sent to the laboratory *before treatment is begun*. The doctor will probably start therapy with a sulphonamide drug, though he may change this in the light of the report he receives in about 48 hours from the laboratory.

It cannot be stressed too strongly that the patient is not necessarily cured because her symptoms go away. She still needs at least one further test of the urine.

Recurrent urinary infections in a girl or woman need full investigation including special X-rays. So does *any* urinary infection occurring in a male, since very often some important structural abnormality will be found to be a contributory factor.

URINE is the fluid produced by the kidneys (see **kidneys**). It contains many of the body's waste products which, if they were allowed to accumulate, would poison the body.

The kidney is essentially a structure which, under pressure, filters off fluid from the blood into millions of tiny tubules. From these the important chemicals are reabsorbed into the bloodstream. Eventually, all these tubules come together, and deliver the urine into the region of the kidney called the pelvis.

From there, the urine passes down the thin tube called the ureter (see **ureter**) into the bladder (see **bladder**), in which it collects. From time to time, when a sufficient quantity has accumulated, the urine is voluntarily expelled to the exterior through the urethra (see **urethra**).

Urine is a golden yellow fluid under normal conditions, though it may become much paler, and, in fact, more or less clear, when a person drinks a great deal of liquid. It is darker and more concentrated in conditions where there is fever; this is because fluid is being lost through perspiration from the skin rather than the kidneys.

'Smoky', *blood-stained* urine always needs prompt medical investigation, though it may not necessarily be due to a very serious condition. This topic is dealt with under the heading **haematuria.**

Extremely *frothy* urine may indicate the presence of protein. This too needs investigation. The subject is discussed under the heading **proteinuria.**

Very *dark* urine is seen in a number of disorders, and commonly in the condition called obstructive jaundice (see under **jaundice**). However, the colour of urine must be interpreted in conjunction with the other features of the condition, and an odd coloration is not necessarily anything to be alarmed about. There are, for instance, a number of dyes contained in sweets which can discolour the urine; a similar effect is produced by rhubarb, and drugs such as senna.

The normal volume of urine passed by an adult in the course of a day is about 1500 ml, or roughly $2\frac{1}{2}$ to 3 pints. This quantity may be considerably affected by factors such as the weather (less being passed in hot climates) and the actual body temperature; little may be passed when the patient is feverish.

The persistent passage of large quantities of urine (polyuria) may simply be due to excessive intake of water — this sometimes occurs in psychologically disturbed people. However, polyuria may also be a feature of diabetes mellitus (see **diabetes mellitus**), or of the much rarer condition diabetes insipidus (see **diabetes insipidus**). It can also be a symptom of certain types of nephritis (see **nephritis**).

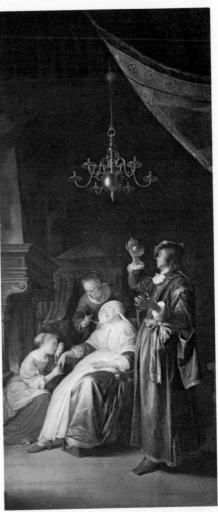

Carlo Bevilacqua

Examination of the urine to diagnose disease in mediaeval times. Specimens were also tasted.

389

Pain on passing urine (*dysuria*) is also a very frequent symptom of urinary infection, but in men (in whom such infections are rare unless there is some structural abnormality present — see below), urethritis (see **urethritis**), usually due to gonorrhoea, is a more common cause. Among women, urethritis should be considered if there is also a pus-like discharge from the urinary passage.

The commonest structural abnormality which may be associated with pain and difficulty in passing urine in men is enlargement of the prostate gland (see **prostate**). Among boys, congenital abnormalities of the bladder and urethra may cause trouble, and predispose to infection.

The normal routine urine tests carried out by a doctor in his surgery (i.e. for life insurance examinations, or for 'checkups') are simply for protein (see under **proteinuria**) and for sugar. The presence of sugar is frequently, but by no means invariably, indicative of the presence of diabetes mellitus (see **diabetes mellitus**). Other conditions in which sugar may be present in the urine include renal glycosuria (a completely harmless variant of normal kidney function), and 'lag storage' (a mild and relatively unimportant chemical abnormality). Sugar is also found in the urine of many healthy expectant mothers, and its presence can sometimes be due to treatment with certain drugs.

URINE — STOPPAGE OF. Acute retention, as it is medically termed, is very common among elderly men. In the vast majority of cases, it is due to enlargement of the prostate gland (see **prostate**), but other causes include stricture of the urethra (see **urethra**), and stones jammed in the exit of the bladder.

Among women, absolute stoppage of urine is rare, but can be due to stones, disease of the urethra, or swellings in the pelvis (e.g. a large fibroid) pressing on the bladder and urethra.

In almost all circumstances, this painful and uncomfortable condition can be relieved as soon as the patient reaches hospital by passing a sterile rubber catheter into the urethra (see **catheters**) and drawing off the urine.

390

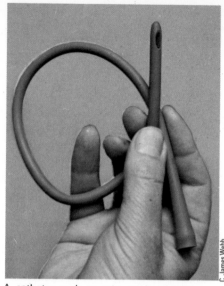

A catheter such as this, made of rubber or plastic, is used to relieve urinary retention.

The urine is then allowed to drain off slowly, usually into a sealed jar, to reduce the risk of infection. In a few patients, it is necessary to give a general anaesthetic in order to produce sufficient relaxation to pass the catheter; very rarely the doctor may insert a needle directly through the wall of the abdomen instead of passing a catheter up the urethra.

Persistent failure to produce more than a little urine over a period of some days is a serious symptom which, if untreated, would lead to the disorder known as uraemia (see **uraemia**); if an adult patient passes not more than half a pint or so for two or three days and seems increasingly ill, then medical advice is essential.

Where failure to pass urine is associated with painful enlargement of the bladder, the condition is known as acute retention and demands immediate attention.

The frequent passage of smallish quantities of urine frequently indicates an infection in the urinary tract (see **urinary infections**), and laboratory investigation may be necessary to determine the cause and appropriate treatment. In women, the symptom can also be due to *traumatic urethritis* ('honeymoon cystitis'), (see under **urethritis**).

UROLOGY is the branch of surgery which deals with disorders of the urinary tract (the kidneys, ureters, bladder and urethra) in both sexes, and usually with disorders of the genital tract in the male. Disorders of the female genital tract are normally dealt with by specialists in gynaecology.

In investigation of disorders of the urinary tract, many different methods of examination may be employed. Specimens of urine are tested for the presence of blood, protein and sugar, as well as bacteria, all of which may indicate disease. The lower reaches of the tract can be inspected by means of a cystoscope (see **cystoscope**), and the kidneys and ureters by means of X-rays, which can be used to follow the excretion of special dyes into the urine from the bloodstream, and to demonstrate the presence of calculi (stones) which sometimes form within the tract. Treatment is dependent upon the results of these tests.

URTICARIA is an inflammatory condition of the skin, caused by an allergic reaction (see **allergy**). It is frequently referred to in lay terms as 'nettle-rash', though it may, in fact, be caused by a very wide variety of substances, and only rarely by nettles. (The appearance of urticaria does, however, bear a slight resemblance to the rash produced in an ordinary, i.e. non-allergic, person when he touches a nettle.)

The characteristic feature of urticaria is the 'weal'; this is a raised, reddish area of skin, often whiter in colour near the centre, and with a sharply defined margin.

Basically, this 'weal' is due to vasodilatation (widening of the blood vessels) in the affected area, and to fluid leaking out of these blood vessels and producing the typical raised, puffy appearance of the skin.

Very frequently, it is quite impossible to identify the 'allergen' which caused the condition. However, sometimes urticaria follows injection of serum (see **serum**), as, for instance, when patients are given ATS (anti-tetanus serum) to give temporary protection against tetanus (see **tetanus**).

Foods which may provoke urticaria include eggs, strawberries and shellfish, though (for reasons that are not understood) the patient may have eaten these foods often in the past with no ill-effects. Among drugs which may produce urticaria, penicillin is far the most important, but many others may provoke a similar response. Insect bites may also sometimes cause urticarial reactions. So too can the presence of certain parasitic worms in the body, though this is an uncommon cause of the condition.

Giant urticaria, or angio-neurotic oedema, is a particularly severe form of the disorder, in which the loss of fluid from the blood vessels produces a really gross swelling of the tissues, particularly around the eyes and mouth.

In a single short-lasting episode of urticaria, if there is no obvious precipitating cause, then there is little point in searching for one. If urticaria is recurrent, however, it is important to try to find the allergen, so that the patient can avoid it, if possible, in future.

Antihistamine drugs such as mepyramine (see **mepyramine**) are often helpful in treating urticaria, because they combat the effects of histamine, a substance released during the course of allergic

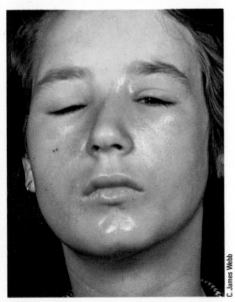

C. James Webb

Severe urticaria, or angio-neurotic oedema, producing swelling of the tissues of the face, which feels tense, hot and itchy during the attack.

reactions. Giant urticaria may require the careful administration of adrenaline by injection, or possibly therapy with steroids (see **steroids**).

URTICARIA PIGMENTOSA should not be confused with ordinary urticaria (see **urticaria**), as it is a quite different and far less common condition.

'Weals' are found on the skin in this condition as they are in urticaria, but they occur in the region of pigmented (i.e. dark) spots which are always present, and which are probably a congenital abnormality. These dark patches contain cells which release large quantities of histamine (a chemical which plays an important part in allergic reactions) whenever they are rubbed or otherwise irritated. Sometimes, the bones and internal organs as well as the skin may be affected by urticaria pigmentosa.

UTERUS is the medical name for the womb. It is situated just above the vagina (see **vagina**), into which the cervix (see **cervix**) or neck of the womb protrudes.

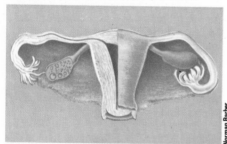

Norman Barber

The uterus, with the fallopian tubes extending on either side towards the ovaries, and the cervix, or neck, opening into the vagina, below, and protruding slightly into it.

In its non-pregnant state, the uterus is about three inches long and an inch thick; at the upper end (which is its widest part), it is about two inches across, but it tapers down to a width of about an inch in the region of the cervix. During pregnancy, this small organ undergoes a remarkable increase in size, eventually attaining a length well over a foot: yet, a few weeks after delivery, it has contracted quite dramatically and returned to its normal size.

The uterus is, of course, a hollow structure, but in the non-pregnant state, the cavity within it is little more than a slit, with most of the bulk of the organ being taken up by its thick muscular walls. In pregnancy, these walls stretch enormously, so that by the time of delivery, the capacity of the cavity of the womb is very great – being enough to contain the baby, the afterbirth (see **placenta**) and a very considerable quantity (usually one to two pints) of amniotic fluid ('the waters').

At its two upper corners, the uterus is joined by the Fallopian tubes (see **Fallopian tubes**), which carry eggs downward from the region of the ovaries (see **ovaries**). It is probable that conception (see **conception**) occurs in one or other Fallopian tube, when one of the sperms deposited in the region of the cervix during intercourse (see **intercourse**), having made its way up through the uterus, enters the Fallopian tube and unites with a ripe egg, or ovum, newly released by the ovary. The fertilized ovum then embeds itself in the lining of the uterus. This lining is prepared for the reception of such a fertilized egg each month, under the influence of the hormones called oestrogens (see **oestrogens**), during the course of what is called the menstrual cycle. If a fertilized ovum does not reach the lining of the uterus, then this lining is shed in the process of menstrual bleeding. (See **menstruation**.)

Disorders of the uterus include fibroids (see **fibroids**), infection (see **endometritis**), prolapse (see **prolapse**), metropathia haemorrhagica (see **metropathia haemorrhagica**), endometriosis (see **endometriosis**), and cancer.

Cancer of the body of the uterus (as opposed to the cervix) is commonest among women in their forties. The most frequent symptom is bleeding after the change of life. Other types of abnormal bleeding are discussed under the heading **menopause**. If such symptoms occur, or if, before the menopause, there is bleeding between the periods, consult a doctor immediately, as full investigation is absolutely vital.

The cervix is actually a part of the uterus, but its disorders are dealt with under the heading **cervix**.

UVEITIS is a type of inflammation which affects the middle of the three layers of tissue in the eye. This layer has three parts – the iris (see **iris**), which is the coloured disc that surrounds the pupil; the ciliary body, from which the lens of the eye is suspended; and the choroid (which forms a cover for the retina (see **retina**)), the screen on which light is focused by the lens.

Uveal tract inflammation, as it is often called, may be due to infection by a wide variety of germs, and also to other causes, such as sarcoidosis (see **sarcoidosis**). The symptoms vary, but often include pain, blurring of vision, and redness of the eye. Treatment depends on the nature of the underlying disorder.

UVULA is the small, globular mass of tissue which hangs down from the middle of the soft palate, at the back of the throat.

The uvula varies considerably in size from person to person, but such variations are of no importance. It is also common to find that a person has a completely split uvula – that is, there are two masses instead of one hanging at the back of the palate. This condition is quite harmless, and is merely an indication that the uvula and the soft palate are formed before birth by the joining together of two processes of tissue from the right and the left side. Of course, if complete failure of fusion occurs, the condition of cleft palate results. If this failure of fusion extends far enough forward, it will involve the third process of tissue that makes up the upper jaw, and there will be a cleft in the hard palate, and possibly a hare-lip as well. This subject is discussed further under the heading **hare-lip.**

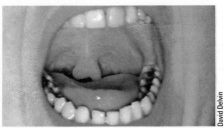

A split uvula is harmless: the condition indicates how the uvula and palate are formed.

VACCINATION in the strictest sense means immunization against smallpox by inoculation with material derived from calves with cow-pox, or vaccinia (see **cow-pox**). However, the term has become rather ambiguous, and nowadays it is often applied to other kinds of immunization as well.

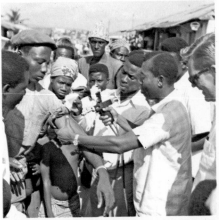

Here, Ghanaians are vaccinated against smallpox. Mass-injections may forestall an epidemic.

Vaccination against smallpox was first attempted by the English surgeon Edward Jenner in 1796. It was widely known at that time that inoculation of material from the pustules of mild cases of smallpox usually provided protection against the disease, but often had disastrous results.

However, Jenner hit on the idea of inoculating people instead with material from the pustules of the very mild condition called cow-pox (vaccinia). He is said to have got the idea from a West country belief that milkmaids who had acquired cow-pox from the udders of infected cows were never affected by smallpox.

The new technique was an immediate success, and since that time it has led to an enormous reduction in smallpox deaths in countries where it is widely practised.

Nowadays, vaccination is usually carried out during the first two years of life. For purposes of international travel, revaccination is necessary every three years, and although immunity probably in fact lasts longer than this, it is normally wise to keep protection against smallpox

393

up to date, because of the ever-present danger (in these days of fast air travel) of infection being brought even into countries where smallpox used to be considered rare.

The most commonly used method of vaccination nowadays is by *multiple pressure*. Through a drop of fluid placed on the skin, the doctor makes a series of 'pressures' with the side (not the tip) of a needle, over a small area of the skin. This technique is absolutely painless.

In a primary (first) vaccination, a firm lump develops on the skin four days later, and two or three days afterwards this lump forms a fluid-filled 'head'. In re-vaccination, the whole process is much quicker, and there may be no fluid-formation. The mild constitutional upset seen after primary vaccination does not occur after revaccination.

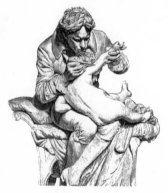

Edward Jenner, shown here inoculating his son, was the first doctor to attempt vaccination.

Serious complications of vaccination are very rare. Encephalitis (see **encephalitis**) is said to occur once in 100,000 vaccinations, and to be commoner where the first vaccination is postponed till adulthood. Generalized vaccinia (cow-pox) is also believed to occur in about one case in 100,000.

However, children or adults with active eczema, and mothers in early pregnancy should not, as a rule, be vaccinated. If there is any doubt, the family doctor will advise (see also **smallpox**).

Other types of vaccination. As mentioned above, the word vaccination is now

often applied to immunization against other diseases as well. In Britain, for instance, it has been the practice since 1958 to refer to all agents which confer *active* artificial immunity (see under **immunity**) as 'vaccines'.

Vaccination, in this sense, is available against a wide variety of diseases. In temperate climates, routine vaccination is normally carried out against diphtheria, whooping-cough, tetanus, poliomyelitis, measles, and tuberculosis, as well as smallpox. A schedule showing the ages at which these vaccinations may be carried out will be found in the tables at the end of the dictionary.

A vaccine against German measles is also being developed, and will probably soon come into routine use.

VACCINE – see under **vaccination**.

VACCINIA – see **cow-pox**.

VAGINA is the front passage which leads from the vulva (see **vulva**) up to the cervix (see **cervix**) or neck of the womb. It lies between the bladder in front, and, the rectum behind.

The vagina is a muscular tube which is about 3 to $3\frac{1}{2}$ inches long in the un-distended state, though it can be expanded considerably during intercourse. The walls are moistened by a thick whitish fluid secretion which is acid in nature, and therefore forms an effective barrier to the entry of infection.

Vaginal discharge. The presence of the ordinary type of secretion (the flow of which may be greatly increased by sexual excitement) does not constitute a vaginal discharge, and requires neither treatment nor the application of the expensive 'cosmetic' preparations so popular in some countries (especially the USA). A brown or blood-stained discharge, however, requires immediate gynaecological investigation, as does a pus-like discharge. A white, semi-solid, irritant discharge is likely to be due to vaginal thrush, or monilia (see **monilia**). A yellowish irritant discharge is most frequently due to the trichomonas organism (see **trichomonas vaginalis**).

VAGINISMUS literally means 'spasm of the vagina'. Women who are nervous about sex are sometimes so completely unable to relax that intercourse is more or less impossible.

Under normal circumstances, the muscles around the opening of the vagina are fairly taut, but relax under the stimulus of sexual excitation so that it is possible for the man's penis to enter. At the same time, the lubricant fluids secreted by various parts of the female genital tract greatly facilitate entry.

In vaginismus, however, there is no relaxation of the muscles, and little secretion of fluid. Attempts at intercourse cause pain, and make the muscles contract even more tightly. In extreme cases, the patient may be so frightened of intercourse that the mildest attempts at lovemaking cause her, quite involuntarily, to clamp her legs together and hunch her whole body up self-protectively.

This tragic state of affairs, with its almost inevitable legacy of marital disharmony and ill-will, was apparently exceedingly common in Victorian brides, and was still very often encountered some years ago. In the last decade or so, however, vaginismus seems to have been much less of a problem than formerly. The reasons for this are fairly obvious — the most important one being that young women nowadays have a much more enlightened attitude to the sexual side of marriage, while their husbands are much more likely to be aware of how to arouse them (see **love play**).

Treatment of vaginismus consists first of all in making sure there is no painful vaginal disorder present which might be responsible for precipitating attacks. Next, the doctor will probably have a frank talk with both husband and wife, and discuss with them ways in which they can overcome the difficulty. In addition to general advice on sex technique, he may suggest the use of a lubricant, or possibly a cream containing a mild local anaesthetic, which will make things easier for the wife.

These measures are usually very successful after a period of time. If they are not, it will often be best for the wife to have psychiatric help (for instance, desensitization — see **desensitization**). Some doctors obtain good results with the traditional treatment of giving the wife metal or glass dilators of progressively increasing size to insert each day. Others feel that the benefits of this therapy are entirely psychological, though this is, of course, of no importance whatsoever if the patient gets better.

VAGINITIS means inflammation of the vagina. This is usually associated with some form of vaginal discharge (see under the heading **vagina**).

Senile vaginitis occurs in women of 45 years of age and upwards (and not just in the old, as the name implies). It is due to the reduced output of female hormones after the menopause, and it responds to administration of these hormones, together with acid douches.

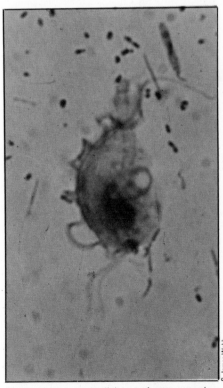

C. James Webb

Trichomonas vaginalis, a minute organism which causes the complaint vaginitis in women, inflammation of the vaginal lining.

395

VAGITUS UTERINUS is the Latin term for a baby's cry heard prior to delivery.

This phenomenon is not uncommon in the last minutes before the infant's head is born, but cannot occur until well on in labour, because there is no air normally present in the womb for the baby to expel from its lungs.

VAGOTOMY is an operation in which the left and right vagus nerves, which supply the stomach (among other structures), are cut through. The object of this procedure is to reduce the output of acid from the stomach.

Vagotomy is of considerable value in the treatment of duodenal ulcers, which are normally associated with a high acid output. It is also effective in the quite common condition in which a gastric ulcer recurs at the site where a stomach (previously operated on for ulcer) has been joined surgically to the small intestine. In the more usual type of gastric ulcer, however, the results of vagotomy are less satisfactory.

The operation of vagotomy is usually combined with some sort of drainage operation on the lower end of the stomach, since otherwise this organ, deprived of its nerve supply, would be unable to empty properly. The most commonly performed drainage procedure at present is called *pyloroplasty*; essentially, it is simply a way of enlarging the outlet from the stomach to the duodenum.

After vagotomy and pyloroplasty, a small number of patients are troubled by severe diarrhoea. A rather larger number have weight loss, flatulence, anaemia and other relatively minor side-effects. However, over 90 per cent of patients are completely satisfied with the results.

VARICELLA is another, text-book, name for chicken-pox (see **chicken-pox**).

VARICOCELE, or varicocoele, means a dilatation (widening) of the group of veins which carry blood away from the testicles (the male sex glands). These veins pass upwards from the scrotum as part of the spermatic cord, before joining together successively into a single vein on each side (the testicular vein).

The left testicular vein empties into the left renal vein, which carries blood away from the left kidney. This latter blood vessel is very susceptible to compression by other structures in the abdomen, or (rarely) by a tumour of the kidney. The result is back pressure on the veins draining the left testicle. On the right side, the anatomical arrangements are different, and back pressure is unlikely to occur. Not surprisingly, therefore, the majority of all cases of varicocele are left-sided.

It is said that up to 10 per cent of all men aged 15–35 have a varicocele. Most of them are quite unaware of it, and since mild cases are entirely harmless and produce no symptoms, this does not matter.

In more severe cases, the patient notices the widely-dilated veins, which are usually described as being like a 'bag of worms' in the scrotum. He may also complain of a 'dragging' pain. Under certain circumstances, an operation may be advisable to relieve the condition, but the surgeon may feel that it is only necessary to prescribe a support.

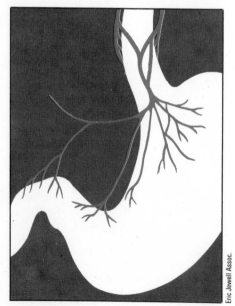

Eric Jewell Assoc.

In vagotomy, the stomach's vagus nerves are cut to reduce the flow of acid from the stomach, valuable treatment for stomach ulcers.

VARICOSE VEINS are among the most common human afflictions. A vein is said to be varicose when it is abnormally dilated (widened), lengthened, or tortuous. Such varicosities occur at various sites in the body − notably in the rectum (see under **haemorrhoids**), in the scrotum (see **varicocele**), and at the lower end of the gullet, where they may cause vomiting of blood (haematemesis). Varicose veins are also seen at the vulva in pregnancy. Most commonly, however, they occur in the legs.

Varicose veins of the legs are due to leakage of the valves which normally prevent back-flow of blood. Such back-flow is made much worse by obesity or repeated pregnancies.

Many people have no symptoms from their varicose veins, except for the ugly appearance − and in men, this is often effectively camouflaged by the hairs of the legs.

Severe varicose veins may, however, be associated with a tired, aching feeling in the calves, with ankle-swelling, and with varicose ulcers (see under **ulcers**).

Mild cases are treated by weight reduction, and, if necessary, the use of a supportive stocking or bandage. More severe cases may respond to injection of 'sclerosants' (which block the vein up completely), but whether this method will work or not depends on the exact site of the affected vein.

Very frequently, the varicose vein may either be tied off or 'stripped' − that is, pulled out completely. The latter operation usually results in complete cure.

VARIOLA is another name for smallpox (see **smallpox**).

VAS DEFERENS is the tube which carries seminal fluid up from each testicle, in the scrotum, to the urethra (see **urethra**). This sperm-containing fluid is first collected by a tightly-coiled tube called the epididymis, and delivered into the vas deferens. The vas carries it upwards, and into the trunk itself through a small aperture in the groin region of the body wall. From there, the vas deferens runs through the pelvic region, and finally joins

the urethra at the site of the prostate gland, which itself makes a contribution to the fluid that is produced from the urethra at ejaculation (see **ejaculation**).

Cutting across the vas deferens (**vasectomy**) is a simple, painless, and effective method of sterilization (see **sterilization**).

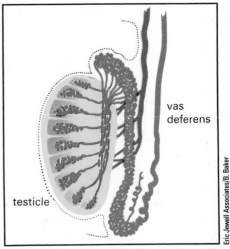

vas deferens

testicle

Eric Jewell Associates/B. Baker

Vas deferens is the tube which carries seminal fluid from the testicles to the urethra.

VEGETARIANS are people who do not eat meat or fish, or the products of these foods. Although Man is a carnivore (meat-eater) by nature, it is perfectly possible to remain healthy on a very carefully thought-out vegetarian diet. The main problem is, of course, to ensure an adequate supply of protein (see **proteins**).

A very small number of vegetarians refuse to eat anything at all which comes from animals, including, for instance, milk and butter. This type of diet is likely to lead to serious illness.

VEINS are the blood vessels which return blood in the direction of the heart (unlike the arteries, which carry blood away from the heart). Apart from the pulmonary veins, which carry 'fresh' (i.e. oxygen-rich) blood from the lungs to the heart, all the veins of the body contain 'stale' (i.e. de-oxygenated) blood, which they return through the great veins (or venae cavae) so that it may be re-oxygenated. The subject of circulation of blood through the arteries and veins is discussed more fully under the heading **blood.**

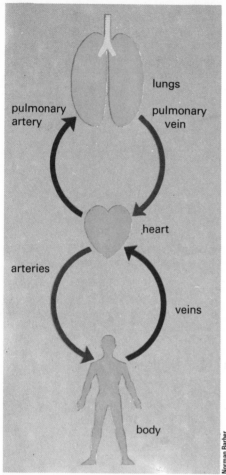

Veins are the blood-vessels that return blood to the heart, which re-pumps it to the body.

VENA CAVA is the term applied to either of the two great veins of the body (see **veins**).

VENEREAL DISEASES are those passed on during sexual activity.

By far the most serious type of VD is syphilis (see **syphilis**). The two commonest examples of these diseases, however, are gonorrhoea (see **gonorrhoea**), and non-specific urethritis (see under **urethritis**). Both have potentially serious complications.

398

Chancroid (see **chancroid**), or soft chancre, is fairly common in the warmer parts of the world, and in the sea-ports of temperate countries.

Lymphogranuloma venereum (lymphogranuloma inguinale) is mainly seen in the tropics and in the southern states of the USA. It is caused by a virus, and is characterized by the development of tender swollen glands in the groins, with eventual abscess formation.

This disorder should not be confused with the similarly named granuloma venereum (granuloma inguinale), a chronic ulceration of the skin of the genital regions, caused by a germ known as the *Donovan body*. It occurs in much the same regions of the world as does lymphogranuloma venereum, and is thought to be a venereal disease of low infectivity.

All the other types of VD are, however, highly infectious. It is therefore essential that anyone who even suspects that he or she has any of these conditions should refrain from intercourse and see a doctor as rapidly as possible. In the UK and certain other countries, 'Special Clinics' at hospitals see patients without prior appointment or doctor's letter, and under conditions of complete anonymity. Although there is still a tendency to try to sweep the complex problem of VD under the carpet as though it did not exist, such clinics can be found in most large towns, though it may be necessary to look for a discreet notice in a public toilet or elsewhere to discover where and when they are held.

VD does not go away by itself, and its long-term effects are very serious. Any delay is dangerous. Prompt treatment, however, offers a certainty of cure.

VENOM – see under **bites.**

VENTILATION is the term doctors use to describe the intake and output of air from the lungs, whether by ordinary breathing, by artificial respiration, or by use of a machine.

VENTRICLE is one of the two lower chambers of the heart – see **heart.**

VENUPUNCTURE, or venepuncture, means inserting a needle into a vein, e.g. as in the ordinary process of taking blood off in a syringe for tests.

It is very much easier and safer to use a vein than an artery for this purpose, since (a) there are usually many prominent veins close under the skin, e.g. on the back of the hand, or at the elbow; (b) there is no pain when a needle enters a vein, but the walls of arteries are richly supplied with nerves, so that puncturing them is somewhat painful; (c) placing a needle in an artery can sometimes be dangerous as, under certain circumstances, gangrene of the part of the body supplied by the artery may follow.

The normal method of venupuncture is as follows. The skin over the vein is cleaned, usually with surgical spirit, and the tip of a sterile needle, attached to a sterile syringe, is pushed carefully through the skin and into the underlying vein; blood can then be withdrawn. As soon as the needle is taken out, downward pressure is applied to the puncture site; bleeding should cease within a minute or two.

A similar technique is used when it is necessary to enter a vein in order to give a patient an intravenous infusion of fluid (a 'drip').

In people who are fat, or who have collapsed veins because of shock, or whose veins have already been extensively used for venupuncture, it may be very difficult to

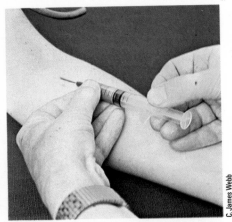

Inserting a needle into a vein, to draw off blood for example, is known as venupuncture.

insert the needle correctly. Where it is absolutely essential to enter a vein (for instance, in the case of a blood transfusion), the doctor may have to 'cut down'. This minor operation involves making an incision in the skin over a vein, dissecting the vein free, opening it and inserting the needle. The skin is then stitched together, and the transfusion of blood is possible.

VERRUCA is the Latin word for 'wart' (see **warts**).

VERTEBRA is one of the bones which together make up the vertebral column, or spine (see under **back**).

The spine contains 33 or these small, irregular bones. They are all connected to each other, but movement between them is possible, so that the spine can very readily bend forwards. Backward and sideways movement is much more limited, except in trained gymnasts.

The vertebrae are classified into various types, depending on the region in which they lie. The cervical vertebrae are those of the neck, the thoracic vertebrae are those of the chest region, the lumbar vertebrae are found in the small of the back, and the sacral and caudal vertebrae are at the base of the spine.

The *cervical* vertebrae are seven in number; the topmost two of these are known as the atlas and the axis (see **axis**); and it is on these that the head rotates. Through a large hole (the vertebral foramen) which is found in each of the vertebrae passes the spinal cord (see **spinal cord**), which is thus contained in a protective bony tunnel for its entire length.

This tunnel is continued through the twelve *thoracic* vertebrae. These can be distinguished from the cervical vertebrae by the fact that they are larger and have strong projections (or 'processes') to which the powerful muscles of the back are attached. They also have special articulating surfaces (or 'facets') at the points where the ribs join them.

The five *lumbar* vertebrae are very large indeed compared with the other types, and they too have thick 'processes' for the attachment of the back muscles. In adults, the spinal cord ends at the second lumbar

C. James Webb

vertebra, and so the protective 'tunnel' of bone is greatly narrowed in the region of the *sacral* vertebrae, which are five in number. In adults, they are fused together to form one bone, the sacrum.

Finally, below the sacrum is the coccyx, the very lowest part of the spinal column, which can be felt just under the skin at the top of the cleft of the buttocks. It is usually composed of four very small vertebrae, which are, in fact, the remnants of the tails of our long-distant ancestors.

Injuries to vertebrae are dealt with under the heading **back.**

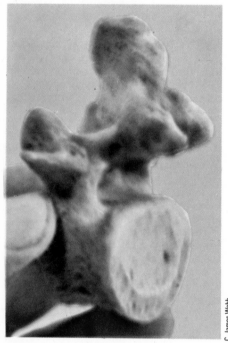

One of the five lumbar vertebrae, the largest of the bones which make up the spine.

VERTIGO means dizziness or giddiness, but doctors restrict the use of the word to the particular type of dizziness in which the patient's surroundings seem to him to be spinning round. Causes of this symptom ('true vertigo', as it is often called) are discussed elsewhere under the heading **dizziness.**

VESICAL means pertaining to the bladder (see **bladder**). Although pronounced

similarly, it should not be confused with the word vesicle (see below).

VESICLE means a small localized collection of fluid in the skin – as, for instance, in the 'spots' of chicken-pox or smallpox. When the fluid is pus (as is, for instance, the case with septic 'spots', or pimples), then it is customary to use the word *pustule* instead of *vesicle*.

VIABLE means capable of life. In medicine, the word is most commonly used in connection with the foetus (or unborn baby) to indicate that it is capable of *independent* life, i.e. outside its mother's womb.

It is specified in the law of many countries that a child is not viable until the 28th week of pregnancy. (A normal pregnancy lasts 40 weeks). Termination (natural or otherwise) of a pregnancy before the 28th week is called abortion, or miscarriage (see **miscarriage**).

However, these definitions were drawn up some considerable time ago, and nowadays, thanks to the great improvements which have been made in the care of premature babies, even a 26 week foetus can occasionally be viable. It may be that this fact will necessitate some redrafting of abortion laws (see also **abortion**).

VIBRIO is the name applied to the comma-shaped bacterium (see **bacteria**), that is responsible for the deadly disease, cholera (see **cholera**).

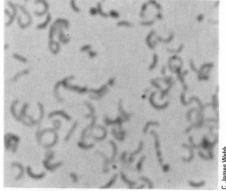

Vibrio is the name given to the comma-shaped bacteria which cause the disease cholera.

VICHY WATER is a mineral water originating from Vichy in France. This type of spring water, like literally hundreds of others, used to be said to be of value in various types of disorder, because of the numerous impurities which give them all a rather pungent taste. However, this belief is no longer held.

VILLUS is the name given to one of the tiny projections of tissue which are found in the small intestine. There are tens of thousands of these projections, and their presence has the effect of greatly increasing the surface area of the intestinal lining. This makes the absorption of digested food very much easier.

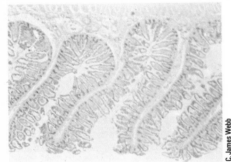

Villi are tiny projections of tissue which aid the intestine's absorption of food.

VIRILISM means the development of male physical characteristics in a female. True virilism (or virilization) is not very common, though young women frequently get alarmed about the possibility if they develop a little excess facial hair — this is nothing to worry about, and can readily be dealt with by cosmetic electrolysis.

In true virilism, the patient usually not only develops a strong facial growth of hair (in the same area as a man's beard), but also has the male pattern of body hair. This is particularly obvious in the abdominal region where normally a woman has little obvious hair above the pubic area. The periods may cease, the voice usually deepens, the body becomes more muscular, and the clitoris (see **clitoris**) enlarges. There may also be the features of Cushing's syndrome (see **Cushing's syndrome**).

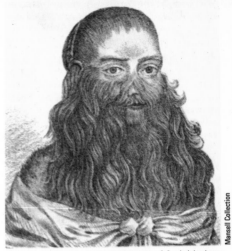

This woman owes her excess of facial hair to the uncommon disorder known as virilism.

These changes are often due to overproduction by the adrenal glands of certain steroid hormones called androgens — these hormones are discussed further under the heading **steroids.**

This excessive production may be caused by simple overactivity of the adrenal glands (see **adrenal**), by the presence of an adrenal tumour (which is usually benign, i.e. non-cancerous), or, occasionally, by overstimulation of the adrenals by the pituitary gland. Depending on the cause, either hormone therapy or surgical removal of part of the adrenal will be effective.

Virilization may also sometimes be due to disorder of the ovary (see **ovary**), in which case treatment will probably be surgical.

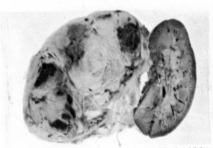

An adrenal tumour, shown here with the kidney attached, is one of the causes of virilism. Such a tumour may overproduce male hormones.

401

It should be stressed that for every woman who has a serious glandular disorder of this type, there are probably a hundred who are worrying unnecessarily about the possibility. Such fears are particularly common among teenagers who have read lurid stories of 'sex change' operations, and similar worries occur, of course, in teenage boys. A consultation with the family doctor will rapidly allay these totally unnecessary fears.

VIRILITY literally means 'manliness', but it has over the years, acquired the additional connotation of male sexual potency. Due to a complete confusion, the word is widely misused simply to mean 'interest in sex,' so that women patients sometimes complain to their doctors of 'not being very virile'.

The male obsession with virility, in the sense of sexual potency, is a curious feature of Man's make-up. This would not matter very much if it were not for the fact that many men (particularly in middle age) are, as a result, convinced that they are somehow lacking in virility and may, therefore, become anxious or depressed, or perhaps be unfaithful to their wives in an effort to 'prove themselves'. In addition, a number of strange and potentially harmful myths have grown up around the whole subject of virility.

Firstly, it should be understood that success in this aspect of marriage is dependent not on some sort of inborn sexual ability on the part of the husband, but on the fact that husband and wife not only love each other but also have a full knowledge of how best to enrich their love-making (see **intercourse**, and **love-play**).

Furthermore, a husband should realize that women do not expect a man to be some sort of sexual athlete capable of making love many times in a single night; although a high proportion of women have the capacity for repeated climaxes (perhaps as many as 20) during love-making, the same does not apply to men. (See **climax**.)

It is also important to realize that the output of the male sex glands diminishes very rapidly during the teenage years, and very much more slowly thereafter. Unfortunately, many middle-aged and elderly men become very worried because they find that the desire for intercourse is not as frequent as it was 20 or 30 years previously. This is perfectly natural, and no amount of expensive 'tonics,' 'vigour-restoratives,' or 'hormone preparations' will change the situation. However, the reduction in sexual activity should normally be very slow indeed (and, in fact, many men in their eighties still have regular intercourse). If there is a *sudden* loss of sexual desire, or if actual impotence (see **impotence**) occurs, the cause is almost invariably psychological, and not due to any hormone deficiency. A doctor's advice should, of course, be sought so that any underlying problems can be resolved.

One of the most widely-believed of all myths is that sexual virility is directly related to the size of the male organ. This is nonsense, and yet many men believe it firmly: an appreciable number of the male population go through life convinced that their genitals are smaller than normal and that this makes them less than adequate lovers. It has, however, been clearly shown that the size of the penis is not a factor in sexual capability. Furthermore, although the size of the flaccid (i.e. non-erect) organ does vary greatly from one man to another, it has been shown that in erection (see **erection**), these differences tend to disappear, and all erect male organs are actually very much the same size.

Linked with the above myth is the even more bizarre one, firmly believed in by men of European stock, that negroes (and, indeed, coloured men in general) have much larger genitals than white men, and are thus better lovers. All this is complete rubbish. The male organs of coloured people are no different in size from those of white men; even if the legend were true, this would not make the coloured man any more virile. Yet psychologists hold that the existence of this fantasy (particularly in the southern states of the USA) plays an important part in maintaining the irrational fear of the black man which is the prime motivation of racial prejudice and causes so much unrest.

VIRUS is the name given to the smallest known type of germ — so small, in fact, that, unlike bacteria, viruses can be filtered through unglazed porcelain.

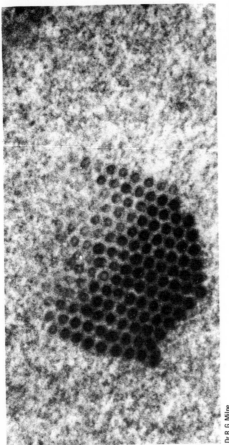

A virus crystal in the salivary gland of an insect, magnified thousands of times.

Dr R. G. Milne

Viruses cause many infections, including the common cold, influenza, smallpox, chicken-pox, measles, mumps, and polio.

From the point of view of treatment, the main difference between bacteria and viruses is that while the former are susceptible to antibiotics, the latter are not. The only exceptions are a very few larger viruses, mainly encountered in the tropics, notably those responsible for trachoma, psittacosis and lymphogranuloma venereum (see **trachoma**, **psittacosis**, and **venereal diseases**).

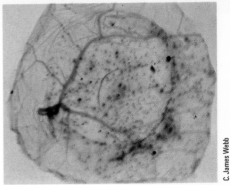

C. James Webb

This smallpox virus is being grown on the live membrane of a chicken's egg.

In all other virus conditions, antibiotics are useless. This fact is not widely appreciated, and many doctors find that they are asked for treatment with penicillin and similar drugs by patients who are suffering from virus infections such as colds.

However, it is possible to give protection against certain virus diseases (such as poliomyelitis, smallpox and measles) by actively immunizing the patient (see **immunity**) — that is by giving him killed or weakened strains of virus which will do him no harm, but which will stimulate the production of antibodies (see **antibodies**) against a future attack of the disease.

Certain chemicals which interfere with the growth of viruses have been isolated in recent years. The best known of these is interferon (see **interferon**). There is some hope that use of such compounds against virus diseases will be possible in the future.

VISCERA is a general term applied to all the organs lying within the cavities of the trunk (i.e. the thoracic and abdominal cavities). An organ such as the stomach or the liver is commonly referred to as an abdominal viscus (the word 'viscus' being the singular of the word 'viscera').

VISION – see **eye**.

VITAMIN means one of a group of chemicals (first isolated at the beginning of this century) which are only present in minute quantities in food, but which are

403

vital to the body's workings. This is because certain of the chemical reactions essential to life require their presence.

Public interest in vitamins was so enormous in the years following their discovery that many people became quite obsessed with them. There are still a lot of people who take vitamin pills or vitamin-containing 'tonics' (see **tonics**) in large quantities, even though they are not in the remotest danger of any type of vitamin deficiency. It should be remembered that, under certain circumstances, taking vitamins, especially in large doses, may actually be harmful. Furthermore, the diet of an adult in most Western countries is likely to be so rich in vitamins that deficiency is practically impossible. There are of course, exceptions — people who are very poor or very old may not always get an adequate diet. Naturally, babies and young children need vitamin supplements, but these should be prescribed by a doctor. Vitamin A is found in carrots and other vegetables, and in eggs, liver, milk, butter, and cheese. Deficiency of the vitamin affects the eyes, and is dealt with under the heading **deficiency diseases.** In the Second World War, attempts were made to improve the night vision of British pilots by giving them extra vitamin A, but this experiment does not seem to have succeeded.

Halibut liver oil and cod liver oil are rich sources of vitamin A, though the main reason why they are given to young children is because they also contain large quantities of vitamin D.

There is no single vitamin B, but a number of different chemicals which used to be called B_1, B_2 and so on. When it became apparent that even 'vitamin B_2' consisted of at least four entirely different compounds, this system began to break down, so that doctors tend more and more to refer to the B group vitamins by their actual chemical names.

The more important B vitamins are as follows. Thiamine (also known as B_1, or aneurine) is essential to prevent beri-beri (see **beri-beri**). Nicotinic acid is needed to prevent pellagra (see **pellagra**). Riboflavin (or riboflavine) is necessary for the health of the skin and mucous membranes,

particularly in the mouth, tongue and eye regions. Rather similar changes to those of riboflavin deficiency are said to be produced by lack of pyridoxine, though little is known about this member of the B group, or about another B vitamin, pantothenic acid. (See also **deficiency diseases.**)

Vitamin B_{12}, or cyanocobalamin, is essential for blood formation. People who have the disorder called pernicious anaemia (see **pernicious anaemia**) need regular injections of this vitamin. Normal persons cannot suffer from deficiency of the chemical, and do not need such injections.

Finally, another substance which is often classed as a B-group vitamin is folic acid (see **folic acid**), lack of which produces what is called a megaloblastic anaemia (see under **anaemia**). It is very important to distinguish folic acid deficiency from pernicious anaemia, as the administration of folic acid is dangerous in the latter condition.

Vitamin C is needed to prevent scurvy (see **scurvy**), which is why young children are routinely given supplements of fruit juice.

Vitamin D is essential to prevent rickets (see **rickets**) and osteomalacia (see **osteomalacia**).

Vitamin E is a chemical factor which was found many years ago to be essential to fertility in rats. In the 1920s and 1930s, it was widely believed to bear some relationship to human fertility. Such was the mood for enthusiasm for vitamins at that time that the compound gained a popular reputation as a restorer of virility (see **virility**), and it was also thought that it might prevent miscarriages. However, it is now felt that vitamin E has no significant effect on the human body.

Vitamin K is one of the essential factors which enable normal blood clotting to take place. In cases of obstructive jaundice (see **jaundice**), lack of bile (see **bile**) in the intestine leads to failure to absorb the vitamin, and supplementary injections may be needed. A similar failure of absorption (but without jaundice) often occurs in new-born children, and causes bleeding from various sites during the first few days of life.

VITILIGO is a disorder in which ivory-white patches appear on the skin. The cause is unknown. Treatment is difficult but some dermatologists obtain good results with drugs called psoralens. Otherwise, a tanning preparation may be used.

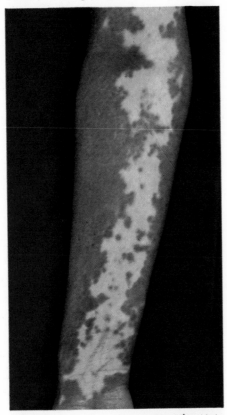

This arm shows an example of vitiligo. Little is known about the cause of this disorder.

VOICE is the sound we produce by expelling air from the lungs through the vocal cords which are situated in the voice-box, or larynx (see **larynx**). After passing through the voice-box, the sounds are modified by the tongue, the teeth and the lips.

No two people's voices are identical, and though it is occasionally difficult to distinguish between two voices by ear, it is, in fact, possible with special equipment to produce a 'voice-print' on paper. Just as is the case with finger-prints, no two persons have the same voice-prints, and this fact has already been made use of for legal purposes – for instance, where there are doubts as to the authenticity of tape recordings.

Where the ordinary voice is lost because of surgical removal of the larynx for cancer, speech therapists can teach a person to produce a very adequate voice using air brought up from the gullet instead.

VOLVULUS means a twisting of the intestines, with resultant obstruction.

In newborn babies, it sometimes happens that the whole of the small intestine is twisted tightly round on itself. This usually occurs because part of the gut has failed to take up its correct position inside the abdomen, and is 'floating' loose in the abdominal cavity. The symptoms are persistent vomiting (often of bile-stained material) starting after birth, coupled with severe dehydration. There may also be abdominal distension. An X-ray may be helpful in distinguishing the condition from other causes of obstruction (see under **obstruction of the bowels**) but, in any case, an operation will be necessary to save the child's life.

VOMITING is caused by violent contractions of the stomach against the diaphragm (the muscular septum that divides the chest from the abdomen). It is usually necessary for the diaphragm to be held rigid for this mechanism to operate; if a person keeps his diaphragm moving up and down, by concentrating on breathing deeply in and out, then it may be possible for him to suppress the urge to vomit.

The causes of vomiting generally lie either within the abdomen, or in the brain and middle ear. An upset of the balance mechanisms of the middle ear (for instance, in sea sickness – see **sea sickness** – or in Menière's disease – see **Menière's disease**) stimulates the vomiting centres of the brain. These centres can also be affected by drugs, by brain disorders in which the pressure inside the skull is raised, and by nerve impulses from the back of the throat: this is why pressing anything down the throat is liable to cause gagging.

Abdominal conditions that cause vomiting include gastritis (see **gastritis**) and gastro-enteritis (see **gastro-enteritis**), appendicitis (see **appendicitis**) and many other conditions which, like appendicitis, cause irritation of the peritoneum, or membrane lining the abdominal cavity (see **peritonitis**). Intestinal obstruction (see **obstruction of the bowels**) can also cause vomiting.

Women and children are more prone to vomit than men. In fact, a young child may vomit in almost any illness, and even if he has overeaten. However, the most common illnesses causing vomiting in childhood are probably tonsillitis (see **tonsillitis**) and gastritis or gastro-enteritis (see **gastritis** and **gastro-enteritis**). In newborn babies, persistent vomiting or regurgitation may be a serious sign, since it can indicate intestinal obstruction (see **obstruction of the bowels**) or blockage of the gullet (see **gullet**). Severe vomiting in a baby of three to ten weeks may be due to pyloric stenosis (see **pyloric stenosis**).

Among women, morning sickness of pregnancy is, of course, a very common cause of vomiting. It usually starts about the sixth week of pregnancy, and should be more or less over six or eight weeks later.

Mild cases usually respond very well to simply having a cup of tea and a biscuit before getting up in the morning; slightly more severe ones may require the prescription of an anti-emetic drug; however, it sometimes happens that an expectant mother becomes so ill with repeated vomiting (hyperemesis) that she has to be temporarily admitted to hospital, where fluid replacement by an intra-venous 'drip' may be needed.

VULVA is the term applied to the external female genitals.

The vulva is the entry to both the vagina (see **vagina**) and the urethra (see **urethra**). It consists of the two sets of labia (lips) and the mons veneris (all of which are dealt with under the heading **labia**), the clitoris (see **clitoris**), and the vestibule, the cleft between the two inner labia into which both the vagina and the urethra open. At the innermost part of the

406

vestibule, and partly closing off the vagina, is the hymen or virgin's veil (see **hymen**).

WARFARIN in an anticoagulant drug which is sometimes used as an alternative to dindevan (see **dindevan**).

WARTS, or verrucas, are small, benign growths on the skin. Many of them are believed to be caused by viruses. It is easy to remove warts surgically or by 'burning' them off chemically. However, if left alone, they do no harm and will usually disappear of their own accord. In older people, it is easy to mistake a wart for a mole, and vice versa, which does not usually matter. It should, however, be borne in mind that moles may sometimes undergo malignant change (see **moles**), when removal is absolutely essential.

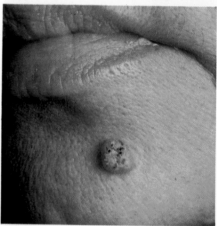

Although warts will generally disappear if left alone, they can be surgically removed.

WASP STINGS are not usually very painful, though they may be extremely distressing to young children, whose pain may be eased by aspirin, and by a cold compress at the site of the sting. Some people think that bathing the skin with a mild acid (e.g. vinegar or lemon juice) is helpful. Very rarely, collapse due to anaphylactic shock (see **anaphylactic shock**) may occur, and necessitate urgent transfer to hospital. Mouth to mouth artificial respiration should be used if necessary.

WASSERMANN REACTION, or WR, is a test for syphilis (see **syphilis**). Blood Wassermann reaction tests are performed routinely on all expectant mothers in most countries; in many parts of the USA, they are carried out on all persons who want to get married.

It should be stressed that a positive Wassermann reaction does not necessarily indicate the presence of syphilis. Such a result can sometimes be caused by other conditions, such as glandular fever.

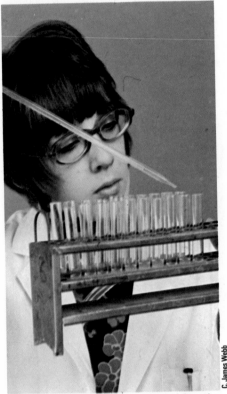

Tubes of serum being prepared for the Wasserman Reaction, a test for syphilis.

WASTING is a term which tends to be used in two senses — loss of weight, and muscle wasting.

Wasting in the sense of loss of weight may be due to tuberculosis, cancer of various types, over-activity of the thyroid gland, or diabetes mellitus. It can also be associated with loss of appetite, due to psychological reasons. However, it should be stressed that weight loss of only a few pounds is a quite meaningless symptom. Where a person loses, say, ten pounds or more without some obvious cause (such as dieting), it is important to consult a doctor as soon as possible.

Wasting of individual muscles or groups of muscles may occur after injury — for instance, the inactivity caused by cartilage injuries of the knee joint almost invariably causes gross wasting of the thigh muscles in an astonishingly short time.

Where there is no such injury, however, muscle wasting is likely to be due to a disorder either of the nervous system or of the muscles themselves. These disorders are very numerous, but all need prompt medical attention.

WATER, or H_2O, is, after oxygen, the most important chemical needed for the continuance of life. It is impossible for an adult to survive long without it, and young children and babies who are suffering from dehydration (e.g. in attacks of gastroenteritis) can die from lack of water within an alarmingly short time.

The maintenance of hygienic water supplies is essential to the health of the community. In the most developed countries, tap water is carefully purified by a special process of filtration. Regular tests are carried out to ensure that there is no significant contamination by germs. It is still true, however, that in most countries of the world, tap water is liable to contamination, and should not be drunk unless it has been boiled first. Almost invariably, this contamination consists of germs from the bowel (for instance, typhoid or cholera), which have a quite extraordinary ability to find their way into water supplies. Careful control of sewage disposal must therefore go hand-in-hand with the development of a pure water supply (see also **wells**).

WATER CLOSETS were probably first developed in Elizabethan times, but they were primitive and insanitary devices. It was not until the middle of the last century that the modern WC was invented by Sir Thomas Crapper, who was plumber-royal to Queen Victoria. This type of WC has a

407

water seal in the U-bend to prevent germs returning up the pipe.

One problem with the current design of WC is that when flushed, it sprays tiny droplets of germ-containing fluid all around it. This can, of course, be dealt with by having a lid or cover, and in recent years practically all WCs have been manufactured with such a cover. Ideally, this should be made of some material, such as plastic, which can be washed down with a household disinfectant, and which will not form a resting-place for germs.

In America, it is customary for hotels to 'sanitize' WC seats and then to seal them with paper, so that they can only be used by one person. This is not normally considered necessary in other countries, but it is obvious that it is an elementary precaution to avoid touching public WC seats which could possibly have been contaminated by some infectious discharge.

Rather more important, but not as widely recognized as it might be, is the fact that all WC fittings are likely to be intermittently contaminated with germs, so that it is so important to prevent infection by washing the hands after visiting the toilet.

WATER-HAMMER PULSE is the name given to a very sudden and 'collapsing' pulse which is found in a particular type of valvular heart disease.

WATER ON THE BRAIN is an old term which was generally employed to mean hydrocephalus (see **hydrocephalus**), the condition in which, in the unborn child, the head enlarges because of an excess of fluid in the brain. The term also seems to have sometimes been used, however, to mean meningitis (see **meningitis**).

WAX in the ears is one of the commonest causes of deafness (see **deafness**). Often people do not realize that their ears are blocked by wax, and assume that their hardness of hearing is due to some other cause, such as advancing age. The great improvement in hearing after syringing of the ears is often quite startling. Preparations are available which can be instilled into the ears to soften the wax, but far

408

better results are produced by expert syringing.

WEANING is the process of taking a child off breast milk (or bottle feeds) and introducing solid food. Provided the introduction is very gradual, i.e. over a period of several weeks, problems are not likely to be encountered. It is obviously unwise to suddenly switch a baby to a diet principally composed of solids.

It is possible that abdominal upsets due to weaning may cause the condition called intussusception, which is quite common at this time (see **intussusception**).

WEBBED FINGERS, like webbed toes, are a common but seldom serious deformity. In the majority of cases, the bones of the fingers are quite normal, and hence it is possible for a plastic surgeon to correct the deformity by operation. Surgery is often postponed until well after babyhood, so that the fingers are larger and easier to work with.

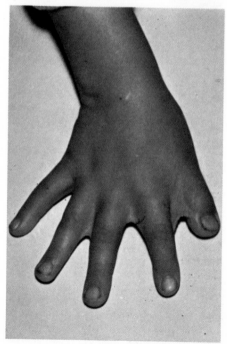

Webbed fingers are a relatively common deformity which can usually be corrected by surgery.

WEIGHT increases throughout childhood until the late 'teens. A table of heights and weights will be found at the end of the dictionary, but it is important to remember the advice given under the heading **development in children** – that both babies and older children vary greatly, so that parents should not be too concerned if their offspring vary a little from the normal figures given.

Contrary to what was widely believed until quite recently, weight should not increase very much after the age of about 20, and the development of a 'middle-aged spread' is not a desirable thing. Tables of weight for adults will also be found at the end of the dictionary, and it should be realized that any significant increase on the figures given is likely to be deleterious to health. Well over two thousand years ago, the Greek physician Hippocrates is said to have remarked that those who are very fat are more liable to sudden death. This is just as true today; furthermore, it can be shown statistically that the more a man exceeds the desirable weight for his height, the shorter is his life expectancy.

WEIL'S DISEASE is a form of leptospirosis – that is, infection by a germ of the group called Leptospira. There are a number of species of this group which can cause disease in Man. Most of them are basically infections of rats and other animals; Man tends to become ill if his work brings him into contact with infected animals or their excreta. Thus, leptospirosis is seen most frequently in sewer-workers, veterinary surgeons, miners, and slaughterhouse employees.

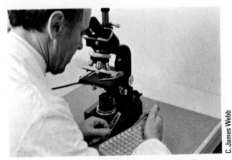

The presence in the blood of antibodies to leptospirosis indicates Weil's disease.

The commonest species of these germs to infect Man is *Leptospira icterohaemorrhagiae* (or *icterohaemorrhagica*). This very often produces only a relatively mild illness, characterized by fever, headache, redness of the eyes, nausea, and prostration. It may, however, cause the full picture of Weil's disease. In this condition, there is severe jaundice, and a marked tendency to bleed from many parts of the body. There may also be kidney failure.

Most cases of leptospirosis respond to antibiotics, but in Weil's disease itself the patient will be very ill, and intensive hospital treatment may be needed to save his life, particularly if kidney failure is present.

WELLS still provide a considerable proportion of the water supply in much of the world. Where well water consists only of rain which has percolated through uncontaminated soil, it is likely to be absolutely pure. However, it must be borne in mind that contamination of the soil by human excreta (particularly in cess-pools) anywhere in the region of a well may very frequently also lead to contamination of the well water. Outbreaks of infection are likely to result.

WET DREAMS – see **emissions.**

WHEEZING is produced by narrowing of the air passages within the chest. It may be a feature of asthma (see **asthma**), chronic bronchitis (see **bronchitis**) and obstructive airway disease (see **obstructive airway disease**). It may also occur in one type of heart failure, called left ventricular failure, which is discussed under the heading **congestive cardiac failure.**

WHISKY, or whiskey, is a spirit produced from grains such as barley and rye, or, occasionally, from potatoes. Like brandy (see **brandy**), it has no medicinal value, except as a means of promoting sleep in the elderly. Contrary to long-held popular belief, it is not a 'stimulant,' and its only value in cases of fainting is likely to be psychological.

WHITE LEG used to be a common condition in pregnancy and the lying-in period,

409

but for some reason is now far less frequently encountered. It is due to thrombosis (clotting) in a particular large vein in the leg. The potential complications are serious, and so it is important to try to prevent this type of thrombosis occurring. The subject is discussed further under the heading **phlebitis.**

WHITES is the popular name for leucorrhoea – a thick, whitish vaginal discharge. Although a moderate amount of white vaginal secretion is perfectly normal, a doctor's advice should be sought if the amount is very large, or, more important, if the secretion is yellowish, offensive, brownish or blood-stained, or if it is semi-solid in nature (see also **vagina**).

WHITLOW is a term which is popularly applied to all infections around the tip of the finger. The commonest of these is called a paronychia (or a 'run around,' as it is known in America).

Germs (usually staphylococci – see **staphylococci**) penetrate the skin through a crack or a hang-nail, and cause pus formation just to one side of the nail. Very often, the abscess spreads around the base of the nail as well. Treatment usually consists of a minor operation to let the pus out.

WHOOPING COUGH, or pertussis, is an infectious disease which occurs mainly in childhood. It is caused by a bacterium known as *Haemophilus pertussis* or *Bordetella pertussis.*

Whooping cough is not a very serious disease when it occurs in adults or older children, but it can be a killer in the very young: in Britain, for example, it causes about 100 deaths a year. Four-fifths of these deaths are said to occur in the first year of life, which is why immunization (usually in the form of 'triple vaccine') should be carried out at an early age.

At first, the features of whooping-cough are those of a persistent cold, but the cough becomes a more and more prominent feature, until eventually the child has recurrent paroxysms. These may occur a dozen times or so in 24 hours, and are worst at night: the child's whole body is shaken by half a dozen or more coughs in rapid succession. He is unable to breathe between each one, and only when the paroxysm ends is he able to take a great gasp of breath, which produces the characteristic noise known as a whoop. He then usually brings up a blob of mucus. Paroxysms may go on for a week or more.

Doctors differ about whether the use of antibiotics is necessary. These drugs will, however, be employed if the child develops complications such as pneumonia or infection of the middle ear (see **otitis media**). Other complications include a bleeding tendency (particularly affecting the eyes), and convulsions (which may be caused by encephalitis – see **encephalitis**). A long term chest complication which should be watched out for is bronchiectasis (see **bronchiectasis**); X-rays should be carried out if the child's cough is slow to clear up.

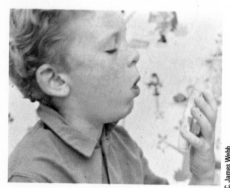

This child is coughing on to a jelly plate to isolate the whooping cough germs.

410

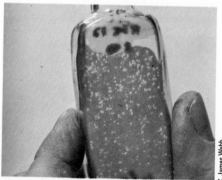

The germs, taken from the plate and grown in a bottle, can then be identified.

WILSON'S DISEASE, also called hepato-lenticular degeneration, is a familial disorder which is characterized by a form of cirrhosis of the liver, together with brain degeneration. The latter feature may cause mental defect and a type of Parkinsonism (see **Parkinson's disease**). Unlike other types of Parkinsonism, this disorder comes on quite early in life — usually in adolescence.

The diagnosis of the condition can be difficult, but may be aided by finding characteristic coloured rings in the eyes. Once the cause of the condition is established, the patient can be considerably helped by being given a drug which lowers the concentration of copper in the tissues. It is believed that Wilson's disease is caused by an inherited defect in the way the body deals with this metal, so leading to a deposition of copper in the brain and liver.

WINDPIPE, or trachea, is the main tube which carries air in and out of the lungs. It starts at the larynx, or voice-box (see **larynx**), and runs downwards in front of the gullet, to a point in the upper part in the chest where it divides into two slightly smaller tubes called bronchi, which supply the right lung and the left lung. The windpipe is about four inches long. Its upper part can be felt in the front of the neck, where a number of the bands of cartilage that are found in its wall are easily palpable under the skin. It is at this site that the operation of tracheotomy (see **tracheotomy**) is performed.

WINE is a form of alcoholic drink made by fermenting grape juice. Fortified wines (e.g. port, sherry and Madeira) contain added spirits as well, and are thus stronger than ordinary wines. Like other forms of alcohol, wines have no medicinal use, except as a night-time sedative. Some wines, including claret and red Burgundy, are, however, said to contain iron, and this is possibly the reason why red wines are widely regarded as having some sort of tonic properties.

In certain medical conditions, drinking wine is inadvisable. In particular, people who take anti-depressant drugs should seek their doctor's advice on this point.

WINTERGREEN is a plant which produces an oil containing methyl salicylate. Preparations of this oil are still sometimes rubbed on the skin over painful joints, torn muscle fibres and so on. They produce a pleasant warmth of the skin, though it is highly doubtful whether this is particularly beneficial.

Wintergreen preparations are often rubbed on the chest of a patient who has a cold or cough. This can, of course, have no conceivable effect on the interior of the chest, but the pleasantly aromatic fumes rising toward the nose certainly do no harm, and may even help the patient's nose to clear.

WISDOM TOOTH is one of the four teeth which come through behind the ordinary molar teeth in early childhood. While most wisdom teeth come through without much trouble, a proportion of young people suffer considerable pain because one of these teeth becomes impacted — that is, jammed against the backmost molar. There may also be difficulties because of the fact that a flap of gum often remains overhanging the top of the wisdom tooth, offering a ready site for infection. For these reasons, wisdom teeth frequently have to be removed.

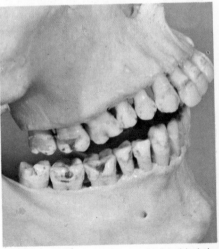

C. James Webb

The four wisdom teeth are sited behind the ordinary molar teeth, at the back of the jaw.

411

WOMB – see **uterus.**

WOOLSORTER'S DISEASE is anthrax, or malignant pustule, the infectious disorder caused by a bacterium called *Bacillus anthracis*. It occurs in sheep, horses, goats and cattle, and readily affects Man. People who are especially liable to the condition include woolsorters, people who work with sheep and cattle, and those who deal with hides, with bone-meal, or with animal carcasses,

The characteristic feature of this condition is an ugly looking blackish ulcer which develops from a lump on the skin. There may be associated enlargement of the lymph glands. If the infection spreads, a very serious and often fatal illness may result. However, treatment with antibiotics, if started in time, is likely to be curative.

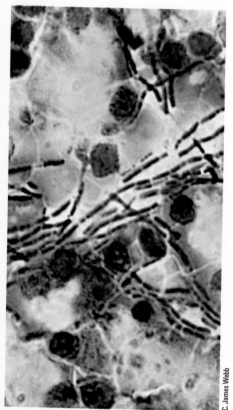

This smear of a spleen shows *Bacillus anthracis*, the bacterium which causes anthrax.

412

It is therefore essential that anyone who works with untreated wool or hides, or who is in any way likely to be exposed to this disease, should consult his doctor at once if an unexplained lump or ulcer develops on the skin.

WORD BLINDNESS is a form of difficulty in reading which may affect even the most intelligent children. It is essential that a child who seems otherwise bright but who cannot make normal progress with reading should have an expert opinion to see if he is suffering from word blindness. The subject is discussed further under the heading **dyslexia.**

WORMS of various types are among the most widespread creatures in nature. Some worms are parasitic on Man, and these fall into two classes, the flatworms and the roundworms. These are dealt with under the heading **parasites** and also under the names of the individual types of worm.

WOUNDS – see **stab wounds, bleeding, head injuries, first aid, shock** and **fractures.**

WRIST is a word of slightly ambiguous meaning. Many people use the term to indicate the lower part of the arm, including the wrist joint. In this sense, for instance, fractures of the wrist may actually mean fractures of the forearm bones (the radius and the ulna), the commonest example of which is a Colles' fracture (see **Colles' fracture**). Other types of injury which may occur in this region include Smith's fracture (which is similar to a Colles' fracture except that the displacement of bone is in the reverse direction) and greenstick fracture (see **greenstick fractures**).

Anatomists, however, tend to use the term 'wrist' to mean the carpus – the region of the palm nearest the forearm, which contains eight tiny bones bound together by strong ligaments. These bones too are very susceptible to fracture, especially from a fall on an outstretched hand. Damage to the blood supply often causes delay in healing.

WRIST-DROP is a condition in which the hand becomes floppy and limp as the result of weakness in the wrist region. This is normally due to a peripheral neuritis (see under **neuritis**), or inflammation of nerves supplying the forearm muscles.

The initial symptoms are often numbness and tingling of the hands, but soon afterwards the patient finds that his power to 'make a fist' and flex the wrist is diminished. Eventually, the hand flops limply at the wrist joint. In generalized disorders, a similar phenomenon (foot-drop) may be seen in the feet.

Causes include the absorption of poisons, such as lead or arsenic, infections such as diphtheria, and deficiency of the B group vitamin thiamine — or to give the condition its more common name, beriberi (see **beri-beri**).

Sometimes, wrist-drop may occur as a feature of a rather mysterious illness called the Guillain-Barré syndrome, but then it is likely to be associated with other symptoms such as difficulty in walking. The cause of this condition is unknown, though it has been suggested that it may be due to a virus infection. Most cases get better, and recovery may be hastened by treatment with steroid drugs (see **steroids**).

Wrist-drop can also be due to injury to the nerves. This can sometimes happen if an unconscious patient's arm is allowed to rest unsupported across the sharp edge of an operating table, for example.

WRITER'S CRAMP, or 'scrivener's palsy' as it used to be called, is a spasm of the muscles of the hand and forearm.

Although a cramped feeling comes on in anyone who writes for a long time at a stretch, some people who do a great deal of writing find that cramp eventually affects them whenever they try even to begin to write. This condition seems to occur not in authors (as the name might perhaps imply), but in those whose writing always involves repetitive and non-flowing movements of the hand and fingers. Typically, therefore, writer's cramp is seen in ledger clerks, comptometer operators and typists.

The sufferer may get round his disability for a while by using different methods of holding the pen (or of striking the typewriter keys) but often the progressive lack of co-ordination eventually makes all writing impossible.

In a small proportion of cases, there is a psychological basis to the disorder, and these people can be helped by psychiatric means. In most patients, however, the doctor has to advise giving up trying to write altogether (at least for the time being). Various types of massage and exercise will often prove helpful.

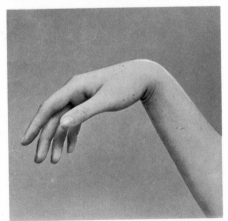

An example of wrist-drop, caused by weakness in the wrist region. It is usually curable.

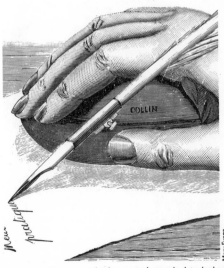

This cumbersome device was intended to help people suffering from writer's cramp.

413

WRY NECK, or spasmodic torticollis, is a disorder in which the head is turned to one side. There is associated spasm of the neck muscles. Sometimes the spasm is continuous, but it may also be rapidly intermittent, so that the patient keeps making odd twisting movements.

The neck should be X-rayed, as occasionally the disorder may be due to structural abnormality of the vertebrae (see **vertebrae**) in this region. Sometimes, it may be possible to demonstrate that the patient has some eye abnormality which makes him keep turning his head to the side in order to see clearly. Sometimes, too, it is evident that a psychological dis-

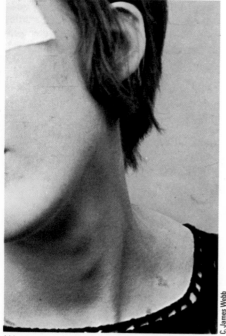

Wry neck, when the head is turned to one side, is usually treated by massage and exercise.

turbance of a hysterical nature (see **hysteria**) may be the cause of the patient's odd posture, and in these instances he can be treated by psychiatric means.

Most cases, however, are treated by massage and exercise. Sometimes, encasing the neck in a plaster collar for some weeks may be helpful. Occasionally, surgery is undertaken on the nerves supply-
414

ing the affected muscles, but not all doctors agree that this treatment is justifiable.

In newborn children, the situation is rather different, as wry neck may be due to a birth injury to one of the sternomastoids, the pair of very large muscles which lie one on either side of the front of the neck. Usually, there is a large swelling in the affected muscle. In early childhood, the deformity of the neck vertebrae mentioned above is also a likely cause.

X-RAYS, or Röntgen rays (so called after their discoverer, Professor Röntgen of Wurzberg) have been known since 1896.

X-rays are actually a form of electro-magnetic radiation, just as visible light is. This electro-magnetic radiation consists of rays of varying wavelengths. The very longest rays (those with a wavelength of anything up to several miles) are wireless waves; much shorter than these are the infra-red (heat) waves. The wavelength of visible light is less than that of infra-red radiation, and shorter again than this are ultra-violet waves.

X-rays, however, are of very short wavelength indeed (about one hundred millionth of a centimetre), and they have great penetrating power, which enables them to pass easily through the soft tissues of the body. They do not pass quite so readily, however, through more dense tissues, and bones, for instance, provide a considerable obstacle to their passage. This is because bone contains the mineral calcium. Calcium has a heavier atom than those found in most tissues of the body, which are largely made up of 'light-weight' atoms like hydrogen, oxygen and carbon.

It is thus easy to take X-ray pictures of bone, and fairly straightforward to obtain clear radiographs of parts of the body where thick tissues (e.g. the heart) are contrasted with thin ones (e.g. the lungs). Where an X-ray of soft tissues only is required, it may be necessary to outline the structure to be studied with an opaque dye — this is, for example, the technique used in barium X-rays (see **barium meal**, and **barium enema**), and in X-rays of the kidneys (pyelograms) and gall-bladder (cholecystograms). Similar methods are used to study the spinal cord and brain.

XANTHOMATA are small yellowish lumps in the skin. They tend to occur particularly on the eyelids and the hands. Xanthomata are a feature of several disorders of fat metabolism, but, in particular, they may indicate the presence of a familial chemical defect in which a failure to break down fat in the normal way is associated with a greatly increased liability to coronary heart disease.

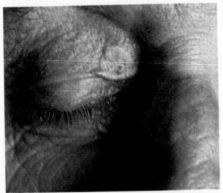

Xanthomata, small yellowish lumps in the skin, often warn against coronary heart disease.

XEROPHTHALMIA is a disorder of the outer layers of the eyeball. It is caused by deficiency of vitamin A, and is characterized by atrophy and eventual ulceration of the 'white' of the eye.

XYLOCAINE is a local anaesthetic drug; the official name is lignocaine (see **lignocaine**).

YAWS is an infectious tropical disease caused by a germ known as *Treponema pertenue*. Although this organism belongs to the same group as that of syphilis (the spirochaetes), yaws is not a venereal disease.

Practically all cases of yaws are seen in the warm regions of the world — mainly equatorial Africa and the South Pacific. The disease was very common in the West Indies until the Second World War, but since then has been practically eradicated from most of the islands.

Yaws is most frequently seen in young children, who often acquire it through contact with their mothers. After an incubation period of several weeks, the first sign of the disease appears; this is usually a reddish lump on the skin of the legs. It may heal up, but two or three months later the patient develops a secondary eruption, which consists of similar swellings all over the body. They often affect the soles of the feet, where they may develop into ulcers, thus making walking very painful.

Some years later, the disease may produce considerable destruction of the bones and skin, with very severe ulceration and deformity.

Fortunately, penicillin provides an immediate cure for yaws, except in cases of several years' standing where deformity and ulceration have developed. The World Health Organization's eradication campaigns have involved the treatment of some 50 million people, and as a result of these measures, and probably the improvement in living standards in many parts of the tropics, the incidence of yaws is now rapidly diminishing.

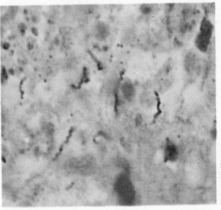

C. James Webb

The spirochaete organisms that cause yaws: a disease which attacks the bones and skin.

YEAST is a primitive organism whose principal importance to Man is that it can be used in the making of both bread and beer. It does, however, contain certain vitamins of the B group (see **vitamins**). While deficiency of these vitamins is most unlikely to occur in the temperate zones of the world, yeast extracts may be a useful food additive in parts of the tropics. These extracts often contain a substance called

415

'tyramine', which makes them highly dangerous to people who are taking antidepressant drugs called monoamine oxidase inhibitors.

YELLOW FEVER is a virus disease which is transmitted to Man by mosquitoes. At the present time, it is found only in West Africa and South America, but this has not always been so. In the eighteenth and nineteenth centuries, the disease often occurred far north in the United States. In Europe, yellow fever was occasionally seen in the Spanish ports, but never spread very far, because of the absence of suitable mosquitoes to pass it on.

It was not until 1881 that Carlos Finley was the first man to suggest that the mosquito *Aedes aegypti* was the carrier of the disease. Later, as a result of the high rate of infection among United States troops in Cuba during the Spanish-American war, the American army set up a yellow fever commission under Major Walter Reed. Experiments carried out on volunteers during 1900 and 1901 enabled the commission to demonstrate that the organism carried from man to man by the mosquito was a virus.

Control of yellow fever now seemed to be quite a straightforward business, and an enormous eradication programme launched against the mosquito rapidly banished the disease from the southern United States, much of the Caribbean, and South and Central America. One result of this was to enable the Panama Canal to be built at long last.

However, in 1928, a mysterious outbreak occurred in Rio de Janeiro. This did not seem to have resulted from the usual man-mosquito-man cycle of infection, and research eventually demonstrated the very disappointing fact that yellow fever was unlikely to be wiped out after all, since another source of infection existed. This source is the vast monkey population of the South American jungles, from whom the virus can be carried to Man by the bite of various species of forest mosquitoes.

Since then, yellow fever has at least been contained, and the number of cases occurring outside the jungles is now relatively small. There has, however, been

a tendency in recent years for the disease to spread northward from the jungles of Latin America, and immunization is therefore a wise precaution for anyone visiting the Caribbean or the area of the Gulf of Mexico. Though the risk is very small, the effects of the disease are so terrible as to make protection essential.

The first symptoms of yellow fever come on about 5 days after infection. There is fever, headache and backache, followed by nausea and vomiting. Jaundice and bleeding from various sites occur a day or two later. Haemorrhage into the stomach is common, and causes the vomiting of black material. The temperature falls after a while, and the patient feels better; he then relapses, however, and may die of kidney complications. There is no specific treatment, but skilled nursing increases the patient's chance of recovery. He must, of course, be kept under a net, lest a mosquito bite him and pass the disease on to someone else.

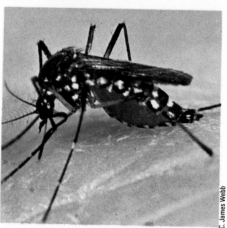

This mosquito, sucking blood from a finger, is a carrier of the virus disease yellow fever.

YOGHURT is a sour milk preparation. It has no medicinal value, and no advantage over ordinary milk (see **milk**).

ZOONOSES are diseases of animals which can be transmitted to humans.

ZOSTER is a shortened form of the term herpes zoster, meaning shingles (see **herpes zoster**).

416

GUIDE TO PRONUNCIATION

Below appears a list of some medical words which commonly give rise to difficulties in pronunciation. Remember that medical words can be pronounced in several different ways. The most commonly used pronunciations are given here.

A

ABDOMEN	— ab-doh-men or ab-doh-men.
ACHALASIA	— ay-kal-ay-see-ah.
ACHOLURIA	— ay-kol-yew-ree-ah.
ACHONDROPLASIA	— ay-kon-dro-play-see-ah.
ACROMEGALY	— ak-ro-meg-ah-lee.
ADENITIS	— add-en-eye-tis.
AEROPHAGY	— air-off-ah-jee.
AETIOLOGY	— eat-ee-oll-o-jee.
ALLANTOIS	— al-an-toe-is.
AMOEBIC	— am-ee-bic.
ANAEMIA	— an-ee-me-ah.
AORTA	— ay-or-tah.
ASCITES	— ass-eye-tees.

B

BACTERIURIA	— back-ter-your-ee-ah.
BILHARZIA	— bill-hart-zee ah.
BIOPSY	— bye-op-see.
BRACHIAL	— bray-kee-al.
BRADYCARDIA	— brad-ee-card-ee-ah.
BRONCHIECTASIS	— bron-kee-ek-tah-sis.
BRUCELLOSIS	— broo-sell-o-sis.

C

CAECUM	— see-cum.
CAESARIAN	— sez-ay-ree-an.
CANTHARIDES	— kan-thar-eye-dees.
CERVICAL	— sir-vie-kal.
CHANCROID	— shan-kroyd.
CHIROPODIST	— kirr-op-o-dist.
CHIROPRACTORS	— kye-ro-prak-tors.
CLITORIS	— klit-or-is.
COELIAC	— see-lee-ack.
COR PULMONALE	— kor-pull-mon-ah-lay.

CROUP	— kroop.
CURARE	— kyoo-rah-ray.

D

DEMENTIA	— duh-men-shah.
DENTINE	— den-teen.
DIURETICS	— dye-your-et-icks.
DUODENUM	— dyoo-o-dee-num.

E

ECHINOCOCCUS	— eck-eye-no-kok-us.
EMPHYSEMA	— em-fizz-ee-mah.
EMPYEMA	— em-pie-ee-mah.
ENURESIS	— en-your-ee-sis.
EROGENOUS	— er-rodge-enn-us.

F

FAECES	— fee-sees.
FLATUS	— flay- tuss.

G

GESTATION	— jest-ay-tion.
GLAUCOMA	— glaw-ko-mah.
GONADS	— go-nads.
GYNAECOLOGY	— guy-nee-kol-o-jee.

H

HAEMATURIA	— hee-mat-you-ree-ah.
HALITOSIS	— hal-ee-toe-sis.
HOMOSEXUAL	— hom-o-sex-you-al. (NOT home-o-sex-you-al.)
HYDRAMNIOS	— high-dram-nee-os.

I

IATROGENIC	— yat-ro-jen-ick.
ILEITIS	— eye-lee-eye-tis.
IMPETIGO	— im-pet-eye-go.
IMPOTENCE	— im-pot-ense. (NOT im-po-tense.)
INFARCTION	— in-fark-shun.
ISCHAEMIA	— is-keem-ee-ah.

K

KETONES	— kee-tones.
KYPHOSIS	— kye-fo-sis.

L

LABIA	— lay-bee-ah.
LEUKAEMIA	— lyew-keem-ee-ah.

LUPUS	– loo-puss.

M ━━━━━━━━━

MAMMOGRAPHY	– mam-og-raff-ee.
MANTOUX	– man-too.
MASOCHISM	– mas-o-kism.
MELAENA	– mel-ee-nah.
MENARCHE	– men-ar-kay.
MYXOEDEMA	– mix-uh-de-mah.

N ━━━━━━━━━

NAEVUS	– nee-vus.

O ━━━━━━━━━

OEDEMA	– uh-dee-mah.
OESOPHAGUS	– uh-soff-ah-guss.
OESTROGENS	– ee-stro-jens.
OPISTHOTONOS	– op-is-thot-on-os.
ORTHOPAEDICS	– or-tho-pee-dix.
OSMOSIS	– os-mo-sis.
OTITIS MEDIA	– o-tie-tis mee-dee-ah.
OTOSCLEROSIS	– o-toe-skler-o-sis.

P ━━━━━━━━━

PAEDIATRICS	– pee-dee-at-rix.
PARANOIA	– parr-ah-noy-ah.
PETIT MAL	– pet-ee mal
PHENYLKETONURIA	– fee-nile-kee-tonn-you-ree-ah.
PHIMOSIS	– fie-mo-sis.
PLACEBO	– plah-see-bo.
PLEURA	– ploo-rah.
PNEUMOCONIOSIS	– new-mo-kone-ee-o-sis.
POLYCYTHAEMIA	– poll-ee-sigh-theme-ee-ah.
PROSTATE	– pros-tate
PSITTACOSIS	– sit-ah-ko-sis.
PTOMAINE	– toe-main.
PUERPERIUM	– poo-er-pee-ree-um.
PULMONARY	– pull-mon-ah-ree.

S ━━━━━━━━━

SALMONELLAE	– sal-mon-ell-ee.
SAL VOLATILE	– sal vol-at-il-ee.
SCABIES	– skay-bees.
SCHISTOSMIASIS	– skis-to-som-eye-ah-sis.

SCHIZOPHRENIA	– skit-zo-free-nee-ah.
SCIATICA	– sigh-at-ick-ah.
SEBACEOUS	– seb-ay-shus.
SEMEN	– see-men.
SPIROCHAETES	– spy-ro-keats.
SPONDYLITIS	– spon-dill-eye-tis.
STILBOESTROL	– still-bees-troll.
STRYCHNINE	– strick-neen.
SUBARACHNOID	– sub-ah-rack-noyd.
SYNAPSE	– sigh-napse.
SYNCOPE	– sin-ko-pee.
SYNDROME	– sin-drome.
SYNOVIAL	– sigh-no-vee-al.

T ━━━━━━━━━

TABES	– tay-bees.
TACHYCARDIA	– tack-ee-card-ee-ah.
TENOSYNOVITIS	– tee-no-sigh-no-vie-tis.
TESTOSTERONE	– tes-toss-ter-one.
THIAMINE	– thigh-ah-mean.
TINNITUS	– tin-it-us.
TOURNIQUET	– tour-nee-kay.
TOXAEMIA	– tox-ee-mee-ah.
TRACHEA	– truh-kee-ah.
TRICHINIASIS	– trick-in-eye-ah-sis.
TSETSE	– set-see.
TULARAEMIA	– tyew-lah-ree-mee-ah.

U ━━━━━━━━━

UMBILICUS	– um-bill-eye-cuss.
URAEMIA	– you-ream-ee-ah.
UREA	– you-ree-ah.
URETER	– your-it-er.
URETHRA	– your-ee-thra.
UVEITIS	– you-vee-eye-tis.
UVULA	– you-view-lah.

V ━━━━━━━━━

VAGOTOMY	– vay-got-om-ee.
VENA CAVA	– vee-nah-cave-ah.
VERRUCA	– ver-oo-ka.
VISCERA	– vis-er-ah.
VITILIGO	– vit-ill-eye-go.
VOLVULUS	– vol-view-luss.

Average heights and weights in boys and girls, from birth to age eighteen.

Note: both height and weight may vary considerably from the figures given, even in perfectly healthy children. If in doubt, parents should consult the family doctor or infant welfare clinic. The tables assume that the child is measured without shoes or clothes. Before a child learns to stand, height cannot be accurately measured without special techniques.

Age/years	Height/inches		Weight/pounds	
	Boys	Girls	Boys	Girls
Birth	—	—	7	7
1	30	29	22	22
2	34	34	28	27
3	38	38	32	32
4	41	41	36	36
5	44	43	43	41
6	46	46	48	47
7	49	49	54	52
8	51	50	60	58
9	53	52	66	64
10	55	55	72	70
11	57	57	78	79
12	59	60	84	88
13	61	62	93	99
14	64	63	108	108
15	66	63	120	114
16	68	64	130	117
17	68	64	136	119
18	69	64	139	120

Ideal weights for men and women.

Note: these are not average but *ideal* weights. In most western countries, average weights are often much higher (particularly among the middle aged) because people tend to be heavier than they should be. Separate figures are not given for different age groups, as nowadays, it is realized that a healthy person's weight should not increase by more than a few pounds after reaching adulthood. (Weights are in pounds, measured with clothes and shoes on. Heights are measured in feet and inches, with shoes off.)

MEN

Height	Type of Build		
	Small	Medium	Large
5–4	126	133	140
5–6	133	140	147
5–8	140	150	161
5–10	150	161	168
6–0	160	168	180
6–2	168	182	196
6–4	182	196	206

WOMEN

Height	Type of Build		
	Small	Medium	Large
4–10	100	105	112
5–0	105	112	119
5–2	110	116	126
5–4	112	119	130
5–6	118	126	135
5–8	126	133	140
5–10	130	140	149

Incubation periods of infectious diseases.

Note: the incubation period is the time that elapses between exposure to the disease and the appearance of its symptoms. In many cases, the incubation period will be appreciably longer or shorter than the time shown under the heading 'average'; very occasionally it may fall outside the figures given under the heading 'usual limits'.

Disease	Average (days)	Usual limits (days)
Chicken-pox	17	14–21
Diphtheria	4	2–5
Dysentery (bacillary)	3	1–7
Erysipelas	4	1–8
German measles	14	12–21
Glandular fever	11	8–15
Infective hepatitis (infectious jaundice)	40	15–45
Measles	10	8–15
Mumps	21	14–28
Paratyphoid	6	2–10
Poliomyelitis	9	5–15
Scarlet fever	3	2–7
Smallpox	12	7–16
Typhoid	11	6–21
Whooping-cough	12	7–21
Yellow fever	5	3–7

Schedules of Immunization and Vaccination for Children.

Note: There are a number of different immunization programmes in use in various parts of the world, depending not only on the diseases prevalent in those countries, but on the views of the doctors practising there as to the best time to give immunization. In addition, it should be stressed that, for individual children, the doctor may have very good reasons for departing from standard schedules. Two programmes are shown below: the first has been in use in many countries during the last decade, while the second was recently adopted as the standard programme in Great Britain.

Whatever programme of immunization a child has, it is important for the parents to keep a full record.

Boyd Committee Schedule (1959)

Age	Vaccine	Interval
2–6 months	'Triple' (Diphtheria, tetanus, whooping-cough)	
3–6 months	Second 'triple'	4 weeks
4–6 months	Third 'triple'	4 weeks
7–10 months	Polio (by mouth)	
7–10 months	Second polio	4 weeks
15–18 months	Fourth 'triple' and third polio	
1–2 years	Smallpox vaccination	
School entry	Diphtheria and tetanus	
8–9 years	Smallpox revaccination. Diphtheria and tetanus	
10–15 years	BCG (anti-TB)	

Current UK Schedule

Age	Vaccine	Interval
1–12 months	'Triple' (3 doses) Polio (3 doses)	7 weeks & 6 months
12–24 months	Measles	3 weeks
	Smallpox vaccination	3 weeks
5 years	Diphtheria and tetanus Polio	
	Smallpox revaccination	
10–13 years	BCG (anti-TB)	
15–19 years	Polio Tetanus Smallpox revaccination	